INTRODUCTION TO
CRITICAL CARE SKILLS

INTRODUCTION TO
CRITICAL
CARE SKILLS

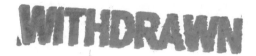

Janet-Beth McCann Flynn, RN, PhD

Nurse Consultant
Great Falls, Virginia

Nancie Pardue Bruce, RN, DNSc

Assistant Professor
College of Nursing
Florida Atlantic University
Boca Raton, Florida

with 227 illustrations

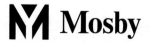 Mosby

St. Louis Baltimore Boston Chicago London Philadelphia Sydney Toronto

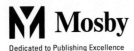
Mosby

Dedicated to Publishing Excellence

Editor: Robin Carter
Developmental Editor: Winnie Sullivan
Production Editor: Catherine Schwent
Designer: Jeanne Wolfgeher
Illustrators: Jack Tandy, Eric Lubbers
Cover photograph: ©Peter A. Simon/PHOTOTAKE, NYC.

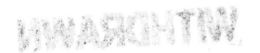
Printed in the United States of America.

Mosby–Year Book, Inc.
11830 Westline Industrial Drive
St. Louis, MO 63146

Library of Congress Cataloging-in-Publication Data

Flynn, Janet-Beth McCann
    Introduction to critical care skills/Janet-Beth McCann Flynn,
Nancie Pardue Bruce.
      p. cm.
      Includes index.
      ISBN 0-8016-2455-X : $29.95
      1. Intensive care nursing. I. Bruce, Nancie P. II. Title.
      [DNLM: 1. Critical Care--methods--nurses' instruction. WY 154
F648i]
RT120.I5F59 1993
610.73'61—dc20
DNLM/DLC
for Library of Congress
                            92-48815
                               CIP

93 94 95 96 CL/MV 9 8 7 6 5 4 3 2 1

Contributors

Nancie Pardue Bruce, RN, DNSc

Chapters 1, 5, 6, 8, 11, 15, 16, 17

Assistant Professor
College of Nursing
Florida Atlantic University
Boca Raton, Florida

Pamela B. DeLoach, RN, BSN, CCRN

Chapter 12

Nurse Manager
Neuro Trauma Acute Care Unit
Maryland Institute for Emergency Medical Services
    Systems
Baltimore, Maryland

Deborah Duncan*, RN, MSN, CCRN

Chapter 18

Lieutenant Colonel, Army Nurse Corps
Formerly at U.S. Army Institute of Surgical Research
Fort Sam Houston, Texas

Janet-Beth McCann Flynn, RN, PhD

Chapters 1, 2, 3, 4, 6, 10, 13, 14, 20

Nurse Consultant
Great Falls, Virginia

Barbara A. Goldrick, RN, PhD, CIC

Chapter 17

Director, Center for Nursing Research and Scholarship
School of Nursing
Georgetown University
Washington, D.C.

Phyllis B. Heffron, RN, MSN

Chapter 1

Faculty Facilitator, RN-BSN Program
College of Nursing
University of Iowa
Iowa City, Iowa

Debra L. Joseph, RN, BSN

Chapter 11

Manager, Clinical Support Services
Datascope Corporation
Montvale, New Jersey

Walter A. Laukaitis, Jr., RN, BSN

Chapter 20

Clinical Supervisor, Medical/Psychiatric/Obstetrical
    Clinical Nursing Division
Washington Hospital Center
Washington, D.C.

Linda Manglass, RN, MSN, CS

Chapter 3

Private Practice
Washington, D.C.

Douglas Mayers, MD

Chapter 10

ACLS Affiliate Faculty
National Naval Medical Center
Research Physician
Infectious Disease Department
Naval Medical Research Institute
Assistant Professor of Medicine
Department of Medicine
Uniformed Services University of the Health Sciences
S. Edward Hibert School of Medicine
Bethesda, Maryland

Nancy C. Molter*, RN, MN, CCRN

Chapter 18

Colonel, Army Nurse Corps
Former Chief Nurse
U.S. Army Institute of Surgical Research
Fort Sam Houston, Texas
Cardiovascular Clinical Nurse
Specialist-Telemetry
St. Luke's Lutheran Hospital
San Antonio, Texas

---

*The opinions or assertions contained herein are the private views of the
authors and are not to be construed as official or as reflecting the views
of the Department of the Army or Department of Defense.

Cynthia Ann Ondra, RN, BSN

Chapter 12

Former Primary Nurse III
Neuro Trauma Center
Maryland Institute for Emergency Medical Services
    Systems
Baltimore, Maryland

E. Francine Roberts, RN, MSN

Chapter 6

Assistant Professor
School of Nursing
George Mason University
Doctoral Candidate
George Mason University
Fairfax, Virginia

Lois Shurig, MSA, RN, CCRN

Chapters 7, 9

Director of Cardiology
Oakwood Hospital
Management Consultant in Health Care
Clinical Consultant in Cardiology
Dearborn, Michigan

Elizabeth C. Suddaby, RN, MSN, CCTC

Chapter 21

Heart Transplant Coordinator
Children's National Medical Center
Washington, D.C.

Melissa B. Zerbe, RN, DNSc

Chapter 19

Associate Professor
School of Nursing
Georgetown University
Washington, D.C.

Reviewers

Charold L. Baer, RN, PhD, FCCM, CCRN
Portland, Oregon

J. Ann Brooks-Brunn, DNS, RN
Indianapolis, Indiana

Jacqueline J. Clibourn, RN
Braintree, Massachusetts

Lynne Hutson Danekas, RN, MS
Wheaton, Illinois

Elenita F. Diaz, RN, BSN, MEd, CCRN
Baltimore, Maryland

Patti Eisenberg, RN, MSN, CS
St. Louis, Missouri

Ann Fagerness, RN, BSN, CNRN, CCRN, C
Seattle, Washington

Terry M. Foster, BSN, RN, CEN, CCRN
Cincinnati, Ohio

Deborah Gayer, RN, MS, CPNP
Columbia, Missouri

Barbara Habermann-Little, RN, MN
Oakland, California

Eva Kresge, RN
Seattle, Washington

Julie Marcum-Guest, RN, MS, CCRN
Oklahoma City, Oklahoma

Lisa M. Martin, RN, CCRN
Dallas, Texas

Edwina A. McConnell, RN, PhD
Madison, Wisconsin

Mary Courtney Moore, RN, RD, MSN
Nashville, Tennessee

Colleen Pfeiffer, RN, PhD
Ridgeway, Wisconsin

Timothy A. Philipp. RN, PhD
Chicago, Illinois

Michael Schroyer, RN, MSN, CCRN, CNA
Chicago, Illinois

Robert E. St. John, RN, RRT, BSN
St. Louis, Missouri

Roberta Strohl, RN, MN
Baltimore, Maryland

*To my husband **Jim***
for his sacrifice in giving up our time together

*To my children **Carlton and Elizabeth***
who were both born during the writing of this book

*To my mother **Elizabeth Pardue***
for her encouragement, baby-sitting, and financial support.

— N.P.B. —

*To my husband **Ed***
for his steadfast support and encouragement

*To my daughter **Erin***
for her patience in waiting for my presence

*To my mother **Mabel McCann***
for raising me to be the person I am

— J-B.McC.F. —

*From both of us to all of the **nurses***
who care for critical care patients

Preface

One can identify with the novice nurse who walks on a critical care unit feeling amazed and threatened by the sights and sounds of the high-tech machinery and monitors. Many experienced nurses have seen the fear and inadequacy on the faces of student nurses and have often wished to erase such fear. Finding good resources to use for teaching the technical aspects of critical care nursing was always very difficult. It was difficult to find in the nursing literature current critical care skills written out in a step-by-step format. For that reason many original skills were written exclusively for this textbook. What began as a desire to teach our own students grew into a collection of handouts and then a project for a book. We have designed this book, *Introduction to Critical Care Skills,* to present a simple approach to understanding and performing critical care skills, within the framework of the nursing process. The complexity level of this book is appropriate for undergraduate nursing students taking a course in acute care nursing, graduate students specializing in critical care, staff nurses wanting to enter the field of critical care, and nurses currently working in critical care units.

This book is organized into 21 chapters. The first three chapters are broad in scope and contain topics relevant to the other 18 chapters. Chapter 1 introduces the nursing process since this is viewed as the framework for delivering nursing care. Chapter 2 provides a broad overview of patient teaching. Each of the following chapters then presents further information for teaching patients with problems that relate specifically to the chapter topic. Chapter 3 details information on crisis intervention since many patients (and their families) who require critical care nursing are in a state of crisis. Nurses, too, can experience crises as a result of the critical care environment and related stressors. Chapters 4 through 21 present a wide variety of concepts and skills ranging from general skills, such as hemodynamic monitoring, to specific skills such as those needed to care for the organ donor. An attempt was made to focus on higher level skills more unfamiliar to the nurse already schooled in basic skills. Due to space constraints, some of the emergency and shock-trauma nursing skills could not be included in the book.

Each chapter is designed to be a modular learning unit and can (with some cross-referencing) be used independently of the other chapters. This permits flexibility in choosing the sequencing of the readings. Each chapter begins with a list of learning objectives to direct the reader through the chapter. The major concepts are introduced and developed as a theoretical background for the skills that follow. This provides the nurse with the theoretical knowledge to understand the rationale behind performance of the skills. Since this book follows a nursing process format, the conceptual development of the chapter topic is followed by an assessment section reflecting the chapter content. For example, the ECG chapter contains the cardiac assessment, the intracranial monitoring chapter includes a neurological assessment, and the enteral feeding chapter contains a nutritional assessment. Each chapter then lists a selection of sample nursing diagnoses and patient outcomes that might apply in a patient situation. These lists are by no means all-inclusive. They are to be used as examples to aid readers in designing their own individual nursing care plans. Each chapter contains skills presented in a detailed step-by-step format, with rationales included in the steps. Skills are preceded by a list of equipment and supplies that will be needed for that skill. Additionally, the book includes many helpful tables, figures, charts, and formulas that were specifically designed to help critical care nurses organize and retrieve information quickly.

Chapters 2 to 21 include sections on pediatric considerations. Pediatrics was included in this textbook in order to integrate knowledge throughout the lifespan, pointing out the differences and similarities of pediatric and adult procedures. Since nurses with a critical care background are now being hired to perform complex skills in the home, a home health care section has been added to each chapter of the book. Presently the trend is for patients to be discharged home with high-tech equipment. The home health care information was included since these highly technical skills are rarely found in traditional home health care textbooks.

It is our hope that this book will enable the critical care nurse to feel more comfortable with advanced technology so that there is energy left over to treat the patient as a person who deserves human caring. Beyond technological support, human care is one of the most powerful and essential forces to help people to survive and recover from critical illnesses. It is important to the authors that this book not be considered as strictly a technical skills resource. We hope that some of the information in the chapter sections on psychosocial considerations and patient and family teaching will help the nurse to consider the person behind the technological support systems.

Introduction to Critical Care Skills is a book of selected concepts and procedures designed to be used as a companion to theory textbooks of critical care nursing. It is not intended to be used as the sole source for learning to care for the critically ill patient. The technologies used in critical care units change very rapidly. We have made an attempt to ensure that these critical care skills appropriately reflect results of current research and practice. Our challenge now to our readers is to develop a research-based practice and to continue to update these skills when indicated by current research findings.

Janet-Beth McCann Flynn
Nancie Pardue Bruce

Acknowledgements

No book of this diversity and complexity could ever have been completed without the support, encouragement, and assistance of others. We would like to acknowledge Rick Weimer and Don Ladig for their faith in our ability to accomplish this project. We wish to express a sincere thank you to Robin Carter and Winnie Sullivan who provided expert assistance, working long hours editing highly technical material and keeping us on track. We also thank Catherine Schwent for her patient editorial support throughout detailed revisions. We are indebted to our artists, Jack Tandy and Eric Lubbers, for their talent in preparing detailed original art to illustrate nursing concepts. We would like to thank our contributors for sharing their knowledge and expertise with us. It takes hundreds of hours to research, write, and rewrite skills steps, a job that few writers were willing to assume, so we gratefully acknowledge their diligence. Nurse experts were selected by the publisher to review chapters in this book. We wish to thank them for their guidance and suggestions. In this day and age it is rare to find a book written without the aid of word processing. We would like to thank Brenda Hundley for her expert help in carefully and accurately typing many of the chapters. We offer a sincere thank you to our past professors at Vanderbilt University and The Catholic University of America for providing us with the knowledge and inspiration to continue growing and contributing to the nursing profession. Finally, no book can ever be completed without the love and support of the people closest to us. We, authors, appreciated having each other through many years of work, frustration, and time away from family. We wish to thank our parents, husbands, and children. Words cannot convey our appreciation for their endurance of our time and resources spent on this project.

Contents

CHAPTER 1

The Nursing Process and the Critical Care Patient

Objectives

After completing this chapter, the reader will be able to:

- Describe the nursing process and its use in nursing practice.
- Describe the assessment phase of the nursing process in critical care nursing.
- Compare and contrast the initial assessment, the admission assessment, the complete assessment, and the ongoing assessment.
- Discuss nursing diagnosis.
- Differentiate between behavioral and collaborative nursing diagnoses.
- Plan patient care goals and outcome criteria in critical care nursing situations.
- Describe nursing intervention for the critical care patient and its relationship to assessment and nursing diagnosis.
- Discuss methods of evaluating patient care outcomes in critical care nursing.
- Design a nursing care plan using the components of the nursing process: assessment, nursing diagnosis, formulation of patient outcomes, planning, intervention, and evaluation.
- Use the nursing process in the critical care setting.

In the past 20 years, critical care nursing has evolved into a prominent specialty requiring highly sophisticated levels of skilled nursing care and theoretical knowledge. Critical care nurses provide high technological care to patients with complex multisystem problems. This advanced level of nursing care is both a formidable responsibility and an exciting challenge.

The nursing process was formally introduced by Yura and Walsh[28] in 1967 when the first edition of their classic textbook, *The Nursing Process,* was published. They iden-

tified four steps in the nursing process: assessing, planning, implementing, and evaluating. Since 1967, the nursing process has continued to evolve as a result of changes in nursing and the health care system. Advances in quality assurance programs, nursing audits, policy statements, and nurse practice acts have strengthened the nursing process. In the 1970s, two additional steps were added to the nursing process—nursing diagnosis and patient outcomes. The nursing process now consists of six steps (see box on p. 2).

Over the years, the significance and impact of the nursing process has grown tremendously, and it is now well-accepted as the core of nursing practice. In simple terms, it is a systematic, theory-based method of determining the patient's health problems, planning the best way to achieve designated outcomes, delivering the appropriate care in a timely manner, and evaluating how well the care has actually achieved the patient goals.[17] The process is composed of input from the nurse, the patient, and family and can be used in any health care setting for any type of need the patient may have, including the fast-paced, highly technical environment of the critical care setting.

Some hospitals are now combining the nursing care plan with the nursing progress notes in one standardized form (Fig. 1-1). These forms can then serve as a legal base for verifying that nursing care has been provided according to accepted standards of professional practice. Combined progress note-care plans are used to validate the costs of care for insurance claims, Medicare, and home health care and also serve as a basis for assessing fees of nursing care.

Many challenges exist in critical care nursing. Critically ill persons are often unable to communicate with their caregivers. The critical care team is frequently under intense pressure for long periods of time. The psychological and social aspects of a critical illness may be inadvertently overlooked, and the challenge of successfully communicating with anxious relatives can be overwhelming at times.

BOCA RATON COMMUNITY HOSPITAL
Department of Nursing

Stamp

PROGRESS NOTES

Date and Time	NRS, Dx # and Initials	APPRAISAL Objective/Subjective Data Reflecting Current Status	GOALS Short Term Outcomes For The Patient	PLAN Nursing Interventions	EVALUATION Stated Goals
9-6-90 8AM	28 nn	"I've been short of breath for a couple weeks" Resp 26 labored-crackles bilateral bases- 3+ ankle edema bi- laterally - anxious	demonstrates respiratory rate between 22-24 c̄ exertion in 4 hrs - urinates >1000 ml by end of shift- states breathing easier- demonstrates bilateral clear breath sounds	HOB ↑ 30° - Assess lungs g4°-accurate I+O restrict fluid intake 1000ml/24 hrs- maintain O₂ at 4 L - elevate edematous extremities-daily wts	12ᴺ-this oxygen helps my breathing" R 22 - few scattered crackles 2 PM Output 1200 ml
(red line)					
9-6-90 5 PM	28 BC	Lungs-few scattered crackles in bases Resp 22 c̄ minimal exertion. SOB persists on exertion	demonstrates normal resp pattern 20/min by end of shift - lungs clear to auscultation within 24 hrs.	Auscultate breath sounds for crackles g4°.assess for A complaints of SOB ↑notify MD	9PM Resp 20/min even and unlabored- few scattered crackles
(red line)					

Init.	Full Signature	Title	Init.	Full Signature	Title	Init.	Full Signature	Title	Init.	Full Signature	Title
nn	Nancy Nurse	RN									
BC	Betty Clay	RN									

Fig. 1-1   Sample patient care plan. *(Courtesy Boca Raton Community Hospital, Boca Raton, Florida).*

▼ **Steps of the Nursing Process**

ASSESSMENT

Assessment is the ongoing, systematical collection and organization of information used to determine patient needs for nursing care. Assessment data comes from numerous sources, including the patient interview, written records, physical examination, and observation. This information is integrated into an organized format called a *data base.*

NURSING DIAGNOSIS

Nursing diagnosis is a statement of an actual or potential nursing care need of a patient. The nursing diagnosis constitutes a nursing judgment, derived from the analysis and integration of information in the data base, and serves as the basis for the remaining steps of the nursing process.

PATIENT OUTCOMES

Patient outcomes are statements of the expected behaviors the patient is expected to achieve as a result of nursing care. Patient outcomes are measurable statements developed for each nursing diagnosis.

PLANNING

Planning involves making a determination, based on the nursing diagnosis, on how to meet the patient's needs for nursing care. The plan includes patient goals, expected outcomes, and nursing interventions. The *nursing care plan* directs the nursing interventions and serves as documentation regarding the kind of care the patient is receiving.

IMPLEMENTATION

Implementation is the action phase of the nursing process where the nurse carries out the plan to meet the needs of the patient. By implementing the nursing care plan, the nurse endeavors to reach the patient outcomes.

EVALUATION

Evaluation is studying the actual patient outcomes and making a judgment on the efficacy of nursing interventions, that is, do the expected outcomes match the actual outcomes, and, if not, what are the possible explanations. The means for evaluating nursing care is "built-in" to the nursing process by specifying outcome goals in the nursing care plan. Evaluation becomes an ongoing process during the life of a nursing care plan.

But within the highly technical critical care setting, it is essential that the nurses practice within a caring perspective. Caring means that persons, events, projects, and things matter to people.[1] Caring is the moral ideal of nursing, whereby the end is protection, enhancement, and preservation of human dignity.[27] Experienced nurses in this specialty assume a high degree of individual responsibility and depend on the guidance and organization of the nursing process to help them provide the best possible care. A rapid and orderly assessment followed by the appropriate nursing diagnoses can, in a matter of seconds, make a major difference in the life of a patient.

ASSESSMENT

Assessment is the first step of the nursing process and serves as the foundation for the other steps. During the assessment phase, data are systematically collected, analyzed, interpreted, and validated to formulate a nursing diagnosis. In 1986, Johnson and Brown[18] identified three types of assessment for the critical care patient. This has now been refined and expanded into the following four different types of nursing assessment performed at varying times during the patient's stay on the unit:

* Initial assessment.
* Admission assessment.
* Complete assessment.
* Ongoing assessment.

The Initial Assessment

The initial assessment is performed when the nurse first comes in contact with the patient. This may occur when the patient is arriving at a shock-trauma receiving area, when the nurse greets the patient at the beginning of a shift, or when the nurse reenters the room after a period of time. The initial assessment is completed within several minutes and is crucial for discovering life-threatening conditions. It is based on specific priorities of care that include: assessing the patient's airway, breathing, circulation, and basic neurological functioning (see box on Guidelines for Conducting the Initial Assessment p. 10, top). When a patient is admitted to a trauma or emergency department, the initial assessment is divided into a primary and secondary survey. The secondary survey is actually a head-to-toe assessment that is also known as a complete assessment.

The Admission Assessment

The admission assessment is performed on the patient's initial admission into the critical care unit. It is similar to the format used in standard health care assessments carried out in noncritical care settings. The admission assessment is essentially a review of all the body systems and includes psychosocial aspects and demographic data. The goal is to collect patient data using a systematic process that gives comprehensive health status information (see box on p. 10, bottom). Fig. 1-2 is an example of a nursing assessment tool helpful for collecting patient data. The nurse's effectiveness in conducting the admission assessment depends on a familiarity with the components of a complete assessment and the sources of data, knowledge of interviewing principles, and skills in collecting the medical history and performing a physical examination.

Sources of data

Sources of data include the patient, family members, significant others, other health care providers, and written past health records. For those patients who are unable to communicate, a medical history must be obtained from family members, friends, or old records.

Subjective and Objective Data. Data collected can be classified as subjective or objective. *Subjective data* is in-

Text continued on p. 11

WASHINGTON ADVENTIST HOSPITAL
Department of Nursing
PATIENT HISTORY AND ASSESSMENT

Section I (To be filled out by patient/family, NA, NT, LPN, RN)

Date_____ Time of admission: _____ Informant: _____

Admitted/transferred from:_____ Via:_____ Male: _____ Female: _____

Language spoken: _____ Religion: _____

Special communication needs: _____ No _____ Yes (explain) _____

Marital status: _____ Single _____ Married _____ Divorced _____ Widowed

Telephone: (H) _____ (W) _____

Family member/friend 1) _____

2) _____ Telephone: (H) _____ (W) _____

Who would you like to give consent for procedures/tests should you be unable? _____ Telephone: _____

Do you have a living will? Yes _____ No _____

Do you have a durable power of attorney? _____

ALLERGIES (medication, food, environment): _____

Chief complaint: _____

Recent hospitalizations/outpatient procedures (date, place, reason):_____
_____

Surgical history:_____

Are you being treated or have you ever had any other illness/condition such as:

HEALTH HISTORY

____ Heart disease   ____ Hyper/hypotension   ____ Dizziness   ____ Cancer   ____ Falls

____ Respiratory disease   ____ Asthma   ____ TB   ____ Seizures   ____ Sexually transmitted

____ Blood disease   ____ Bleeding tendency   ____ Anemia   ____ Mental illness   disease

____ Liver disease   ____ Hepatitis   ____ Diabetes   ____ Injury   ____ Other

____ None of the above

If any of the above checked, please explain: _____
_____

Habits (smoking, alcohol, nonprescription drugs): _____

Rest/sleep hours: Day/night _____ Naps _____ Pain: _____ No _____ Yes (Date: _____ Other test: _____

Blood transfusion: _____ No _____ Yes (Date: _____ Reaction: _____ No _____)

CURRENT MEDICATIONS

DRUG	DOSE	FREQUENCY	DRUG	DOSE	FREQUENCY

AIDES AND DEVICES

DENTURES   **VISUAL AIDS**   **PROSTHESIS**   **AIDES**

____ Uppers   ____ Glasses   ____ Joint replacement   ____ Braces/crutches

____ Lowers   ____ Contact lens   (type)_____   ____ Cane

____ Partials   ____ Artificial eye R/L   ____ Artificial limb   ____ Walker

                       ____ Implanted lens R/L   ____ Breast prothesis R/L ____ Hearing aide R/L

____ No devices or equipment

Section II (To be filled in by NA, NT, LPN, RN)

(Include jewelry, watch, rings, purse, wallet, money, credit cards)   Sent Home _____

VALUABLES LIST

ITEM   DISPOSITION (where placed)   To Safe _____
_____
_____
_____

VITAL SIGNS:

_____ BP _____ T _____ P _____ R   _____ HT. _____ WT. (Actual, Estimate)

ADMITTING GUIDE FOR PATIENTS (Explain)

____ Visiting hours   ____ Phone   ┌─────────────────────
____ Call system   ____ Siderails   │ ADDRESSOGRAPH
____ Bed controls   ____ Introduction to roommate │
____ Smoking policy   ____ TV   │
____ Room lights   ____ Educational channels   │

Fig. 1-2   Nursing assessment tool. *(Courtesy Washington Adventist Hospital, Tacoma Park, Md.).*

Section III (To be filled in by LPN I, RN)

NEUROLOGICAL
- ____ Alert
- ____ Oriented
- ____ Disoriented
- ____ Neurodeficits
- ____ (List) _____
- ____ Semicomatose
- ____ Comatose
- ____ Other _____
- ____ Visual loss R____ L____
- ____ Hearing loss R____ L____
- ____ Speech deficit
- ____ Aphasic ____ Slurred

PULMONARY
- ____ Respirations appear normal
- ____ regular rate
- ____ Congestion
- ____ Productive cough
- ____ Short of breath
- ____ Wheezing R____ L____
- ____ Rales R____ L____
- ____ Rhonchi R____ L____
- ____ Decreased BS R____ L____
- ____ Tracheostomy
- ____ Other _____

CARDIOVASCULAR
- ____ Regular pulse
- ____ Irregular pulse
- ____ Chest pain
- ____ Pacemaker
- ____ IV ports
- ____ Grafts/shunt
- ____ Other
- FALLS PRECAUTIONS ___ No ___ Yes
- (Orange Band/Dot System Initiated)

GASTROINTESTINAL
- ____ Bowel sounds +/−
- ____ Incontinence of stool
- ____ Nausea
- ____ Vomiting
- ____ Constipation
- ____ Diarrhea
- ____ Abdominal distention
- ____ Ostomy (Type) _____
- ____ Feeding tube (Type)
  _____
- ____ Other _____
- ____ No problems noted
- Bowel routine: _____
  _____
- Last BM: _____

UROLOGICAL
- ____ Frequency
- ____ Urgency
- ____ Burning on urination
- ____ Incontinence
- ____ Foley
- ____ Ostomy (Type) _____
- ____ Other _____
- ____ No problems noted

REPRODUCTIVE
- ____ Last menstrual period
- _____ Pap smear _____
- ____ Gravida ____ Para
- ____ Vaginal itching
- ____ Vaginal bleeding
- ____ History of prostate
  problems
- ____ Other _____
- ____ No problems noted

MUSCULOSKELETAL
- ____ Steady on feet
- ____ Arthritis
- ____ Weakness R____ L____
- ____ Non-wt bearing R____ L____
- ____ Disability _____
- ____ Fracture _____
- ____ Paralysis R____ L____
- ____ Other _____

DERMATOLOGICAL
- ____ Skin color
- ____ No skin breakdown
- ____ Dry skin/rash
  (location) _____
- ____ Red area _____
- ____ Edema _____
- ____ Motiling/cyanosis
- ____ Jaundice
- ____ Varicosities
- ____ Lesions _____
- ____ Pressure sore (location)

NOTE: If patient has any skin breakdown, initiate PRESSURE SORE FLOW SHEET Skin Care Precaution Initiated: ____ No ____

PSYCHOLOGICAL/EMOTIONAL
- ____ Calm/cooperative
- ____ Anxiety present
- ____ Agitated/uncooperative
- ____ Depressed
- ____ Mental impairment
- ____ (Type) _____
- ____ Other _____

SYSTEMS ASSESSMENT (Admitting Status)

☐ See Critical Care Flow Sheet

Describe general appearance: _____

Section IV (To be filled in by RN)

HOME ENVIRONMENT
Lives:
- ____ Alone
- ____ With spouse
- ____ With children
- ____ With other

Specify: _____

- ____ Nursing home
- ____ House
- ____ Apartment
- ____ Other _____
- ____ Stairs _____
- ____ Elevator

LEVEL OF CARE/ADL
- ____ Independent
- ____ Needs assist
  _____
- ____ Dependent

MOBILITY
- ____ Ambulatory
- ____ Needs assist
- ____ Bedridden

MEANS OF SUPPORT
Occupation _____
Full-time ____ Part-time ____
Retired ____ Unemployed ____
Social Security ____
Other _____

Community agencies currently using:
_____

DISCHARGE ASSESSMENT

Person(s) to assist at discharge: _____
Environmental needs (Include ability to return home, support system, financial concerns): _____
_____
Equipment needs (Health care supplies, assist aides, devices): _____
Compliance with past health care regime: _____
Referral: ____ Social service ____ Dietary ____ PT/OT ____ Chaplain ____ Home health ____ ET ____ Other _____
    Reason for referral: _____
Educational needs: ____ Cardiac ED ____ Diet teaching ____ Diabetic ED ____ Medications ____ Wound care
    ____ PreOP/PostOP teaching ____ Other _____
Nursing diagnosis: 1.) _____
(Problem list)   2.) _____
    3.) _____

Fig. 1-2 cont'd. Nursing assessment tool.

Continued.

VITAL PARAMETERS				0700-1500					VITAL PARAMETERS				1500-2300					DATE
TIME	0700	0800	0900	1000	1100	1200	1300	1400	TIME	1500	1600	1700	1800	1900	2000	2100	2200	CODES
TEMP									TEMP									IV:
A. Pulse									A. Pulse									NB - new bag/bottle
Resp									Resp									DC - discontinued
BP (cuff)									BP (cuff)									
BP (A-line)									BP (A-line)									
MAP									MAP									* (Asterisk):
15 minutes									15 minutes									See patient progress record for further detail/explanation.
30 minutes									30 minutes									NOTE: This code pertains to all pages of this flowsheet.
45 minutes									45 minutes									
CVP									CVP									DAILY WEIGHT
PAP S/D									PAP S/D									
PAMP									PAMP									
PAWP									PAWP									
C.O./C.I.									C.O./C.I.									TYPE SCALE
SVR/PVR									SVR/PVR									
mv02/Sat.									mv02/Sat.									BSA
Recal									Recal									
11-7 Total	0700	0800	0900	1000	1100	1200	1300	1400	7-3 Total	1500	1600	1700	1800	1900	2000	2100	2200	3-11 Totals 24°
1									1									1
2									2									2
3									3									3
4									4									4
5									5									5
6									6									6
7									7									7
8									8									8
9									9									9
10									10									10
11									11									11
12									12									12
13									13									13
							8° Total Intake									8°/24° Total Intake		
1									1									1
2									2									2
3									3									3
4									4									4
5									5									5
6									6									6
7									7									7
8									8									8
9									9									9
10									10									10
							8° Total Output									8°/24° Total Output		

Fig. 1-2 cont'd.   Nursing assessment tool.

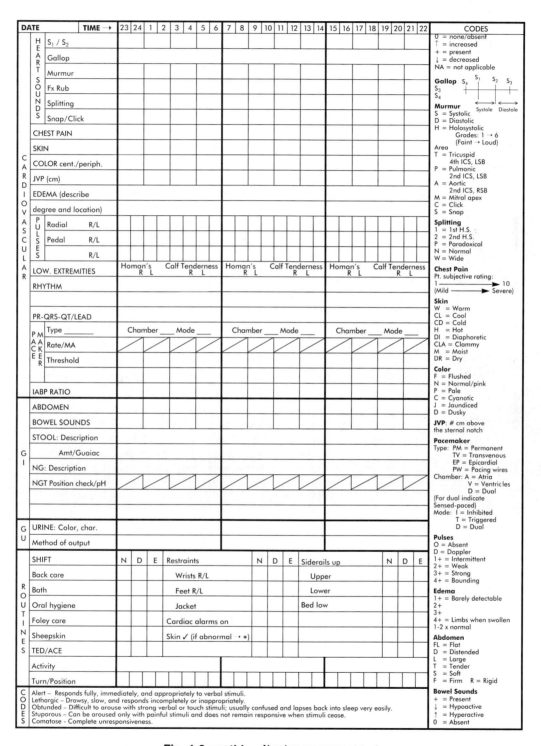

Fig. 1-2 cont'd.   Nursing assessment tool.

Continued.

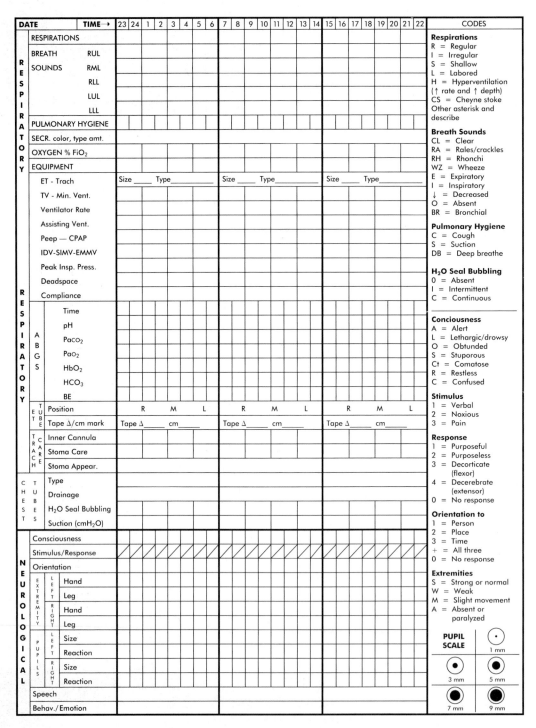

Fig. 1-2 cont'd.   Nursing assessment tool.

Date:							INVASIVE LINE CARE				VITAL PARAMETERS		2300-0700						
LAB TEST RESULTS							**CHECK WHEN CHG'D** N D E				TIME	2300	2400	0100	0200	0300	0400	0500	0600
Time							P #1 Dressing				TEMP								
Na							E Tubing				A. Pulse								
K							R #2 Dressing				Resp.								
Cl							I Tubing				BP (cuff)								
CO$_2$							P #3 Dressing				BP (A-line)								
BUN							H Tubing				MAP								
Creat.							C Cordis				15 minutes								
Glucose							E Prox. Tbg.												
S/A							T Middle				30 minutes								
FS Gluc.							A Distal												
WBC							L Dressing				45 minutes								
Hb							A Dressing												
Hct							I Tubing				CVP								
PT patient							E Solution				PAP S/D								
% act.							S Dressing				PAMP								
PTT patient							W Prox. Tbg.				PAWP								
% act.							A Prox. Inj.				C.O./C.I.								
Platelets							G Distal				SVR/PVR								
CPK							Z Solution				mv02/Sat.								
MB							C S Tubing												
LDH total							O T Solution				Recal								
LDH 1							**I & O**				TIME	2300	2400	0100	0200	0300	0400	0500	0600
SGOT							1												
Digoxin							2												
Theophy							3												
Dilantin							4												
							5												
							6												
							7												
							8												
							9			** cc µg								
TIME	SPECIAL TEST DONE/RESULTS						10			** cc								
							11			** cc								
							12												
							13 Diet:												
							**If peripheral, ✔ site q 1°:												
NAME:							1 True Urine Output				8° Total Intake								
							2 Urine + G.U. Irrigant												
							3 Specific Gravity												
							4												
							5 Chest Tube												
							6												
							7 NG Tube												
							8												
							9												
							10				8° Total Output								

Fig. 1-2 cont'd. Nursing assessment tool.

Guidelines for Conducting the Initial Assessment

When performing an initial assessment, the nurse must carry out the emergency interventions as needed while assessing the patient. While performing the initial assessment, obtain a brief history from the transferring staff. Maintain cervical spine control for all patients with a questionable trauma history.

EQUIPMENT AND SUPPLIES
In room:

- Stethoscope
- Blood pressure cuff
- Bag-valve mask with oxygen supply
- Suction bottle and tubing
- Suction catheters and mouth suction
- Oral and nasal airways
- Gloves and masks
- Emergency drugs

On unit:

- Intubation tray
- Chest tube insertion tray and setup
- Central catheter tray
- IV bottles or bags, tubing, and intracatheters
- Emergency crash cart
- Defibrillator

NURSING INTERVENTIONS
Airway

1. Observe for patency of the airway. Look, listen, and feel for stridor, foreign bodies, drooling, edema, and soft tissue damage.
2. If patient is intubated or has tracheostomy, ensure that the airway is properly secured and patent. Verify placement.
3. Assess the need for suctioning an oral or nasal airway, jaw thrust/chin lift, or emergency intubation.

Breathing

1. Observe for adequacy of ventilation by watching for rise and fall movements of the chest wall. If necessary, place your hand on the chest to feel for movement.
2. Auscultate breath sounds.
3. Assess the effectiveness of ventilation, noting: cyanosis, respiratory pattern, rate and depth of respirations, retraction, use of accessory muscles, subcutaneous emphysema, sucking chest wound, tracheal shift from midline, and decreased level of consciousness.

Breathing—cont'd

4. Note functioning of respiratory assistive devices. Check ventilator settings and patient responses.
5. If necessary, provide for assisted ventilation with either a bag-valve mask on high-flow oxygen or a mechanical ventilator.
6. Prepare to intervene for life-threatening conditions and assist with chest tube insertion or needle thoracostomy, if appropriate.

Circulation

1. Palpate pulses for quality, location, rate, and rhythm.
2. If no pulse, begin advanced cardiac life support (see Chapter 10).
3. Quickly observe for uncontrolled external bleeding, or bleeding through dressings, casts, or chest tubes. Provide for direct pressure, elevation, or return of patient to operating room.
4. Observe for circulation indicators, such as poor capillary refill, cool skin temperature, pallor, cyanosis, and diaphoresis.
5. Be prepared to administer IV fluids through large bore (14-18 gauge) catheters. If the patient shows signs of shock (e.g., drop in blood pressure and increased pulse rate), insert an IV catheter in each arm.

Neurological

1. Perform a brief neurological assessment using the Glasgow Coma Scale (see Chapter 12).
2. Evaluate the patient's verbal response as either oriented, confused, inappropriate words, incomprehensible words, or no response.
3. Assess the patient's motor response as to purposeful movement, withdrawal, flexion, extension, or no response when obeying commands or responding to pain.
4. Observe pupillary response by noting bilateral equality and responsiveness to light.
5. Report a sudden deterioration in neurological status. This change may be because of changes in perfusion or metabolism.

Guidelines for Conducting the Admission Assessment

The admission assessment usually begins with an interview where the nurse elicits information relating to the health history. Often the patient is too ill to provide information. Much of the information obtained will be from family and friends and, at times, may be incomplete. A substantial portion of the admission history will be obtained over time. A common format for the admission assessment that helps the nurse to collect data necessary for determining nursing diagnoses includes the following:

- *Biographical and demographic data.*
- *Reason for admission (chief complaint).*
- *History of present illness;* also known as present health status, presented as a narrative, beginning with the onset of chief complaint and its progression to the present.
- *Past health status*—a review of childhood illnesses, mental health illnesses, past hospitalizations, surgeries, injuries, blood transfusions, immunizations, habits (alcohol, drugs, and smoking), allergies (to food and drugs), and medications, both prescription and over-the-counter.

- *Family history*—includes inquiry about close blood relatives with ages and states of health or causes of death and the presence of any significant genetic or familial diseases.
- *Review of physiological systems*—questions about each system of the body, including visual and hearing deficits and use of prosthetic devices.
- *Psychosocial history*—questions about life style, sexuality, sleep patterns, occupation, work habits, coping methods, values, and substance abuse.
- *Health maintenance efforts*—questions about exercise, rest, sleep, regular medical checkups, and dental care. Questions for the psychosocial history and health maintenance efforts can be organized through the Functional Health Patterns framework articulated by Gordon (see box on p. 11). This framework is helpful in collecting data necessary for identifying nursing diagnoses.
- *Physical assessment*—performed in a manner similar to that of the complete assessment.
- *Current health data and diagnostic studies.*
- *Potential complications*—the most common complications for patients with the identified condition are listed.

▼ **Functional Health Patterns**

---

1. HEALTH PERCEPTION-HEALTH MANAGEMENT PATTERN

- Perceived pattern of health and well-being.
- General level of health care behavior (how health is managed).
- Health status related to future planning.

2. NUTRITIONAL-METABOLIC PATTERN

- Food and fluid consumption relative to metabolic need.
- Pattern, types, quantity, preferences of food and fluids
- Skin lesions and healing ability.
- Indicators of nutritional status (skin, hair, and nail condition).

3. ELIMINATION PATTERN

- Patterns of excretory function.
- Routines and devices used.

4. ACTIVITY-EXERCISE PATTERN

- Exercise, activity, leisure, and recreation.
- Activities of daily living.
- Sports.
- Factors interfering with activity.

5. SLEEP-REST PATTERN

- Pattern of sleep, rest, and relaxation.
- Perception of quantity and quality of rest.
- Energy level.
- Sleep aids and problems.

6. COGNITIVE-PERCEPTUAL PATTERN

- Adequacy of sensory modes.
- Pain perception and management.
- Cognitive functional ability.

7. SELF-PERCEPTION–SELF-CONCEPT PATTERN

- Attitudes about self.
- Perception of abilities.
- Body image, identity, and general emotional pattern.
- Pattern of body posture and speech.

8. ROLE-RELATIONSHIP PATTERN

- Role engagements—family, work, and social.
- Perception of responsibilities.

9. SEXUALITY-REPRODUCTIVE PATTERN

- Satisfaction or disturbances in sexuality.
- Reproductive stage.
- Reproductive pattern.

10. COPING-STRESS TOLERANCE PATTERN

- General coping pattern and effectiveness.
- Perceived ability to manage situations.
- Reserve capacity and resources.

11. VALUE-BELIEF PATTERN

- Values, goals or beliefs that guide choices.
- Conflicts related to health status.

Adapted from Gordon M: *Nursing diagnosis: process and application,* ed 2, New York, 1987, McGraw-Hill; Holloway NM: *Medical surgical care plans,* Springhouse, Pa, 1988, Springhouse.

formation derived directly from the patient (if possible), family, and friends. Subjective data is only what the patient, family, or friends report, not what the nurse can observe or validate. Examples of subjective data include feelings of pain, anxiety, or dizziness, a description of how a previous symptom was treated at home, or a statement about a current family relationship. *Objective data* is information nurses gather directly through observing, listening, smelling, feeling, and/or measuring, such as body temperature, blood pressure, degrees of swelling, laboratory findings, and x-rays.

Establishing an effective communication system through the use of good interviewing skills assists the nurse in taking the medical history and eliciting subjective data.

The Complete Assessment

Within the critical care unit the complete assessment is performed after the initial assessment and when the patient is stabilized. Nurses in most critical care units perform a complete head-to-toe assessment of each patient on admission to the unit and then every 4 to 8 hours (see box on Guidelines for Conducting a Complete Assessment pp. 12

and 13). This assessment should usually take the whole first hour of the shift and should not be delayed much beyond the first hour of the shift. The nurse's complete assessment is expected to be customized to the patient's chief complaint. Critical care nurses will need to focus on only the most important physical signs and symptoms.

The Ongoing Assessment

The ongoing assessment of the critical care patient will occur at intervals usually prescribed by the patient's physician and will depend on the critical nature of the patient's illness. The ongoing assessment consists of recording all of the patient's vital signs, hemodynamic variables, intracranial pressure, respiratory variables, ventilator settings, and intake and output at specific intervals. Equipment checks should be performed regularly. The ongoing assessment focuses on the chief complaint and accompanying problems as they occur, including potential problems, such as hazards of immobility. During the ongoing assessment the nurse refers back to admission data as necessary to compare or confirm new findings. Psychosocial status may be assessed at this time (see box on Guidelines for Conducting the Ongoing Assessment on p. 14).

EQUIPMENT AND SUPPLIES

- Stethoscope
- Pen
- Penlight or flashlight
- Blood pressure cuff
- Cotton-tipped sticks
- Gloves

PREPARATION

1. Carry assessment tools or ensure that they are in the patient's room.
2. Obtain the patient's history, either through a verbal report or by reading the chart.
3. Wash hands and observe Universal Precautions.
4. Introduce self to patient and explain plans.
5. Rapidly perform initial assessment to detect any life-threatening emergencies.
6. Look for general data first, then specific.

DRUGS AND DIET

1. Check the diet, drugs, and IV fluids the patient should be receiving, noting their actions, how they will be interacting, their compatibility, and when they are to be administered.

EQUIPMENT

1. Inspect equipment, such as pacemaker, bedside defibrillator, ECG monitor, intraaortic balloon pump, enteral feeding pump, IV lines and infusion pumps, oxygen equipment, ventilator settings, wall suction equipment, chest tubes and drainage container, and endotracheal cuff pressure.
2. Ensure that all equipment is working well and at the prescribed levels before continuing with the complete assessment. Check that all tubes are actually attached. Double-check stopcocks.
3. Ensure that all IV sites have fluids infusing appropriately or have heparin locks. Inspect for the need to label lines.
4. Calibrate and balance monitoring equipment.

VITAL SIGNS AND PHYSIOLOGICAL VARIABLES

1. Measure temperature, pulse, respirations, blood pressure, and weight (if a weight measurement is appropriate at this time).
2. Check and record physiological monitoring variables (i.e., intracranial pressure, respiratory, and hemodynamic variables) where appropriate. Obtain and analyze an ECG rhythm strip.

URINE PARAMETERS, FLUID BALANCE, AND LABORATORY REPORTS

1. Obtain urine sample, observing for mucous strands and sediment. Test for sugar, acetone, protein, hematuria, pH, and specific gravity.
2. Observe hourly urine output trend on flow sheet and compare with fluid intake.
3. Record and review recent medical studies, laboratory values, culture reports, and chest x-ray.

GENERAL HEAD-TO-TOE SURVEY

1. Observe patient's general appearance and state of health, including nutritional status. Note body type (thin, fragile-appearing, robust, stocky), developmental level of maturity, gait, and other body movements.
2. Observe general demeanor and behavior (friendly, tense, talkative, quiet, anxious, unconscious).

Psychosocial

1. Assess emotional status, perception, interaction with family and staff, grief behaviors, coping skills, and level of cooperation.

Skin and mucous membranes

1. Inspect and palpate for rashes, petechiae, pressure areas, edema, contusions, abrasions, pallor, cyanosis, moisture and temperature differences; evaluate skin turgor and texture.
2. Inspect incisions and sutures, noting redness, swelling, odor, bleeding, pain, and tenderness.

Head and face

1. Note the shape and scalp integrity and color. Assess for changes in hair texture (dryness or brittleness), quantity, and distribution.
2. Test facial nerves by observing the symmetry of the patient's face.
3. Ask patient to raise and lower eyebrows, close eyes tightly, smile, and puff out cheeks so the facial muscle strength can be assessed.
4. Have patient close eyes while the nurse touches the jaw, cheek, and forehead bilaterally to test the sensory division of the trigeminal nerve. Ask the patient to compare and describe the sensations on both sides.
5. Percuss facial sinuses.

Eyes

1. Compare alignment of the eyes. Are they alike? Check for complete lid closure because exposure of the cornea may cause drying and uleration.
2. Inspect the conjunctiva and sclera by separating the eyelids. Observe for foreign bodies, inflammation, conjunctival redness, jaundice, or a pale lid.
3. Assess the pupils, which indicate the function of cranial nerves II and III. Turn down the lights and observe the size, shape, equality, and reaction to light of the pupils. Shine a penlight from the outer aspect of one eye inward and observe for pupil constriction in this eye (direct response) as well as in the opposite eye (consensual response).
4. Test the patient's corneal reflex with a cotton wisp.

Ears, nose, mouth, and throat

1. Inspect and palpate the auricles and surrounding tissue for warmth, tenderness, deformities, lesions, pressure areas, cysts, or swelling.
2. Inspect the ear canal for drainage. If discharge is present, note color, odor, and consistency. Obtain an order for a specimen culture. Test drainage for glucose.
3. Inspect the nostrils for pressure areas, especially in patients who have nasotracheal airways or nasogastric tubes. Observe for discharge.
4. Inspect for pressure areas in the mouth and throat from an endotracheal tube. The tube may need to be retaped or adjusted.
5. Using a tongue depressor and penlight, inspect the patient's oropharynx, buccal mucosa, gums, and tongue for inflammation, color changes, white patches, exudate, ulcerations, bleeding, and lesions.
6. Press both sides of the patient's posterior pharynx with a cotton-tipped applicator to test gag reflex.

Neck

1. Inspect the trachea for midline position, and observe for any use of accessory neck muscles in breathing. Any deviation of the trachea to either side indicates deformity and requires further investigation.
2. Inspect and palpate the neck over the trachea for subcutaneous emphysema or other swelling that might obstruct breathing. Make sure that tracheostomy ties are not too tight.
3. Check the range of motion in the patient's neck. Observe for any nuchal rigidity or neck contractures.

Neurological system

1. Determine the patient's orientation to person, place, and time by asking, "What's your name? Where are you? What day is this?"
2. Assess intellectual performance by having patient add several numbers or answer specific questions such as "How is the job of an airplane pilot different from a police officer?" Be creative when formulating immediate recall questions.
3. Assess memory of recent and past events. Ask patient to name the recent presidents or the last major holiday. Show the patient some items to recall a few minutes later.
4. Assess motor function by having patient give the examiner a hand squeeze with each hand. Have patient raise the legs while pressing the feet forcefully against the examiner's palms. Note if the patient is able to move and reposition self in the bed.
5. Assess sensory function by checking for loss of any peripheral feeling.
6. Record neurological findings using the Glasgow Coma Scale (see Chapter 12). If the patient does not respond to speech, use nailbed pressure to determine response to pain. Place a pen across the nailbed and squeeze the finger. The stimulus causes minimal tissue injury.

Breasts, chest, and respiratory system

1. Inspect for the shape and symmetry of thorax and breasts, respiratory rate, rhythm, and depth and use of accessory muscles.
2. Percuss over the patient's chest for changes in resonance, flatness, and dullness.
3. Palpate for diaphragmatic excursion, position of the trachea, crepitation, tenderness, masses, and edema.
4. Auscultate for normal breath sounds and adventitious sounds.

Cardiovascular system

1. Inspect for bulging, depression, precordial and juxtaprecordial pulsation.
2. Palpate for point of maximum impulse (PMI), friction rubs, thrills, thrusts, and heaves.
3. Auscultate with diaphragm of stethoscope for heart rate and rhythm, character of S_1 and S_2, comparison of S_1 in aortic and S_2 in major auscultatory areas, presence or absence and description of extra heart sounds (S_3, S_4), bruits, pericardial friction rub, or murmurs.

Peripheral vascular system

1. Palpate radial pulse, noting rate, rhythm, quality, and tenderness of arterial wall. Compare with apical pulse and ECG tracing.
2. Palpate the amplitude and character of peripheral pulses: superficial temporal, brachial, femoral, popliteal, posterior tibial, and dorsalis pedal.
3. Palpate the carotid pulses for equality, amplitude, thrills, and bruits.

Venous pulses and pressures

1. Place patient at 45 degree angle and identify internal jugular vein. Determine highest level of visible pulsation. Measure pressure levels in fingerbreadths of distension above the clavicle. Characterize neck veins as mildly, moderately, or severely distended. Neck veins should not be prominent if right heart function is normal.

Abdomen

1. Inspect for scars, lesions, pulsations, umbilical abnormalities, bulging movements, size, and contour. The abdomen is not touched during this inspection.
2. Auscultate for bowel sounds using diaphragm of stethoscope. If peristaltic sounds are not heard, listen for 5 minutes to confirm absence of bowel sounds, possibly indicating peritonitis or paralytic ileus.
3. Using bell of stethoscope, auscultate over the midline for vascular bruits, noting any dilation or constriction of vessels.
4. Note condition of wounds and dressings, suture lines, and drainage from abdominal tubes. Measure the pH and presence of occult blood in gastric drainage tubes.
5. Percuss the borders of the liver, beginning at right iliac crest, percussing up right midclavicular line.
6. Palpate the abdomen for tenderness (local, referred, rebound), rigidity, guarding, masses, character of liver, and presence of distended bladder.

Extremities and musculoskeletal system

1. Inspect upper and lower extremities. Compare both sides for equal size and color. Inspect for masses, edema, and varicosities.
2. Check condition of IV and arterial line dressings, noting insertion dates. Inspect casts and traction. Observe for pressure areas or misalignment.
3. Palpate for masses, tenderness, equal or abnormal temperature, muscle tone and strength, and joint range of motion, noting deformities and limitations.
4. Palpate back for tenderness, lateral bend, extension, and rotation, noting sacral edema and presence of pressure points.

Nails

1. Inspect color of nailbeds. Assess for clubbing and nicotine stains.
2. Palpate nail texture and determine capillary refill time.

Rectal area

1. Using gloves, inspect anal area for skin breakdown and hemorrhoids.
2. Perform rectal examination to check for sphincter tone and fecal impaction, noting color and consistency of stool. Perform test for occult blood.

Male genitalia

1. Wearing gloves, inspect penis and scrotum for edema and skin erosion.
2. Check for position, color, leakage, and proper anchoring of Foley catheter. Palpate catheter for sediment with gloved hands.

Female genitalia

1. Wearing gloves, inspect labia, Bartholin's glands, and urinary meatus. Observe for edema, skin erosion, and discharge. Inspect Foley catheter.

Guidelines for Conducting the Ongoing Assessment

1. Note patient's physiological parameters and perform equipment checks at appropriate intervals as ordered.
2. Instead of looking for normal values, observe for trends and changes in what is normal for that patient.
3. Analyze and interpret the results of data collection, reporting problems or improvements. Compare current and previous findings.
4. Repeat assessment of selected systems as needed.
5. Review chief complaint.
6. Record data.

NURSING DIAGNOSIS

The nursing diagnosis is the second step of the nursing process. It is a diagnostic statement based on the patient assessment. In disciplines other than nursing, or previously when the nursing diagnosis format was not used, this component of care was often referred to as the *patient problem list*.

Nursing diagnosis has not always been a separate step in the nursing process and acceptance of the terminology has been relatively recent. Before the 1970s, for example, nurses did not commonly use the word diagnosis except in reference to the medical diagnosis. When the nursing process was introduced in the literature and in practice, formulation of patient needs was integrated as a part of the assessment step. During the 1970s, many changes in nursing were taking place and there was a strong focus on identification of patient nursing needs. Nurses were also acquiring more sophisticated physical and general health assessment skills. Additionally, there was an increased emphasis on building a distinct nursing knowledge base that differentiated from medicine. In 1973 a group of nurse theorists, most notably Gebbie and Lavin,[8] formed the National Group for the Classification of Nursing Diagnosis and convened a conference to develop a taxonomy of nursing diagnosis. This group has since been renamed the North American Nursing Diagnosis Association (NANDA). NANDA completed their tenth major conference in 1992 and have provided important leadership in promoting the use of the nursing diagnosis model and fostering consistency in nursing terminology.

Definition and Distinction of Nursing Diagnosis

Traditionally, the term *diagnosis* has almost exclusively been associated with the practice of medicine. The medical diagnosis is characterized by a specific pathological condition, such as a disease or an illness, and focuses on symptoms, physical examination findings, and outcomes of diagnostic tests. Examples of medical diagnoses are appendicitis, fractured hip, and leukemia. Although the classification of medical diagnoses is revised according to research findings and biomedical/environmental changes, the bulk of diagnostic terms have a time-honored, historical acceptance attached to them. Medical diagnoses tend to be very concise and may be used throughout the patient's illness or hospitalization, regardless of the patient's condition. The nursing diagnosis, on the other hand, is a recent development and different from a medical diagnosis. The focus is generally described as based on the patient's responses to a particular health problem, illness, injury, or disease. The definition of a nursing diagnosis is related only to those conditions that professional nurses are educationally and experientially capable and licensed to treat. Numerous nursing authors and professional groups have asserted views over the years regarding the definition of nursing diagnosis. One of the more accepted definitions was given by Gordon[9] in 1976 stating the following:

> A nursing diagnosis is a clinical diagnosis made by a professional nurse that describes an actual or potential health problem which the nurse, by virtue of education and experience, is licensed to treat.

Nursing diagnoses tend to reflect the holistic orientation of nursing and the relationship between psychosocial and physiological entities; they include a wide variety of patient responses, such as activities of daily living, coping mechanisms, behaviors and feelings, and role functioning. A patient with a single medical diagnosis may have a number of nursing diagnoses because responses to health problems are multiple and varied. Nursing diagnoses also reflect potential and actual health problems. Actual problems are those the patient is presently experiencing and represent an area in which a need is not being met. Potential problems represent those that will most likely occur in the future unless certain actions are taken to prevent them.

Nursing Diagnosis Formulation

Nursing diagnosis is both a product and a process. The terms *diagnose* and *diagnosing* refer to the process of arriving at a judgment or conclusion, whereas the term *diagnosis* refers to the concluding statement or product.[30] The nursing diagnostic process is a series of steps the nurse goes through as information from the assessment data base is analyzed to correctly identify the patient's health need. This process of data analysis consists of organizing the information, separating relevant from irrelevant data, identifying inaccurate data or inconsistencies and gaps in data, establishing patterns within the data, and comparing the data with norms, standards, and theories.[23] Specifics of the cognitive process used in formulating a nursing diagnosis have been described by several nursing authors, most notably Carpenito,[6] Gordon,[10] Carnevali,[4,5] Newman,[22] and Ziegler.[30] Although the cognitive process is complex and requires a sophisticated knowledge base, the nurse acquires the ability to think rapidly and accurately through experience and familiarity with patient situations. In the critical care setting, the nursing diagnosis may change so rapidly nurses are unaware of the mental steps they go through in assessing, discriminating, and distinguishing signs and symptoms and transforming this information (data) into nursing diagnoses.

Writing Nursing Diagnoses

The written nursing diagnosis is usually referred to as the *diagnostic statement.* Carnevali[5] defines the diagnostic statement as a concise, precise classification label for a cluster of related presenting data. The diagnostic statement is formed by connecting the problem statement and the etiology with a phrase, such as "related to." For legal reasons, the term *related to* should be used rather than other terms, such as *caused by* or *due to,* since cause and effect for most nursing diagnoses have not been established by nursing research.[19] The first part (Part I) of the statement is the patient's actual or potential problem, and the second part (Part II) is the contributing factors or etiology as to the probable cause for the problem. Besides these basic components of the diagnostic statement, there are additional refinements that can be used. The following examples illustrate nursing diagnostic statements:

- Potential impaired of skin integrity related to uremic rash secondary to renal failure.
- Anxiety related to impending heart surgery.
- Impaired glucose metabolism related to sepsis: hyperglycemia.

NANDA has formalized a specific method for assisting nurses in identifying and describing patients' problems. This method, called Problem-Etiology-Signs and Symptoms (P-E-S), is a simple formula that can be applied to assist in correctly labeling factors associated with the patient problem, which also helps to formulate the diagnostic statement.

Problem

The *problem* can be an actual or potential problem, or one for which the patient is at high risk.[10] The problem, as specified in the nursing diagnostic statement, must be one that the nurse is licensed and legally allowed to identify and treat. It should be clearly and concisely stated.[14]

The list from the Tenth National Conference on Nursing Diagnoses contains all of the currently accepted nursing diagnoses from previous conferences, including refinements of nursing diagnoses from the previous conferences and newly accepted diagnoses (see the box on p. 16).

Etiology

The *etiology* is the probable cause of the actual or potential health problem.[14] It should be clearly and concisely stated so that it can be easily understood and useful at the bedside. The etiology serves to identify what is creating or maintaining the problem. It guides the nurse in developing the plan of care in that it conveys what must change for the patient to achieve a healthy state.[20]

Signs and symptoms

Signs and symptoms refer to those defining characteristics that are discerned during the assessment phase.[14] These characteristics are specific for each diagnosis and therefore are termed *critical defining characteristics.* When these occur in a patient, a nursing diagnosis can be

made. Partial listings of signs and symptoms for each approved nursing diagnosis are available.[11,20,21] The list for most diagnoses, however, is still being developed. After completing the assessment, if the symptoms match those on the list, the nursing diagnosis is confirmed. If the symptoms do not appear on the list or are unclear or incomplete, then the nurse must use education and experience to judge if the noted signs and symptoms indicate actual or potential problems.[16] If they do, then the nursing diagnoses can be made and written as a part of the nursing care plan.

Various approaches to the P-E-S format have been identified in nursing literature.* Nurses using nursing diagnoses may find that a variation of these styles suits their specific needs.

The P-E-S format can be written in one statement.[16] The problem and etiology are written together along with the signs and symptoms. The signs and symptoms can appear before, with, or after the diagnostic statement.[16]

1. Signs and symptoms that *precede* the diagnostic statement: Edema related to capillary leakage secondary to sepsis.
2. Signs and symptoms written *with* the diagnostic statement: Decreased cardiac output related to mitral stenosis manifested by orthopnea, dyspnea, left arterial enlargement, apical premature beats, paroxysmal supraventricular tachycardia (PSVT), and atrial fibrillation.
3. Signs and symptoms can *follow* the diagnostic statement: Decreased cardiac output related to decreased contractability:
   - Orthopnea.
   - Dyspnea.
   - Tachycardia.
   - Juglar vein distortion.
   - Decreased urine output.
   - Dependent edema.

Two or more problems can be used in one diagnostic statement if they are highly related and are responsible for the same problem.[13] For example, "anxiety and depression related to impending cardiac surgery."

Related etiologies can be written together if they contribute to the same problem.[13] For example, "impaired skin integrity related to immobility and decreased cardiac output."

Health maintenance nursing diagnoses can be written to identify healthy behaviors. For example, "maintenance of low sodium diet related to patient compliance with medical regime."

Occasionally, only the problem will be identified. Additional data may be needed to determine the etiology. This is especially true of the psychological etiologies that are rooted in the subconscious or unconscious. Diagnosis statements such as these may be written: "anxiety, as manifested by tachycardia, diaphoresis, and elevated blood pressure. The box on p. 17, top, summarizes the steps in writing the nursing diagnosis.

---

*Refs 3, 11, 12, 15, 24-26.

NANDA-Approved Nursing Diagnoses

Acitivity intolerance
Activity intolerance, high risk for
Adjustment, impaired
Airway clearance, ineffective
Anxiety
Aspiration, high risk for
Body image disturbance
Body temperature, high risk for altered
Breastfeeding, effective
Breastfeeding, ineffective
Breastfeeding, interrupted
Breathing pattern, ineffective
Cardiac output, decreased
Caregiver role strain
Caregiver role strain, high risk for
Communication, impaired verbal
Constipation
Constipation, colonic
Constipation, perceived
Coping, defensive
Coping, family: potential for growth
Coping, ineffective family: compromised
Coping, ineffective family: disabling
Coping, ineffective individual
Decisional conflict (specify)
Denial, ineffective
Diarrhea
Disuse syndrome, high risk for
Diversional activity deficit
Dysreflexia
Family processes, altered
Fatigue
Fear
Fluid volume deficit
Fluid volume deficit, high risk for
Fluid volume excess
Gas exchange, impaired
Grieving anticipatory
Grieving, dysfunctional
Growth and development, altered
Health seeking behaviors (specify)
Home maintenance management, impaired
Hopelessness
Hyperthermia
Hypothermia
Incontinence, bowel
Incontinence, functional
Incontinence, reflex
Incontinence, stress
Incontinence, total
Incontinence, urge
Infant feeding patterns, ineffective
Infection, high risk for
Injury, high risk for
Knowledge deficit (specify)

Management of therapeutic regimen (individual), ineffective
Mobility, impaired physical
Noncompliance (specify)
Nutrition, altered: high risk for more than body requirements
Nutrition, altered: less than body requirements
Nutrition, altered: more than body requirements
Oral mucous membrane, altered
Pain
Pain, chronic
Parental role conflict
Parenting, altered
Parenting, altered, high risk for
Peripheral neurovascular dysfunction, high risk for
Personal identity disturbance
Poisoning, high risk for
Posttrauma response
Powerlessness
Protection, altered
Rape-trauma syndrome
Rape-trauma syndrome: compound reaction
Rape-trauma syndrome: silent reaction
Relocation stress syndrome
Role performance, altered
Self-care deficit, bathing/hygiene
Self-care deficit, dressing/grooming
Self-care deficit, feeding
Self-care deficit, toileting
Self-esteem, chronic low
Self-esteem, disturbance
Self-esteem, situational low
Self-mutilation, high risk for
Sensory, perceptual alterations (specify type: visual, auditory, kinesthetic, gustatory, tactile, olfactory)
Sexual dysfunction
Sexuality patterns, altered
Skin integrity, impaired
Skin integrity, impaired, high risk for
Sleep pattern disturbance
Social interaction, impaired
Social isolation
Spiritual distress (distress of the human spirit)
Spontaneous ventilation, inability to sustain
Suffocation, high risk for
Swallowing, impaired
Themoregulation, ineffective
Thought processes, altered
Tissue integrity, impaired
Tissue perfusion, altered (specify type: renal, cerebral, cardiopulmonary, gastrointestinal, peripheral)
Trauma, high risk for
Unilateral neglect
Urinary elimination, altered
Urinary retention
Ventilatory weaning response, dysfunctional (DVWR)
Violence, high risk for: self-directed or directed at others

Adapted from the *Proceedings of the Tenth National Conference of the North American Nursing Diagnosis Association*, April 1992.

Guidelines for Writing the Nursing Diagnosis

1. Complete the patient assessment.
2. Review medical and nursing orders previously written.
3. Analyze and interpret the data obtained from the assessment.
4. Based on the assessment, formulate tentative nursing diagnoses.
5. Refer to approved nursing diagnoses list for assistance. Use the P-E-S format.
6. Formulate the problem.
7. Select modifiers to the problem (see the box below). For example:
   - Disturbance in, e.g., disturbance in comfort.
   - Ineffective, e.g., ineffective breathing pattern.
8. Use the connecting phrases "related to" and "secondary to" to help clarify the etiology.
9. Formulate and write the etiology. Avoid using medical diagnosis if possible.
10. Support nursing diagnoses with signs and symptoms using the expression "as evidenced by" or "as manifested by."
11. Write the nursing diagnostic statement clearly and within the realm of nursing.
12. Write diagnoses with legal implications in mind. Do not write such statements as, "Skin breakdown related to inadequate turning."
13. Avoid value judgments, such as "Impaired health maintenance related to refusal to take medications." Use a more appropriate phrase, such as "related to lack of knowledge regarding importance of medications."
14. If an identified nursing diagnosis is not on the accepted list, word the problem clearly, identify the problem cause, and write out the diagnostic statement.[19]

Problem Modifiers

Altered	Disabling	Increased
Compromised	Disruption	Ineffective
Decreased	Dysfunctional	Overload
Deprivation	Excesses	Perceived
Deficiency	High risk	Potential
Deficit	Impaired	Uncontrolled

Nursing Diagnosis and Critical Care Nursing

Traditionally, nursing diagnoses were developed and accepted based on the premise that nursing diagnoses must describe only those activities that are within the domain of independent nursing actions those actions nurses are licensed to perform. In the area of critical care nursing, there are longstanding, unresolved issues related to the use of nursing diagnosis. To date, few nursing diagnoses have been validated with empirical research.[7] An additional concern revolves around the issue of differentiating medical diagnoses from nursing diagnoses. When there are overlapping areas of assessment and intervention or when the medical and nursing diagnoses are the same, e.g., cardiac

arrest, critical care nursing leaders have expressed concern as to the suitability of nursing diagnoses to the domains of critical care nursing.[2,5,19,27,29] Carpenito[6] lists the following three problems with nursing diagnosis in the critical care areas:

1. Nursing diagnosis may result in independent *and* dependent nursing interventions.
2. Nurses may formulate some patient goals (as a result of nursing diagnosis) that may be legally more appropriate for the physician to accomplish.
3. The inevitability of some diagnoses being joint (between nursing and medicine) leads to confusion.

Nursing diagnoses that were developed by NANDA for the nurse generalist, although useful to some extent in critical care, are not always specific enough for critical care nurses who must care for patients with life-threatening physiological problems that require high levels of specialized knowledge.

Currently there is support in the literature for nursing diagnoses more clearly suited for critical care. These are called *physiological* and *collaborative nursing diagnoses*.[24,25] An example of physiological-collaborative nursing is: "serum electrolyte deficit: low potassium." Collabortive nursing diagnoses are problems that the nurse will treat in conjuction with the physician.

Critical care nursing diagnosis leaders have proposed a solution for the limited usefulness of the current NANDA approved list of nursing diagnoses.[6,25,26] They differentiate between behavioral nursing diagnoses and collaborative nursing diagnoses. *Behavioral nursing diagnoses* (BND) are those that are formulated based on the assessment of the patient's psychosocial needs. BNDs do not require medical intervention unless the patient needs medication therapy. Examples of BNDs are: anxiety, loneliness, denial, anger, grieving, and sensory deprivation. *Collaborative nursing diagnoses* (CND) are diagnoses that focus on the physiological needs of the patient and require both nursing and medical interventions to treat or correct. Examples of collaborative nursing diagnoses can be found in the box below. The role of the critical care nurse is not to diagnose medical conditions, such as pulmonary embolism or adult

Examples of Physiological or Collaborative Nursing Diagnoses

Potential for organ failure: brain, related to decreased tissue perfusion.
Decreased atrial conduction: premature atrial contractions.
Potential blood volume deficit.
Decrease in pulmonary perfusion: emboli.
Serum glucose excess.
Nutritional deficit.
Aberrant cellular growth.
Potential disturbance in bowel motility.
Acid-base disturbance: respiratory acidosis.
Ineffective airway clearance: crackles.
Extracellular fluid volume excess: pulmonary-alveolar edema.
Potential infective phlebotic complications related to prolonged IV therapy.

respiratory distress syndrome (ARDS) but to recognize the biological and psychological response generated by these conditions. Within the diagnosis of ARDS the critical care nurse can make several CNDs and BNDs for example: ventilation-perfusion imbalance (CND), and anxiety (BND).

There are controversies surrounding the concept of using CNDs. One school of thought suggests that nursing diagnoses should only be used when nurses treat patients independently, applying the knowledge and the skills that they are licensed to use.[5,11] The other school of thought leans toward the use of CNDs.[6,13,20]

This controversy is becoming less significant as the NANDA-approved nursing diagnoses list includes more physiological nursing diagnoses. Since managing critically ill patients is a responsibility shared by nursing and medicine, the use of CNDs allows the nurse to clearly state the patient's problem in terms that are readily understood by all members on the health care team.

The challenge in the critical care nurse's role in nursing diagnosis is becoming clearly articulated, and resolution in this area will benefit from interdisciplinary efforts. In current practice, the extent to which nursing diagnosis is employed in the area of interdependent and jointly dependent/independent nursing interventions will be determined by each institution and its critical care nursing service.

PATIENT OUTCOMES

Developing patient outcomes is the third step in the nursing process.[14] Patient outcomes are specific measurable behaviors that the nurse and the patient expect the patient will develop as an outcome of care. Patient outcomes should be written using terms that clearly define the desired patient behaviors (see the box on the upper right for a list of suitable terms). One or more patient outcomes are written for each nursing diagnosis.

Patient outcomes with specific measurable criteria serve many purposes. They provide a framework for the subsequent steps in the nursing process. Formulation of outcomes is an opportunity for the patients to participate in their own health care. Outcomes serve as guideposts for the selection of specific nursing interventions. They specify positive patient behaviors that are a direct result of good nursing care. They enhance communication and continuity of care. They may serve as possible criteria for nursing outcome audits. Since it is possible that outcomes will serve as a means of a nursing audit, they should be carefully written and time-limited so that they can be clearly evaluated.

The following characteristics describe well-written patient outcomes:

- Patient-centered and achievable.
- Clear, concise.
- Directive.
- Observable.
- Measurable.
- Time-limited.

> ◢◣
>
> ### List of Selected Objective Words
>
> **WEASEL WORDS***
>
> Knows
> Acquires knowledge of
> Fully understands
> Realizes
> Becomes familiar with
> Appreciates
> Values
> Feels
> Demonstrates knowledge
>
> **CLEARLY DEFINED WORDS†**
>
> | | |
> |---|---|
> | Describes | Writes |
> | Identifies | Expresses |
> | Defines | Verbalizes |
> | Compares | Articulates |
> | Contrasts | Displays |
> | Lists | Exhibits |
> | States | Evidences |
> | Recalls | Manifests |
> | Differentiates | Voids |
> | Recites | Excretes |
> | Demonstrates | Ingests |

*Words open to interpretation.
†Words open to little interpretation.
Adapted from Flynn J-BMcC: *Teaching-learning.* In Flynn J-BMcC, Heffron PB: *Nursing: from concept to practice,* ed 2, Norwalk, Conn, 1988, Appleton-Century-Crofts.

- Realistic.
- Mutually determined.
- Positive.

Outcomes should be written with a focus on improving the patient's abilities and lessening disabilities. They should be designed for each patient, maintaining that person's individuality. They should be *patient-centered.* This can be extended to the patient's family where appropriate. Consider, for example, a 29-year-old man with third degree burns covering 40% of his body. A significant nursing diagnosis might be: Potential for ineffective airway clearance related to laryngeal edema. A patient outcome could be written as follows: "Patient will exhibit a patent airway throughout hospitalization." Specific patient outcomes (statements that delineate behaviors) could then be designed as follows. Patient evidences the following:

- Lungs clear to bases on auscultation.
- Bilateral equal breath sounds to bases.
- Spontaneous unlabored respirations (of normal respiratory pattern), 12 to 20 times per minute.
- Arterial blood gases within desired limits for patient (usually Pao_2 60 to 100 mm Hg and $Paco_2$ 35 to 45 mm Hg).
- Chest x-rays within normal limits for patient.

These outcomes identify the criteria by which this patient will demonstrate improvement.

Outcomes should be written clearly and concisely. This will enable all health care personnel who use the outcomes to understand them. For example, "The patient will discuss postoperative expectations (cough, turn, deep breathe)."

Outcomes should set the direction. They should provide guidelines for all those individuals using the outcome criteria.

Patient outcomes must be stated in measurable terms. They should address what the patient will do and to what extent. There are many words and phrases that are open to a wide range of interpretation to those who read them. Examples of these include: to know, to understand, and to appreciate. These terms and phrases are unclear and cannot be demonstrated or observed. How can one assess a patient's appreciation? When outcomes are stated in measurable terms, an evaluation can be made about improvement. The following examples show incorrect and correctly stated outcomes:

Incorrect: Patient knows the need for clear lungs.
            Patient appreciates need for IPPB.
Correct: Patient lists causes of orthostatic pneumonia.
            Patient turns at least every 2 hours.

Patient outcomes must be measurable. What are the blood pressure, pedal pulses, arterial blood gasses, etc.? Can the patient and family list signs and symptoms of the disease and discuss infection control correctly? Can they perform treatments without error?

State the time for attaining the outcome, for example, "within two hours, by postoperative day 1, or by the time of discharge." Outcomes in critical care should consider the frequent physiological changes in these extremely ill patients. Setting a deadline or time limit helps the nurse during the evaluation phase. If a patient has not reached the predicted outcome within the deadline established, the plan of care will need to be revised. Setting a time limit is also helpful for legal reasons if a patient's chart is audited. The nurse is able to indicate when a patient did not improve within standard time limits, the case received special attention and more efforts were extended to solve the problems.

State outcomes realistically. A goal that is realistic can be obtained with some effort. Outcomes that are unrealistic are usually not obtainable and serve to decrease the patient's motivation.

Outcomes should be determined mutually by the nurse and the patient and family, when possible. Unfortunately, in critical care there is often no time for this step because of the life-threatening nature of the patient's condition or the ethics of care.

Write positive outcomes as opposed to negative ones. Instead of writing, "The patient expresses an absence of pain," write, "The patient expresses a feeling of comfort and relaxation." This state of mind helps the nurse to look for positive improvements rather than focusing on the potential negative results. The box, top right, reviews the steps in writing patient outcomes.

PLANNING

Planning is the fourth step in the nursing process. In this step, the nurse uses the patient outcomes to determine the nursing interventions that are required to assist the pa-

Guidelines for Writing Patient Outcomes

1. Determine priorities. Life-threatening situations receive highest priority.
2. Complete the patient assessment.
3. Formulate the nursing diagnoses.
4. Determine how much patient and/or family participation will be possible for determining mutual outcomes.
5. List behaviors to be attained.
6. Decide which approximating behaviors will best attain the patient outcomes. Terms such as "absence of," "lack of," or "free from" should not be used when writing patient outcomes since attainment can be difficult to measure. Instead, write positive outcomes that can be observed or measured.
   - Poorly written: The patient evidences lack of skin breakdown.
   - Well-written: The patient evidences dry, intact skin of normal color, temperature, and turgor.
7. Write outcomes in terms of patient's behavior. For example:
   Nursing Diagnosis[6]:
   Decreased cardiac output related to myocardial depression and relative hypovolemia.
   Patient Outcomes: Patient evidences the following:
   Blood pressure ± 20 mm Hg preshock level.
   Oriented to person, place, and time.
   Urine output greater than 0.5 ml/kg/hr.
   Full, strong pulses present bilaterally.
   Pulmonary artery wedge pressure: 6-15 mm Hg.
   Cardiac index: 2.5-4.0 L/min.^{2}
8. Write statements clearly and concisely.
9. Use action verbs (measurable terms).
10. Identify time element. For example: Breath sounds following suctioning will be clear.
11. Determine outcomes mutually (if possible).
12. Evaluate the patient outcomes.
13. Refine the list of outcomes, clarify any vagueness, and avoid duplication.

tient and/or family. Planning involves developing strategies to correct, minimize, or prevent patient problems identified by the nursing diagnosis and directed by the patient outcomes.

In the planning phase, the nurse must involve the patient when appropriate. Patients who can communicate effectively should always be involved in their own care and involved in making decisions regarding the priority of their problems. If the patient is experiencing a life-threatening event, however, the nurse must make a judgment, giving the life-threatening event the highest priority. During the planning phase, the nurse also determines the problems that can be solved by nursing activities, and the problems that can be solved with the help of patient and family.

Written Nursing Care Plan

A clear, concise, written plan of nursing care can provide all the information needed to communicate the indi-

Guidelines for Establishing the Nursing Care Plan

1. Complete the assessment.
2. Determine the nursing diagnoses.
3. Set priorities.
4. Determine patient outcomes with specific patient outcomes.
5. Determine the limits on outcomes.
6. Determine the nursing interventions that will most effectively achieve the desired outcomes.

Guidelines for Conducting Evaluation

1. Review assessment.
2. Review nursing diagnosis.
3. Review patient outcomes and outcome criteria.
4. Review plan.
5. Consider the following key points:
   - Have the outcomes been written in measurable terms?
   - Has the patient demonstrated behaviors (physiological, as well as psychological) to achieve the outcomes?
   - Were the outcomes realistic?
   - Were the outcomes specific?
   - Should the plan be modified as a result of the evaluation?
   - Is more data needed?
   - Has the priority order of the nursing diagnoses changed?
   - Are new patient outcomes needed?
   - Are new nursing interventions needed?
   - Are new time limits needed?

vidualized plan to nursing personnel involved in the patient's care. The written nursing care plan contains a summary of the problems, the nursing diagnoses in priority order, the patient outcomes with outcome criteria, nursing interventions designed to achieve the patient outcomes, and space for evaluation. See Fig. 1-1 for an example of a nursing care plan and the box above on Guidelines for Establishing the Nursing Care Plan.

The plan of nursing care, directed by the patient outcomes, is developed in the form of instructions, or nursing orders, that detail the selected nursing interventions. They are based on the etiology component of the nursing diagnostic statement and are carried out during the implementation phase of the nursing process.

Nursing interventions may be classified as dependent, independent, or interdependent—a distinction that rests on the source of authority for the action. *Dependent* nursing interventions are those that relate to the implementation of medical orders. *Independent* nursing interventions are activities that nurses are licensed to perform by virtue of their education and experience. *Interdependent* nursing interventions describe the activities that nurses carry out in cooperation with other health team members, such as physical therapists, respiratory therapists, nutritionists, and physicians.

Many times in the critical care setting, the nursing plan is being devised as it is being carried out because of a life-threatening event. Once the patient has been stabilized, the nursing plan can be written completing the planning phase.

IMPLEMENTATION

Implementation is the action phase of the nursing process. It is during implementation that the nursing care plan is initiated and completed. The selected nursing interventions are executed to benefit the patient in a predicted way relating to the nursing diagnosis and the patient outcomes. Depending on the condition of the patient and the nature of the problem, the nurse, the patient, or the family (or any combination of these) may carry out the nursing care plan. Whenever possible, the patient should be incorporated as an active participant in the implementation of planned interventions.

The success or failure of the implementation depends on the nurse's intellectual, interpersonal, and technical abilities.[29] This includes the nurse's ability to continually collect new data that is then related to existing nursing diagnoses, outcome criteria, and the nursing care plan.

EVALUATION

The final phase in the nursing process is evaluation. This is the phase where the changes in the patient's measurable outcomes are appraised (see box above). Evaluation is considered in terms of how the patient achieved the outcomes. The goal of evaluation is not to determine if the nursing interventions were completed but instead to determine if the patient has achieved the outcomes and to what degree. Evaluation is viewed in terms of behavioral expectations of the patient relative to the patient outcomes.[14]

Careful evaluation can provide information on the degree that the nursing diagnoses and selected nursing interventions have been on target and may pinpoint omissions during other steps of the nursing process. The nurse, patient, and the family are all agents in the evaluation and should be involved whenever possible. All of those involved in this process have an opportunity to learn from it and to set new directions for the future.

The nursing process is a dynamic one, and evaluation is the key to its cyclical flow. Since the patient's health state can change, evaluation is ongoing; identifying those areas where reassessment, redirection, and the reordering of priorities may be necessary. Objective evaluation helps determine the need for new nursing diagnoses, patient outcomes, and strategies for intervention.[29]

REFERENCES

1. Benner P, Wrubel J: *The primacy of caring: stress and coping in health and illness,* Menlo Park, Calif, 1988, Addison-Wesley.
2. Breua C, Dracup K, Walden J: Integration of nursing diagnoses in critical care nursing literature, *Heart Lung* 16:6, 1987.
3. Carlson J, Craft C, McGuire A: *Nursing diagnoses,* Philadelphia, 1982, WB Saunders.

4. Carnevali DL: *Nursing care planning: diagnosis and management,* ed 3, Philadelphia, 1983, JB Lippincott.
5. Carnevali DL: A daily living functional health status perspective for nursing diagnosis and treatment in critical care nursing, *Heart Lung* 14:5, 1985.
6. Carpenito LJ: Nursing diagnosis in critical care: impact on practice and outcomes, *Heart Lung* 16:6, 1987.
7. Fehring R: Methods to validate nursing diagnosis, *Heart Lung* 16(6):625, 1987.
8. Gebbie KM, Lavin MA: *Classification of nursing diagnoses,* Proceedings of the First National Conference held in St. Louis, Oct 1-5, 1973, St Louis, 1975, CV Mosby.
9. Gordon M: Nursing diagnosis and the diagnostic nursing process, *Am J Nurs* 76:1298, 1976.
10. Gordon M: Nursing diagnosis: process and application, ed 2, New York, 1987, McGraw-Hill.
11. Gordon M: *Manual of nursing diagnosis: 1984-1985,* New York, 1985, McGraw-Hill.
12. Guzzetta CE, Forsyth GL: Nursing diagnosis pilot study: psychophysiological stress, *ANS* 2:27, 1979.
13. Guzzetta CE Dossey BM: Nursing diagnosis: framework, process, and problems, Heart Lung 12(3):282, 1983.
14. Guzzetta CE Dossey BM: *Cardiovascular nursing: holistic practice,* St. Louis, 1992, Mosby-Year Book.
15. Guzzetta CE: Nursing diagnoses in nursing education: effect on the profession, *Heart Lung* 16(6):595, 1987.
16. Guzzetta CE: *Nursing diagnosis.* In Flynn JM, Heffron PB: *Nursing from concept to practice,* ed 2, Norwalk, Conn, 1988, Appleton and Lange.
17. Hickey PW: *Nursing process handbook,* St Louis, 1990, Mosby-Year Book.
18. Johnson MM, Brown MA: *Assessment.* In Zschonche DA, editor: *Mosby's comprehensive review of critical care,* St. Louis, 1986, CV Mosby.
19. Kerner CV, Guzzetta CE, Dossey BM: *Critical care nursing: body, mind, spirit,* ed 2, Boston, 1985, Little, Brown, and Co.
20. Kim MJ, McFarland GK, McLane AM: *Pocket guide to nursing diagnosis: proceedings from the fifth national conference,* St Louis, 1984, CV Mosby.
21. Kim MJ, McFarland GK, and McLane AM: *Pocket guide to nursing diagnosis,* St. Louis, 1991, Mosby-Year Book.
22. Newman MA: Nursing diagnosis: looking at the whole, *Am J Nurs* 84:12, 1984.
23. Pinnell NN, deMeneses M: *The nursing process: theory, application, and related processes,* Norwalk, Conn, 1986, Appleton-Century-Crofts.
24. Roberts SL: The role of the collaborative nursing diagnosis in critical care, *Crit Care Nurse* 7(4):81, 1987.
25. Roberts SL: Physiologic nursing diagnoses are necessary and appropriate for critical care. *Focus Crit Care* 15(5):81, 1987.
26. Steele D, Whalen J: A proposal for two nursing diagnoses: potential for organ failure and potential for tissue destruction, *Heart Lung* 14(5):426, 1985.
27. Watson J: *Nursing: human science and human care. A theory of caring,* New York, 1988, National League for Nursing.
28. Yura H, Walsh MB: *The nursing process,* New York, 1967, Appleton-Century-Crofts.
29. Yura H, Walsh MB: *The nursing process,* ed 5, Norwalk, Conn, 1987, Appleton and Lange.
30. Ziegler SM, Vaughn-Wroebel BC, Erlen JA: *Nursing process, nursing diagnosis, nursing knowledge,* Norwalk, Conn, 1986, Appleton-Century- Crofts.

CHAPTER 2

Patient Teaching

After completing this chapter, the reader will be able to:

- Discuss the principles of learning.
- Explain the teaching guidelines for the critical care patient.
- Formulate behavioral objectives.
- Compare and contrast the nursing process and teaching process.
- Design a teaching care plan including objectives, content, and teaching methods.
- Develop the components of the assessment step in the teaching-learning process for the critical care patient.
- Evaluate methods of teaching.
- Discuss rationale for using teaching tools.

Patient education benefits critical care patients by providing information and fostering learning about their illnesses. It reduces anxiety by providing an atmosphere of caring and by correcting misinformation.[1,2] The critical care setting—often an unfamiliar and frightening experience—evokes anxiety and fear in many patients. The ongoing interaction between the patient and the nurse as educator creates an atmosphere in which the patient and family have an opportunity to ask questions and have them answered.

LEARNING
Domains of Learning

Learning is grouped into distinct areas, called *domains.* The cognitive domain includes intellectual behaviors, such as knowledge of facts, knowledge of behavior, processing of information, and the recollection of information. The affective domain encompasses attitudes, values, and emotions. An individual's family beliefs, ethnic beliefs, and lifestyle form part of the affective domain, thus making it a difficult domain in which to teach. The psychomotor domain includes motor or physical skills. Learning to take a

pulse is an example of a psychomotor skill. The perceptual domain includes sensation, figure perception, symbol perception, perception of meaning, and perceptive performance.

Within the domains, behavior is arranged from simple to complex (see the box on p. 23). Progression in the affective domain is toward increasing internalization and individualization.

Principles of Learning

The principles of learning provide the rationale for what to teach, when to teach, and how to teach. It is important for the nurse to know each principle to formulate a comprehensive teaching plan for the patient (see the box on p. 24).

TEACHING

Teaching is a purposeful, planned activity. There are a variety of methods for effective teaching, most of which can be adapted to an individual's situation and environment. The box on p. 24 contains Guidelines for Teaching.

Patient teaching in the critical care setting is difficult given the physical and emotional condition of the patient. Effective patient teaching begins on admission and continues through the entire hospitalization of the patient.

ASSESSMENT

Assessment of learning requires the collection of data about the patient's learning needs, ability to learn, learning style, barriers and facilitators,[5] self-concept, and learning needs of the family.[8] Identification of learning needs enables the nurse to tailor teaching activities for the patient and family (see box on the right of p. 24).

Family Involvement

Caring for critically ill patients includes meeting the learning needs of their family members. This is especially true when the patient is comatose or severely ill.

The nurse engages in an ongoing assessment of the family's learning needs and readiness to learn. The nurse must identify what learning needs the family perceives as important for the patient and for themselves.

▼ **Taxonomies of Educational Objectives**

COGNITIVE DOMAIN
Knowledge

Defines terms.
Identifies specific facts.
Recalls information.

Comprehension

Translates information into own words.
Identifies meaning of abbreviations and scientific terms.
Summarizes information.
Interprets information.
Defines implications and consequences of action.

Application

Applies facts to situations.
Identifies steps in procedures.

Analysis

Distinguishes facts from hypotheses.
Identifies relationships between ideas and facts.

Synthesis

Describes personal experiences, ideas, and feelings.
Prepares plan of action using facts.

Evaluation

Evaluates behaviors using internal standards.

AFFECTIVE DOMAIN
Reception

Expresses awareness.
Expresses willingness to receive information.

Response

Responds with facts but not internalized material.
Responds with commitment.
Responds with total commitment and is satisfied with the change.

Valuation

Accepts a value.
Prefers a set of values.

Organization

Places values into a framework.
Compares the relationships of values.
Identifies prominent values in the framework.

Characterization by a value or value complex

Acts consistently according to value set.
Contrasts values.
Discusses a philosophy of life.
Discusses a philosophy of health.

PSYCHOMOTOR DOMAIN
Perception

Observes skill.
Identifies and describes skill.
Recalls the skill.

Readiness

States readiness to perform skill.
Demonstrates the ability.

Response

Performs skill independently.

Adaptation

Adapts the skill correctly to meet own needs.
Performs the skill correctly without prior demonstration.
Performs the skill correctly after a specific lapse of time.

PERCEPTUAL DOMAIN
Sensation

Detects and expresses awareness of change.
Specifies that an attribute has changed.
Specifies the direction of a change.
Describes extent of change.

Figure perception

Evidences awareness.
Judges distance of light and sound.
Detects tactile qualities, such as hardness and sharpness.
Perceptual organization
Evidences awareness of relationship of parts to a whole.
Resolution of detail
Judges size.
Judges shape.
Interprets successive bits of information.

Symbol perception

Reads.
Detects color.
Responds correctly to verbal instructions.
Responds correctly to written instructions.
Recognizes people and identifies them by name.
Recognizes items and identifies them by name.

Perception of meaning

Comprehends language.
Makes mental associations (e.g. pain medication reduces pain).
Expresses insight into cause and effect relationships (e.g., exercise may precipitate angina).
Makes decisions.

Adapted from Bloom BS, Englehart MD, Furst CJ et al: *Taxonomy of educational objectives: the classification of educational goals, handbook I: Cognitive domain*, New York, 1956 David McKay; Krathwohl DR, Bloom BS, Masia BB: *Taxonomy of educational objectives: the classification of educational goals, handbook II: Affective domain*, New York, 1964 David McKay; Flynn J-BMcC, Heffron PB: *Nursing: from concept to practice*, ed 2, Norwalk, Conn, 1988, Appleton & Lange; Moore MR: The perceptual-motor domain and a proposed taxonomy of perception, *Aud Vis Comm Rev*, 18:379-413, 1970.

▼ **Principles of Learning**

1. Learning is more likely to occur in the following situations when the learner:
   - Perceives a need to learn.
   - Believes the subject matter is helpful in meeting personal needs.
   - Is motivated to learn.
   - Is ready to learn.
   - Perceives both a learning need and a way to meet that need.
   - Is actively participating in the learning experience.
   - Is physically, emotionally, and mentally stable.
   - Does not perceive learning or change as a threat.
   - Views experience as rewarding.
2. Retention of learning is increased in the following situations when learning:
   - Occurs over time rather than in one massed exposure.
   - Is used and applied immediately and frequently.
   - Is encouraged by positive reinforcement.
3. Material that is integrated into the learner's prior knowledge and experience is more likely to be retained.

▼ Guidelines for Teaching

1. Present content by progressing from what the individual knows to what the individual does not know. Approaching material to be taught in this way helps alleviate the patient's anxiety and helps the patient to transfer the application of information from a known to an unknown situation.
2. Teach from the simple to the complex. Providing the patient with the basic concepts initially establishes a firm knowledge base.
3. Proceed from concrete to abstract content. Individuals learn better when their senses can be used to learn new material. Therefore defining concepts by incorporating as many senses as possible makes learning the abstract content easier.
4. Limit teaching to concise, brief explanations.
5. Provide new information and answers to questions in easily understood terminology.
6. Explain each procedure before carrying it out.[1] Limit teaching in the critical care setting to what is relevant to a given patient at a particular time. Giving information provides the patient with a sense of what is happening, increases security, and decreases anxiety.
7. Determine short-term goals with concise objectives.
8. Repeat explanations frequently.
9. Be specific, especially when giving instructions.

▼ **Assessment of Learning Needs**

SOCIOCULTURAL

- What is the patient's age?
- What is the patient's level of education?
- Can the patient read and write?
- Is the patient employed and what are the work responsibilities?
- What is the patient's ethnic background?
- Are there cultural differences that can interfere with treatment?
- What is the patient's socioeconomic status including housing and transportation?

EMOTIONAL STATUS

- How is the patient adapting to the illness?
- What fears does the patient have about the illness?
- Does the patient express concerns about the present condition?
- How does the patient usually cope with problems?
- Does the patient have available, effective support systems?
- How is the patient coping at the present time?

PHYSIOLOGICAL STATUS

- Is the patient alert and oriented to time, place, and person?
- Can the patient see and hear?
- Does the patient wear glasses or a hearing aid?
- Does the patient have any pain?
- Is the patient weak or fatigued?
- Is the patient experiencing any respiratory difficulty?
- Does the patient complain of nausea?

READINESS TO LEARN

- What is the patient's knowledge base about the present condition?
- What would the patient like to know about the illness?
- Has the patient accepted the condition?
- Is the patient asking questions or nonverbally relaying an interest in learning?
- What has the patient's past learning experience been like?
- Is the patient emotionally mature enough to take responsibility for learning?

MOTIVATION TO LEARN

- Is the patient willing to participate in the treatment regimen?
- Does the patient use nontraditional or home remedies?
- What is the patient's belief about health care?
- What is the patient's attitude toward life?
- Is the patient complying with the prescribed medical regimen?
- Where is the patient's information about health and illness gained?
- How is this information applied?

Family participation enhances the teaching-learning process in a variety of ways.[3] Family members can validate and clarify assessment data. They can help the patient remember information and carry out prescribed orders.

NURSING DIAGNOSIS

Examples of appropriate nursing diagnoses within the teaching-learning process could include the following:
- Knowledge deficit related to limited understanding of newly diagnosed myocardial infarction (MI).
- Potential knowledge deficit related to denial of situation, secondary to fear.
- Potential knowledge deficit related to lack of motivation.
- Noncompliance with prescribed medication regime related to poor vision.
- Disturbance in health maintenance related to limited ability to hear systolic and diastolic blood pressure sounds.

PATIENT OUTCOMES

Patient outcomes (or learning goals) are statements that explain the behavior to be demonstrated after learning has occurred (see sample patient outcomes in the box on the right). The nurse and patient collaborate to formulate mutually attainable goals. Family members may be included in goal setting; however, this depends on the patient's desires and the subject being taught. It is prudent to establish both short- and long-term patient outcomes. In the critically ill, short-term outcomes are used most frequently. The patient's unstable condition makes it difficult to set long-term goals. Goals change as the patient becomes an active participant in the health care plan (see Chapter 1 and box on Writing Behavioral Objectives at bottom right).

PLANNING

Planning is initiated as soon as the patient's learning needs are identified and the nursing diagnoses and outcomes are formulated. In the planning phase, the critical care nurse formalizes the strategy for what is to be taught, how it is to be taught, who will teach, and where and when teaching will occur.[4] A teaching plan is developed to address each of these issues.

Development of a Teaching Care Plan

The development of the teaching care plan is a vital element in the planning phase of the teaching-learning process. The teaching plan is an organized, written document representing the patient's learning needs (Fig. 2-1).

IMPLEMENTATION

Teaching methods refer to the way the nurse will conduct the teaching-learning sessions.[3,4] They include impromptu, one-to-one, group instruction, lecture, role-playing, demonstration, and practice.

▼ **Sample Patient Outcomes**

The following patient outcomes were written for a patient in a coronary care unit (CCU) who has a knowledge deficit related to limited understanding of his newly diagnosed MI. These patient outcomes would be fulfilled through separate teaching sessions and each has a subset of lesson objectives. These outcomes could also be written to include the family in the teaching.

During the CCU stay, the patient will be able to do the following:
- State the purpose for admission.
- Describe treatment details of the CCU regimen.
- State the rationale for prompt reporting of chest pain.
- Identify personal habits harmful to recovery (for example, straining at stool and excessive fluid intake).
- Discuss the signs and symptoms, healing process, and risk factors associated with an MI.

Before discharge, the patient will be able to do the following:
- Discuss risk factor modifications.
- Describe stress reduction techniques.
- Identify dietary restrictions.
- Explain medication regimen.
- State progressive exercise schedule.
- Demonstrate pulse taking.
- State when sexual intercourse can safely be resumed.

The following patient outcomes were written for a patient who has a knowledge deficit related to limited understanding of the preoperative and postoperative coronary artery bypass graft (CABG) surgical period.

The patient will be able to do the following:
- Discuss what will be experienced and what can be expected during the preoperative and immediate postoperative periods.
- Demonstrate coughing and deep breathing, incentive spirometry, and leg and arm exercises.
- Articulate fears and anxieties related to the surgical experience.

The following patient outcomes were written for the CABG patient a week after surgery.

The patient will be able to do the following:
- Discuss the surgical procedure and underlying disease process, methods of risk factor modifications, medications, and schedule for return visits to the surgeon or nurse practitioner.
- Describe the integration of presurgical dietary practices with the prescribed dietary regimen.
- Specify the relationship of exercise to normal coronary function, the disease process, and prescribed limitations.
- Demonstrate the ability to palpate the radial pulse for 1 minute and record findings.
- Describe performance of self-care activities within the limitations of the prescribed medical regimen.
- Articulate expected emotional responses and coping abilities.

▼ **Writing Behavioral Objectives**

1. Write objectives using behavioral terms (see Chapter 1).
2. Prepare each objective with only one outcome, otherwise it is difficult to evaluate objective attainment.[4]
3. Formulate realistic and obtainable objectives.
4. Set priorities.
5. Determine teaching content based on objectives.[6]

PATIENT EDUCATION PROGRESS NOTES (KNOWLEDGE DEFICIT)

DON'T FORGET: Problem needs to be addressed every 48 hours until resolution.

LEARNER
- Patient
- Spouse
- Significant other

GOALS (Learner will . . .)
- Demonstrate proper technique
- List signs and symptoms
- Describe side effects
- Demonstrate proper use

METHOD/PLAN
- Video/Television
- Verbal explanation
- Demonstration
- Handout (list title)
- Written explanation

POSSIBLE TOPICS
- Medication/IVs
- Diagnostic procedures
- Wound/Skin care
- Tube/Drain care
- Diet/Tube feeding
- Activity
- Assistive devices

Date/Time and Initials	APPRAISAL OF LEARNER Specific Objective/Subjective Data Reflecting Current Status of Selected Topics	GOALS Learner's Expected Outcome After Educational Process	PLAN Specific Content and Methods Used in Educational Process	EVALUATION Did Learner Achieve Stated Goals?
9-6 8 PM mn	c/o SOB - denies SOB for past couple of weeks - denies noticeable weight gain - states has gained some weight - clothes tighter (red line)	list 3 "danger" signs requiring notification of MD this shift	Verbal explanation of signs of impending reoccurence weight gain > 2 lb ↑ ankle swelling ↑ SOB c̄ activity or at night	9 PM Able to state signs of impending reoccurence c̄ minimal assist

Init.	Full Signature	Title	Init.	Full Signature	Title	Init.	Full Signature	Title	Init.	Full Signature	Title
mn	Nancy Nurse	RN									

Fig. 2-1   Sample teaching care plan. *(Courtesy Boca Raton Community Hospital, Boca Raton, Fla.)*

There are no special rules on the selection of a teaching method. However, there are factors that the nurse should consider when selecting a teaching method.[4] More than one strategy can be used during the course of teaching a patient and/or family. This is actually recommended, since a variety of learning experiences increases interest and enhances learning. The following factors should be used when selecting a teaching method.

- Select methods most appropriate for the learning domain that each behavior represents.
- Consider all available teaching methods.
- Determine when each method is most effective.
- Consider the content to be taught.
- Consider the patient's strengths, learning style, and familiarity with each teaching method.

Teaching methods include the following:

- Impromptu teaching.
- One-to-one teaching.
- Group discussion.
- Lecture.
- Role playing.
- Demonstration and practice.

Teaching Tools and Instructional Media

Teaching tools and instructional media are used to provide information to patients and families. These teaching devices assist the patient and family to achieve the behavioral objectives.

Teaching tools do not replace the teaching methods but instead are used to complement the chosen teaching methods. Teaching aids enhance learning by actively engaging the learner in multisensory learning experiences.[3,7] This makes learning more interesting for the patient and increases retention. The selection of instructional media is based on the patient's learning needs and abilities.

Printed Material

A major concern when using printed material is the patient's and family's reading ability. For printed material to be effective, it must match the patient's ability to read and comprehend information.[6] Determining the patient's reading ability can be difficult. Generally, the patient is embarrassed about not being able to read and may not admit a lack of ability. The nurse should incorporate the following questions in the admission assessment: "Do you like to read?" and "What kinds of things do you regularly read?" These questions provide insight into the patient's motivation to read and reading level. The nurse can also observe the patient reading.

The nurse must determine the reading level of the printed material to be distributed to the patient. This is relatively simple and involves the application of a readability formula. These formulas focus on the grammatical components of the material. Examples of readability formulas are FOG, FRY and SMOG (Table 2-1).

Table 2-1   SMOG Conversion Table*

The easiest method to use for calculating the readability index of textual material using SMOG is the following:
- Count the number of polysyllabic words in 30 sentences (including repetitions of words and abbreviations)
- Look up on chart below

Total polysyllabic words	Approximate grade level (+1.5 grades)
0-2	4
3-6	5
7-12	6
13-20	7
21-30	8
31-42	9
43-56	10
57-72	11
73-90	12
91-110	13
111-132	14
133-156	15
157-182	16
183-210	17
211-240	18

*Developed by Harold C. McGraw, Office of Educational Research, Baltimore County Schools, Towson, Md, 1982.

Audiovisual Aids

Audiovisual aids represent a combination of sight and sound and sometimes touch and smell. Chalk boards, bulletin boards, flannel boards, graphics, transparencies, slides, film strips, audiocassettes, videocassettes, and closed-circuit television programs are examples of audiovisual aids. Audiovisual aids are useful for presenting facts, illustrating psychomotor skills, and fostering attitude changes.[3]

EVALUATION

Evaluation is the final phase of the teaching-learning process. It determines what the patient has learned and if the patient's behavior has changed as a result of the learning experience.[4]

Evaluation is not limited to the patient, however. The teacher should be evaluated along with the teaching methods and audiovisual material. This feedback is used to identify strengths and weaknesses of the methods and to alter the plan accordingly.

The most effective evaluations are performed as an ongoing process. The nurse uses the findings to reinforce desirable behavior, refocus undesirable behavior, and individualize the teaching plan.

The patient is evaluated against the behavioral objective written during the planning phase of the nursing process. It is extremely important that the behavioral objectives be written in observable and measurable terms; otherwise, the evaluation will be difficult and vague. Types of evaluation tools include written and oral tests, checklists, rating scales and interviews, observations, and health records.

Table 2-2   Learning Characteristics, Cognitive Development, and Teaching Methods for Children

Age	Learning characteristics	Cognitive development	Teaching methods
Infancy-3 yr	Sensorimotor	Short attention span Limited vocabulary Respond to one-step-at-a-time commands Experience time only in association with events Have difficulty delaying gratification Cannot distinguish fact from fiction Magical thinking common Cannot understand cause and effect Fear of strangers Separation anxiety	Manipulation of objects Short sessions lasting 2 to 5 min Short sentences with simple explanations Soothe, comfort, hold, and cuddle infants Tactile stimulation Allow toddlers to hold and manipulate some equipment (for example, stethoscope, syringe without needle) Pictures Dolls and puppets Same nurse
4-6 yr	Social interaction Modelling	Motor skills somewhat developed Egocentric; interpret world through their own feelings Beginning to use symbols Highly curious Longer attention span Begin to perceive cause and effect	Play with equipment Answer questions Use words children understand Games Puppet shows Dolls and dollhouses Storytelling Children's books Coloring in specially prepared books Encourage drawing
7-11 yr	Concrete reasoning Inductive reasoning	Learn from reality Lack ability to transfer Learn immediately, since learning tied to situation Increasing use of symbols Longer attention span	Manipulation of equipment Answer questions Reading materials, games, models, board displays (felt and chalkboards, particularly useful) Puppet shows Dolls Encourage cooperation with intrusive and painful procedures Promote coping behaviors Encourage problem solving
12+ yr	Abstract Deductive reasoning	Can conceptualize Understand cause and effect Symbol mastery Analyze problems Can problem solve	Encourage questions Use reading materials Encourage art work Encourage problem solving

PEDIATRIC CONSIDERATIONS

Teaching strategies must be adapted to the patient's level of development and understanding. Teaching activities for a child must include the child's parents because they need to be well-informed to make health care decisions.

Developmentally, young children tend to conceptualize on a concrete or functional level. They engage in egocentric and, often, magical thinking. Older children may regress to this behavior in times of high stress. During adolescence, children progress to the level of abstract conceptualization. Because there is variation and unevenness in the advance of this process, the learning needs of children cannot be identified by age alone and must, for each child, be assessed individually. Other factors, such as behavior, should also be considered when formulating a teaching plan for a child (Table 2-2).

The development of teaching objectives for infants and toddlers requires parental involvement. Parental presence fosters and reinforces learning and helps to dispel the anxiety children may experience when they encounter strangers or are separated from their parents.

Toddlers may feel threatened by the hospital setting, so a safe, secure environment should be established for teaching-learning encounters. Many institutions have policies that painful procedures be performed only in a treatment room not the child's bed. This establishes the child's bed as "safe" territory. Most pediatric units also have a playroom. Playrooms are never to be used for painful procedures so that children can view them as a shelter from the general hospital environment.

The nurse should take advantage of play as an effective learning tool. Children learn through the sensorimotor activity, the active participation in a learning event, and the manipulation of objects that play affords.

Young children (to 3 years old) lack a sense of the passage of time. To facilitate an association between teaching and the learning need, teaching sessions should be conducted as close as possible to the time of the event to which the teaching relates. The sessions should be brief—lasting from 2 to 5 minutes—to accommodate the young child's short attention span and learning must be continually reinforced.

The preschooler (4 to 6 years old) is very curious and interested in learning. Language ability of the preschooler is somewhat limited and children learn best with physical and visual stimuli. A safe environment is needed for the child to feel secure. The preschooler has a longer attention span. Teaching sessions of about 15 minutes are appropriate.

The school age child can be an active participant in the teaching-learning process. They can be engaged in learning activities for about 30 minutes. Safe environments are helpful to reduce anxiety. Children of this age like to have some control over learning activities and can be given choices.

Adolescents are in transition from concrete to abstract thinking. Adolescents may have misconceptions about health and illness. It is helpful to establish what they know before teaching begins. Misconceptions can be clarified. Adolescents are concerned about privacy, about physical appearance and possible disfigurement, and, the opinions of their peers.

HOME HEALTH CARE CONSIDERATIONS

As the lengths of hospitalizations grow shorter, more teaching is being performed in the home. Also, many quite ill individuals are now choosing to return to their own homes for care. This may require the patient or the family to change central line dressings, monitor IV infusions, and perform ventilator care, suctioning techniques, and many other sophisticated procedures.

In home health care, teaching is viewed as one of the most important responsibilities of the home health care nurse. The patient and family members are the designated learners in the home situation. The nurse in the home begins by assessing the patient and family for prior learning on the topic and determines what adaptations are needed in the home. Many times, once returning home out of the structured environment of the hospital, retention of learning diminishes.

When teaching in the home, the nurse should assess the environment and establish a setting that is conducive to learning. Teaching should be adapted for ease of application within the home. For example, cardiac risk factors could be taught in a living room, washing and sanitizing ventilatory equipment in the kitchen or bedroom, and TPN dressing changes in the bedroom. Distractions that may interfere with learning (for example, the television) should be reduced or removed.

When teaching at home, the nurse must determine what supplies the patient needs to perform skills. Reading materials and audiovisuals can be important tools for teaching in the home.

Teaching the patient at home can be challenging and rewarding. The more extensive the nurse's knowledge and skill, the easier it is to teach and the more interesting the teaching-learning process becomes.

REFERENCES

1. Bille DA: *Patient/family teaching in critical care.* In Kenner C, Guzzetta C, Dossey B: *Critical care nursing: body-mind-spirit,* Boston, 1985, Little, Brown.
2. Bille DA: Process-oriented patient education, *Dimens Crit Care Nurs* 2:108, 1983.
3. Boyd MD: *The teaching process.* In Whitman NI et al, editors: *Teaching in nursing practice,* Norwalk, Conn, 1986, Appleton-Century-Crofts.
4. Flynn J-BMcC: *Teaching and learning.* In Flynn J-BMcC, Heffron PB: *Nursing from concept to practice,* ed 2, Norwalk, Conn, 1988, Appleton and Lange.
5. Ford RG, editor: *Patient teaching: manual I, nursing '87,* Springhouse, Pa, 1987, Springhouse.
6. Redman BK: *The process of patient education,* ed 6, St. Louis, 1988, Mosby-Year Book.
7. Rorden JW: *Nurses as health teachers: a practical guide,* Philadelphia, 1987, WB Saunders.
8. Whitman NI: *Assessment of the learner.* In Whitman NI et al, editors: *Teaching in nursing practice,* Norwalk, Conn, 1986, Appleton-Century-Crofts.

CHAPTER 3

Ineffective Coping Requiring Crisis Intervention

Objectives

After completing this chapter, the reader will be able to:

- Define crisis.
- Assess the critical care patient and family.
- Identify the characteristics of patients and family members in crisis in the critical care setting.
- Describe crisis theory and crisis intervention techniques to maintain adaptive functioning for the nurse in the critical care setting.
- Apply crisis intervention techniques to promote positive adaptation with the patient and family in crisis.

Patients and their families requiring critical care nursing are typically faced with profound disruptions in equilibrium and their ability to cope. A *crisis* is a period of emotional disequilibrium.

A crisis occurs when a person faces obstacles to life goals that appear insurmountable, using customary methods of problem solving. Usual coping methods are unavailable or not working. Helplessness and increased anxiety are experienced.[4]

A crisis state can be precipitated by the following:
- Disruption in physiological integrity and functioning.
- Critical care setting itself.
- Alteration in family roles and responsibilities.
- Fear and anxiety associated with hospitalization.
- Illness.

Crisis theory and crisis intervention techniques, within the framework of the nursing process, provide the critical care nurse direction to assess the patient and family's ability to cope and adapt to this critical care experience.

A crisis is composed of the following characteristics[4]:
- A threat or danger to life goals.
- Mounting tension or anxiety where the effects of fear, guilt, or shame are felt.

- Unresolved problems from the past.
- A turning point in which the person may achieve emotional growth or become further disorganized.

A crisis does not occur automatically as a result of a particular set of circumstances. There are identifiable phases of development that lead to an active state of crisis. Caplan[4] describes the following four phases in the development of extreme anxiety and, finally, crisis[1,2,13]:

Phase I. The individual is faced with a crisis-provoking situation. Attempts are made to cope with the anxiety and tension by using behaviors that have worked in the past.

Phase II. The crisis-provoking situation continues to cause anxiety and tension as usual coping mechanisms and problem-solving techniques fail. The person feels increasingly upset and perplexed. At this stage, since there is greater stress, the possibility of a crisis state occurring increases but is still not inevitable, depending on what happens next.

Phase III. Emergency problem-solving mechanisms are brought into play; the individual searches for assistance and calls on all reserves of strength. As a result, the problem may be solved and equilibrium restored.

Phase IV. If the problem is not solved, an active crisis state will result. A person in crisis feels helpless and does not know where to turn or what to do. Internal strength and social supports are unavailable or lacking. Unbearable anxiety and tension are experienced.[4]

A person cannot stay in crisis indefinitely. The feelings experienced are too uncomfortable and distressing. It is generally accepted that there is a limitation to the amount of time an individual can remain in a crisis state. The emotional discomfort stemming from the extreme anxiety moves the person to reduce the anxiety to a more manageable level as quickly as possible. The acute emotional upset can last from a few days to a few weeks. The following outcomes are possible for the individual experiencing a crisis state:

- The person can return to a precrisis state. This happens as a result of effective problem solving, made possible by one's internal strength and supports.
- The person may not only return to the precrisis state but also can grow from the crisis experience through discovery of new resources and ways of solving problems.
- The person reduces intolerable tension by lapsing into maladaptive patterns of behavior. For example, the individual may become very withdrawn, suspicious, or depressed. Others in crises may reduce their tension, at least temporarily, by impulsive, disruptive behavior. Others may resort to extreme measures, such as suicide.

Crises have inherent growth-producing potential. People who master crisis situations have had the opportunity to develop a broader repertoire of coping skills that will help them deal more effectively with life situations in the future.

STAGES OF CRISIS

Resolution of a crisis evolves through several stages. These stages include the following:

Shock. The shock stage begins with the onset of the crisis. Individuals may experience shock or disbelief at what has happened. Individuals may describe feeling numb or very calm. They may function in a mechanical fashion and appear to be in control of the situation. They may minimize what has happened. Individuals may be inappropriately calm or even cheerful. All of these behaviors are defense mechanisms.

Realization. The defense mechanisms give way in this stage and individuals become aware of the situation and its impact on the future. The reality of the situation seems to overwhelm individuals. This stage is characterized by high anxiety, panic, depression, anger, and helplessness. It is a stage of disorganization. Individuals experience an inability to plan, reason, or understand the situation.

Reorganization. In reorganization, individuals attempt to reestablish their identities and identify ways in which to rebuild their lives. At times they may retreat, questioning whether the struggle is worth the effort. Periods of despair may be interspersed with renewed determination.

Acknowledgment. In this stage, individuals admit that the event occurred. This stage may be characterized by depression.

Adaptation. Individuals accept the results of the crisis and adapt behaviors to make the necessary changes. A new identity appears along with hope and a renewed sense of personal worth. This stage is characterized by a reduction in anxiety.

THE INDIVIDUAL IN CRISIS

Individuals in crisis are experiencing emotional discomfort, disequilibrium, and a reduced ability to cope. Aguilera[1] identified balancing factors that may determine the state of equilibrium. Weakness in any one of these areas can be directly related to whether a crisis is precipitated, the intensity of the crisis experience, and its resolution (Fig. 3-1).

These balancing factors are the individual's perception of the event, the presence of adequate support systems, and adequate coping mechanisms. A knowledge of the balancing factors as they relate to each patient can be used by the nurse as a guide in assessing the intensity of a crisis. This information helps formulate a nursing plan to assist the individual and family in adapting to the crisis.

Perception of the Event

In the critical care setting, admission to the unit is the event that most commonly precipitates a crisis. The nurse must identify the event that precipitated the crisis, and more important, the patient's perception of it. In the critical care setting, the crisis is generally caused by the physiological insult. The patient's perception of this illness includes knowledge, understanding, fantasies, and misconceptions. The event itself is compounded by the need for hospitalization, the intensity and nature of the critical care setting, separation from supports, and potential changes in role.[24] A change in the patient's physical state or a change in the family stability might also precipitate a crisis.

Determining the patient's perception of the experience is necessary to establish meaningful communication with the patient and family. How does the patient view what is happening? What is of most concern and importance right now? What are the patient's previous experiences with the health care system? What is the predominant mood? What feelings are evident? How does the patient see this illness affecting family roles and relationships?

The patient and the family may not perceive the event in the same manner as the nurse or others. This is especially true after the initial stabilizing of physiological systems. Additionally, determining if the patient is viewing the experience realistically or in a distorted manner is useful. If the events and experiences are perceived realistically, there will be a recognition of the relationship between the event and the emotional distress. Interventions can then be directed toward relief of anxiety and fear, and successful resolution will be more probable.[1] If the patient is unable to supply this information, family members may be helpful.

Support Systems

Identification of support systems is necessary in determining the patient's response to the crisis experience and provides information helpful in predicting the patient's ability to resolve the crisis. If possible, assess who is important to the patient. Who does the patient look for and ask for? Who visits and calls? How will these people be able to provide support to the patient? Adequate situational support is a crucial determining factor in the patient's ability to adapt to the crisis-provoking event.

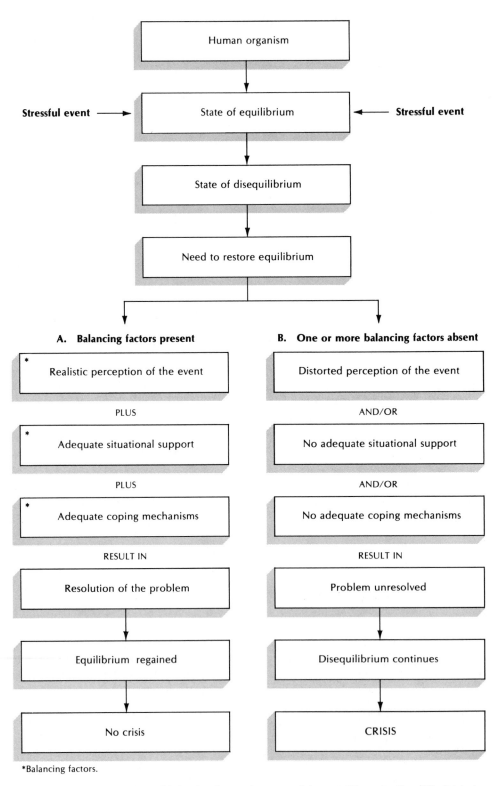

Fig. 3-1   Paradigm: effect of balancing factors in a stressful event. (From Aguilera DC: *Crisis intervention: theory and methodology,* ed 6, St Louis, 1990, Mosby–Year Book.)

Coping Mechanisms

Coping behaviors usually available to the patient are commonly not available in the critical care setting. Coping mechanisms are conscious or unconscious ways of relieving and dealing with anxiety and fear.

Anxiety can be viewed as a state of disequilibrium or tension that prompts attempts at coping. It is manifested at different levels ranging from mild to severe (Table 3-1).

Individuals cope in a variety of ways; some methods of coping are helpful, others are deleterious. Successful attempts at coping reduce tension and promote a sense of well-being.[3] The critical care patient may attempt to control or diminish anxiety and fear by employing defense mechanisms, and the specific form of these defenses may be observed by the critical care nurse. Defense mechanisms include the following:

- Compensation.
- Denial.
- Displacement.
- Identification.
- Projection.
- Rationalization.
- Regression.
- Repression.
- Sublimation.
- Suppression.
- Reaction formation.
- Introjection.
- Conversion.

In the coronary care unit the most common reactions are anxiety, depression, issues of behavioral management, hostility, and delirium.[5] In the surgical care unit, delirium, depression, and anxiety about weaning from the ventilator are the major psychological problems. In the respiratory intensive care unit, depression, anxiety about weaning from the ventilator, and issues surrounding behavioral management are the most common problems.[28]

THE FAMILY AND CRISIS

A crisis affecting any family member affects all members. The crisis produces shifts in family equilibrium. Having a family member acutely ill in a critical care unit represents a sudden crisis event, without time for preparation. Such an intense crisis is demanding and chaotic for all persons involved. The threat of death or a prolonged, debilitating illness is a major precipitating factor for crisis in the family. Required role changes, financial concerns, transportation issues, and time away from home and work are other sources of stress for family members.[22] A family with a profoundly ill member requiring critical care could be experiencing more than one crisis simultaneously. Fam-

Table 3-1   Levels of Anxiety

Level	Behavior patterns
Mild anxiety	Alertness Quick eye movements Increased hearing ability Increased awareness
Moderate anxiety	Decreased awareness of environmental details Focus on selected aspects of self (or illness)
Severe anxiety	Disturbances in thought patterns Incongruency of thoughts, feelings, and actions
Panic	Distorted perceptions of environment Inability to see or understand situation Unpredictable responses Random motor activity

From Long BC, Phipps WJ: *Essentials of medical-surgical nursing*, St Louis, 1985, Mosby–Year Book.

▼   **Perceived Needs of Families of Critical Care Patients in Order of Priority[17,18,23,25]**

1. To feel there is hope.
2. To have questions answered honestly.
3. To know the prognosis.
4. To know specific facts concerning the patient's progress.
5. To have explanations given in terms that are understandable.
6. To receive information about the patient once a day.
7. To be called at home about changes in the patient's condition.
8. To feel that the hospital personnel care about the patient.
9. To see the patient frequently.
10. To know why things were done for the patient.
11. To have the waiting room near the patient.
12. To be assured that the patient is receiving the best care possible.
13. To know exactly what is being done for the patient, and experience relief from initial anxiety.
14. To know how the patient is being treated medically.
15. To visit at any time, to be with the ill person.
16. To have visiting hours changed for special conditions.
17. To have a place to be alone while in the hospital.
18. To feel accepted by the hospital staff.
19. To receive explanations about the environment before going into the critical care unit for the first time.
20. To ventilate feelings, such as guilt and anger.
21. To receive directions about what to do at the bedside.
22. To have visiting hours start on time.
23. To be told about transfer plans while they are being made.
24. To be assured that it is alright to leave the hospital for awhile.
25. To talk with the doctors every day.
26. To be alone at any time.
27. To have friends nearby for support.
28. To be encouraged to cry.
29. To talk about the possibility of the patient's death.
30. To have a readily accessible telephone.

ily members often become disorganized and feel unable to cope. The family will experience fluctuating levels of anxiety, confusion, and helplessness. Family members' attention is focused on the ill member, therefore they are less attentive to their surroundings. They experience the same stages of crisis as the patient and are affected by the same set of balancing factors.

Perception of the Event

Determining the family's perceptions of the event and experience is necessary in establishing meaningful communication. Assess their perceptions of the impact of this crisis on family functioning and their role in the hospitalization and recovery process. What cultural and spiritual factors influence their perceptions?

A significant portion of nursing time is spent working through communication and perception issues.[10,12] Family members may hear the same information, but each perceives it differently. If families are not communicating and perceiving events realistically, they will have a more difficult time adapting to and resolving the crisis successfully.

Support Systems

It is constructive and healthy to use available systems of support in a crisis situation. Are other family members, neighbors, friends, church acquaintances, and clergy available to offer support? Is this particular family more in need of logistical support, such as help with transportation, baby sitting, shopping and meal preparation, or is their need more for emotional support, such as talking, sharing, grieving, and spiritual guidance? It is helpful to identify the "strong" one in the family, since this person is least likely to give expression to their own emotional needs or to seek support because of the time and energy they are expending to support others.

Coping Mechanisms

Several coping behaviors have been identified in families of critical care patients, such as minimization, intellectualization, repetition, emergence of a family leader, and desire to remain near the patient.[2,11]

Nurses in critical care settings are sometimes reluctant to interact with families because of what they feel is a lack of knowledge about families. Nurses should be realistic about the support that they can provide families and should not hesitate to make appropriate referrals, for example, to psychiatric clinical nurse specialists, clergy, social workers, or support groups.[17]

Families have increasingly become the focus of critical care nursing research and education. Various researchers[18,23,25] have conducted interviews with patients and their families to determine their perceived needs. Family needs have been identified and ranked in order of priority (see box on p. 33).

ASSESSMENT

Assessment begins before or on initial contact with the person. It is often possible to anticipate that an individual may be experiencing a crisis because of the events that caused hospitalization. Family and friends who accompany patients may also be in crisis. Serious illness, injury, or death brings fear of the unknown and of the possibility of disfigurement, pain, and disability.

Conveying a caring attitude is necessary in establishing an alliance with the individual. The goal of care is to reestablish psychological equilibrium as quickly as possible. The first step in crisis assessment is to identify events that led to the person's distress.

The crisis may be anticipated or unanticipated and may be related to maturational or situational events. To determine the precipitating event, the patient should be asked about what it is that immediately preceded the decision to seek care. The process of talking about the event and recalling time sequences, circumstances surrounding it, and others involved is often helpful for the patient and family. The opportunity to put the events in order and make some sense out of what is often chaos has a calming effect and gives a sense of control. Simple, direct questions and clarifying comments are useful in assisting the patient. In attempting to identify the precipitating event, look for themes of loss. Often a recent loss will trigger or reawaken feelings of another loss (for example, death of a mother a few months earlier). On occasion, individuals will not make the connection between a crisis event in their lives and problems they are experiencing. Through careful assessment the nurse can help patients relate the current crisis to other life events and can determine the level of intensity of the crisis (see the box on p. 35).

NURSING DIAGNOSIS

Analysis of the data gathered during the crisis assessment allows the nurse to proceed to the problem-solving stage, which begins with formulation of the nursing diagnoses. The following samples of appropriate nursing diagnoses for the patient and family in crisis are given below:

Patient
- Diversion activity deficit related to intensive care unit (ICU) environment.
- Ineffective individual coping related to a new diagnosis of myocardial infarction (MI).
- Powerlessness related to inability to speak secondary to endotracheal (ET) tube.
- Denial related to fear of death.
- Social isolation related to decreased contact with family secondary to hospitalization.
- Sleep disturbance related to change in life style.
- Disturbance in self-esteem related to dialysis.

Family
- Ineffective family coping related to critical condition of the patient.
- Disturbance in role performance related to spouse's stroke.
- Anxiety related to head of household's illness and loss of income.
- Anticipatory grieving related to impending death in family.

▼
Crisis Assessment

1. Assess the patient and family's perception of the event.
   • How does the patient view the event?
   • What influences the perception?
   • What are the implications and their significance?
   • What does it mean now?
   • What is the impact of the event now and in the future?
   • Is the precipitating event being viewed realistically by the patient?
   • Are perceptions validated by others as realistic?
   • Are perceptions of the present situation influencing other aspects of life?
2. Identify situational supports.
   • Who are the significant persons in the patient's life and in the family system?
   • Has the event been discussed with them? If not, why?
   • If so, how did they respond?
   • Who is available to discuss feelings and share concerns?
   • With whom does the patient feel comfortable?
   • Who serves as leader of the family? Who makes decisions?
   • Who helps the family?
3. Identify coping mechanisms.
   • Has the patient or family experienced crisis before?
   • How was it handled?
   • Is the present situation similar or different?
   • What coping mechanisms are being used?
   • What coping mechanisms were used in the past (coping history)?
   • Is the patient identifying coping mechanisms?
4. Assess anxiety level (Table 3-1).
5. Determine defense mechanisms.
6. Assess ability to communicate.
7. Assess the patient's ability to follow orders.
8. Determine the following about the patient:
   • Ability to concentrate.
   • Level of awareness.
   • Memory level.
   • Change in thought processes, for example, hallucinations and delusions.
9. Survey the environment for distractions and stimulation.
10. Monitor vital signs.
11. Record findings of the following:
    • Status on admission.
    • Significant stress-related physiological responses.
    • Perception of events.
    • Support systems.
    • Coping mechanisms.
    • Coping history.

• Hopelessness related to family member's heart failure.

PATIENT OUTCOMES

The process of crisis intervention is directed by the plan of care that follows the identification of nursing diagnoses. The plan is directed toward specific desired outcomes that, when attained, should aid crisis resolution. The following are examples of such outcomes for the patient and family:

Patient
• If conscious and able to speak, verbalizes anxiety.
• If conscious but not able to speak, communicates wants and feelings through alternative routes.
• Demonstrates adaptive coping behaviors.
• Identifies the threat that causes fear.
Family
• Verbalizes feelings of depersonalization, helplessness, and hopelessness.
• Identifies anxious feelings.
• Assists in patient care.
• Expresses realistic hopes.
• Expresses anxiety.

CRISIS INTERVENTION

Crisis intervention is a process aimed at assisting the patient and family to regain and maintain adaptive functioning. The essential element of crisis intervention is the intensive nature of support required to help the ego maintain its integrity and its ability to use coping mechanisms. A crisis, according to Caplan,[4] is self-limiting. Early intervention can assist the individual to emerge as a stronger person. The outcome of a crisis is governed by the kind of interaction that occurs between the individual and the nurse during the time of crisis.

Often usual methods of coping are ineffective and render the individual helpless. A state of disequilibrium produces a need to reduce anxiety.

In a crisis, help should be immediate. Staying with the person, talking through the situation, and encouraging catharsis facilitate recognition and expression of feelings and subsequent relief of guilt (see the box on p. 36 for crisis intervention guidelines.). Strengthening of coping mechanisms is crucial in preventing the formation of symptoms. Personal growth is facilitated by using problem-solving skills and a hierarchy of needs framework to help the person set priorities. (Fig. 3-2 shows a model of crisis intervention.)

Many times, particularly with initial crisis work, assessment and crisis intervention are carried out simultaneously. The nurse initially focuses on concurrent assessment and intervention regarding the following: (1) how disrupted the patient is and will be in the future, (2) what available internal coping mechanisms exist, (3) who is currently available to provide support, and (4) what other external resources can be mobilized. Possible alternatives are explored; very specific directions are frequently necessary in this stage regarding what should be tried and what should be done by the family.

Stress Management

Some approaches to stress management require special training or equipment. Stress management therapists help persons design and implement a structured program of change to enable the individual to control and deal more effectively with stress. Stress management methods include the following:

Guidelines for Conducting Crisis Intervention

PATIENT:

1. Quickly establish support and engage in eye contact. Sit down. Touch the patient.
2. Determine the patient's level of orientation.
3. Establish and maintain consistency in care by having the same nurses work with the patient to promote a therapeutic one-to-one relationships.
4. Allow and support participation in decision-making and choices no matter how small to decrease feelings of helplessness and lack of control.
5. Keep the patient informed of routine care, progress, and developments of condition and care. Knowledge reduces anxiety and fear of the unknown.
6. Maintain a calm, hopeful attitude.
7. Offer alternative cognitive messages, such as handling pain one day at a time. Offer hope and focus on strengths to assist patient in thinking positively and enhancing confidence.
8. Use relaxation techniques and guided imagery techniques to assist the patient in eliciting the relaxation response that will reduce tension, pain, and negative effects of stress.
9. Manipulate the environment to control noise, decrease isolation, provide privacy, control sights, and adjust lighting. Explain equipment.
10. Maintain the patient's outside interests by informing and discussing current events, sports, and hobbies.
11. Allow opportunities for ventilation of feelings, including grief, about illness and this experience. Convey empathy and unconditional positive regard. This promotes awareness and reduces tension. Acceptance and validation of feelings by the nurse as normal enhances self-esteem and decreases anxiety.
12. Allow and support through grieving and anger.
13. Encourage use of situational supports as healthy and adaptive coping behaviors.
14. Continue to clarify communications and perceptions, for example, patient's perception of recovery process, complications, and long-range concerns.
15. Use therapeutic verbal and nonverbal skills, such as attending behaviors and showing care, concern, and respect. Emphasize, clarify, summarize, validate, and acknowledge. Avoid unhelpful communications, such as superficial reassurance, checking equipment too often, ignoring the patient when carrying out a procedure, rushing, contradicting other personnel, and ignoring questions or concerns that tend to be uncomfortable.
16. Help the patient identify problems and explore alternatives.
17. Discuss new ways to deal with the problem. Offer suggestions and provide opportunities to try new behaviors if possible.
18. Provide repeated explanations about the critical care setting.
19. Support the patient's self-esteem.
20. Restore control to the patient as appropriate.
21. Encourage the patient to participate in self-care when able.
22. Help the patient establish short-term goals.

FAMILY:

1. Establish rapport with the family.
2. Locate a quiet area for interaction.
3. Orient the family to the unit including a tour, introductions to the critical care team, and unit routine, especially nurse assignments. Explain equipment and technologies before seeing the patient and prepare the family for visiting. Offer to accompany family to the bedside on the first visit.
4. Meet the family's need to be with the patient by finding out where the family members can be reached, clarifying visiting policies, and being flexible.
5. Facilitate family communication with other members of the critical care team and with the health care system by serving as liaison and patient advocate.
6. Assist the family in identifying needs. Explore alternatives. Problem solve. Offer suggestions. Give "permission" to take time off and focus on other concerns. Assist the family in nurturing each other.
7. Foster realistic hope.
8. Determine the desire of the family to be involved in patient care and allow assistance in daily care.
9. Introduce family to resources available, including support groups and community resources. Assist in forming a family support group.
10. Support coping behaviors that appear to be working for the family. Comment on positive aspects of adaptation and functioning that you observe. Focusing on the positive and on strengths enhances family self-esteem and confidence.
11. Assist the family in using support systems. Suggest extended family, friends, and clergy be contacted. Make telephone calls and elicit more involvement if the immediate family are unable. Suggest ways friends can be of assistance to the family if they seem unsure how to be of help. This promotes maximum support system involvement and enhances effective coping.
12. Allow time for and assist family to communicate their feelings, concerns, fears, and anxieties. Use empathy and unconditional positive regard. Ventilation of feelings promotes awareness and reduces tension.
13. Provide information in understandable terms. Check effectiveness of communications. Patiently answer repeated questions. Assure family of the patient's comfort. Inform of impending death.

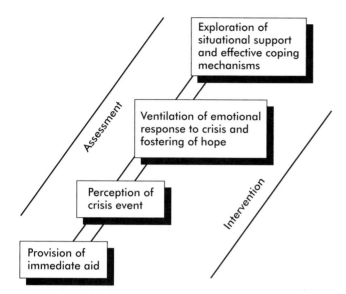

Fig. 3-2 A model for crisis intervention. (From Braulin JLD, Rook J, Sills GM: Families in crisis: the impact of trauma, *Crit Care Q* 5:38, 1982.)

1. Biofeedback—learning voluntary control over autonomically regulated body functions.
2. Behavioral change programs—behavioral conditioning to eliminate a specific stress-related behavior, such as smoking or overeating.
3. Systematic desensitization—providing specific stressful stimuli (such as those related to phobias) in increasing doses while the individual acquires relaxation skills.
4. Autogenic training—teaching cognitive behavior change together with physiological behavior change through passive concentration.

Nurses can help patients prevent or minimize the effects of stress by assisting in the following: (1) identifying existing or potential stressors, (2) recognizing the effectiveness of responses to stressors, (3) developing and testing new behaviors, such as problem solving, and (4) learning ways to minimize the effects of stress, such as by deep breathing or relaxation exercises.[26]

Relaxation techniques

Relaxation exercises are developed from the concept that stress with anxiety does not and cannot exist when the muscles of the body are relaxed. Relaxation exercises do not "cure" stress but do help to minimize the effects of stress and give the person a sense of control. A daily program of relaxation exercises has been shown to have an effect on physiological responses to stress (for example, lowering of elevated blood pressure or elevated blood sugars) and in psychological responses to stress (for example, decreased level of anxiety). They are also helpful on a short-term basis when anxiety is present.

The four basic components of relaxation techniques are the following[13]:

1. Quiet environment—deleting all possible noise and distractions.

2. Comfortable position—sitting with no undue muscle tension.
3. Passive attitude—emptying all thoughts from the conscious mind.
4. Mental device—focusing on a sound, word, phrase, mental image, object, or breathing pattern to shift the mind from logical, externally oriented thoughts.

The important factor is that the person empties the mind of all thoughts and concentrates on the mental device. It is natural for the mind to wander. When this occurs, the person simply redirects the mind back to the mental device.

Progressive relaxation consists of tensing and relaxing muscle groups and focusing on the feelings of relaxation. The systematic application of progressive relaxation has three major effects, which are as follows:

1. Muscle groups are relaxed more and more with each practice.
2. Each of the major muscle groups is relaxed one after the other. As a new muscle group is added, the previously relaxed portions also relax.
3. More total body relaxation is experienced as the person moves into the relaxation phase (see the box below).

Benson's relaxation response (see the box on the top left of p. 38) omits the muscle tensing. It is particularly helpful for muscle relaxation in patients who are experiencing pain or discomfort. It is important to remain with the patient to coach and encourage the relaxation.

PEDIATRIC CONSIDERATIONS

The admission of a child to a critical care unit is usually because of an unplanned event. It is stressful for both parents and child and may precipitate a crisis situation. The outcome may be unknown, and this uncertainty adds to the anxiety experienced by the family.

▼ **Progressive Relaxation**

1. Assume a comfortable position in a quiet room.
2. Begin by focusing on easy breathing.
3. Tense specific muscle groups (see step 5) for 5 to 7 seconds, then relax quickly.
4. Concentrate for 10 seconds on the sensations of the relaxed muscles.
5. Follow a sequence, repeating each muscle group, tensing 2 or 3 times:
   • Hand and arm: clench fist, pull elbow tightly to sides (dominant arm first).
   • Face: wrinkle forehead, close eyes tightly, wrinkle nose, purse lips, smile with teeth tightly clenched.
   • Neck: pull chin to chest.
   • Trunk: pull shoulder blades together, tighten stomach and buttocks.
   • Leg and foot: push down with leg, point toes upward (dorsiflexion) (dominant leg first).
6. Repeat process in any areas in which increased tension has been identified.

From Long GC, Phipps WJ: *Essentials of medical-surgical nursing*, St Louis, 1985, Mosby–Year Book.

▼
Benson's Relaxation Response

1. Assume a comfortable sitting position in a quiet room.
2. Close eyes.
3. Relax body muscles (i.e., "let go").
4. Concentrate on breathing. Repeat a word or sound, such as "one" or "umm" after each exhalation.
5. Continue for about 20 minutes.
6. Open eyes.
7. Take time to adjust to surroundings before moving.

From Long BC, Phipps WJ: *Essentials of medical-surgical nursing,* St Louis, 1985, Mosby–Year Book.

The child is exposed to unfamiliar, invasive, painful, and frightening equipment and procedures. The parents are aware that they cannot control the situation. All of this adds to feelings of powerlessness, hopelessness, and helplessness.

During a crisis event, overwhelming stress can severely impair organized behavior and reduce parental functioning. However, this overwhelming stress often allows parents to more readily accept assistance and crisis intervention that will reduce stress levels and strengthen coping behaviors.

Parental intervention techniques include teaching parents about the critical care setting and the child's condition. Teaching should be expanded to include the feelings of guilt and alterations in parenting roles. Consistency in staffing is important during the child's stay in the critical care unit.

Defining diversional, comforting, caretaking, and monitoring tasks will help to identify activity that parents might feel comfortable doing. When parents are ready, they should be invited to participate in their child's care. Communication, mutual trust, and support in this process is essential.[9]

When the child's critical care admission is unplanned, therapeutic interventions need to be initiated as soon as possible. This is unrealistic at times when the immediate survival needs of the child take priority over the supportive needs of parents.[9]

Crisis events in children are triggered by their developmental stages and the fears associated with each stage (see box, top right). These fears can be used as a guide to anticipate a child's concerns (see the box on the Guidelines for Crisis Intervention with Children on p. 39).

HOME HEALTH CARE CONSIDERATIONS

Care of an ill family member at home is a stressful event. This increase in stress can provoke a crisis state within the family. There are several adaptive things families must do to maintain equilibrium and avoid a crisis state. Families must cope effectively as a means of managing stress.

When the family first encounters the idea of caring for a family member at home, often there is a period of shock and disbelief followed by denial. These coping strategies

▼
Developmental Stages of a Child's Concerns and Fears in the Critical Care Unit

Desertion (4 months to 2 years)—Separation from mother evokes protest, grief, and despair. Frequent visiting is essential.

Dismemberment (2½ to 5 years)—Concerns about separation are still prominent, but fear of bodily hurt increases, magnified by a special sensitivity to pain, wounds, blood, and procedures. Magical thinking, florid fantasy life, and nightmares make informed preparation essential.

Death (5 to 6½ years)—Concerns about death, disappearing, people not returning, oneself being lost or gone forever. A special vigilance develops for the fate of oneself, loved ones, and other patients in the critical care unit.

Displacement (7½ to 8½ years)—Concerns about losing one's place in the critical care unit; concerns about being tied and trapped forever, away from home, school, friends; fears of being left out.

Disability (8½ to 10 years)—School-aged concerns about loss of intellectual, social, and physical abilities, resolving around assertion, competence, and competition. Loss of physical function and loss of school time (getting behind) become stressful critical care issues.

Disgrace (11 to 13 years)—Prepubertal embarrassment over bodily functions, body products, body exposure with staff and other patients, and then anticipation of humiliation with friends.

Disfigurement (13 to 18 years)—Although concerns about disability, pain and disgrace are still present, adolescents develop an intense preoccupation with bodily appearance, proportion, intactness, differences, and dysfunctions, which stimulates depression, acting out, and medical noncompliance at times.

From Ravenscroft K, Finklestein C: *Psychosocial aspects of pediatric intensive care.* In Shoemaker WL, Holbrook RR et al, editors: *Textbook of critical care,* ed 2, Philadelphia, 1988, WB Saunders.

are effective while the family adjusts to the idea and gathers the necessary energy to deal with the event. Once denial is resolved, another useful coping mechanism is information gathering. This strategy enables the family to determine what is needed and to begin to set priorities and allocate resources.

Support systems are also important in helping to prevent crisis in the home. Groups such as Mended Hearts bring together people who have experienced similar situations and have adjusted to the demands.

Once the family brings the patient home, there are many sacrifices and adjustments to be made. These produce a variety of unanticipated problems that can provoke a crisis state within the family. One such problem is the caregiver burden. This usually occurs because one member in the family is designated to assume responsibility for providing care of the patient at home. The strain of this responsibility is often compounded by the accompanying problem of role conflict. Everyone has a variety of roles in life to fulfill and when one's time is occupied as the primary caregiver, it becomes difficult to perform at a maximal level in other roles. Role fatigue develops as the caregiver uses more energy to meet everyone's needs and ful-

Guidelines for Crisis Intervention with Children

1. Establish rapport. Call child by name. Be sure the child knows your name.
2. Approach child at eye level. Minimize use of face masks if possible.
3. Avoid leaving the child alone.
4. Allow the parents to remain with the child. Separation from parents is a major source of anxiety and fear. Parental presence (when practical) during procedures may lessen the child's anxiety. Parents should also be permitted and encouraged to participate in the child's care, as appropriate, to decrease feelings of helplessness.[25]
5. Provide the child with simple explanations that can be understood. Children 1- to 3-years-old understand language and simple information. Children over the age of 5 can more fully understand information concerning procedures, injuries, and equipment. School-aged children may cope with anxiety by avoiding or denying the situation or by becoming actively involved in their own care. The amount of information needed and desired depends on the coping strategy in use. Anxiety may decrease when simple, honest explanations are provided and when the child feels comfortable asking questions. Children avoiding or denying their situation may become more anxious or worried if offered too many or too-detailed explanations.[25]
6. Avoid placing the child in an area where critical care activities can be seen. This can add to the child's anxiety level, since the child may think that he or she will be subject to these procedures next.
7. Do not discuss the child's condition at bedside. Although the child may be unable to comprehend the words of such conversations, he or she may detect the tone of voice used. The active imagination of a child may easily lead to misinterpretation and increase anxiety.[25]
8. Provide the child with honest answers, especially about painful procedures. The worst possible situation for a child is to hear someone say, "This won't hurt a bit" and then proceed with a painful procedure. Gentle warnings about pain promote a sense of trust and allow the child to believe that what the nurse says is reliable.
9. Encourage independence and autonomy to reduce feelings of powerlessness and helplessness.
10. Allow the child to make choices when possible; this further supports independence and autonomy.
11. Establish a consistent routine and sleep patterns.
12. Allow the child to keep a favorite toy, book, game, blanket, or other object, if possible. If this object cannot be left in bed with the child, position it where it can be seen and allow the child to hold it when possible. These objects allow the child to feel more secure in the strange hospital environment.

fill obligations. The stress associated with the caregiver role is often exacerbated by confinement and other restrictions in personal freedom that impede the ability of that family member to meet personal needs.

CRITICAL CARE NURSES AND CRISIS

Critical care nurses are exposed to high stress levels daily at work.[16] Early research carried out with critical care nurses focused on the stress of working in the critical care setting.[6,27] More recent research has shown how critical care nurses perceive the critical care setting and how they adapt to this setting. Results showed critical care nurses differed from noncritical care nurses in the following ways. Critical care nurses[14,15]:

- Felt less powerful and more controlled by the environment; this seemed to be related to the emergency aspect of the setting.
- Were more detached; detachment seemed in response to the environment's heavy stimuli and served as a defense mechanism to decrease anxiety.
- Were more adventurous and thus attracted to the challenging critical care setting.
- Scored lower than noncritical care nurses on somatic complaints, personal and family problems, and workload dissatisfaction.

Because of the high attrition rate of critical care nurses, many studies have been conducted in the past 15 years that have examined critical care nurse stress.[19-21,26] Major sources of stress are the following:

- Conflict and communication problems in interpersonal relationships.
- The critical care setting and management of it, including equipment, noise, and space.
- The patient and the nature of the patient care, especially death.
- Heavy workload.

Interestingly, the following major sources of satisfaction for critical care nurses are similar[27]:

- Nature of direct patient care.
- Interpersonal relationships.
- Acquisition of knowledge.
- Performance and use of skills.
- The critical care setting.
- Reward systems.

It is generally accepted that the critical care setting is a stressful environment in which to work, and, although some studies suggest critical care nurses cope well with the stress, they are still subject to the stress and its potentially negative effects. Critical care nurses must assess their stress levels and coping abilities and make every effort to bring about and maintain adaptive levels of functioning. Any one of the sources of stress identified could precipitate reduced coping and possibly a crisis for the critical care nurse. As with the patient and family, consideration of the balancing factors provides an index of the nurse's ability to avoid or constructively adapt to a crisis.

Perception of the Event

Nurses' perception of a situation, whether it is perceived as a stressor or source of satisfaction, is essential in understanding their response to the situation.[8]

Support Systems

An adequate support network is the social context from which nurses derive reassurance about their ability to cope with the stress of the critical care setting. Support systems can include family and staff members.

Coping Mechanisms

How can nurses assess how well they are coping? One can cope in the critical care setting only as well as one copes in other areas of life. The nurse's self-assessment of coping skills (see the box on p. 40) includes a look at the following[6]:

- One's level of functioning in relation to expectations.
- Degree to which challenge, goal orientation, and enthusiasm characterize one's attitude toward work and family life.
- Nature of one's interpersonal relationships and the satisfaction they offer.
- Extent to which one engages in enjoyable and relaxing leisure activities.
- Whether the above and other factors combine to afford a sense of peace, balance, and contentment in life.

Examining one's coping behaviors and adaptation outside of work, as well as in the work environment, provides a thorough measure of coping ability.

Preventing Work Environment Stress

Self-evaluation may reveal a need to improve the ability to cope with the stress of the critical care setting. Strategies recommended for achieving that end include the following:

- Increasing knowledge and skill to maximum ability.
- Recognizing that the major satisfiers for critical care nurses are similar to what have been identified as stressors; one can exercise choice in how these are perceived and experienced.
- The stress of the critical care setting is often administratively determined. Be assertive with administration and review the following five basic rights for health care professionals[7]:
  1. The right to be treated with respect.
  2. The right to a reasonable workload.
  3. The right to an equitable wage.
  4. The right to determine your own priorities.
  5. The right to ask for what you want.
- Requesting and participating in a support group for your unit's nurses. This group should meet regularly with an objective, qualified person from outside the unit to discuss critical care issues, such as grief and loss, intrastaff conflicts, and emotional management of patients and families.

▼ **Coping Skills Self-Assessment**

1. Assess perception of the event:
   - How do you perceive yourself in the critical care setting—your reactions, your patients, other staff?
   - What influences your perceptions?
   - Are your perceptions validated by others as accurate and realistic? Realistic perceptions allow for recognition of the relationship between the events, sources of stress, and your response.
   - Are perceptions of the work situation influencing perceptions of life in other areas and vice versa? Perceiving other areas of your life with dissatisfaction, frustration, or boredom affects your outlook at work. Similarly, perceiving the work environment with anxiety, dissatisfaction, or burnout will affect other areas of your life.
2. Determine support systems:
   - Assess supports.
   - Who do you have available to discuss feelings and share concerns?
   - Who are the support people in your work environment?
   - Have you identified them and do you use them? (It is not unusual for people under increased stress or in crisis to refrain from using support systems that are available.)
   - Assess your social supports, as well as your family supports.
3. Identify coping behaviors:
   - Are you associating exclusively with critical care nurses and critical care staff members because others seem "difficult" to relate to?
   - Are you so tired and lacking in energy after work that you don't want to do anything? (Positive adaptive functioning and effective coping require a balance of work and play.)
   - Is behavior such as lateness, illness, or unfinished work being brought to your attention?
   - Are you becoming a technical expert and ignoring the patient?
   - When family and friends remark about how different you seem, do you ignore them, rationalize, or deny their observations?

- Consistently assessing stress management at and away from work; using stress management and relaxation techniques as appropriate.

REFERENCES

1. Aguilera D: *Crisis intervention: theory and methodology,* ed 6, St Louis, 1990, Mosby–Year Book.
2. Busch KD: *Stages of illness: the patient's response.* In Hudak C et al, editors: *Critical care nursing,* ed 4, Philadelphia, 1986, JB Lippincott.
3. Caplan G: *An approach to community psychiatry,* New York, 1961, Grune & Stratton.
4. Caplin MS, Sexton DL: Stresses experienced by spouses of patients in a coronary care unit with myocardial infarction, *Focus Crit Care* 15(5):31, 1988.
5. Cassem NH, Hackett TP: *The setting of intensive care,* In Hackett TP, Cassem NH, editors: *Massachusetts General Hospital handbook of general hospital psychiatry,* ed 3, St Louis, 1991, Mosby–Year Book.
6. Cassem NH, Hackett TP: Sources of tension for the critical care unit nurse, *Amer J Nurs* 8:72, 1972.

7. Chenevert M: *Special techniques in assertiveness: treatment for women in the health profession,* St Louis, 1978, Mosby–Year Book.

8. Cleland VS: The effect of stress on performance, *Nurs Res* 14:292, 1965.

9. Curley MAQ: Effects of the nursing mutual participation model of care on parental stress in the pediatric intensive care unit, *Heart Lung,* 17(6):682, 1988.

10. Halm MA: Effects of support groups on anxiety of family members during critical illness, *Heart Lung* 19(1):62, 1990.

11. Jacono J, Hick G, Antonioni C et al: Comparison of perceived needs of family members between registered nurses and family members of critically ill patients in intensive care and neonatal intensive care units, *Heart Lung,* 19(1):72, 1990.

12. Kupferschmid B: Families of critically ill patients, *Crit Care Nurs Curr* 5:2, 1987.

13. Long BC, Phipps WJ: *Essentials of medical-surgical nursing,* St Louis, 1985, Mosby–Year Book.

14. Maloney J: Job stress and its consequences on a group of intensive and non-intensive care nurses, *Adv Nurs Sci* 4:31, 1982.

15. Maloney J, Bartz C: Stress tolerant people: intensive care nurses compared with non-intensive care nurse, *Heart Lung,* 12:4, 1983.

16. McCraine EW, Lambert VA, Lambert CE: Work stress, hardiness, and burnout among hospital staff nurses, *Nurs Res* 36(6):374, 1987.

17. Meijs CA: Care for the family of the ICU family, *Crit Care Nurse* 9(8):42, 1989.

18. Molter N: Needs of relatives of critically ill patients: a descriptive study, *Heart Lung* 8:332, 1979.

19. O'Keefe B, Gilliss CL: Family care in the coronary care unit: an analysis of clinical nurse specialist intervention, *Heart Lung* 17(2):191, 1988.

20. Robinson JA, Lewis DJ: Coping with ICU work-related stressors: a study, *Crit Care Nurse* 10(5):80, 1990.

21. Robinson KM: Predictors of depression among wife caregivers, *Nurs Res* 38(6):359, 1989.

22. Simpson T: Needs and concerns of families of critically ill adults, *Focus Crit Care* 16(5):388, 1989.

23. Stanik JA: Caring for the family of a critically ill surgical patient, *Crit Care Nurse* 10(1):43, 1990.

24. Stockdale LL: Person-centered counselling: application in an intensive care setting, *Heart Lung* 18(2):139, 1989.

25. Strange JM: *Shock trauma care plans,* Springhouse, PA, 1987, Springhouse.

26. Topf M, Dillon E: Noise-induced stress as a predictor of burnout in critical care nurses, *Heart Lung* 17(5):567, 1988.

27. Vincent P, Billings C: Unit management as a factor in stress among intensive care nursing personnel, *Focus Crit Care* 15(3):45, 1988.

28. Zschoche DA, editor: *Mosby's comprehensive review of critical care,* St Louis, 1986, Mosby–Year Book.

CHAPTER 4

Respiratory Care: Artificial Airways and Oxygenation

Objectives

After completing this chapter, the reader will be able to:

- Describe the appropriate methods of examining the respiratory system.
- Formulate several nursing diagnoses for the patient with a respiratory dysfunction.
- Identify the sites for arterial punctures.
- Describe the procedure for an arterial puncture.
- Check the adequacy of circulation in an upper extremity artery.
- Interpret arterial blood gas values.
- Compare and contrast low flow and high flow oxygen administration devices.
- Describe the use of the closed multiuse–suction catheter and the directional-tip catheter.
- Discuss methods of airway intubation and maintenance.
- Describe postural drainage positions and chest physical therapy.
- Compare the pediatric respiratory care with adult respiratory care.
- Adapt respiratory care to home health care.

Oxygen therapy is a supportive treatment used in conjunction with other medications and treatments to prevent or reverse tissue hypoxia. *Hypoxia* is a condition in which oxygen is insufficient to meet the metabolic needs of the body. Hypoxia is caused by *hypoxemia,* a deficiency of oxygen in the arterial blood. Severe hypoxemia is present when the Pa_{CO_2} is below 40 mm Hg. Moderate hypoxemia is present when the Pa_{O_2} is below 60 mm Hg. Oxygen therapy may be needed as the Pa_{O_2} falls beneath 80 mm Hg (mild hypoxemia).[16]

ASSESSMENT

Assessment of respiratory status is extremely important for critical care patients. Inspection, palpation, percussion, and auscultation are used when assessing respiratory status. The anterior and posterior chest are examined bilaterally.

Patient History

Although difficult to obtain, a detailed patient history is necessary for the critical care patient. The respiratory ability of the patient determines the speed and focus of the assessment. For persons in acute distress, the history and interview is limited to a small number of questions related to the onset, course, and the nature of the presenting symptoms. When the patient is too ill to respond, information can be obtained from family, friends, or previous hospital records.

The following material should be included in the patient history:
- Chief complaint.
- Medical history (particularly noting recurrent pulmonary infections, tuberculosis, spontaneous or traumatic pneumothorax, pulmonary edema, pulmonary embolus, pulmonary infarction, asthma, and fungal respiratory diseases).
- Family medical history (particularly noting lung cancer, emphysema, and tuberculosis).
- Date of last chest x-ray and result.
- Date of last tuberculosis test and result.
- Occupational history (particularly noting exposure to chemical irritants, such as dust, fumes, asbestos, or smoke).

Present medical history should include the following:
- Shortness of breath.
    Onset and duration
    Constant or intermittent
    Alleviating or aggravating features
    Associated signs and symptoms
    How is it relieved

Worse at a particular time of the day

How many pillows used for sleeping

- Cough.

    Onset and duration

    Frequency

    Change in frequency

    Alleviating or aggravating features

    Nature of cough (dry or wet)

    Sputum characteristics, such as amount, color, odor, viscocity, presence or absence of blood

    How is cough relieved

- Wheezing.

    Onset

    Cause (e.g., plants, stress, or exercise)

    Allergies

- Chest pain.

    Location and radiation

    Severity and character (i.e., crushing or shooting)

    Onset and duration (i.e., constant or intermittent)

    Alleviating and aggravating factors

- Night sweats
- Temperature elevation
- Any recent contact with persons having tuberculosis
- Frequent colds, bronchitis, croup, or allergies
- Skin changes (i.e., grayness, blueness, or excessive redness)
- Any changes in contour of the chest or fingers
- Numbness or tingling in feet or hands

Respiratory Assessment
Inspection

1. Assess the patient's general appearance, ability to breathe, and ability to clear airway.
2. Assess the skin for cyanosis, grayness, or excessive pinkness (prolonged hypoxemia can lead to erythrocytosis and produce a ruddy appearance).
3. Assess the fingers for nicotine staining, clubbing of the fingers, and cyanosis. Nicotine staining is generally indicative of heavy smoking. Cyanosis and clubbing indicate hypoxemia.
4. Inspect the thorax for size, shape, movement, scars, development, and skin and hair distribution. The normal shape is symmetrical, with the anteroposterior (AP) diameter being less than the lateral diameter. In the normal adult, this ratio ranges from 1:2 to 5:7. In infants, the elderly, and patients with emphysema, this ratio may be 1:1. Any skeletal disorders should be noted (e.g., kyphosis, scoliosis, funnel chest, and barrel chest). These are important to note since they may alter the mechanics of respiration or affect the transmission of breath sounds.
5. Inspect the slope of the ribs and the costal angle for shape and symmetry. The ribs are normally situated at about a 45 degree angle to the vertebrae. In the healthy adult, the costal angle is less than 90 degrees, widening with inspiration.

6. Inspect the intercostal spaces for bulging during expiration or for retractions during inspiration. Note other muscles used in respiration (i.e., the diaphragm, abdominal muscles, and muscles of the neck and shoulders).
7. Observe rate, depth, and rhythm of breathing. Men and children breathe diaphragmatically; women breathe thoracically or costally. Changes in these patterns may be significant. A normal adult breathes 12 to 20 times per minute. The respiratory rhythm has regular cycles, with the inspiratory phase slightly longer than the expiratory phase. The ratio of respiration to pulse rate in the healthy adult is 1:4.

Palpation

1. Palpate the trachea to determine its position.
2. Assess skin temperature and palpate for masses, swelling, or lesions.
3. Palpate lung excursion from the anterior or posterior chest.
4. Feel the amount of thoracic expansion during quiet and deep respirations. Observe the divergence of the thumbs during inspiration and convergence during inspiration. Expansion should be bilateral. Ask the patient to take a deep breath. Note ease of respirations.
5. Palpate the chest for vocal or tactile fremitus with palmar and ulnar aspects of the hand or hands. If one hand is used, move from one side of the chest to the corresponding area on the opposite side. If two hands are used, place simultaneously on the thorax, one on each side. Ask the patient to repeat a word or phrase (if able) that creates resonance. A commonly used phrase is "ninety-nine." Tactile fremitus is generally present in adults. Palpable vibrations have the greatest intensity near the origin of the sound and decrease toward the periphery.
6. Palpate soft tissue of the thorax near the top of the chest wall or neck. *Crepitus* is a palpable sensation caused by the presence of small air bubbles in the subcutaneous tissue. It has a characteristic crackling feeling or popping sound when palpated. Crepitus can be caused by air leaking into the tissue after neck or chest surgery or as a result of a trauma to the chest.

Percussion

1. Percuss the chest to determine relative amounts of air, fluid, or solid material in the lungs and the position and boundaries of organs. There are five basic percussion notes heard over the chest.
2. Percuss the chest downward from the apices. The upper borders of the lungs extend anteriorly 3 to 4 cm (about 1½ inches) above the clavicles and extend posteriorly to the level of the seventh cervical vertebra.

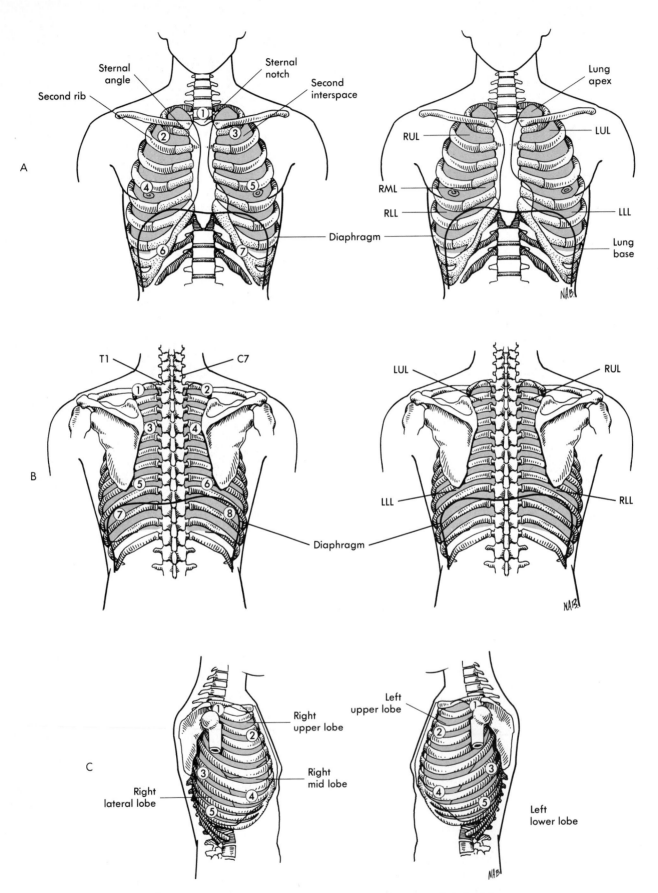

Fig 4-1   Auscultation sites: **A,** Anterior thorax. **B,** Posterior thorax. **C,** Lateral thorax.
(From Phipps WJ, Long BC, Woods NF, et al: *Medical-surgical nursing: concepts and clinical practice,* ed 4, St Louis, 1991, Mosby–Year Book.)

Auscultation

1. Auscultate the chest in a systematic side-to-side manner, moving the stethoscope lightly from top to bottom. At each point of auscultation, assess both inspiration and expiration. Auscultate the anterior and posterior chest. Both lateral chest walls are auscultated at the intercostal spaces (Fig. 4-1).

   The absence or decrease of normal breath sounds may indicate a pathological condition.

2. Auscultate normal breath, adventitious, and voice sounds (Table 4-1). Identify vesicular, bronchial, and bronchovesicular breath sounds.

3. Listen for adventitious breath sounds. Assess for several breaths. If adventitious breath sounds are heard, do the following:
   - Determine if sound is continuous (wheeze) or interrupted (crackles).
   - Determine if sounds are heard on inspiration or expiration.

Table 4-1 Common Assessement Abnormalities of the Thorax and Lungs

Findings	Description	Possible etiology and signifance
Adventitious sounds		
Fine crackles	Series of soft, short, explosive, high-pitched sounds heard just before the end of inspiration; result of rapid equalization of gas pressure when collapsed alveoli or small, terminal bronchioles suddenly snap open; similar sound to that made by rolling hair between fingers just behind ear.	Interstitial fibrosis (asbestosis), interstitial edema (early pulmonary edema), alveolar filling (pneumonia), loss of lung volume (atelectasis).
Coarse crackles	Series of short, low-pitched sounds caused by air passing through airway intermittently occluded by mucus, unstable bronchial wall, or fold of mucosa; evident on inspiration and, at times, expiration; similar sound to blowing through straw under water; increase in bubbling quality with more fluid.	Congestive heart failure, pulmonary edema, pneumonia with severe congestion, chronic obstructive pulmonary disease (COPD).
Rhonchi	Continuous rumbling, snoring, or rattling sounds resulting from obstruction of large airways with secretions; most prominent on expiration; change often evident after coughing or suctioning.	COPD, cystic fibrosis, pneumonia.
Wheezes	Continuous high-pitched squeaking sound caused by rapid vibration of bronchial walls; first evident on expiration but possibly evident on inspiration as obstruction of airway increases; possibly audible without stethoscope.	Bronchospasm (caused by asthma), airway obstruction (caused by foreign body or tumor).
Stridor	Continuous musical sound of constant pitch; result of partial obstruction of larynx or trachea.	Croup, epiglottitis, vocal cord edema after extubation, foreign body.
Absent breath sounds	No sound evident over entire lung or area of lung.	Pleural effusion, mainstem bronchi obstruction, large atelectasis.
Pleural friction rub	Creaking or grating sound caused by roughened, inflamed surfaces of the pleura rubbing together; evident during inspiration and expiration and no change with coughing; usually uncomfortable, especially on deep inspiration.	Pleurisy, pneumonia, pulmonary infarct.
Voice sounds		
Bronchophony, whispered pectoriloquy	Spoken or whispered syllable more distinct than normal on auscultation.	Pneumonia.
Egophony	Spoken "e" similar to "a" on auscultation because of altered transmission of voice sounds.	Pneumonia, pleural effusion.

From Lewis SM, Collier IC: *Medical surgical nursing*, 1992, St. Louis, Mosby–Year Book.

- Differentiate between wheezes and crackles.
- Determine if present bilaterally.
4. Ask patient to cough. Reassess for presence of adventitious breath sounds.
5. Assess voice sounds (if possible). Ask patient to say "ninety-nine" while auscultating. If bronchophony is heard do the following:
  - Assess for whispered pectoriloquy. Ask patient to whisper "one, two, three" while auscultating the chest.
  - Assess for egophony. Ask patient to repeat "e-e-e" while auscultating.

Sputum

Production of sputum is abnormal. The normal respiratory tract does not manufacture it and produces it only in the presence of an underlying pathophysiological state. When the patient is coughing up sputum, it should be examined as a part of the complete assessment.

Arterial blood gases

Analysis of arterial blood gases (ABGs) has become an integral part of the physiological diagnosis and therapeutic treatment of critical care patients (Table 4-2 shows normal ABG values). ABGs provide information about a patient's acid-base balance, alveolar ventilation, tissue oxygenation, and arterial oxygenation. ABG analysis is the measurement of Pao_2 and $Paco_2$ in the blood and determination of blood plasma pH concentration. Additionally, nonrespiratory (metabolic) components are included in an ABG analysis. The most useful of these are actual HCO_3^- and the base excess for normal ABG values.

To get an accurate ABG analysis, care must be taken in drawing, transporting, storing, and analyzing the specimen.

Pulse oximetry

Pulse oximetry is a reliable, easy, and noninvasive method to continuously monitor hemoglobin oxygen saturation (Sao_2), pulse rate, and pulse amplitude.[32] A pulse oximeter measures the absorption, or amplitude, of two wavelengths of light (red and infrared) passing through body parts with high perfusion of arterial blood.[1] Pulse oximetry is based on the principle that well-oxygenated (red) hemoglobin absorbs and reflects different frequencies of light than reduced (blue) hemoglobin. Well-oxygenated blood absorbs a small amount of red light waves, while reduced hemoglobin blood absorbs more. The pulse oximeter sensor calculates the ratio of red to infrared absorption to determine Sao_2 values.

Pulse oximetry has many uses in critical care. It can be used to monitor critical care patients at risk for poor perfusion related to congestive heart failure, COPD, adult respi-

---

Skill 4-1   Interpreting ABG Results

▼ **NURSING INTERVENTIONS**

1. Examine pH.
   - Is it normal, acidotic, or alkalotic? A pH below 7.35 represents acidosis.
   - A pH above 7.45 indicates alkalosis.
   - A normal pH with an abnormal HCO_3^- level and Pco_2 indicates a compensated acid-base disorder.
2. Examine $Paco_2$ in relation to pH. Is it normal, elevated, or decreased?
   - Elevated $Paco_2$ with a decreased pH indicates respiratory acidosis.
   - Decreased $Paco_2$ with an elevated pH indicates respiratory alkalosis.
   - Increased $Paco_2$ with a pH greater than 7.40 indicates compensation for metabolic alkalosis.
   - Decreased $Paco_2$ with a pH less than 7.40 indicates compensation for metabolic acidosis.
3. Examine HCO_3^- level. Is it normal, elevated, or decreased?
   - Elevated HCO_3^- with an elevated pH indicates metabolic alkalosis.
   - Decreased HCO_3^- with a decreased pH indicates metabolic acidosis.
   - Elevated HCO_3^- with a pH less than 7.40 indicates respiratory acidosis.
   - Decreased HCO_3^- with a pH greater than 7.40 indicates respiratory alkalosis.
4. Determine the cause of the acid-base disorder by assessing the patient's history and present physiological status. (Fig. 4-2).

Table 4-2   Normal ABG Parameters

	Arterial		Mixed Venous	
	Normal	Range	Normal	Range
pH, units	7.40	7.35-7.45	7.36	7.31-7.41
$Paco_2$, mm Hg	40	35-45	46	41-51
Pao_2, mm Hg	100	80-100	40	—
Sao_2, %	97	95-100	75	—
HCO_3^-, mEq/L	24	22-26	24	22-26
Tco_2	25	23-27	25	23-27
BE, mEq/L	0	±2	0	±2
Oxygen content (vol %)	20	—	15	—

From Oakes D: *Clinical practitioners pocket guide to respiratory care*, Rockville, Md, 1988, Health Educators.

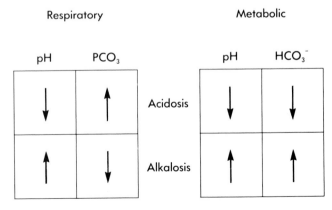

Fig. 4-2   Acid-base imbalances.

Table 4-3 Pulse Oximetry: Correlation of Arterial Oxygen Saturation with Pao_2

Pao_2(%)	Sao_2(%)	Considerations
≥70	≥94	Adequate unless patient is hemodynamically unstable or has oxygen-unloading problem: With a low cardiac output, dysrhythmias, a leftward shift of the oxyhemoglobin dissociation curve, or carbon monoxide inhalation, higher values may be desired. Benefits of a higher blood oxygen value need to be balanced against the risk of oxygen toxicity.
60	90	Adequate in almost all patients: Values are at steep part of oxygen-hemoglobin dissociation curve. Provides adequate oxygenation but with lesser margin of error than above.
55	88	Adequate for patients with chronic hypoxemia if no cardiac problems occur: These values are also used as criteria for prescription of continuous oxygen therapy.
40	75	Inadequate but may be acceptable on a short-term basis if the patient also has carbon dioxide retention: A high Pao_2 may cause CO_2 narcosis. In this situation, respirations are stimulated by a low Pao_2. Thus the Pao_2 cannot be raised rapidly. The nurse may use low-flow, low-concentration oxygen therapy to gradually increase the Pao_2. Monitoring for dysrhythmias is necessary.
<40	<75	Inadequate: Tissue hypoxia and cardiac dysrhythmias can be expected.

From Lewis SM, Collier IC: *Medical surgical nursing*, St. Louis, 1992, Mosby–Year Book.

ratory distress syndrome (ARDS), head trauma, stroke, and open heart surgery.[5] The oximeter can also be used to monitor patients during and after endotracheal (ET) intubation, suctioning, postural drainage, mechanical ventilation adjustments of Fio_2, and positive end-expiratory pressure (PEEP). Additionally, it has audible and visual alarms to provide an alert system for a potentially life-threatening hypoxemia.

The pulse oximeter has been shown to reliably detect changes in the 70% to 100% Sao_2 range in infants, children, and adults.[20] It is not accurate below 70% Sao_2, but values still provide important clinical information[31,32] when used in conjunction with other clinical signs (Table 4-3).

Many factors influence the accuracy and reliability of pulse oximetry, such as high-intensity fluorescent lamps, surgical lights, infrared heating devices, hypothermia, hypotension, vascular disease, edema, and strong venous pulsations[10,21]

NURSING DIAGNOSIS

The following are possible nursing diagnoses for patients with respiratory problems:
- Impaired gas exchange: respiratory acidosis related to hypoventilation secondary to pneumonia.
- Impaired gas exchange: respiratory alkalosis related to hyperventilation secondary to fever.
- Impaired gas exchange related to partial airway obstruction.

- Ineffective breathing pattern related to acute head injury.
- Ineffective airway clearance related to diminished cough reflex.
- High risk for acid-base imbalance related to respiratory deficits.
- Ventilation/perfusion imbalance related to inadequate ventilation.
- Impaired gas exchange related to poor diffusion secondary to ARDS.
- Anxiety related to ET tube.
- Impaired verbal communication related to artificial airway.

PATIENT OUTCOMES

The following are examples of expected outcomes for patients with respiratory problems:
Patient evidences:
- Bilateral breath sounds clear and equal in all areas.
- Both lungs clear and fully aerated on chest x-ray.
- ABG values within normal limits for patient.
- Normal skin color for patient.
- Unlabored respirations.
- Respiratory rate between 12 to 20 breaths per minute (or within normal limits for patient).
- Negative sputum culture and sensitivity results.
- Normal temperature 36° to 38° C (97° to 100.5° F).
- Serum electrolytes within normal limits for patient.
- Alertness and orientation to person, place, and time.

HAZARDS AND COMPLICATIONS OF OXYGEN THERAPY

Administration of oxygen is not without hazards and complications. Careful monitoring and assessment may prevent some of the complications or detect them in an early stage (see box on p. 48). Complications include the following:
- Absorption atelectasis.
- Oxygen-induced hypoventilation.
- Dehydrated mucosa.
- Oxygen toxicity.

METHODS FOR ADMINISTERING OXYGEN THERAPY
Low Flow Systems

A low flow system is one that administers oxygen while the patient also inspires room air. The concentration of oxygen varies as the patient's ventilatory pattern changes and is only effective for patients with an intact upper respiratory tract. Low flow devices are comfortable and economical but do not supply an accurate or fixed concentration of oxygen. The Fio_2 is therefore dependent on the respiratory rate, tidal volume, and liter flow. This method of administration is contraindicated when patients require carefully gauged concentrations of oxygen. The nasal cannula, nasal catheter, simple face mask, partial rebreathing mask, and nonrebreathing mask are low flow devices (Table 4-4).

Guidelines for Initial Fio₂ Selection

Oxygen is delivered in liters per minute (L/min) or as a concentration of oxygen. The concentration is expressed as a fraction of inspired oxygen (Fio_2), such as 0.4, or as a percentage, such as 40%. One of the goals of oxygen therapy is to treat hypoxemia using the lowest Fio_2 possible. Selection of the appropriate Fio_2 is based on the patient's medical history, clinical picture, and probable baseline ABGs. The following guidelines are suggested for selecting initial Fio_2 flow:

- For patients with no history of CO_2 retention and mild-to-moderate respiratory distress, exact Fio_2 is not critical. If hemoglobin desaturation is mild, an intermediate oxygen concentration (40%) may be appropriate.
- For patients with no history of CO_2 retention and severe hypoxemia, an initial Fio_2 of 50% to 100% is indicated.
- Patients with chronic CO_2 retention in severe exacerbations of COPD should receive an Fio_2 of 24% and must be monitored closely. They may require mechanical or artificial ventilation.
- Intubated patients require an Fio_2 that results in ABGs that closely match their baseline Fio_2.

No matter what the patient's condition, however, oxygen therapy must be evaluated by clinical assessment and by ABGs. The amount of oxygen is adjusted to the patient's response to oxygen therapy and the individual need.

EQUIPMENT AND SUPPLIES

- Oxygen source
- Flowmeter
- Oxygen tubing
- Simple face mask or oxygen breathing device
- Humidifier filled with sterile, distilled water
- *No Smoking* sign
- Sterile gloves, sterile water soluble lubricant, tongue depressor, and tape for nasal catheter

NURSING INTERVENTIONS

1. Check physician's order. Introduce self to patient, identify patient, and explain procedure.
2. Ensure privacy.
3. Wash hands.
4. Assemble equipment.
5. Post *No Smoking* sign. Caution patient and visitors not to smoke.
6. Fill humidifier with sterile distilled water to appropriate mark.
7. Attach humidifier to flowmeter.
8. Attach oxygen tubing to humidifier.
9. Adjust flowmeter to prescribed flow rate.
10. Ensure flow of oxygen through oxygen device.
11. Apply mask over the nose and mouth. Tighten the headstrap so that it holds the mask on securely but not so tightly that the mask leaves an indentation in the patient's skin.
12. Adjust oxygen flow as appropriate.
13. Cleanse beneath mask frequently. Assess skin for breakdown or redness.
14. Change mask and tubing according to agency policy. Provide alternate means for oxygen therapy when patient is eating.
15. Assess function of equipment frequently.
16. Assess patient's response.
17. Record data.

Table 4-4 Oxygen Administration Devices

Equipment	Objectives	L/min	Fio₂ (%)	Advantages/Disadvantages
Low flow systems				
Nasal cannula	Provides oxygen through a low flow oxygen delivery system.	1	24	Can be used with mouth breathers
		2	28	Convenient
		3	32	Comfortable
		4	36	Good low flow
		5	40	Allows for talking and eating
		6	44	Fio₂ not really accurate because it depends on patient's respiratory pattern
				May cause sinus pain
				>2 L/min requires added humidity
				Easily displaced
				Nasal passages must be patent
Simple face mask*	Provides oxygen through a mask and low flow oxygen delivery system.	5	40	Simple set-up; good for emergency situations
		6	50	Can get uncomfortable
		8	60	Poor patient tolerance
				Fio₂ not really accurate because it depends on patient's respiratory pattern
				Cannot provide enough humidity for prolonged use

*A minimum flow rate of 5 L/min to flush expired carbon dioxide from the mask is needed.
†Jet adapters on Venturi masks are color coded.

Table 4-4 Oxygen Administration Devices—cont'd

Equipment	Objectives	L/min	Fio$_2$ (%)	Advantages/Disadvantages
Simple face mask (cont'd)				Must be removed at meals Tight fitting mask can cause pressure sores Aspiration of vomitus is a potential problem
Partial rebreathing mask	Provides a high oxygen concentration through a low flow delivery system.	6 8 10-15	35 45-50 In excess of 60 depending on patient's ventilatory pattern	Simple set-up; good in emergency situations Can be uncomfortable Does not provide adequate humidity for long-term use
Nonrebreathing mask	Provides high oxygen concentration.	6 8 10-15	55-60 60-80 80-90	Delivers the highest possible oxygen concentration (55%-90%) possible from a low flow system Good for short-term therapy and transport Has three one-way valves Requires a tight seal May irritate skin

Humidifying systems

Equipment	Objectives	L/min	Fio$_2$ (%)	Advantages/Disadvantages
Aerosol mask (High humidity face mask)	Delivers a specific Fio$_2$ through an aerosol device.		28-100 (variable)	High humidity Accurate Fio$_2$ Does not dry mucous membranes Can be uncomfortable May need extra equipment for higher Fio$_2$ Moisture build-up in tube
Face tent	Delivers high humidity.		21-55	Used for patients with facial trauma Does not dry mucous membranes Can function as high flow system when attached to Venturi system Interferes with eating and talking Impractical for long-term use Possible to rebreathe CO_2
Trach mask T-tube	Delivers a specific Fio$_2$ through an aerosol system.		28-100 (variable)	High humidity Accurate Fio$_2$ Can control oxygen Does not need vent May need extra equipment for higher Fio$_2$

High flow systems

Equipment	Objectives	L/min	Fio$_2$ (%)	Advantages/Disadvantages
Venturi mask†	Provides high flow oxygen with a precise Fio$_2$ in a selected range.	Blue-4 Yellow-4 White-6 Green-8 Pink-8	24 28 31 35 40	Can provide humidity Accurate oxygen levels Simple set-up; good for emergency situations Well tolerated Can only have Fio$_2$ in selected range Hot and confining Must fit snugly

Continuous positive airway pressure (CPAP)

Equipment	Objectives	L/min	Fio$_2$ (%)	Advantages/Disadvantages
CPAP mask	Provides continual positive airway pressure through a mask without the use of a ventilator.		30-100	Do not need ventilator Do not need to be intubated Can get gastric distension Mask is uncomfortable Not useful if patient becomes apneic

Nasal cannula

The most commonly used oxygen delivery device is the nasal cannula. The nasal cannula permits administration of oxygen to relatively stable patients who have regular breathing patterns.

Simple face mask

The simple face mask consists of a single plastic facepiece and an elastic headband. Exhaled gas is vented through small holes on either side and around a loosely fitted mask. The simple face mask provides minimal increase in oxygen capacitance, therefore it provides a small advantage over the nasal cannula or nasal catheter. To ensure an oxygen accumulation and to prevent a CO_2 build-up in the mask, a minimum of 5 L/min oxygen flow is required. Flows greater than 8 L/min do not increase delivered Fio_2. At settings of 5 to 8 L/min an Fio_2 of 40% to 60% can be expected, depending on the patient's ventilatory status.[13]

Partial rebreathing mask

Partial rebreathing masks are simple oxygen masks with a 750 to 1000 ml oxygen reservoir bag added, enabling the patient to breathe oxygen at moderately high concentrations. The first third of the air exhaled by the patient is returned to the bag; the remaining air is exhaled through the vents in the mask. The air that is returned to the bag is the same oxygen that the patient inhaled and comes from the dead spaces in the respiratory tract (i.e., the trachea and bronchi) where little or no gas exchange occurs. By recycling expired oxygen, the mask delivers oxygen concentrations of about 35% to 60% when the flow rate is set at 6 to 15 L/min. This type of mask is useful when there is a need to raise arterial oxygen. This system should be set at 6 or more L/min. Fio_2 of greater than 60% is not possible with a partial rebreathing mask.

The nonrebreathing mask

The nonrebreathing mask is similar to the partial rebreathing mask but valves are incorporated. Valves prevent exhaled gas from flowing back into the bag. A second set of valves, located on the mask's vents, prevent the patient from inspiring room air, thus controlling the concentration of inhaled oxygen. These valves increase the concentration of oxygen delivery to the patient. The Fio_2 ranges from 55% to 90%.

The flow rate is set between 6 to 15 L/min at the point where the reservoir bag remains one-third full during inspiration. During an emergency, this mask will provide a patient with the highest concentration of oxygen possible from a low flow system.

Humidifying Systems

Supplemental humidity must accompany delivery of oxygen because the gas is totally dry and can irritate the mucous membranes. Humidity can be provided through a nebulizer or humidifier. The large-volume nebulizer delivers 100% humidity with a heated or cool mist and is used for

---

Skill 4-3   Administering Oxygen with a Partial Rebreathing Mask'

▼ ....

EQUIPMENT AND SUPPLIES
- See equipment and supplies for Skill 4-2

NURSING INTERVENTIONS

1. Follow Skill 4-6, steps 1 to 16.
2. Adjust oxygen liter flow by watching the rebreathing bag fill. The bag should receive enough oxygen so that it remains at least half full at the end of each inspiration. If the bag is full at the end of the inspiration cycle, the oxygen delivery is too high and needs to be lowered. Conversely, if the bag is less than half full, the oxygen delivery is too low and needs to be increased.
3. Record data.

Skill 4-4   Administering Oxygen Through Nonrebreathing Mask

▼ ....

EQUIPMENT AND SUPPLIES

- See equipment and supplies for Skill 4-2

NURSING INTERVENTIONS

1. Follow Skill 4-6, steps 1 to 13.
2. Adjust oxygen liter flow by watching bag as patient breathes. The bag should receive enough oxygen so that it remains one-third to one-half full at the end of each inspiratory phase. If bag is more than one-half full, decrease oxygen flow and if less than one-third full, increase oxygen flow.
3. Record data.

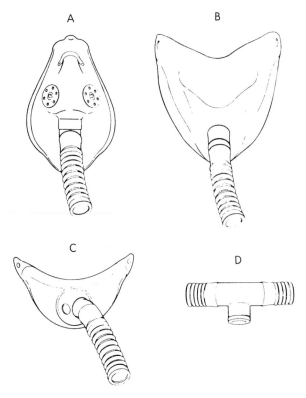

Fig. 4-3   A, Aerosol mask. **B,** Face tent. **C,** Tracheostomy collar. **D,** T-tube. (From Kacmarek RM, Stoller JK: *Current respiratory therapy,* St Louis, 1988, Mosby–Year Book.)

Skill 4-5 **Administering Oxygen by a Large-Volume Nebulizer**

NURSING INTERVENTIONS

1. Fill the water chamber with sterile distilled water.
2. Add a heater and in-line thermometer between the outlet port and the patient, if ordered. Heat mist to 21.1° to 37.7°C (70° to 100°F)
3. Attach flowmeter to oxygen source and screw nebulizer onto flowmeter.
4. Turn flowmeter up to 10 to 14 L/min. This device requires at least 10 L/min to operate. Observe mist coming out of outflow port.
5. Dial in the prescribed Fio_2 at the outlet port.
6. Attach the large-bore tubing to outlet port and connect the mask or T-tube to the distal end of the tubing.
7. Measure the gas flow at the patient's end of the tubing using an oxygen analyzer.
8. Attach the mask or other device to the patient.
9. Monitor large-bore tubing for moisture buildup and monitor gas temperature.

long-term therapy with aerosol masks, tracheostomy collars, T-tubes, and others (Fig 4-3). Nebulizers provide a fine aerosol mist of fluid droplets that settle deep into the lungs; whereas, humidifiers add water vapor to inspired air. Nebulizers can help to mobilize thick secretions and facilitate a productive cough. A humidifier, such as the cold bubble diffuser, delivers only 20% to 40% humidity and should be used with every low-flow oxygen-delivery device except for the nasal cannula, when the flow is 2 L/min or less. To provide the patient who has a high-flow Venturi mask with humidification, entrained room air, rather than the oxygen, is humidified.

Aerosol mask

The aerosol mask or high humidity face mask is used primarily to deliver a high concentration of oxygen with a high degree of humidity. The mist should be visible within the mask at all times. The tubing must be monitored frequently for moisture accumulation.

Face tent

The face tent is an open plastic mask. It delivers high humidity and is used when only small amounts of oxygen are needed. It can be used as a substitute for the face mask if the patient experiences claustrophobia when wearing the face mask and for patients with facial trauma.

Tracheostomy collar (mask)

The tracheostomy collar is used to administer high humidity oxygen to the patient with a tracheostomy. Accurate Fio_2 levels can be provided. (see Table 4-4).

T-tube

The T-tube is a plastic, valveless, T-shaped device used to provide constant oxygen and humidity to patients with

tracheostomies or ET tubes. One side of the device attaches directly to the tracheostomy or the ET tubes while the other end is connected to large-bore oxygen delivery tubing coming from a heated nebulizer. The third port serves as a chimney to vent the excess air and can serve as a partial rebreather. If attached to a Venturi system, a T-tube can serve as a high flow system.

High Flow Systems

High flow systems require use of Venturi adaptors for maintaining consistent precise humidity and Fio_2, and temperature of inspired air is controlled (see Table 4-4).

The Venturi mask is a light-weight plastic mask that delivers precise, constant oxygen. Concentration of oxygen is not affected by the patient's respiratory patterns. Oxygen enters the tubing at a prescribed flow rate. When it reaches the Venturi system, it meets a constricted orifice. To maintain the same flow rate, the velocity increases, resulting in a decrease in pressure on tubing walls and allowing room air to enter the ports. The mask has diluter jets that can be adjusted to change oxygen concentrations. The amount of air entrained is determined by the size of the aperture; the smaller the opening, the higher the increase in velocity, the larger the decrease in pressure, and the larger the amount of room air entrained (Fig. 4-4). The Venturi mask must fit snugly. If it does not fit, if the tubing is kinked, if the ports are blocked, or if less than the recommended flow is used, Fio_2 can be altered.

CHEST PHYSICAL THERAPY TECHNIQUES

Chest physical therapy (CPT) is performed to loosen and remove thick secretions from the airways. CPT is commonly used in prevention and treatment of respiratory complications. CPT includes percussion, vibration, and postural drainage.

Chest percussion is performed by clapping the patient's chest wall in a rhythmical fashion with cupped hands. The chest is percussed moving from the highest to the lowest point. The sudden compression of the air between the hand and the chest wall creates an energy wave that is transmit-

Skill 4-6 **Administration of Oxygen by a Venturi Mask**

NURSING INTERVENTIONS

1. Follow Skill 4-2, steps 1 to 10.
2. Adjust correct-concentration adapter prescribed. (Some ventimasks dial in the oxygen percentage; others are packaged with adapters to allow variation in concentration.)
3. Place mask over nose and mouth. Tighten head strap. Adjust to position of comfort.
4. The mask should be removed frequently, cleansed, and dried to prevent skin breakdown beneath the mask. Change the mask and tubing according to institution policy or more frequently as needed.
5. Add humidity to Venturi stream, if indicated.
6. Assess the patient's response to therapy.
7. Record data.

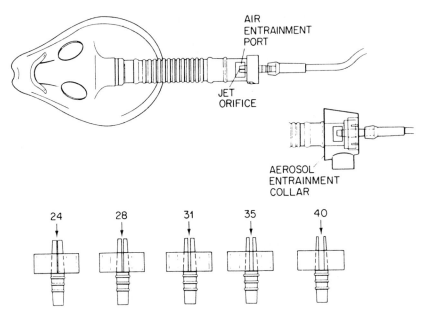

Fig. 4-4   The ventimask. (From Kacmarek RM, Stoller JK: *Current respiratory therapy,* St Louis, 1988, Mosby–Year Book.)

ted through the chest wall to the lung tissue thus loosening secretions in the larger airways. Bronchodilators are generally administered 15 to 20 minutes before percussing the chest. This helps to loosen secretions.

Precautions must be taken so that the patient is not injured during the percussion process. Precautions include the following[26]:

- Percussion of rib cage area only so that soft tissue and organs, such as the kidneys, are not injured.
- Spine, sternum, and female breasts are not percussed.
- Surgical sites are not percussed.
- Open lesions or burns over the rib cage are not percussed.
- Extreme caution must be taken to avoid vigorous clapping on infants and children, the elderly, and persons with a history of fragile bones or chest surgery.
- Patient with low platelet counts are not percussed.

Vibration is an expiratory technique for loosening secretions by vibrating the chest wall with flat hands when the patient exhales. Vibration is used to mobilize secretions in the smaller airways and is generally used in conjunction with percussion.

It is not known exactly why chest vibration enhances the movement of mucus. Several reasons for the effectiveness of vibration have been hypothesized, including the following:

- Generates increased ciliary movement.
- Stimulates responses in chest wall to clear mucus.
- Enhances peak expiratory flow.

Postural drainage is a CPT technique in which the patient is moved into a variety of positions to facilitate secretion drainage by gravity. The patient is tilted into various positions, directing specific airways to the ground. The lung segments supplied by those airways are drained of secretions.

To achieve maximum clearance, each position should be maintained for about 15 to 20 minutes if the positions can be tolerated by the patient. After one segment is drained, the patient is repositioned to drain other segments. Percussion and vibration can be carried out while the patient is in the various positions. Because of the variability and complexity of the tracheobronchial tree, practical postural drainage positioning should be limited to congested lung segments. The time spent in the drainage positions will vary depending on the patient's condition, since many of the postural drainage positions place the head down.

ARTIFICIAL AIRWAYS
Oropharyngeal Airway

The simplest airway is the oropharyngeal airway. This type of airway is a curved tube made of plastic, rubber, or metal. The oropharyngeal airway extends from the lips to the pharynx. It displaces the tongue anteriorly and prevents it from slipping back into the posterior pharyngeal area. It is essential that the oropharyngeal airway be placed properly since improper placement can actually block the airway (Fig. 4-5, *A*). This airway should not be used in a conscious patient, since it can induce vomiting.

The oral airway is sized for adults and children. The sizes vary by length and width. Adult sizes range from no. 3 to no. 10 or small, medium, and large. Most adults require a medium-sized oropharyngeal airway. To determine the correct size of the airway, hold it along the patient's cheek with the flange parallel to the front teeth. The end of the curved portion of the airway should reach the angle of

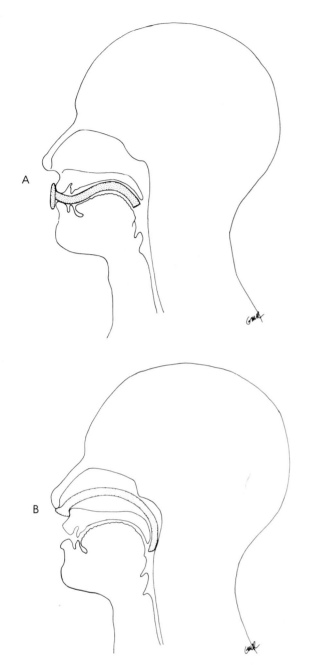

Fig. 4-5   A, Oropharyngeal airway in place. **B,** Nasopharyngeal airway in place. (From Sheehy SB: *Emergency nursing: principles and practice,* ed 3, St Louis, 1992, Mosby–Year Book.)

the patient's jaw. A too large airway can obstruct respiration while a too small airway will not hold the tongue in the proper position.

   The advantages of an oropharyngeal airway include its ease of insertion and its ability to hold the tongue away from the hypopharynx. The disadvantages of this type of airway are that conscious patients have difficulty tolerating it since it stimulates the gag reflex, and it is easily dislodged. Oropharyngeal airways are contraindicated for those patients who have suffered trauma to the lower area of the face or who have undergone oral surgery.

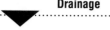

Skill 4-7   CPT–Percussion, Vibration, and Postural Drainage

EQUIPMENT AND SUPPLIES

- Stethoscope
- Towel
- Pillows
- Tissues
- Curved basin
- Suction equipment (if necessary)
- Gloves
- Paper bag

NURSING INTERVENTION

1. Review most recent chest films and ABGs before proceeding.
2. Explain procedure.
3. Auscultate lungs. Note location and degree of retained secretions. Listen for diminished, absent, or bronchial breath sounds that indicate obstructed airways and reduced air passage.
4. If needed, administer pain medication (according to physician's order) 30 minutes before treatment. Suction the intubated patient. Turn off continuous enteral tube feeding 30 minutes before CPT.
5. Inflate trach cuff. Position patient (depending on lobes to be drained and percussed). Use pillows to support patient. Maintain drainage of each segment. Change position for each lung segment to be percussed.
6. Support patient with pillows, as needed.
7. If patient is conscious and alert, ask patient to breathe deeply and exhale using abdominal and diaphragmatic muscles. If patient is receiving oxygen or is on a respirator, these should not be removed.
8. Monitor cardiac rate and rhythm, breathing patterns, and color during procedure. If dysrhythmias, dyspnea, or cyanosis develop, discontinue procedure.
9. A towel or gown may be used to cover area to be percussed.
10. With cupped hands, percuss each affected segment for about 2 to 3 minutes. Preferably begin percussing after 10 to 20 minutes of postural drainage. The percussive force should be adequate to dislodge the secretions in the lung tissue but not hard enough to harm the patient. Clap the chest wall, alternating hands, in a rhythmic fashion. Have the patient take a few deep breaths or sigh the respirator patient 2 to 3 times following percussion.
11. Perform vibration only while the patient is exhaling. Ask patient to inhale (if not on respirator). Place hands (one on top of the other) over the segment to be vibrated. Straighten arms. Ask patient to exhale (or wait for expiratory phase of breathing when on respirator). Gently vibrate the chest wall using a light shaking motion throughout the entire expiratory phase. Vibrate each designated segment 3 to 5 times.
12. Alternate percussion and vibration to maximize the movement of secretions.
13. Encourage patient to cough. Suction the ET tube (if in place).
14. Reposition to drain next segment. Continue procedure until all designated sections have been drained.
15. Auscultate lungs after CPT. Adventitious breath sounds may be louder after clapping and vibration, since secretions have moved to larger airways.
16. Reposition patient. Monitor vital signs.
17. Record data.

Frequent mouth care and oropharyngeal suctioning are important. Further, the airway should be removed every 8 hours to be cleaned and reinserted. A new airway should be used every 24 hours. The mouth should be assessed for any injuries or breakdown every 8 hours as well.

The purposes of the oral airway are to:
- Provide a patent airway for comatose patients and those in respiratory arrest receiving manual bag-valve-mask ventilation.
- Prevent the patient from biting the tongue, grinding the teeth, and biting ET tubes.
- Facilitate secretion removal.

Nasopharyngeal Airway

Nasopharyngeal airways are contraindicated in patients who have had injuries to the nose, nasal obstruction, predisposition to epistaxis, or who have prolonged clotting times (Fig. 4-5, *B*).

Frequent mouth and naris care are needed to maintain good tissue condition. Suctioning is also needed. The airway should be removed and cleaned at least every 8 hours.

The purposes of the nasal pharyngeal airway are the following:
- Aid in maintaining patent airway.
- Provide access for suctioning.
- Prevent nasal trauma from repeated suctioning.

Esophageal Obturator Airway

The esophageal obturator airway (EOA) is used for unconscious, apneic patients (over the age of 16). This type of airway is used as a temporary means for providing positive pressure ventilation. If the patient requires mechanical ventilation, tracheal intubation should be performed as soon as possible. The EOA consists of a mask to seal off the nose and mouth; a tube with perforations at the area of the posterior pharynx and a blind distal end; and a balloon that, when inflated, allows for little or no air passage into the stomach and prevents aspiration of vomitus.

This type of airway is most commonly used outside of the hospital by rescue personnel. ET entubation is the method of choice within the hospital. Nurses most commonly remove the EOA rather than placing one. The EOA is not removed however until the ET tube is in place.

ET Intubation

An ET tube is an airway that is guided into the trachea, usually by a laryngoscope. It is used in situations that require controlled access to the patient's natural airway, in patients who either cannot breathe spontaneously or cannot maintain an adequate gas exchange, and for airway protection with drug overdose comatose patients.[8]

The ET tube allows for positive pressure mechanical ventilation and prevents progressive gastric distention and aspiration of stomach contents. The ET tube is an open-cuffed tube that is placed directly into the trachea through the mouth or nose, past the vocal cords, and guided 2 to 4 cm (1 to 2 inches) above the carina. The tube cuff lies below the vocal cords and is inflated once the tube is in place.

The two types of intubation possible are oral ET intubation and nasal ET intubation (Table 4-5).

ET tubes are the airway of choice when the patient:
- Is in respiratory failure.
- Is unconscious.
- Is areflexic.
- Has an airway obstruction.
- Cannot be ventilated by other means.
- Requires tracheal suctioning.
- Is expected to require prolonged ventilatory support.

If the patient has an upper-airway obstruction, ET intubation may not be possible. In this event, an emergency tracheostomy is performed instead.

Complications during intubation include the following:
- Tracheal injuries.
- Dental injuries.
- Vocal cord trauma.
- Improper tube placement.
- Hypoxia.
- Cardiac dysrhythmias.
- Laryngeal edema.
- Oronasopharyngeal erosion and hemorrhage.
- Increased airway resistance if tube is too small relative to anatomical airway or to minute ventilation.

There are different sizes of tubes and types of cuffs available. Oral tubes are slightly larger than nasal tubes. The tube chosen should be three fourths the size of the patient's trachea. Inflatable cuffs made of pliable material surround the lower end of the tube. The inflated cuff provides a seal when against the trachea to prevent air leakage. Tubes without cuffs are available but are rarely used.

Intubation bypasses the body's natural humidifying process performed by the nasopharynx. Humidification must be provided to loosen mucus and secretions and to prevent drying of respiratory mucosa.

Extubating the patient

Generally the ET tube is removed only when the patient no longer requires an artificial airway, ventilatory support, or pulmonary care.

It is necessary to clear the airway of secretions before removing the ET tube. Failure to do so can lead to compromised respiratory status.

Acute and chronic complications may follow extubation. Therefore the patient should be closely monitored and frequently assessed. Acute complications include laryngeal edema or trauma and absence of gag reflex. Chronic complications include tracheal stenosis or granulomas; vocal cord scarring, pupillomas, or paralysis; and hoarseness.

Accidental Extubation. Occasionally accidental extubation occurs. This requires immediate intervention to avoid respiratory failure. If the Fio_2 needed and the number of ventilator breaths required are low, the patient may tolerate

Table 4-5   Advantages and Disadvantages of ET and Tracheostomy Tubes

Tube	Advantages	Disadvantages	Indications
Oral ET	Good for short-term intubations. Larger tubes can be used. Better respiratory toilet can be performed. Bronchoscopy easier. Easy to insert. Shorter length. Less acute angle. Protects lower airway from foreign body aspiration. Avoids introduction of nasal bacteria into the trachea. Minimal gastric distension.	More tongue and tooth injuries. Maximum placement 14 days. Difficult to suction secondary to greater curvature. Difficult to stabilize. Poorly tolerated in a conscious patient. Patient may bite the tube. Hyperextension of head necessary. Oral hygiene more difficult. Requires laryngoscopy. Easy to dislodge. Patients require more sedation. Laryngeal pathology may occur. Vagal stimulation may result from excessive tube movement. Conscious patients cannot be fed orally. Patients unable to speak. Loss of cough reflex. Hemorrhage can occur.	To establish and maintain a patent and accessible airway. To permit positive-pressure ventilation.
Nasal ET	Easier to suction than oral. Easier to stabilize than oral. Better tolerated by patients. Can be inserted blindly. More patient comfort. Accidental extubation less frequent. Able to swallow. Communication possible. Easy to secure. Requires less sedation.	Recommended maximum placement 14 days. Smaller tubes necessary. Less effective pulmonary toilet. Nasal bleeding. Sinusitis. Skilled personnel needed for placement. Tube kinking because of curvature. Laryngeal pathology.	To establish and maintain a patent and accessible airway. To permit positive-pressure ventilation.
Tracheostomy	Best tolerated for prolonged periods. Easy to suction. Easy to stabilize. Most comfortable. Communication possible. Ability to swallow. Reinsertion of trach tube relatively easy with mature stoma. No laryngeal injury. Decreases dead space in the respiratory system.	Surgical procedure. Infection. Stenosis. Innominate artery erosion. May cause necrosis of trachea. May cause tracheoesophageal fistula. Increases risk of mucus plugs. May cause hemorrhage. May cause mediastinal pneumothorax.	To establish and maintain a patent and accessible airway after ET intubation or when the latter is not desirable. With a cuffed tube, to help decrease the possibility of aspiration of regurgitated gastric contents. With a cuffed tube, to permit long-term, positive pressure mechanical ventilation. To reduce the anatomic dead space and relieve the work of breathing. To relieve upper airway obstruction. When ET intubation is impossible. To manage secretions.

the extubation if humidified oxygen is administered by mask. If the patient cannot be oxygenated adequately, emergency ventilatory assistance by means of a bag-valve-mask device and oxygen reservoir is necessary.

The Tracheostomy

The surgical incision into the trachea between the second and third tracheal ring is called a tracheostomy. A tracheostomy tube is placed into the trachea.

Tracheostomy tubes are made of plastic, rubber, or metal. They can be cuffed or uncuffed and can have a sin-

gle or double cannula. Tracheostomy tubes can be fenestrated allowing for speech. The standard cuffed tracheostomy tube is T-shaped and consists of a curved cannula with a flange. Ties are attached to secure the tube.

The cuff is a balloon that encircles an ET tube or a tracheostomy tube. When inflated, the cuff seals off air leaks around the tracheostomy tube using the least amount of pressure. The cuff pressure can be adjusted to reduce injury to the trachea. Cuff pressure should be less than capillary perfusion pressure. There are two types of cuffs: (1) hard (high-pressure, low volume) and (2) soft (low-pressure, high volume) (Table 4-6).

Text continued on p. 59.

Skill 4-8   Inserting the Oral ET Tube

EQUIPMENT AND SUPPLIES

- Laryngoscope with curved (MacIntosh) or straight blade (Jackson-Wilson or Miller) and light source (with new batteries) (at least two sizes of blades and two types of blades)
- ET tube
- Stylette to guide tube
- Magill forceps
- 10 ml syringe to inflate cuff
- Water soluble lubricant
- Suction regulator, cannister, catheter, and sterile gloves
- Oral airway or bite block
- Bag-valve-mask device
- Flowmeter
- Oxygen source
- Adhesive tape
- Gloves
- Tincture of benzoin
- Anesthetic spray or 4% lidocaine jelly for anesthestizing throat
- Intravenous sedation if indicated by physician
- Suction equipment

NURSING INTERVENTIONS

1. Introduce self to patient. Explain procedure to patient. Provide emotional support. Assess patient's ventilatory effort. If necessary, provide manual ventilations with bag-valve-mask.
2. Administer 100% oxygen through mask or bag-valve-mask. Monitor vital signs and ECG monitor for dysrhythmias. Administer IV sedation if prescribed.
3. Remove any dentures. Apply wrist restraints if necessary.
4. Check equipment. Use syringe to inflate cuff. Check for leaks. Completely deflate cuff. Check laryngoscope batteries and light. Various sizes and lengths of ET tubes are available. Choose size and length appropriate for the patient; 21 cm is generally a good length for adults.
5. If using stylette, lubricate entire length and insert into ET tube. Ensure that tip of stylette does not extend beyond the tip of the ET tube.
6. Position patient flat in bed with neck slightly flexed, head elevated slightly higher than shoulders with rolled towel. Wear gloves.
7. Open patient's mouth using crossed-finger technique if necessary. Spray posterior pharynx with local anesthesic.

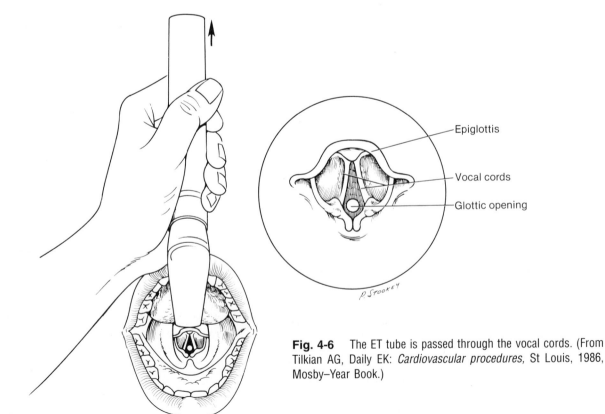

Fig. 4-6   The ET tube is passed through the vocal cords. (From Tilkian AG, Daily EK: *Cardiovascular procedures*, St Louis, 1986, Mosby–Year Book.)

8. Suction if necessary.
9. Hyperoxygenate with 100% Fio_2 for 2 minutes before intubation if airway is not obstructed.
10. With the blade in functioning position on the handle, hold laryngoscope in the nondominant hand.
11. Insert blade into the right of the patient's mouth. Slide blade to center of mouth to displace tongue.
12. Advance blade until the epiglottis can be visualized (Fig. 4-6). If a straight blade is used, advance past the epiglottis. If curved blade is used, position tip of blade anterior to the epiglottis (Fig. 4-7, *A* and *B*). As the tip of the blade slides over the base of the tongue, the laryngoscope will be elevated at a 45 degree angle toward the feet. Do not force the laryngoscope. Pressure to lift the jaw should come from the arm of the person placing the scope. Do not use the teeth as pivots.
13. Pass the lubricated ET tube through the mouth into the larynx between the vocal cords. Do not pass the tube down the lumen of the laryngoscope blade since this will obscure visualization.
14. Advance ET tube until cuff slides beyond the vocal cords. If intubation attempt is unsuccessful, do not wait more than 30 seconds to return patient to ventilation with 100% oxygen on bag-valve-mask.
15. Once the ET tube has passed through the vocal cords,

remove laryngoscope and the stylette (if used) and inflate cuff.
16. Observe for chest expansion and auscultate lungs while ventilating with bag-valve-mask to ensure adequate placement of tube. If breath sounds are heard in right lung but not in left lung, tube may need to be retracted a few centimeters. Then auscultate lungs again to assess placement.
17. Assess for abdominal distention. If this occurs and breath sounds are not heard on auscultation while ventilating, remove tube. Hyperoxygenate. The physician will attempt intubation again with a clean tube.
18. Hyperoxygenate with 100% Fio_2 after successful intubation.
19. Suction through tube and orally.
20. Note position of ET tube at lips in reference to centimeter marking on tube (Fig. 4-8).
21. Secure tube with adhesive tape after using skin prep to ensure adhesion (Fig. 4-9). Tape should be changed every 24 hours or as needed. Move tube to opposite side of mouth when tape is changed.
22. Provide oxygen through T-piece or ventilator if indicated.
23. Explain to patients that they will be unable to speak because of the presence of the tube between vocal cords but speaking will be possible as soon as the tube is removed. Also inform the patients' family of this condition.
24. Ensure that the nurse-call system is within easy reach of patient.
25. Provide support to patient and family and explain equipment and need for suctioning.
26. Obtain chest x-ray to assess tube placement.
27. Obtain ABGs 30 minutes after intubation, as ordered, to assess adequacy of oxygenation.
28. If the patient is confused or attempts to remove the tube, apply soft wrist restraints if necessary to avoid extubation.
29. Obtain sedation order from physician and administer as ordered.
30. Record data.

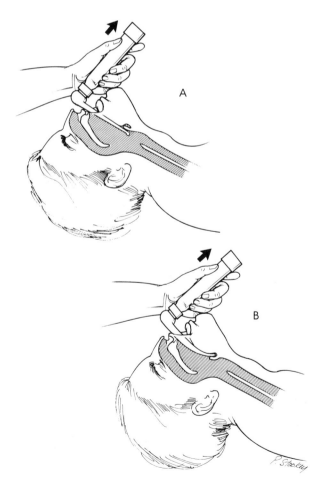

Fig. 4-7   A, If straight blade is used, advance past epiglottis. **B,** If curved blade is used, position tip of blade anterior to the epiglottis. (From Tilkian AG, Daily EK: *Cardiovascular procedures,* St Louis, 1986, Mosby–Year Book.)

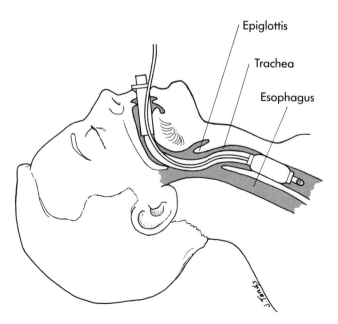

Fig 4-8   The endotracheal tube in place.

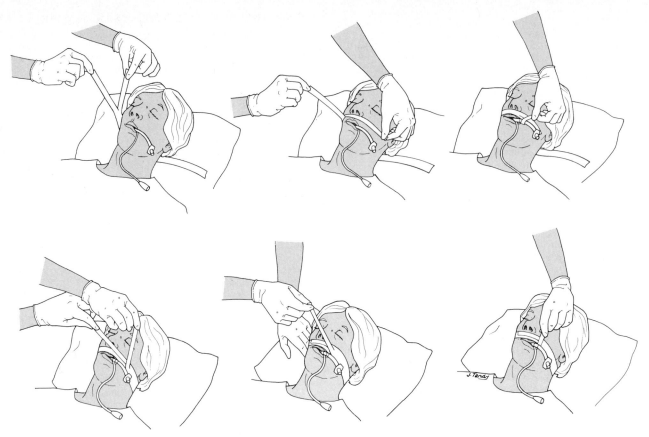

Fig. 4-9   Taping the ET tube in place.

Table 4-6   Types of Tracheostomy Tubes

Tube type	Advantages	Disadvantages
High-pressure, low volume (hard)		
Plastic cuffed	Disposable Cuff bonded to tube (will not detach)	More likely to cause tracheal damage than low-pressure cuff
Plastic double-cuffed	Decreased risk of tissue necrosis with alternate inflation of cuffs (only if schedule is followed)	Rigid inflation/deflation schedule May be difficult to insert If tracheal damage does occur, it covers large area
Low-pressure, high volume (soft)		
Cuffed plastic	Disposable Decreases risk of tracheal necrosis Does not need to be deflated periodically Cuff bonded to tube	Costly
Foam cuff (self-inflating silicone)	Does not require injected air Foam expands from room air (passive inflation, no pressure monitoring required)	If air is inadvertently injected into inflation line, it may lead to tracheal damage
High- or low-pressure		
Metal, cuffed	Available in small sizes Inner cannula can be removed for cleaning Can be sterilized because cuff is removable	Cuff tears easily Inner cannula can be dislodged Cuff can slip off Adapter needed for ventilation
Metal or plastic cuffless tubes	Reduces risk of tracheal damage Available in small sizes Inner cannula can be removed for cleaning	Does not prevent aspiration

Skill 4-9   Extubation

EQUIPMENT AND SUPPLIES

- Bag-valve-mask device
- Oxygen source and nebulizer
- 10 ml syringe
- Suction regulator, cannister, sterile catheter, and sterile gloves
- Appropriate oxygen equipment (aerosol mask) after extubation per physician's order
- Equipment for emergency reintubation at bedside

NURSING INTERVENTIONS

1. Confer with physician regarding readiness for extubation.
2. Introduce self.
3. Explain procedure.
4. Ensure necessary privacy.
5. Assemble equipment.
6. Prepare oxygen administration setup to be used after extubation.
7. Wash hands.
8. Obtain vital signs.
9. Elevate head of bed 30 degrees to 45 degrees, or higher, if tolerated, to allow for optimal pulmonary expansion. Wear gloves.
10. Suction oropharynx to prevent secretions from entering trachea after cuff is deflated.
11. Hyperoxygenate with 100% Fio_2 for 2 minutes.
12. Remove tape.
13. Deflate cuff. (See section on Cuff Deflation.)
14. Advance suction catheter down ET tube and suction, leaving catheter in place. Tell patient to take a deep breath (or inflate lungs manually). Remove the tube at peak inspiration. Tube removal is easier at peak inspiration and less traumatic since the vocal cords are dilated. Withdraw ET tube and suction catheter gently while maintaining suction. Suction oropharynx.
15. Immediately apply humidified oxygen as prescribed.
16. Encourage patient to cough. Remove gloves.
17. Assess vital signs every 15 minutes for 1 hour, then every 30 minutes for 2 hours, or per unit policy.
18. Auscultate lung sounds.
19. Obtain ABGs 30 minutes after extubation, or sooner if patient exhibits signs of respiratory distress.
20. Assess for the following signs of laryngospasm, laryngeal or vocal cord edema, and respiratory distress: cyanotic skin color, diaphoresis, increased respiratory rate, and change in mental status indicating possible hypoxemia. Listen over trachea for tracheal stridor.
21. Record data.

High pressure, low volume cuffs have small surface areas and require high pressures (180 to 200 mm Hg) to inflate. These cuffs tend to distort the trachea. Today, most artificial airways are low pressure, high volume. These cuffs are made of compliant materials that conform to the shape of the trachea. With the low pressure, high volume cuff, deflating the cuff every hour or two is not necessary. Deflation is necessary only at extubation. One of the most important aspects of care is the assessment of cuff pressure. Cuff pressure should be measured at least once every 8 hours to ensure that an adequate pressure is maintained. The cuff seal is maintained at the lowest possible pressure and volume (minimal occlusive volume [MOV] or minimal air leak technique [MLT]). An adequate cuff pressure is between 20 to 25 mm Hg.[13,25] Cuff pressure can be measured with a manometer or by minimal-leak technique. Measurement of cuff pressure can be performed by using a three-way stop clock, syringe, and pressure manometer, or with a cufflator (Skill 4-12).

A leak in the cuff, pilot tube, or one-way valve can result in an emergency situation especially for the patient receiving mechanical ventilation. A leak in the system causes a loss of volume delivered to the patient, and a decrease in peak inspiratory pressure.

A small leak in the cuff system can be discovered by a cuff pressure that decreases over time. A large leak, occurring from a blown cuff, will have a more rapid onset. Cuff leaks can be assessed by the following:

- Decreased breath sounds.
- Air movement through the tube in the spontaneously breathing patient.
- Feeling air flow at the mouth in a patient receiving positive pressure ventilation.

When leaks are detected, attempt to reinflate the cuff while observing the pilot balloon and valve for leaks. If leaks are caused by a blown cuff, the tracheostomy tube will need to be replaced. Leaks at the valve or pilot balloon can be bypassed by placing a needle and stopcock in the pilot tube distal to the leak.

Fenestrated tracheostomy tubes are devices that are designed for weaning and speaking. They are fenestrated in the outer cannula. When the tube is plugged, the patient is able to breathe and speak because air is directed through the upper respiratory tract. When the inner cannula is in place, the tube functions as other tracheostomy tubes. The fenestrated tracheostomy tube is designed to allow the patient to learn to breathe spontaneously and expel secretions before extubation is attempted.

Another type of tracheostomy is the speaking tracheostomy tube. A small tube with an opening above the tube's cuff allows for low flow (2 to 4 L/min oxygen or air) to flow through the vocal cords allowing the patient to speak.

Caring for the patient with a tracheostomy is always a challenge. Since the natural airway is bypassed, the oxygen being administered must be humidified and warmed. The airway must be monitored routinely for patency. To prevent thick secretions, the patient must be kept well hydrated. Since these patients are at risk for infection, careful tracheostomy care and suctioning must be maintained. If the tracheostomy has a cuff, pressure must be monitored to reduce the chance of tracheal damage because of an overinflated cuff.

Skill 4-10   Tracheostomy Tube and Skin Site Care

EQUIPMENT AND SUPPLIES

Tracheostomy care kit or the following:
- Sterile towel to create sterile field
- Sterile cups
- Sterile saline or water
- Hydrogen peroxide
- Sterile gloves
- Mask
- Protective eyewear
- Sterile cotton swabs
- Cotton tape or tracheostomy ties
- Sterile 4 × 4 gauze pads
- Sterile tracheostomy dressing
- Sterile tracheostomy brush or pipe cleaners
- Scissors
- Syringe for cuffed tracheostomy tubes
- Stethoscope
- Hemostat
- Bag-valve device
- Manometer designed to measure cuff pressure
- Small bag for trash
- Several inches of gauze (optional)
- Short length of wire (optional)

NURSING INTERVENTIONS
Double cannula care

1. Introduce self.
2. Check ID band. Assess the need for suctioning. Monitor pulse and respirations. Assess for signs of airway infection (i.e., coughing, purulent mucus production, chest pain, fever, crackles and wheezes, dullness on chest percussion, and chest x-ray that suggest infiltrates or effusion). Assess skin (i.e., erythema, pain, and purulent discharge).
3. Position patient in semi-Fowler's position (if possible).
4. Open tracheostomy set or prepare sterile field and equipment. Pour solutions into sterile bowls.
5. Place clean glove on nondominant hand. Place sterile glove on dominant hand.
6. Remove tracheostomy mask or respirator tubing with nondominant hand. Suction inner cannula before removing with dominant hand (see suctioning technique on p. 63). NOTE: If the patient does not have copious secretions, hyperventilate the lungs by sighing the respirator or with a bag-valve device do the following before suctioning[11]:

- Use nondominant hand to turn on oxygen to 12 to 15 L/min.
- Attach tracheostomy adapter to bag-valve device then to the tracheostomy.
- Compress the bag as the patient inhales or every 5 seconds for an adult (3 seconds for an infant).
- Observe rise and fall of chest.
- Remove bag-valve device.

If copious secretions are present, do not hyperventilate but turn liter flow on oxygen delivery system up for a few minutes before suctioning.

7. Remove tracheostomy dressing with nondominant hand and place in small trash bag. Unlock and remove inner cannula with nondominant hand (Fig. 4-10, A). Place in hydrogen peroxide to soak.
8. Place oxygen tracheostomy mask over tracheostomy, or if patient is on ventilator, reconnect ventilator.
9. Remove soiled glove. Reglove with sterile gloves.
10. Remove inner cannula from soaking solution.
11. Scrub with small brush to remove secretions on the inside and outside of the cannula (Fig. 4-10, B).
12. Rinse inner cannula with sterile saline.
13. Inspect inner cannula for cleanliness. If still soiled, repeat soaking and scrubbing.
14. Dry inside of cannula by pulling gauze through it or use dry pipe cleaners. Place on sterile field.
15. Suction outer cannula (see suctioning technique on p. 63).
16. Cleanse exposed outer surface of outer cannula with hydrogen peroxide or saline with cotton-tipped applicators.
17. Cleanse skin and stoma site with hydrogen peroxide or saline using a circular motion from stoma outward (Fig. 4-10, C). Hydrogen peroxide can be detrimental to the skin so should be used with care.
18. Rinse skin with sterile saline and dry with sterile gauze. Assess stomal site for skin breakdown and infection.
19. Apply bacteriostatic cream to area if ordered.
20. Replace inner cannula and lock (Fig. 4-10, D).
21. Carefully and gently replace tracheostomy dressing under flanges of tracheostomy tube (Fig. 4-10, E). Change tracheostomy ties. Replace ties one at a time. Retie at front side of patient's neck.
22. Remove gloves. Discard trash in appropriate container.
23. Place patient in position of comfort.
24. Remove supplies.
25. Wash hands.
26. Record data.

Plugging a Tracheostomy Tube

In general, tracheostomy tubes are plugged as the patient's condition improves in order to wean the patient (Fig. 4-11, A and B). The tracheostomy is plugged for specified lengths of time several times a day, e.g., 10 minutes every 4 hours. As the patient is able to tolerate the plugging procedure, the length of time is increased, as is the frequency; e.g., 30 minutes every 2 hours. The patient is carefully monitored during the time that the plug is in place. The purpose is to wean patients from the tracheostomy.

Skill 4-11   Plugging a Tracheostomy Tube

EQUIPMENT AND SUPPLIES

- Sterile tracheostomy plug
- Suction equipment (see suctioning procedure on p. 63)

NURSING INTERVENTIONS

1. See double cannula technique, Skill 4-18, steps 1 to 9.
2. Deflate tracheostomy cuff, if ordered.
3. Discard gloves.
4. Reglove with sterile gloves.
5. Fit plug into cannula (inner or outer tube, depending on whether tracheostomy tube has double or single cannula).
6. Remain with patient while tracheostomy tube is plugged.

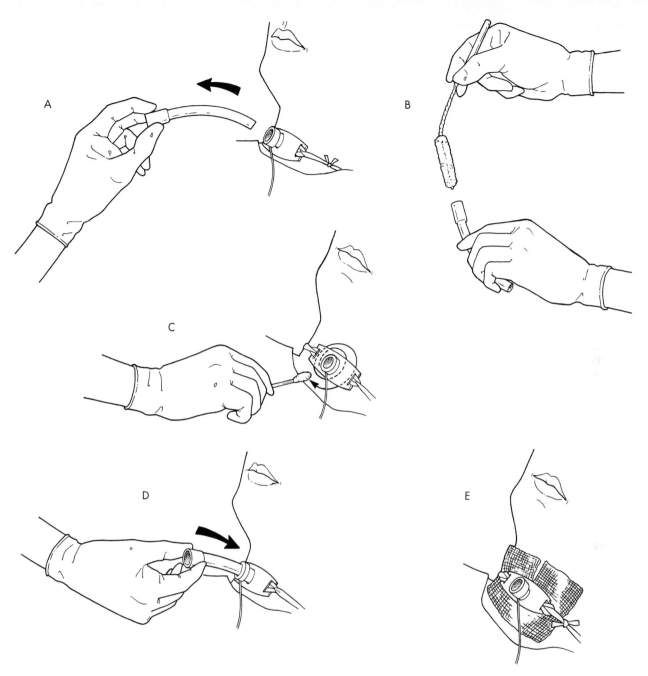

Fig. 4-10   **A,** Unlock and remove the inner cannula with the nondominant hand. Centers for Disease Control recommend wearing gloves for the procedure. **B,** Scrub inner cannula with a small brush. **C,** Cleanse skin around stoma site. **D,** Replace inner cannula. **E,** Replace tracheostomy dressing.

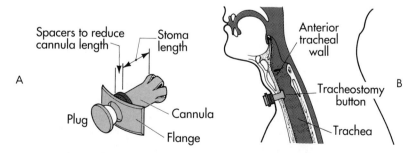

Fig. 4-11   Olympic tracheostomy button. **A,** Tracheostomy button inserted into stoma. The button extends from the stoma opening to the anterior tracheal wall. **B,** Parts of the tracheostomy button. The button consists of a cannula, spacers that adapt the button to the length of the stoma, and a plug that fits into the cannula. The plug is removed for suctioning. (From Lewis SM, Collier IC: *Medical-surgical nursing: assessment and management of clinical problems,* ed 3, St Louis, 1992, Mosby–Year Book.)

Skill 4-12   Initial Inflation of the Cuffed Tracheostomy and Measuring Cuff Pressure

EQUIPMENT AND SUPPLIES

- Mercury manometer
- 3-way stopcock
- 10 ml plastic syringe
- Stethoscope
- Suction equipment

NURSING INTERVENTIONS
Initial inflation

1. After tracheostomy tube is inserted, prepare to inflate cuff.
2. Suction if necessary.
3. Insert syringe into valve on tracheostomy tube.
4. Inflate cuff during the inspiratory phase of breathing.
5. Inject air from a syringe a few ml at a time (check manufacturer's guidelines to determine the amount of air needed) to reach minimal occlusive volume (MOV).
6. Auscultate patient's neck adjacent to the trachea. No air leak should be heard.
7. Withdraw 0.1 ml of air to create small air leak. Minimal air leak reduces the chances of tracheal injury (Fig. 4-12). Auscultate the neck. If leak is not heard, withdraw another 0.1 ml of air. Repeat auscultation.
8. Ask patient to attempt to speak (if able). If cuff is sufficiently inflated, the patient's voice cannot be heard, air is not expelled from the patient's mouth, and a slight leak can be heard on auscultation.

Measuring cuff pressure

1. Measure cuff pressure the following ways
   a. 3-way stopcock method:
   - Attach manometer, cuff inflation line, and syringe to stopcock.
   - Close the stopcock to the cuff pilot balloon so that air cannot escape from the cuff.
   - Inject air from syringe into manometer tubing until the pressure reading reaches 10 mm Hg. This will prevent a sudden deflation of the cuff when the stopcock to the cuff and manometer is opened. Close stopcock to manometer.
   - Auscultate the patient's trachea. A smooth sound indicates a sealed airway while a gurgling sound indicates a leak. If no leak is heard, deflate cuff until leak is heard. When leak is heard, reinflate the cuff until the leak is no longer heard on inspiration. Turn off stopcock to the syringe.
   - Read manometer on expiration. Pressure should not exceed 15 to 20 mm Hg (if Hg manometer is used) or 25 to 33 cm H_2O (Scanlon). Check manufacturer's suggested values since these tend to vary.
   - Note cyclic pressure changes with inspiration and expiration.
   - Turn stopcock to occlude cuff line.
   b. Cufflator techniques:
   - Attach cufflator to the cuff port.
   - Measure the current pressure in cm H_2O. Cuff pressure should not exceed 27 cm of H_2O at end exhalation.
2. Clamp inflation tube either with hemostat (have protectors on hemostats and clamps to cover serrated teeth) or port valve.
3. Remove manometer, syringe, and stopcock.
4. Record the following data: auscultation assessment, presence of minimal air leak, cuff inflation pressure and volume, time of inflation, and inspiratory and expiratory pressure.

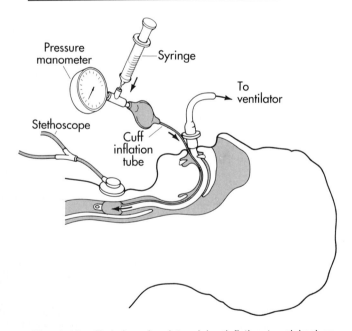

Fig. 4-12   Technique for determining inflation to minimal occluding volume and cuff pressure. The cuff is inflated until no leak is heard on inspiration when a stethoscope is placed over the trachea. Air is injected using a syringe connected to a stopcock and pressure manometer. (From Lewis SM, Collier IC: *Medical-surgical nursing: assessment and management of clinical problems,* ed 3, St Louis, 1992, Mosby–Year Book.)

Suctioning

Retained secretions alter gas exchange, causing dyspnea, hypoxemia, hypercapnia, cardiovascular stress, and fatigue. Over time, retained secretions may damage cilia and interfere with their mucus-raising properties. Additionally, retained secretions may lead to atelectasis and infection. Patients who are unable to expectorate must be suctioned.

Entry of a suction catheter into the trachea will usually initiate coughing, which may help to raise secretions from the lungs. The negative suction pressure removes the secretions. Suctioning may also be used to obtain a specimen for analysis. Suctioning may cause complications such as hypoxia, trauma, bradycardia, tachycardia, dysrhythmias, ischemia, respiratory distress, potential respiratory arrest,[7] and tracheal irritation. Vagal stimulation may occur resulting in bradycardia, heart block, hypotension, syncope, ventricular irritability, ventricular tachycardia, and asystole. Other complications resulting from tracheal irritation include the stimulation of tracheal and carinal reflexes, resulting in paroxysmal cough, which can have an effect on venous return and cardiac output and infection.

To reduce the risk of complications, the patient should only be suctioned when needed. Hyperinflating and oxygenating the lungs reduces the risk of hypoxemia, dysrhythmias, and microatelectasis. It has been recommended that hyperinflation and hyperoxygenation breaths (TV = 1.5 times normal and Fio_2=100%) be administered before and after each catheter pass.[6,29] Hyperinflation can be performed in three ways: (1) asking the conscious patient to deep breathe; (2) using a manual resuscitation bag and mask; and (3) using a ventilator through the "sigh" control. The first of these methods is patient-controlled, therefore variable. In the second method, lung volumes delivered are completely dependent on the skills of the person using the resuscitation bag and vary from one hyperinflation volume to the next. The ventilator, however, is able to deliver approximately the same hyperinflation volume with each sigh.

Maintaining sterile technique throughout the suctioning procedure reduces the risk of infection. Monitoring vital signs before, during, and after suctioning provides data about breathing problems, dysrhythmias, and hypotension.

The type of suction techique used will depend on the presence or absence of an artificial airway. Nasopharyngeal suction requires the use of sterile technique. Oral suction performed through the oral cavity can be performed with clean technique. Nasopharyngeal suctioning is performed through the naris. ET and tracheal suctioning are performed through artificial airways. Sterile technique is maintained throughout endotracheal and tracheal suctioning procedures. Frequency of suctioning depends on individual need. A patient with fulminating pulmonary edema may need to be suctioned every 15 minutes to keep the airway patent while a patient without many secretions may be suctioned only every 2 to 4 hours.

Suction catheters are available in different sizes (8 to 14 Fr are most commonly used). The correct size should be chosen depending on the patient's size and age and the size of the airway. A suction catheter should be no larger than half the diameter of the tracheostomy tube.

Skill 4-13   Suctioning

EQUIPMENT AND SUPPLIES

- Suction regulator and cannister
- Bag-valve-mask device connected to 100% oxygen
- Suction kit (with sterile gloves, catheter, and cup)
- Sterile saline bottle
- Sterile saline (3 to 10 ml) without preservative
- Absorbent pads
- Tissues
- Goggles (or glasses) and mask
- Gown (if necessary)
- Assistant

NURSING INTERVENTIONS

1. Introduce self to patient and explain procedure.
2. Ensure privacy.
3. Wash hands.
4. Assemble equipment.
5. Place patient in semi- or high Fowler's position if not contraindicated. This position allows patient to assist in coughing and expectorating mucus.[2]
6. Assess for the following: excess secretions; excess intratracheal secretions; soiled or wet tracheostomy tapes or dressing; diminished air flow; and signs and symptoms of airway obstruction.
7. Auscultate lung sounds to determine need for suctioning.
8. Turn on suction. Check suction pressure. Occlude the tubing. The suction pressure should not exceed 100 to 120 mm Hg.
9. Open catheter kit package and remove cup. Fill clean cup with sterile saline. Prepare the saline for instillation by drawing up saline in a syringe.
10. Put on goggles, mask, and sterile gloves.[17]
11. Attach catheter to suction tubing, keeping dominant hand sterile.
12. Before suctioning, have assistant hyperinflate the patient's lungs five times (during inspiration) to provide extra oxygen. The oxygen concentration should be 100%. Turn flowmeter up to 10 L/min. Patients with COPD may need to be hyperinflated without increasing the Fio_2.
13. Instill 3 to 5 ml of saline into the trachea (optical, check agency policy.) Ventilate patient again. The saline will promote coughing and liquify secretions for easier removal.

14. Leave vent open to air, lubricate catheter with saliva, and introduce catheter. Warn patients that they may feel short of breath. Do not begin to suction until the catheter reaches the carina. Withdraw the catheter 1 cm before beginning to suction.
15. Occlude vent with thumb of opposite hand slowly withdrawing catheter while rotating it between thumb and finger. This rotating motion prevents tissue trauma. Do not suction for more than 10 seconds. Completely withdraw catheter. Check cardiac monitor. Interrupt suctioning if heart rate slows by 20 beats per minute, increases by 40 beats per minute, if blood pressure drops, or if cardiac dysrhythmias occur. If the patient requires a high level of support, such as PEEP (greater than 10 cm H_2O), insert suction catheter through an adapter but do not disconnect the ventilatory circuit from the airway. This helps to prevent hypoxemia.
16. Hyperoxygenate and ventilate for at least five deep breaths and return to baseline vital signs before repeating procedure.[12]
17. Irrigate catheter with saline.
18. Repeat steps 15 to 17 up to three times, if necessary to remove secretions.
19. Turn off oxygen or return oxygen to ordered rate.
20. If needed, suction tracheostomy stoma and then patient's mouth.
21. Wrap the catheter around the sterile gloved hand and pull the glove over the catheter. Dispose of them with the other gloved hand.
22. Flush the suction tubing with saline to clear away the secretions. Turn off suction.
23. Assist patient to a comfortable position.
24. Change ET tube tape or tracheostomy ties every 24 hours and as needed.
25. Provide mouth care.
26. Assess effectiveness by observing respirations and auscultating lungs. Discuss procedure with patient to determine how comfort can be increased.
27. Empty and rinse suction cannister before it fills completely.

Skill 4-14   Suctioning with the Multiuse Suctioning System[3]

Related to this procedure are several new catheters, such as the multiuse suction catheter (Fig. 4-13). This catheter is incorporated directly into the ventilator tubing and allows for suctioning without disconnecting the patient. This catheter does not increase bacterial contamination if changed every 24 hours.

EQUIPMENT AND SUPPLIES

- See equipment and supplies for Skill 4-13
- Multiuse suctioning system

NURSING INTERVENTIONS

1. Attach control valve to wall suction tubing.
2. Before attaching tracheal suction system to patient, depress thumb control valve and set wall suction to desired level while continuing to depress control valve.
3. Attach T-piece to ventilator circuit. Ensure irrigation port is closed.
4. Attach T-piece to ET tube.
5. Patient lavage may be accomplished by advancing the catheter approximately 6 inches down the ET tube, adding fluid through the irrigation port. Make sure suction is not applied during lavage. Suction as needed after lavage.
6. Grip T-piece with one hand and advance catheter with thumb and forefinger of the opposite hand.
7. Apply suction by depressing control valve as needed.
8. While maintaining grip on the T-piece and control valve, gently withdraw suction catheter to fully extended length of the catheter sleeve until black marking on catheter is visible at back of T-piece.
9. Flush catheter through the irrigation port. Start suction before starting flush solution; introduce flush solution slowly while continuing suction.
10. Lift and turn thumb piece 180 degrees to lock position on control valve for safe off.

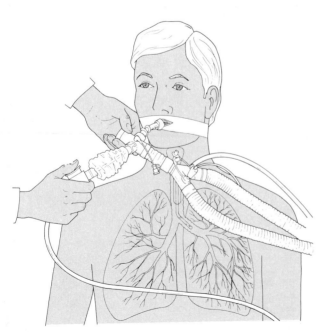

Fig. 4-13   Multiuse tracheal suction system with directional tip.

Skill 4-15   Suctioning with the Directional-Tip Catheter[3]

EQUIPMENT AND SUPPLIES

- See equipment and supplies for Skill 4-14

NURSING INTERVENTIONS

1. To remove tip protector, hold catheter in back of T-piece; with other hand pull tip protector from catheter and discard.
2. Attach control valve to wall suction tubing.
3. Before attaching tracheal suction system to patient, depress thumb control valve and set wall suction to desired level while continuing to depress control valve.
4. Attach T-piece to ventilator circuit. Ensure irrigation port is closed.
5. Attach T-piece to ET tube.
6. Keep T-piece parallel with patient's chin. Radiopaque blue line on catheter indicates direction catheter tip will follow. With patient's head at 12 o'clock, guide catheter into patient's left lung by rotating blue line to 1 o'clock position, and advance catheter while maintaining blue line at 1 o'clock position. Repeat process at 11 o'clock position to enter patient's right lung.
7. Apply intermittent suction by depressing control valve as needed.
8. While maintaining grip on the T-piece and control valve, gently withdraw suction catheter to fully extended length of the catheter sleeve until black marking on catheter is visible at back of T-piece.
9. Flush catheter through the irrigation port. Start suction before starting flush solution; introduce flush solution slowly while continuing suction.
10. Lift and turn thumb piece 180 degrees to lock position on control valve for safe off.

PEDIATRIC CONSIDERATIONS

Initial assessment of the newborn is performed quickly at the time of delivery to determine the general health of the infant. A complete assessment is carried out later. The initial assessment includes the Apgar score.

In 1952, Dr. Virginia Apgar developed a system to provide an objective, quantitative assessment of a newborn's status at birth (Table 4-7). A total score of 0-10 is possible. The more vigorous the infant, the higher the score. The Apgar is performed at 1 minute and 5 minutes after birth. As the pH diminishes, score declines indicating resuscitation interventions may be necessary.

The respiratory system of the newborn is immature. In the first few hours of life, the newborn may exhibit grunting, flaring of the nares, retraction of respiratory muscle, and cyanosis. If these symptoms do not pass after a few hours, they are considered abnormal and indicate underlying pathology. The Silverman-Anderson Index (Fig. 4-22) provides a useful tool for quantifying respiratory status in neonates, infants, and small children. A score of 0 represents no distress while a score of 10 indicates severe distress.

Assess the respiratory rate. In the newborn it ranges from 30 to 60 breaths per minute. A respiratory rate faster

Table 4-7 The Apgar Scoring Chart

Sign	Score 0	Score 1	Score 2
A—Appearance (color)	Blue, pale	Body pink, hands and feet blue	Completely pink
P—Pulse (heart rate)	Absent	Slow (below 100/min)	Above 100/min
G—Grimace (reflex irritability)	No response	Grimace	Cough or sneeze
A—Activity (muscle tone)	Flaccid	Some flexion	Well-flexed
R—Respiration effort	Absent	Weak, irregular hypoventilation	Strong cry

than 60 breaths per minute is considered tachypneic; a rate lower than 30 breaths per minute is considered bradypneic. The breathing pattern of the normal newborn may be slightly irregular owing to the immaturity of the respiratory system.[24] Normally, the diaphragm is used for breathing. The abdomen rises and falls during respiration; the chest remains relatively immobile. Additionally, the newborn breathes through the nose and tolerates mouth breathing poorly.[24]

Palpate and percuss the chest gently. Note flexible ribs, without fractures of clavicles or ribs. Note symmetry and freedom from pain. Note lung resonance. Auscultate the lungs. Fixed crackles may be heard at birth, but they resolve in normal newborns soon after birth. Crackles are abnormal if they continue past the first few hours and may indicate pneumonia or pulmonary edema. Diminished breath sounds may indicate atelectasis or hyaline membrane disease.

Elicit patient medical history from the child's parents, including prenatal medical history, illnesses, immunizations, and medications. Allow adequate time to establish a nurse/patient/family relationship.

The chest circumference is measured as a part of the respiratory assessment of newborns, infants, and children. Configuration of the normal newborn chest is cylindrical with an anteroposterior ratio of 1:1. Chest circumference is about 33 cm (13 inches) at birth and, in general, is about 2.5 cm (1 inch) less than head circumference. The anteroposterior diameter is low; therefore hyperresonance is a normal percussion note heard over the lung fields of infants and young children. Breath sounds of infants are loud and harsh because of the proximity of the trachea and bronchi to the chest walls.

The respiratory system matures as the child grows. By the time the child enters school, the respiratory rate decreases to about 20 to 30 breaths per minute. (Table 4-8 shows age-related normal respiratory variations.)

By adolescence the respiratory rate has decreased to the adult rate. Metabolism increases during this age because of the adolescent growth spurt. Adolescents are generally cooperative during examination and can understand a careful explanation of the examination process. It is during these years that modesty develops. Adolescents may be reluctant to bare their chests for examination. Drapes and gowns should be provided and patience used to complete the examination of the respiratory system.

Table 4-8 Normal Respiratory Rates with Age Variations

Age	Respiratory rate (breaths per min)
Newborn	30-60
2 yr	25-40
4 yr	23-30
6 yr	21-26
8 yr	20-26
10 yr	20-26
12 yr	18-22
14 yr	18-22
16 yr	16-20
18 yr-adult	12-20

Transcutaneous P_{O_2} Monitoring

Transcutaneous oxygen and carbon dioxide monitoring is a relatively new, simple, and noninvasive method of continuously monitoring oxygen pressure at the skin's surface in neonates. It provides an estimate of Pa_{O_2}. This methodology was created to monitor neonates, thereby reducing the need for frequent arterial blood sampling.

Transcutaneous oxygen pressure ($P_{tc}O_2$) is measured by a heated electrode placed on a membrane that adheres to the skin. As heat-induced vasodilation occurs, the heat "arteriolizes" the capillary blood flow and shifts the oxyhemoglobin curve to the right. As oxygen diffuses through the skin from the capillaries, it creates a current through the membrane to the electrode sensor. The current is measured and converted into the partial pressure of oxygen.

Transcutaneous oxygen is not equivalent to arterial oxygen; however they approximate each other, particularly when the values are in the normal range.[14] In patients who present with mild shock (i.e., cardiac index of 2.1 $L/min/m^2$ to 1.5 $L/min/m^2$), the correlation is not as good as with normal cardiac output.[20] The $P_{tc}O_2$ is not accurate at all with patients in severe shock.

$P_{tc}O_2$ is useful with patients who risk a cardiac arrest. A $P_{tc}O_2$ value of less than 25 mm Hg has been shown to precede cardiac arrest in adults by 45 minutes.[30] $P_{tc}O_2$ is also useful during intubation and extubation, during cardiac arrest and resuscitation, and during respiratory arrest.[27]

Oxygen Therapy

The method of oxygen delivery is generally based on the child's age, condition, and the concentration of inspired oxygen needed. The delivery of high concentrations of oxygen (above 40%) requires the use of hoods, isolettes, nonrebreathing masks, or croupettes. Oxygen must be warmed to 31° to 34° C (88° to 94° F) to avoid cold stress and must be humidified. Oxygen concentration lower than 40% can be administered by nasal cannula catheters and masks. However, a nasal cannula is difficult to keep in place in infants and children. There is a method of securing the cannula in place with a small square of stoma adhesive on each cheek. Pediatric equipment is used for administering oxygen therapy to infants and children.

Children receiving oxygen are generally confined to cribs or beds and therefore need sensory stimulation. Pro-

Skill 4-16   Transcutaneous Oxygen Monitoring

EQUIPMENT AND SUPPLIES

- $P_{tc}O_2$ monitor
- Sensor
- Alcohol wipe

NURSING INTERVENTIONS

1. Adjust sensing unit to the selected temperature. Accuracy depends on the proper skin warming temperature. The appropriate temperature is selected for each patient. Premature infants usually require a sensor warmed to 43° to 43.5° C (109° F); full-term infants 44° C (111° F); and older children 44° to 45° C (111° to 113° F).
2. Calibrate the sensor before each use. Then recalibrate at least every 4 hours. This process takes approximately 15 minutes. Therefore if continuous $P_{tc}O_2$ monitoring is needed, a second monitor will be required.
3. Cleanse with alcohol wipe and dry the skin over the area where the sensor is to be placed. The skin must be free of hair, so an area might have to be shaved. Accuracy also depends on correct placement. Usually the chest wall is the site of choice but other sites, such as the abdomen, can be used. The sensor should not be placed over bony prominences or peripheral sites.
4. Place a small drop of ionized water on skin to provide a moist surface for the heating electrode.
5. Place a few drops of electrode solution between the membrane and the electrode.
6. Apply double-sided adhesive ring around sensor collar.
7. Affix collar to skin site. Check placement every hour initially, then every 2 hours, and verify readings with an ABG level.
8. Change membrane daily. Clean sensor with distilled water and dry with lint-free cloth. Cleanse and assess skin site. A mild redness after removal may be seen, but blistering should not occur.
9. Record the following data:
   - Calibration-recalibration
   - Skin condition
   - Sensor placement
   - Sensor temperature
   - Sensor reading
   - ABGs
   - Other relevant data

viding sensory stimulation for the child with a nasal cannula or mask is not really a problem. It is when the oxygen device creates a barrier that this becomes harder. Visual stimulation can be supplied for the child by placing colorful pictures, shapes, or toys in their line of vision. These are placed on the outside of the isolette or tent. Likewise, mobiles can be suspended from the ceiling. The older child can watch television but should not be given the remote control device. Toys can be placed in the tents but must be examined for safety and suitability. Objects that may produce sparks, such as hand-held computer games or friction toys, are not appropriate, since they may be hazardous.

Oxygen content within the oxygen device is monitored frequently to determine the flow rate of oxygen needed to maintain the desired oxygen concentration. This is performed by placing a probe near the child's face.

Oxygen toxicity is a hazard of oxygen therapy for children as well as for adults. In addition to all of the hazards experienced by adults, retrolental fibroplasia is a complication of prolonged exposure to high oxygen tensions. This is a result of excessive delivery of Pao_2 to the retinal artery. In an effort to establish safe guidelines for oxygen use, the American Academy of Pediatrics has issued a set of guidelines for oxygen therapy for the newborn.

A great deal of support and encouragement is needed for the families of children receiving oxygen therapy, since they are frightened and worried about their children. The children during the initial course of oxygen therapy generally present as quite ill, and this supportive treatment increases their fears.

As the neonate improves, Fio_2 should be lowered in 10% intervals based on ABGs. Sudden increases or decreases in oxygen concentration may cause a disproportionate increase or decrease in Pao_2. Therefore Fio_2 must be reduced slowly and the infant weaned from supplemental oxygen cautiously. Oxygen concentration should be returned to previous level if patient exhibits distress.

The oxygen hood

The simplest and most efficient method to deliver oxygen and humidity therapy to a spontaneously breathing infant is with a clear plastic hood that is placed directly over the patient's head. This method is able to supply 100% oxygen to the infant. It also has the ability to warm and humidify the air.

There are two drawbacks to the use of the oxygen hood. It limits mobility and the child must be removed from the oxygen source for feeding. It is used only with cooperative infants and young children.

The isolette

The isolette is designed for use with the newborn infant. It consists of a transparent plastic case allowing the caregivers continuous visualization of the infant. It has a controlled heating unit, a heat-circulating system, a humidity system, and an air-filtering unit. It also has an infant bed, which when adjusted, can provide the Trendelenburg and Fowler's positions. Additionally, there are portholes in the sides of the isolette allowing for rapid access to the infant for feeding, touching, and holding. One great advantage of the isolette over the oxygen hood is that the infant does not need to be removed from the oxygen source while being fed. The main unit is mounted on a cabinet with casters and has storage space for accessory equipment.

Isolettes are used for neonates and infants to control temperature, humidity, and oxygen concentration. Oxygen flow in the isolette can provide an Fio_2 up to 40%. Some isolettes allow for an Fio_2 greater than 40% (up to 85%). If an Fio_2 of greater than that attainable (85%) is required, an oxygen hood can be used inside the isolette. Using the oxygen hood in addition to the isolette constantly controls the Fio_2, compensating for the diluted oxygen mixture that results from opening and closing the access ports.

The croupette and oxygen tent

The croupette or oxygen tent are devices that provide an oxygen concentration of 21% to 60%. Tents can also control temperature and humidity. The croupette is used for children ranging in age from 1 to 10 years old; children older than 10 years old are placed in oxygen tents.

One inconvenience of the croupette or oxygen tent is the moisture buildup. Bed linens and the child's clothing need to be changed frequently to keep the child dry. Stuffed toys cannot be placed in these tents, since they get wet. Patients (and their families) must be warned that electric, battery-operated, or frictionally operated devices cannot be allowed inside the croupette or tent.

Chest Physical Therapy

Percussing the neonate is difficult because the force of the percussion must be great enough to loosen secretions but not so great as to cause injury. The smaller the neonate, the more difficult. Since nurses' hands may be too large for percussing the chest wall in neonates, percussion can be carried out using a small cupped device, such as a padded medicine cup, suction bulb cut in half and padded, a resuscitation face mask, or rubber nipple. The hands are used for larger infants and children.

Percussion of infants should be just firm enough to make the head bob gently. When performed properly, percussion does not hurt. If the child cries, the percussion may be too hard. Do not percuss the bare skin.

For very small or unstable infants, only one segment may be percussed during a treatment. Rotation and treatment of all segments must be noted so that all areas are eventually percussed. Use a finger to mark landmarks on the chest wall to avoid damaging delicate organs. Frequency of percussion varies from 1 to 4 hours depending on the degree of disease, amount of congestion, fatigue level, and general condition.

Vibration can be carried out by placing the fingertips or an adapted padded electric toothbrush on the chest wall (Fig. 4-14).

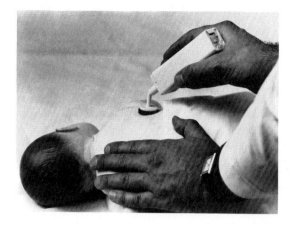

Fig. 4-14 Neocussor—a vibrator used for chest percussion in neonates and infants. *(Courtesy General Physiotherapy, Inc, St Louis.)*

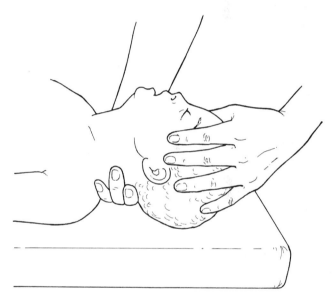

Fig. 4-15 The sniffing position.

Length of treatment will vary according to the condition and age of the child. The time to percuss, vibrate, and position will be shorter in neonates, increasing with age and tolerance.

Postural drainage is an important aspect of CPT for neonates and children. To facilitate maximal percussion and vibration, the child should be positioned 5 to 10 minutes before beginning.

Artificial Airways

Maintaining a patent airway is always a main priority in critical care. Significant differences exist between adult and pediatric patients in regard to airway structure. The child's larynx is located anteriorly and more cephalad than in adults, therefore airway placement is slightly different. The cervical spine is immobilized and the child is placed in a neutral "sniffing" position (Fig. 4-15).

Intubation

Intubation is generally used in infants and children when artificial ventilation will be needed. Indications for placing an ET tube include the following[14]:

- Inability to adequately ventilate the infant or child by resuscitative efforts (i.e., mouth-to-mouth or bag-valve-mask).
- Need for prolonged airway clearance for respirator or prevention of aspiration.
- Need for controlled hyperventilation for children with head injuries.

Careful selection of the appropriate equipment is of special concern for the pediatric patient. Selecting the correct size of ET tube is an important consideration—too large a tube creates extensive mucosal, glottic, or subglottic edema and too small a tube creates rise in airway resistance with an extensive air leak. With a tube of the correct size, the air leak will be detected at 20 to 30 cm H_2O pressure.[15] Generally, the proper size nasal ET tube is one that fits in the nostril comfortably or is about the same diameter as the child's little finger at the level of the nailbed. These simple guidelines are easy to recall in an emergency situation. There is, however, a formula for calculating the ET size. It is as follows[19]:

$$\text{Tube mm} = 16 + \text{age (yrs)}4/*$$

The following specialized pediatric equipment is needed including[28]:

- Medium-sized laryngoscope handles.
- Laryngoscope blades (sizes 0-4, depending on style).
- Straight or curved stylets.
- ET tubes (2.5 to 8 mm internal diameter).

Attempting to intubate infants can be difficult because infants have large tongues, short necks, and high anterior spongy glottises. The trachea is 4 to 5.5 cm long and appears to lie mostly within the chest.

- The child should be positioned and held by another person since a normal conscious infant will fight the intubation procedure. Hyperoxygenate the child for at least 2 full minutes before intubation. Anesthetize the pharynx and cords with a 4% lidocaine spray. Reoxygenate for 30 seconds. Do not interrupt assisted ventilation for more than 30 seconds. If the ET tube cannot be placed in 15 to 30 seconds, the infant or child must be reoxygenated for several minutes before another attempt.[9,19]
- Assess adequacy of ventilation, once the tube has been placed successfully. Watch for bilateral chest movement.
- Auscultate both lungs but since sound readily transmits through an infant's chest, it is not uncommon to hear bilateral breath sounds, even when not present.
- Inspect for bilateral movement and a reduction of respiratory distress symptoms: a chest x-ray should be obtained.

- Secure ET tube once placement is validated. Secure it to the upper lip. If the ET tube has been placed in the nose, tape it in place so that the tip of the nose and the condition of the nares can be assessed.

Extubation

Once the child has been stabilized and no longer needs the tube, the child can be extubated in the following way:

- Extubate when the child's stomach is empty to prevent vomiting.
- Suction the nasopharynx to assure patency.
- Hyperinflate the lungs.
- Remove the tube on inflation to provide adequate lung expansion and to prevent atelectasis; or on expiration so that accumulated secretions on the outside of the ET tube are blown away and thus not inhaled.
- Reassess patient frequently following extubation.
- Evaluate oxygenation 15 to 20 minutes after extubation.

Tracheostomy

Indications for the tracheostomy include the following:

- Mechanical obstruction (e.g., croup, foreign body, laryngeal paralysis).
- CNS difficulties (e.g., head trauma).
- Neuromuscular conditions (e.g., poliomyelitis, amyotonia congenita, Guillain-Barré syndrome).
- Secretional obstruction (e.g., weak cough, chest pain).
- Disturbances of gas diffusion or distribution (e.g., pneumonia).

The reason for the tracheostomy, the outcome, and the approximate length of time that the tube will be in place should be explained to the child and to the parents. In general, parental concern is focused on the often life-threatening events and long-term implications of such a procedure.

Following the procedure, the child will be anxious and frightened when discovering the inability to talk or cry. Parents, too, will be stressed by their child's inability to talk.

Tracheostomy tubes for infants and children are usually made of plastic or Silastic since they can be made with a sharper angle and are more flexible. Most pediatric tracheostomy cannulas have only one cannula. Since the small size of the tube allows for blockage by secretions, they should be monitored frequently and suctioned as needed.

When weaning the patient from the tracheostomy, the diameter of the tube is reduced daily. When a tube several sizes smaller than the original is well-tolerated, the tube is plugged for increasing lengths of time. When the tube has been plugged for 24 hours without difficulty, it is removed. Air leaks through the wound generally close within 24 hours. Surprisingly, weaning from the tracheostomy is as anxiety provoking for the child and parents as the initial placement. They are frightened that the child will not be able to breathe without it.

Some children are discharged from the hospital with the tracheostomy tube still in place. Therefore parents need to be taught how to observe for respiratory distress and how

---

*This formula only applies to children over 2 years of age.

to clean and suction the tracheostomy before the patient's discharge.

Suctioning

Suctioning is stressful and anxiety producing for neonates, infants, and children. The following method should be used when suctioning children:

- Inject saline into the airway (if appropriate), using a few drops to 0.33 ml for neonates and 1 to 3 ml for older children.
- Use suction catheter with a side hole or a Y connector so that the catheter can be introduced without suction and removed while simultaneously applying suction.
- Hyperoxygenate before suctioning. Neonates should receive 10% greater Fio_2 than ventilator setting. Children (older than 6 months old) may be ventilated with 100% Fio_2.
- Suction for a few seconds in the newborn ranging to no more than 10 seconds in the older child.
- Hyperoxygenate between suction passes and at the end of the procedure.
- Assess the response to hyperinflation.
- Determine suction pressure before beginning suctioning (pressures negative 60 to 80 mm Hg for infants and greater than 80 to 100 mm Hg for children).
- Avoid suctioning again for about 30 to 60 minutes (unless necessary).

HOME HEALTH CARE CONSIDERATIONS
Oxygen Administration

Oxygen is frequently administered in the home for persons with respiratory problems, such as COPD. The use of oxygen in the home is not without risk. Patients are carefully evaluated for this type of therapy. Oxygen in the home requires a physician's order specifying the following: L/min, route (e.g., nasal cannula), and time (e.g., as needed for shortness of breath or continuously).

The patient and family must locate a company to supply oxygen and oxygen-support services. Services furnished should include the following:

- Emergency 24-hour service.
- Trained personnel to provide initial setup and instructions on use, care, and treatment.
- At least monthly follow-ups and maintenance.
- Direct billing to insurance coverer.
- Rental cost toward purchase price, if purchase is later desired.

There are three main types of equipment used for home oxygen therapy: cylinders or tanks, oxygen concentrators, and liquid oxygen systems (Table 4-9).

Oxygen in the home is usually administered by nasal cannula, ventimask, or through artificial airways, such as a tracheostomy or ET tube. Also, there is a new method, transtracheal oxygenation (TTO_2) whereby oxygen is delivered through a small flexible, transtracheal catheter (Fig. 4-16). The transtracheal tube is for long-term use. It does not interfere with the cough reflex or with speech. Transtracheal oxygen therapy has advantages over the nasal cannula in that it is more efficient, saves money, requires a lower oxygen concentration, and does not cause breakdown of facial tissues. Additionally, by bypassing the upper airway, the work of breathing is reduced.

Care of oxygen equipment differs in the home from the hospital. In the home, one should do the following:

- Clean humidifiers, tubing, and nasal cannulas (masks, etc.) every 3 days with soap that won't leave a residue. More stringent care may be needed for home care patients who are at high risk for infection; for those patients, the respiratory equipment should be cleansed every 24 hours.
- Rinse thoroughly and disinfect with a quatrinary ammonium compound[18].

Table 4-9 Advantages and Disadvantages of Oxygen Delivery by Tank, Concentrator, or Liquid Oxygen in Home Care

Type of oxygen equipment	Use	Flow rate	Advantages	Disadvantages
Oxygen tanks	Less than 15 hrs per day	High to low flow	Oxygen not lost when in use; economical for low flow, low use; can deliver 100% oxygen accurately; can be used for widest possible range of L/min flow; 100% oxygen accuracy; flow rates adjustable; remaining oxygen can be measured.	Size and weight of tanks; high pressure; limited capacity; large; an extra tank must be kept on hand.
Oxygen concentrators	More than 15 hrs per day	High to low flow	Least expensive for prolonged use; can fill small portable units; remove dust particles from room; manufacture oxygen from room air.	Noisy, electrically powered; adds up to $30/mo to electric bill; must have backup in the event of a power failure; generate heat; large.
Liquid oxygen	Only a few hrs a day	Low flow	Expensive; small, portable unit can be refilled from larger unit; small storage space needed; safe.	Spillage is common when filling small tanks.

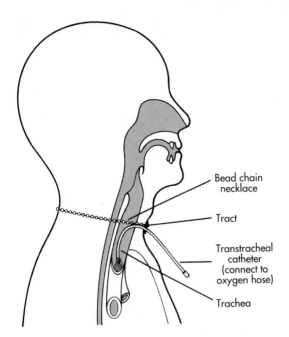

Fig. 4-16 Transtracheal catheter for oxygen administration. (From Lewis SM and Collier IC: *Medical-surgical nursing: assessment and management of clinical problems,* ed 3, St Louis, 1992, Mosby–Year Book.)

- Rinse again following disinfecting.
- Place equipment in a soft, clean towel and allow to air dry. (The patient should have at least three sets of equipment—one to wear, a spare, and the set that is being cleansed.)

Chest Physical Therapy

In the home, patients may need the assistance of family members for CPT. If patients are strong enough, however, or live alone, they may be able to carry out the positioning for postural drainage but will not be able to perform percussion and vibration. The patient will have to be creative in manipulating household items, such as pillows, chairs, and stools, to obtain proper positioning if a hospital bed is not in the home.

It is helpful to give patients charts or diagrams of the procedure so that they won't forget the positions. Also, it may help to set a timer so that sufficient time is spent in each prescribed position. Caution patient not to perform postural drainage immediately before or following meals. Also do the following:

- Teach family members the anatomical landmarks of the thorax.
- Show them where to place their hands for percussion and vibration.
- Caution them to only use cupped hands or percussion devices when performing percussion.
- Describe the hollow sound obtained when percussion is performed properly.
- Demonstrate the procedure and then ask family to perform a return demonstration.
- Teach family how to use a stethoscope and how to distinguish breath sounds and to listen for the presence of mucus in the chest.

Artificial Airway Maintenance

The most common type of artificial airway seen in the home is the tracheostomy. Procedures for care are the same as in the hospital with some adaptations. Portable nebulizers are used for humidification. Carefully instruct the patient and the family about tracheostomy care. Involve the patient and family in tracheostomy care. The more practice and instruction that they have, the more comfortable they will be. Provide detailed and explicit instructions. Written materials are good to reinforce teaching.

Caution patients or home caregivers not to get water into the tracheostomy when bathing. Alert the caregiver to place a bell at the bedside or use some other method to signal that the patient needs help. Assess the home for respiratory irritants and remove them. Keep at least one clean or sterile tracheostomy tube on hand in the event of an accidental extubation. Teach family how to replace tube. Teach family to inflate and measure cuff pressure using minimal leak technique. Allow them to practice.

Encourage the family to take a cardiopulmonary resuscitation (CPR) course. Teach mouth-to-tracheostomy rescue breathing in the event of a respiratory arrest. Teach tracheostomy and skin care. Teach the patient and family how to manipulate the tracheostomy tube and the function of each part. Teach them to remove, clean, and replace an inner cannula.

Establish emergency plans and practice routines. Inform family members that they must have a contact person to call in case of emergency.

Suctioning

Hyperoxygenate the patient before suctioning. Determine whether to use clean or sterile suctioning technique in tracheal suctioning.[4]

If clean technique is being used do the following[4]:

- Rinse the catheter in warm water.
- Wash in warm, soapy water.
- Rinse well.
- Soak in a 1:4 white vinegar and water solution for 30 minutes.
- Rinse in warm water.
- Air dry.
- Shake to remove excess water.
- Wrap in toweling until ready to use.
- Rinse again before use.
- Empty and rinse suction catheter daily to avoid bacterial growth.

Sterile technique is used for those patients who are at risk for infection. When in the home, evaluate the environment for cleanliness. If standard sanitary practices are not used, clean technique cannot be used. Assure that proper handwashing facilities are adjacent to where the suctioning will be carried out. If this is not available, moist towelettes can be used.

PATIENT AND FAMILY TEACHING

Teach patients and family about the purpose and uses of oxygen and the equipment since they are generally frightened when they learn oxygen must be used. Careful explanations of why the oxygen is being used, how it works, and what equipment is used is helpful. This is particularly true when the patient is a child or when the patient is intubated or has a tracheostomy. Explain all procedures to the patient and family as they are carried out. Use easily understood words so that the patient and family understands. Reinforce teaching. When the patient is less critical, the patient and family can be asked to participate in the procedure. See Home Care sections on pp. 69-70 for more information about specific teaching measures.

It is important to teach the family careful handwashing technique, especially if they will be handling oxygen administration or suctioning devices.

Teach the patient and family the basic principles of oxygen use before discharge, including how to do the following[5]:

* Set the correct liter flow.
* Use oxygen administration device (i.e., catheter, cannula, mask).
* Change tanks.
* Adjust flow rate before placing cannula or mask on patient's face.
* Fill a portable system.
* Dust equipment with cotton cloth to prevent sparks.
* Check to determine if portable system has sufficient oxygen.
* Maintain equipment.

In addition to the above factors, the patient and family must learn safety features. These include the following[23]:

* Purchasing sterile distilled water in small amounts and refrigerating it to prevent bacterial growth.
* Ventilating the room where the oxygen is used well.
* Keeping oxygen away from heat sources including pipes and radiators.
* Posting *No Smoking* signs and not permitting smoking within 5 feet of the oxygen source.
* Avoiding tipping or knocking over the tank.
* Keeping fire extinguishers near the oxygen unit.
* Never using oil or grease on the oxygen equipment.
* Never using oily face or hair creams while using oxygen.
* Avoiding nylon materials and woolen blankets, since they may generate static sparks.
* Properly grounding all electrical equipment to be used around oxygen.
* Never using aerosol sprays where oxygen is used or stored.
* Never changing prescribed flow of oxygen, since oxygen should be treated as a drug.

REFERENCES

1. American Heart Association: *Textbook of advanced cardiac life support,* Dallas, 1987, American Heart Association.
2. Ardabel A, Hippert T: *Air and ventilation.* In Flynn J-BM, Hackel R: *Technological foundations of nursing,* Norwalk, Conn, 1990, Appleton & Lange.
3. Ballard Tracheostomy Care: *Closed tracheal suctioning system,* Midvale, Utah, 1987, Ballard Medical Products.
4. Bristol BJ: *Home health considerations.* In Flynn J-BM, Hackel R: *Technological foundations in nursing,* Norwalk, Conn, 1990, Appleton & Lange.
5. Cecil WT, Petterson MT, Lampoonpun S, et al: Clinical evaluation of the Biox II ear oximeter in the critical care environment, *Respir Care* 30:179, 1985.
6. Chulay M: Hyperinflation/hyperoxygenation to prevent endotracheal suctioning complications, *Crit Care Nurse* 7(2):100, 1988.
7. Clark AP, Winslow EH, Tyler DO et al: Effects of endotracheal suctioning on mixed venous oxygen saturation and heart rate in critically ill adults, *Heart Lung* 19(5):552, 1990.
8. Dennison RD: Managing the patient with upper airway obstruction, *Nurs 87* 17(10):34, 1987.
9. Eschar-Neidig JR: Pediatric respiratory arrest: emergency airway management in the critical care setting, *Crit Care Nurse* 8(8): 22, 1988.
10. Gilboy NS, McGaffigan PA: Noninvasive monitoring of oxygenation with pulse oximetry, *J Emerg Nurs* 15(1):26, 1989.
11. Hoffman LA, Maszkiewicz RC: Airway management: the basics of suctioning, *Am J Nurs* 87(1):40, 1987.
12. Hoffman LA, Maszkiewicz RC: Airway management: the specifics of suctioning, *Am J Nurs* 87(1):44, 1987.
13. Kacmarek RM, Stoller JK: *Current respiratory care,* Toronto, 1988, BC Decker.
14. Kram HB: Noninvasive tissue oxygen monitoring in surgical and critical care medicine, *Surg Clin North Am,* 65(4):1005, 1985.
15. Loomis JC: *Pediatric intensive care.* In Gregory GA, editor: *Pediatric anesthesia,* Vol 2, New York, 1983, Churchill Livingstone.
16. Luce JM et al: *Intensive respirtory care,* Philadelphia, 1984, WB Saunders.
17. Mapp CS: Trach care: Are you aware of the dangers? *Nursing* 18(7):34, 1988.
18. Mathews PJ: Changing oxygen setups, *Nursing* 19(5):96, 1989.
19. Mayer TA: Management of the airway in injured children, *Top Emerg Med* 8(4):75, 1987.
20. Melton JD: Noninvasive monitoring techniques, *Emerg Care Q* 3(3):63, 1987.
21. New W: Pulse oximetry, *J Clin Monit* 1:126, 1985.
22. *Nursing '90 IV drug handbook,* Springhouse, Pa, 1990, Springhouse.
23. Openbrier DR, Fuoss C, Mall CC: What patients on home oxygen therapy want to know, *Am J Nurs* 88(2):198, 1988.
24. Parry WH, Baldy MA, Gardner SL: *Respiratory diseases.* In Merenstein GB, Gardner SL: *Handbook of neonatal intensive care,* St Louis, 1985, Mosby–Year Book.
25. Scanlan CL, editor: *Egan's fundamentals of respiratory care,* St Louis, 1990, Mosby–Year Book.
26. Scott AA, Koff PB: *Airway care and chest physiotherapy.* In Koff PB, Eitzman DV, Nev J: *Neonatal and pediatric respiratory care,* St Louis, 1988, Mosby–Year Book.
27. Shoemaker WC, Tremper KK: *Transcutaneous P_{O_2} and P_{CO_2} monitoring in the adult.* In Shoemaker WC: *Textbook of critical care,* Philadelphia, 1989, WB Saunders.
28. Smith RM: *Anesthesia for infants and children,* ed 4, St Louis, 1980, Mosby–Year Book.
29. Stone KS, Vorst EC, Lanham B, et al: Effects of lung hyperinflation on mean arterial pressure of postsuctioning hypoxemia, *Heart Lung* 18(4):377, 1989.
30. Tremper KK: Transcutaneous P_{O_2} measurements, *Can J Anesth* 31:64, 1984.
31. Tyler JA, Seely HF: The Nellcor N-101 pulse oximeter, *Anesthesiology* 41:302, 1986.
32. Yelderman M, New W: Evaluation of pulse oximetry, *Anesthesiology* 59:349, 1983.

CHAPTER 5

Mechanical Ventilation

Objectives

After completing this chapter, the reader will be able to:

- Classify the various types of mechanical ventilators.
- Discuss the indications for intubation and mechanical ventilation.
- Define the various modes, settings, alarms, and special ventilatory modifications used in mechanical ventilation.
- Describe the assembly, start-up, adjustment, and administration of PEEP in a mechanical ventilator.
- Describe the psychomotor skills involved with monitoring the ventilator.
- Troubleshoot the mechanical ventilator.
- Describe the physical complications and assessment of a patient receiving assisted ventilation.
- Formulate the nursing diagnoses and outcomes for patients receiving assisted ventilation.
- Compare and contrast the methods of weaning a patient from mechanical ventilation.
- Discuss the care of a patient receiving independent lung ventilation.
- Explain the psychosocial stressors of patients on mechanical ventilators.
- Differentiate between neonatal and adult-assisted ventilation requirements.
- Discuss assisted ventilation in home health care.

GOALS OF MECHANICAL VENTILATION

The following are the goals of mechanical ventilation:
- Meet the general goals of pulmonary support.
- Use a mode of ventilation that meets the physiological demands of the existing clinical setting.
- Maintain an adequate Pao_2 (hemoglobin saturation > 90%).
- Keep the patient on an $Fio_2 < 50\%$.
- Return the arterial blood gases (ABGs) to the patient's baseline.
- Improve the ventilation-perfusion ($\dot{V}/\dot{Q}$) ratio.
- Improve the distribution of gas.
- Improve alveolar ventilation ($\dot{V}_A$).
- Increase minute ventilation (expired volume per minute) ($\dot{V}_E$).
- Decrease the work of breathing.
- Prevent muscle atrophy.
- Prevent ventilator dependency.
- Wean patient from ventilator as soon as possible.

INDICATIONS FOR INTUBATION AND MECHANICAL VENTILATION

The basic indication for the use of mechanical ventilation in the adult patient is the need to improve the Pao_2 or the $Paco_2$ or to reduce the Fio_2 or the amount of work needed to maintain ABG values at an acceptable level. General guidelines for interpreting the Pao_2 of a patient less than 60 years of age on an Fio_2 of 21% are as follows:
- Pao_2 80 to 100 mm Hg, acceptable range.
- $Pao_2 < 80$ mm Hg, mild hypoxemia.
- $Pao_2 < 60$, moderate hypoxemia.
- $Pao_2 < 40$ mm Hg, severe hypoxemia.
- For each year over 60 years of age, subtract 1 mm Hg for limits of mild and moderate hypoxemia.
- At any age, a $Pao_2 < 40$ mm Hg indicates severe hypoxemia.

Mechanisms that contribute to or cause the development of hypoxemic respiratory failure are the following:
- Ventilation-perfusion ($\dot{V}/\dot{Q}$) inequality—when blood flow and ventilation are mismatched in various regions of the lung, as in pulmonary embolism, severe emphysema, and interstitial lung disease.
- Alveolar hypoventilation—when effective ventilation of the alveoli is no longer adequate for the body's metabolic rate, as in narcotic overdose, neuromuscular diseases, chest wall deformities (e.g., kyphoscoliosis), pneumothorax, and emphysema.
- Diffusion disturbances—processes that physically impair gas exchange across the alveolar-capillary membrane, as in interstitial fibrosis, pulmonary edema, scleroderma, and adult respiratory distress syndrome (ARDS).
- Right-to-left shunt—blood passes from the right side of the heart to the left side, bypassing gas exchange in

Table 5-1 Clinical Measurement Normals and Measurements Indicating Need for Ventilation

Clinical measurement	Normal	May need to institute ventilation
Blood gas tensions		
pH	7.34-7.45	<7.25
$Paco_2$	34-45	>55 with pH <7.25
Pao_2	80-100 (on .21%)	<50 and pH <7.25
Pulmonary function studies		
Tidal volume (TV) (ml/kg)	5-8	<5
Vital capacity (ml/kg)	65-75	<10 or 2 × TV
Forced expiratory volume in 1 sec (ml/kg)	50-60	<10
Respiratory rate	12-20	>40 or absent
Negative inspiratory force	>20-30	<20
Physiological oxygenation studies		
[$P(A\text{-}a)o_2$] breathing 100%	25-65	>350
(Pao_2/PAo_2) ratio	0.75	<0.15
(Qs/Qt)%	<5%	20%-30%
(V_D/TV)%	.25%-.45%	>.50%

From Riggs JH: *Respiratory facts*, Philadelphia, 1989, FA Davis.

the lung. Portions of the lung may not be ventilated, as in atelectasis, pneumonia, and bronchitis.

Criteria for intubation when oxygenation and spontaneous ventilation are adequate include (1) *definite airways obstruction,* such as with tracheal tumor, laryngeal edema, or macroglossia and (2) *threatened airways obstruction* due to deep coma.[27] Criteria for intubation and mechanical ventilation when oxygenation and ventilation are not adequate include: (1) *apnea* such as with neuromuscular disease, muscle relaxants, or depressant drugs; (2) *inadequate oxygenation* such as in ARDS, massive pulmonary emboli, and severe chronic obstructive pulmonary disease (COPD); (3) *impaired alveolar ventilation* such as in drug overdose, flail chest, status asthmaticus, and neurological disease; and (4) *clinical respiratory distress,* whereby in the caregiver's clinical judgment, the increase in work of breathing and a decrease in cardiac reserve caused by respiratory distress will ultimately result in respiratory failure. When ventilation becomes inefficient and exhausting, the patient will have signs and symptoms as listed in Table 5-1. Trends are more important than absolute values. One should take into account the overall clinical picture of the patient along with the respiratory measurements.

CLASSIFICATION OF MECHANICAL VENTILATORS
Negative-pressure Ventilators

Negative-pressure devices mimic the action of the human diaphragm and respiratory muscles of the chest. They apply external negative pressure to the chest wall, causing the rib cage to expand, decreasing intrathoracic pressure, and allowing air to be drawn into the lungs. Inspiration occurs when the subatmospheric pressure is created around the chest and abdomen of the patient. This type of ventilation requires the patient's upper torso and trunk to be completely

enclosed by the device. Passive exhalation occurs when the negative pressure ceases. These ventilators are bulky and provide the nurse with limited access to the patient's torso. Patients have restricted motion, which leads to musculoskeletal, back, or chest pains. These devices can be used for chronic ventilatory assistance, particularly in those patients who are unresponsive to conventional modes of therapy. Such patients can be ventilated without an endotracheal (ET) tube or tracheostomy, resulting in decreased mechanical work of breathing with improved gas exchange. Negative-pressure body ventilation is used primarily to assist patients during slowly progressive neuromuscular diseases, such as muscular dystrophies. They are also being used increasingly for other groups of patients, such as those with chronic restrictive lung disease from kyphoscoliosis who need only intermittent periods of assisted ventilation and those with high spinal cord injury, ARDS, and pneumonia.[3]

Positive-Pressure Ventilators

Positive-pressure ventilators work on the opposite principle from negative-pressure devices. They create a positive, greater-than-atmospheric pressure at the upper airway (e.g., ET or tracheostomy tube) and thus force air into the lungs. Expiration occurs when the positive pressure is removed because of the elastic recoil properties of the lungs and chest wall. Positive-pressure ventilators allow for greater access to the patient and the patient's airway. They are classified according to the mechanism used to terminate the inspiratory phase of each mechanical breath, when the preset pressure time or volume goal is reached, and are described as pressure-cycled, time-cycled, or volume-cycled ventilators.

Pressure-cycled ventilators

Pressure-cycled ventilators produce an inspiratory flow of gas that inflates the lung until a preset pressure is reached. The tidal volume (TV) delivered is determined by the level of peak pressure set on the machine and may vary from breath-to-breath. Any increase in resistance to flow, such as in mucus plugs, secretions, bronchospasm, or obstruction in the circuit, can cause the peak pressure to be reached before an adequate volume is delivered to the patient. Because the delivered TV is variable, positive-pressure ventilators are not the device of choice for prolonged support of the critically ill. This type of ventilation is best suited for short-term ventilatory support, as in postanesthesia units and for patients who have no preexisting pulmonary or thoracic conditions. The primary use of pressure-cycled ventilators is for intermittent positive pressure breathing (IPPB) treatments.

Time-cycled ventilators

Time-cycled ventilators terminate the inspiratory phase after a preset time. These ventilators are used in newborns and premature neonates because they provide precise control over inspiratory time and inspiratory to expiratory (I:E) ratios. Time-cycled ventilators are either volume-preset or pressure-preset ventilators.

Table 5-2 Modes of Mechanical Ventilation*

Mode	Indications	Advantages	Disadvantages
Control—Ventilator totally controls the patient's ventilation. Breaths delivered to the patient will be at the volume and rate set on the ventilator, regardless of the patient's attempts to initiate an inspiration.	Patients whose respiratory muscles are paralyzed (as in Guillain-Barré syndrome), whose respiratory control mechanisms are damaged, or recovering from drug overdose or anesthesia; used in some home care and transport ventilators; rarely indicated.	Operator (machine) controls Pa_{CO_2} and ventilatory pattern.	Patient's respiratory efforts must be suppressed (heavy sedation), overcome (induced hypocapnia), or eliminated (neuromuscular paralysis). The patient will exhibit anxiety if machine is not meeting ventilatory drive. Paralyzed or sedated patient cannot indicate need to adjust ventilator to meet changes in metabolism.
Assist/control (A/C) or continuous mandatory ventilation (CMV)—Ventilator provides all breaths at a set TV and minimal respiratory rate. Patient does not have to make any respiratory effort; but it is possible for patient to trigger the ventilator and receive more ventilator-assisted breaths to increase the respiratory rate.	Short-term ventilatory support; for postoperative patients; to help stabilize the patient after initial intubation; rarely indicated.	Allows patient to choose own respiratory rate while still obtaining an adequate TV with each initiated breath.	Respiratory muscles not fully used, so muscle atrophy can result; if patient breathes too fast due to sepsis, febrile states, pain, or central nervous system (CNS) disorders, respiratory alkalosis can result.
Intermittent mandatory ventilation (IMV)—Preset number of breaths are mandatory and are delivered by the machine at a specific TV. They are delivered on a regular time cycle regardless of when the patient initiates a breath. In between those ventilator breaths the patient may breathe spontaneously at own TV.	Maintenance of the patient who has an intact respiratory center and can accomplish the work of breathing but needs sustained ventilatory support (usually 8 or more breaths/min); weaning chronically ventilated patients from the ventilator (usually 7 or fewer breaths/min).	Patient controls Pa_{CO_2} and ventilatory pattern of spontaneous breaths; patient contributes a portion of ventilation, so weaning essentially starts at the onset of mechanical ventilation; keeps respiratory muscles active and coordinated; lower mean airway pressures and intrapleural pressures than CMV; less barotrauma; lessens psychological dependence; lessens fighting of ventilator.	Mandatory breaths are delivered at a set rate regardless if patient is in inspiration or expiration; increases spontaneous work of breathing; weaning may be prolonged; hypoventilation may occur if patient decreases spontaneous breathing; when the IMV rate is set low, patient must be closely monitored for fatigue.
Synchronized intermittent mandatory ventilation (SIMV)—A preset number of breaths are mandatory and are delivered by the machine at a specific TV. They are delivered when the patient initiates a breath. In between those ventilator breaths the patient may breathe spontaneously at own TV. If the patient does not initiate an SIMV breath, the ventilator will delvier a nonsynchronized breath at the end of the cycle.	Weaning of a patient from a controlled to a spontaneous ventilatory state; maintenance of patient who is spontaneously breathing but is in need of sustained ventilatory support.	Allows synchronization of machine breaths with spontaneous breaths; SIMV starts the weaning process since the patient breathes some unassisted breaths; the mandatory breath can be progressively decreased; helps to strengthen patient's ventilatory muscles.	Minute ventilation is variable, since only the ventilator rate and TV are programmable.
Mandatory minute volume (MMV)—Minimum minute volume is set and whatever portion not breathed spontaneously by the patient will be supplied by the ventilator. If the patient has a significant drop in spontaneous minute volume, backup settings and alarms will be activated. As the patient's spontaneous minute ventilation increases, mechanical support is decreased.	Short-term ventilation when it is anticipated that the patient's spontaneous ventilation will increase within a short period of time, such as after drug overdoses or immediately postoperative.	As the patient increases spontaneous breathing, ventilator assistance decreases, making the weaning process almost automatic; encourages respiratory muscle development by encouraging spontaneous ventilation.	The respiratory pattern is not evaluated. Only the minute volume is evaluated, so rapid, shallow breathing may not be distinguished from slow, deep breathing. If undetected, this could lead to acid-base disturbances or hypoventilation; the minute volume is selected arbitrarily and could be more or less than really needed by the patient.
Inverse inspiratory-to-expiratory (I:E) ratio ventilation (IRV)—Provides inspiration to expiratory times of 2:1 or greater.	Useful in patients with stiff lungs (decreased compliance), as in ARDS; useful in neonates with hyaline membrane disease.	By increasing inspiratory time, the distribution of ventilation improves; the reduced expiratory time prevents collapse of the stiffer alveolar units; achieves higher levels of oxygenation at lower peak airway pressure.	Patients complain of a bloated feeling due to their sense of not being able to fully exhale; requires sedation and/or neuromuscular blockade to remove spontaneous respiratory efforts; hypotension due to decreased venous return to the right side of the heart caused from higher intrathoracic pressures; tachycardias and dysrhythmias; ratios approaching 4:1 result in a significant drop in cardiac output.

*Refs 19, 23, 26, 30, 35, 40.

Table 5-2   Modes of Mechanical Ventilation—cont'd

Mode	Indications	Advantages	Disadvantages
Pressure support ventilation (PSV)—Assists an intubated patient's spontaneous breathing efforts with a clinician-selected amount of positive airway pressure (Fig. 5-1).	Low level PSV augments spontaneous inspiratory efforts when in IMV or MMV modes and supports patients requiring ET tubes only for airway protection or continuous positive airway pressure (CPAP) support. High level PSV used as stand-alone ventilatory support mode; PSV used for weaning of patients (1) with weak ventilatory musculature, such as from cervical spinal cord injury; (2) who tire on SIMV or IMV, due to overcoming high airway resistance of tubing during spontaneous breaths, (3) with COPD; and (4) infants and children.	At low levels (2-10 cm H_2O) pressure support ventilation helps to decrease the discomfort and work of breathing through an ET tube. At high levels PSV may improve comfort and provide a more physiological workload on the ventilatory muscles; weaning in the PSV mode rather than with a T-piece enables the ventilator to safely monitor the patient's condition.	PSV weaning requires that the patient be connected to an expensive, high-tech ventilator; PSV does not deliver consistent volumes in high, normal, and low compliance and airway resistance situations; if the patient has a tendency toward apnea or respiratory muscle fatigue, it may be necessary to provide a backup SIMV mode.
Pressure control ventilation (PCV)—Controls the peak pressure applied to the airways during mechanical ventilation; a pressure plateau occurs until the set inspiratory time elapses (see Fig. 5-1); PCV has been used with inverse I:E ratios.	For use in ARDS in conjunction with inverse I:E ratio to improve oxygenation at lower peak ventilation pressures; useful in patients where mean airway pressure (MAP) is of significance.	The pressure plateau allows filling of poorly ventilated lung units similar to the idea behind a volume hold or plateau; using pressure control rather than volume-limited breaths avoids breath stacking.	Requires sedation of the patient so that there are not assist efforts; has not yet been widely used or tested in the United States.
Airway pressure release ventilation (APRV)—Patient is placed on elevated baseline pressure and allowed to breathe spontaneously, as in CPAP. Brief interruption of CPAP when valve drops circuit pressure, allowing patient to exhale to near functional residual capacity (FRC). Valve is then closed, increasing patient's lung volume to original baseline pressure (see Fig. 5-1).	For use on patients with acute lung injury and markedly decreased lung compliance leading to severe restrictive pulmonary defects.	For patients on CPAP therapy who need augmented ventilation, this mode provides for a lower mean peak airway pressure, avoiding as much barotrauma and depression of cardiac function; the patient can breathe in an unrestricted manner during all parts of the ventilatory cycle and yet receive the partial ventilatory support needed to augment spontaneous ventilation.	Not appropriate for use in patients with increased airway resistance or obstructive lung disease since APRV requires that the peak airway pressure rise and fall rapidly when the release valve opens and closes.
High-frequency positive-pressure ventilation (HFPPV)—High-frequency ventilation characterized by: ventilatory rates between 60-100/min, small tidal volumes, positive airway pressure but with subatmospheric intrapleural pressures throughout the breathing cycle.	Laryngoscopy, bronchoscopy, microlaryngeal surgery, thoracic surgery, correction of tracheal stenosis, and open heart surgery; neonates and infants undergoing plastic surgery for repair of cleft lip or palate; adults and infants in respiratory failure with serious complications; neonates wtih hyaline membrane disease; bronchopleural fistulas.	TV is only slightly larger than dead space, which produces low airway pressure and decreases pulmonary barotrauma and circulatory impairment; the need for sedatives to ensure patient cooperation is reduced.	The catheter used for delivery can kink and become obstructed; if expiratory line becomes blocked, pneumothorax could result; adequate humidification can be difficult to obtain.
High-frequency jet ventilation (HFJV)—High-frequency ventilation characterized by the delivery of pulses of pressurized gas through a small percutaneous transtracheal catheter or through an injector cannula at the end of an ET tube; delivered rates are between 100-200 breaths/min with an I:E radio of 1:2 to 1:3.	Bronchopleural fistula; neuromuscular discoordination resulting in respiratory muscle fatigue; emergency surgical procedures involving the upper airways; acute respiratory failure; infants with pulmonary interstitial edema.	Can maintain oxygenation and CO_2 clearance in presence of large air leaks such as bronchopleural fistulas because lower peak pressures are diffused for shorter periods of time, thus reducing air loss; pulmonary stretch receptor stimulation suppresses the respiratory center, allowing the patient's respiratory muscles to rest when on HFJV; transtracheal cannula can provide ventilatory support with reduced danger of aspiration of debris from upper airway; sedative need is reduced because HFJV can be superimposed on spontaneous breathing; decreases barotrauma risk.	Humidification is difficult; bronchial mucus plugging and necrotizing tracheobronchitis can occur after long-term use; gas delivery catheter can become kinked or obstructed; HFJV is still in the experimental stage; requires specialized ventilator.
High-frequency oscillation (HFO)—High-frequency ventilation characterized by extremely high ventilatory rates (up to 3600/min), with TVs that are much smaller than the anatomic dead space.	Neonates with severe respiratory distress syndrome; potential use for infants with pulmonary hypoplasia and in microsurgery when a stable operating field is required.	Any desired tracheal pressure can be attained by adjusting the bias flow; it is possible to monitor the CO_2 concentration; humidification of inspired gas is relatively easy.	Investigative license from Federal Drug Administration (FDA) required before clinical application; hyperinflation of lungs can occur because of gas trapping; significant reduction in mucus transport.

Volume-cycled ventilators

The volume-cycled ventilator terminates the inspiratory cycle when a preset TV has been delivered. A high-pressure limit control feature can be adjusted to prevent excessive pressures from being delivered to the patient. The peak inspiratory pressure (PIP) may fluctuate according to changes in the patient's airways resistance or compliance. Inspiratory time and I:E ratio can be adjusted in these ventilators by an inspiratory flow rate control. Volume-preset ventilators (both volume-cycled and time-cycled) have the advantage that the TV delivered will remain constant, even with changing lung compliance or airways resistance. Volume-preset ventilators are quite versatile and are the ventilators of choice for adult and pediatric critical care units.

MODES OF MECHANICAL VENTILATION

Even though monitoring and making changes in settings and modes of the mechanical ventilator is the primary role of the respiratory therapist, nurses monitor the patient and must be able to troubleshoot and intervene during life-threatening mechanical ventilation problems. Nurses must also be aware of the implications of changes in ventilator settings and modes so that they can monitor the patient for physical changes and potential problems.

Currently, there are more than 10 ventilator modes that can be applied in varying combinations, in addition to many ventilator settings and special ventilatory modifications (Table 5-2 and Fig. 5-1). The proliferation of new modes complicates the field of mechanical ventilation. It has been predicted that during the 1990s the trend will be toward the unification of existing modes into a smaller group of universally applicable modes considered most beneficial by research studies.[10]

FUNCTIONS OF CONTROLS, DISPLAYS, AND INDICATORS

Nurses need to be able to locate and identify the various functions of the controls, displays, and indicators on the mechanical ventilator.[8] Becoming familiar with the display panel will help the nurse conceptualize the extensive capabilities of the mechanical ventilator. Nurses caring for ventilator patients will need to be able to interpret data and respond appropriately to alarms. The Puritan-Bennett 7200 microprocessor ventilator will be used as an example (Figs. 5-2 and 5-3).

Several new ventilators have been introduced that use computer- or microprocessor-control systems, multiple modes of ventilation, computer-capable monitoring, and extensive data collection capabilities. Examples include the Siemens Servo Ventilator 900C, the BEAR-5, the Hamilton Veolar, and the Puritan-Bennett 7200 Microprocessor ventilator. It is important for the nurse to become familiar with the control panels of these new ventilators. The Puritan-Bennett 7200 Microprocessor ventilator with its computerized electronic circuit design controls all ventilator functions and monitors patient and ventilator performance (Fig. 5-3). This ventilator has an extensive memory and can re-

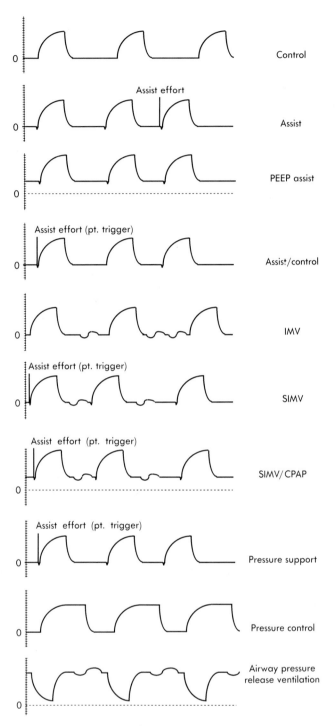

Fig. 5-1   Pressure curves for common modes of ventilation. (From McPherson SP, Spearman CB: *Respiratory therapy equipment,* St Louis, 1990, Mosby–Year Book.)

spond to operator-selected instructions or switch to its special memory, which activates the emergency or backup systems. It also provides the operator with digital monitoring of performance data. If faulty operating conditions occur, the computer's special memory overrides the operator-controlled set-up.

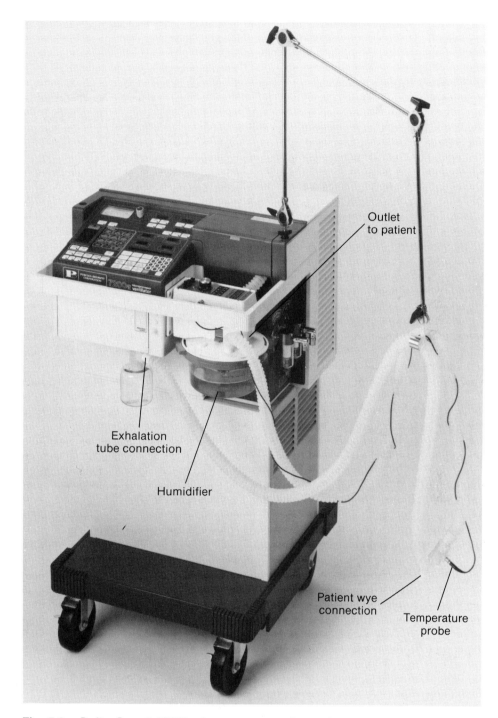

Fig. 5-2 Puritan-Bennett 7200A microprocessor ventilator. *(Courtesy Puritan-Bennett Corporation, Kansas City, Mo.)*

Safety Features

The Bennett 7200 Microprocessor ventilator's safety systems include the following:

- *Self-diagnostic tests.* These tests provide the operator with information regarding whether the ventilator is functional.
- *Emergency ventilation modes.* In disconnect ventilation, apnea ventilation, and back-up ventilation, the ventilator continues to operate, using factory-preset parameters.
- *Alarm system.*

MEASUREMENT OF TUBING COMPLIANCE

Tubing compliance should be calculated for each circuit used to ventilate the patient. This measurement is performed using a rubber test lung and is useful in establishing an accurate corrected TV delivered to the patient (Skill 5-1).

ESTABLISHING INITIAL VENTILATOR SETTINGS

Initial ventilator settings most appropriate for a patient will be established by the physician and are based on patient's needs. They are usually determined by established guidelines and formulas as discussed in the following pages[43,44]:

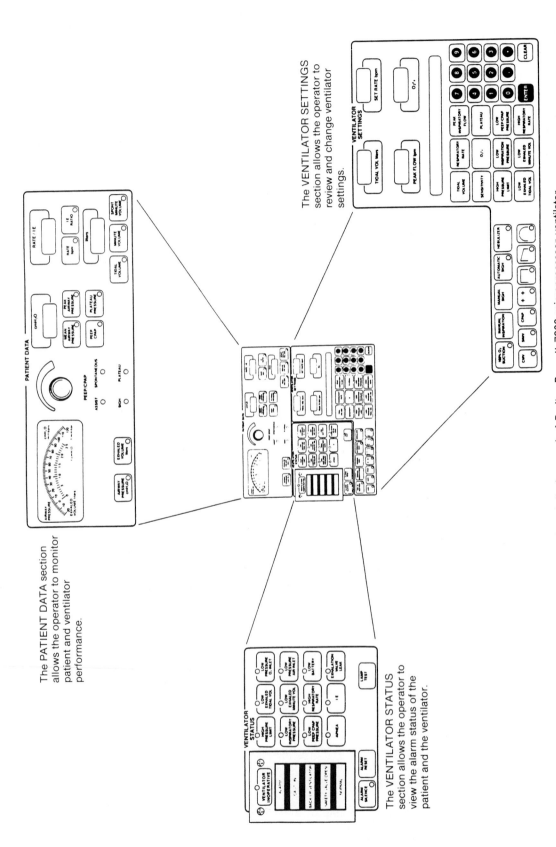

The PATIENT DATA section allows the operator to monitor patient and ventilator performance.

The VENTILATOR SETTINGS section allows the operator to review and change ventilator settings.

The VENTILATOR STATUS section allows the operator to view the alarm status of the patient and the ventilator.

Fig. 5-3   Sections of keyboard display panel of Puritan-Bennett 7200 microprocessor ventilator. *(Courtesy Puritan-Bennett Corporation, Kansas City, Mo.)*

Skill 5-1   Measurement of Tubing Compliance

EQUIPMENT AND SUPPLIES

- Bennett MA-1 or MA-2 ventilator with test lung attached
- Ventilator tubing circuit
- Oxygen and air sources at 50 psi
- Electrical source (110-volt AC current)
- Mainstream humidifier
- Thermometer
- Spirometer
- Respirometer (volume measuring device)
- Sterile distilled water
- Sterile gauze
- External disconnect alarm, if one is not provided

NURSING INTERVENTIONS[43]

1. Set the control panel to the following settings:

Tidal volume	200 ml
Respiratory rate	12/min
Peak flow	40 L/min
Pressure limit	Highest setting
All other controls	Off

2. Remove the tube leading from the exhalation port to the spirometer collection bottle. Attach a respirometer to outlet of exhalation valve to measure the exhaled volume.
3. Use a sterile gauze to cover the patient's Y-tube. The palm of the nurse's hand is then positioned to totally occlude the Y-tube outlet.
4. Press the manual normal volume button to initiate inspiration.
5. Note the pressure achieved on the pressure manometer. It may take several breaths to record the pressure accurately.
6. Read the respirometer and record the TV delivered with each breath. This volume represents the volume compressed in the circuit, since no volume was actually delivered.
7. Divide the following volume recorded with the respirometer by the pressure measured on the pressure manometer:

$$\frac{\text{Tidal volume}}{\text{PIP}} = \text{Compliance}$$

8. The amount obtained in ml/cm H_2O pressure will be the amount of volume lost in the tubing during inspiration per cm H_2O pressure generated by the machine, known as tubing compliance.

Settings

Mode

In the majority of cases the mode will be assist/control (A/C) or synchronized intermittent mandatory ventilation (SIMV) mode. The most common initial mode used is A/C, since it allows patients to regulate their own $Paco_2$ levels should the ventilator rate be set too low.[33] However, patients may trigger the ventilator too fast because of anxiety.

Fraction of inspired oxygen

For an intubated critical care patient, an Fio_2 of 100% is used until oxygen concentration can be made based on the ABG results. There is no known risk of oxygen toxicity at high concentrations when used for 1 to 2 hours. An ABG performed when the patient is breathing 100% oxygen also gives an accurate alveolar-arterial (A-a) gradient.

Table 5-3   Recommended Breathing Frequencies and Tidal Volumes[44]

Patient type	Frequency (breaths/min)	Tidal volume ml/kg
Adults		
Normal lungs	8-12	12-15
Chronic obstructive disease	8-10 or less	10-12
Chronic restrictive disease	12-20 or more	10 or less
ARDS	12-20 or more	10 or less
Children		
0-8 yrs	30-40	6-8
8-16 yrs	20-30	8-10

▼ Corrected Tidal Volume

The following formula is used to determine the actual tidal volume delivered to the patient:

$$\text{TV corrected} = \text{TV} - (\text{PIP} \times \text{Ct})$$

Where
- TV corrected = corrected tidal volume
- TV = measured tidal volume
- PIP = peak inspiratory pressure
- Ct = tubing compliance

For example, assume the following values:
- Volume control setting = 1100 ml
- Measurement at exhalation port = 1000 ml
- PIP = 25 cm H_2O
- Tubing compliance = 4 ml/cm H_2O
- Corrected TV = 1000 ml − (25 cm H_2O × 4 ml/cm H_2O) = 900 ml

The TV control should be adjusted so that the corrected TV is within 50 ml of the ordered TV.

Tidal volume

The tidal volume setting is established based on the patient's age, weight, breathing frequency, clinical condition, and the mode of ventilation chosen (Table 5-3). For example, if a male patient weighing 75 kg is started on mechanical ventilation, the tidal volume he should receive is 900 ml (12 ml/kg × 75 kg = 900 ml). Some of the volume is lost because of compression in the circuit. To determine the actual volume delivered to the patient (corrected tidal volume), a calculation must be performed (see box above).

Respiratory rate or frequency

The respiratory rate (RR) times the TV equals the minute ventilation (MV). The MV determines alveolar ventilation. The RR and TV are adjusted according to the patient's $Paco_2$ level. Increasing the MV decreases the $Paco_2$ and decreasing it increases the $Paco_2$. Patients with head injuries may need to be hyperventilated so they will develop respiratory alkalosis, promoting cerebral vasoconstriction[18]. COPD patients will need to be hypoventilated to maintain them at their baseline $Paco_2$, since they have chronically high CO_2 levels. Lowering their CO_2 levels

Skill 5-2 Initiating Mechanical Ventilation

EQUIPMENT AND SUPPLIES

- Manual resuscitation bag and oxygen flowmeter
- Two ET tubes (size appropriate for patient) (see Chapter 4)
- Syringe appropriate for cuff size
- Adhesive tape
- Intubation tray
- Tracheostomy tray present on unit
- Chest tube insertion tray present on unit
- Suction supplies and sterile normal saline
- Stethoscope
- Equipment for ABG sample
- Clipboard or other means of communication for the patient
- Ventilator flow sheets
- Oxygen analyzer

NURSING INTERVENTIONS[31]

1. Wash hands.
2. Connect ventilator to appropriate oxygen source and electrical outlet.
3. Turn on ventilator and adjust settings as ordered (see section on initial ventilator settings on p. 79).
4. Explain procedure to patient, if awake and alert.
5. Assist with intubation procedure, inflate cuff, tape tube securely, and suction patient's airway (see Chapter 4).
6. Provide ventilatory support with manual resuscitation bag for emergency intubation when ventilator is not at patient's bedside.
7. Connect the ventilator tubing to the patient's artificial airway.
8. Monitor the pressure gauge on the front of the ventilator; if the needle does not rise smoothly, increase the flow rate until it does.
9. Set all alarms based on the manufacturer's manual. Each ventilator will have different locations of available alarms.
10. Determine the maximal inspiratory pressure and set the high-pressure alarm 10 to 15 cm H_2O above that pressure.
11. Set the low-pressure alarm 10 to 15 cm H_2O below the maximal inspiratory pressure.
12. Monitor the exhaled volume for machine-generated breaths; it should be within 100 to 200 ml of the set TV.
13. Set the exhaled volume alarm within 200 ml of the actual exhaled volume.
14. Analyze the oxygen concentration and compare it to the setting.
15. Set the positive end-expiratory pressure (PEEP) level, if ordered.
16. Stay with and help the patient to relax. Provide patient with a clipboard for written communication.
17. If the patient is confused, apply soft arm restraints.
18. Monitor the patient's breath sounds to ensure bilateral, equal ventilation. Ensure that the ET tube is not in the esophagus or right mainstem bronchus.
19. Arrange to have a chest x-ray performed immediately to check for proper tube placement.
20. Draw an ABG sample after the patient has been on the ventilator for about 20 minutes. This time period allows for gas exchange to equilibrate.
21. Based on the ABG results or pulse oximetry, adjust the initial ventilator settings as ordered.

rapidly may result in seizures. Patients with restrictive diseases will need to have lower TV and higher RR levels (see Table 5-3).

In the control or A/C modes, the rate is set based on the selected tidal volume, so that the resulting minute volume will achieve a satisfactory $Paco_2$ and pH. In the A/C mode, the backup rate is set based on the patient's assist rate. If the patient has an adequate spontaneous rate, the backup rate should be set at two to four breaths below this value to prevent hypoventilation in the event of a significant rate reduction. For the SIMV mode, the initial frequency should be set close to that of the patient's own spontaneous breathing rate, at the preselected tidal volume. The SIMV frequency can then be modified based on subsequent ABG results.

I:E ratio

The I:E ratio is the duration of inspiration compared to the duration of expiration. The I:E ratio may be determined by a specific I:E ratio dial or by controls that determine inspiratory time or inspiratory flow rate, ventilatory rate, and expiratory time. If the I:E ratio is maintained at 1:2 or greater, sufficient time for a full exhalation without compromising the venous return or causing cardiovascular complication is permitted. In special circumstances the I:E ratio may be set differently. Patients with obstructive airways disease (e.g., emphysema, asthma) may be ventilated with I:E ratios of 1:3 to 1:4. Short inspiration with longer expiration allows obstructed lung units to fully empty, resulting in a more even distribution of ventilation with each new breath. Those with ARDS, resulting in decreased compliance, may be ventilated with I:E ratios of 2:1. A prolonged inspiratory time allows equilibration between lung units and a more even distribution of ventilation. Once reinflation occurs rapidly after a short expiratory phase, fewer lung units will collapse since they are reexpanded before attaining their closing volumes.[15]

Inspiratory flow rate

The inspiratory flow rate (IFR) is the speed that the TV is delivered. In the A/C mode, inspiratory flows are adjusted to provide the desired inspiratory time, I:E ratio, and breathing pattern. For adult patients, the flow rate control is set within the 40 to 60 L/min range. A high IFR (>40 L/min) shortens inspiratory time, increases turbulence, causing less uniform distribution of ventilation, and interferes less with venous return. A low IFR provides better distribution of ventilation, but the inspiratory time is prolonged (increased I:E ratio). This increases mean intrathoracic pressure, which may impair venous return and decrease cardiac output. Ideally, the IFR is set to deliver an I:E ratio of 1:2. As the tidal volume or respiratory rate increases, the IFR must also be increased to keep the I:E ratio near 1:2.

Pressure limit

This setting limits the highest pressure that will be delivered in the ventilator circuit on volume-cycled ventilators. The control should be set 10 to 15 cm H_2O greater than the peak inspiratory pressure (PIP) in continuous mandatory ventilation (CMV) or IMV modes and 5 cm H_2O above the baseline pressure in the continuous positive airway pressure (CPAP) mode. If the high pressure limit is reached, the inspiration will be immediately terminated and an alarm will sound. This control prevents the administration of dangerous pressures that could lead to pulmonary barotrauma and alerts one to changes in the patient's condition. Reaching the pressure limit could be caused by the following:

- Kinked inspiratory tubing.
- Obstruction in tubing, e.g. from patient lying on it.
- Fluid in tubing.
- Right mainstem bronchus intubation.
- Accumulation of secretions requiring airway suctioning.
- Coughing.
- Severe bronchospasm.
- Patient holding breath as ventilator delivers breath.
- Patient fighting the ventilator.
- Biting on an oral ET tube.
- Pneumothorax.
- Decreasing pulmonary compliance because of ARDS, bronchopulmonary dysplasia, or hyaline membrane disease.

Sensitivity

The sensitivity setting determines the amount of inspiratory effort required of the patient to initiate an inspiration. This setting should be adjusted so that only a negative 1 to 2 cm H_2O change registers on the pressure gauge before the ventilator responds. A too-sensitive machine will self-cycle and cause hyperventilation. A machine that is too-insensitive will also increase the work of breathing and will promote atelectasis, pulmonary edema, and patient discomfort. If PEEP is added, the sensitivity level will need to be readjusted.

Humidification and airway temperature

Humidifier temperatures should be kept close to body temperature, 35° to 37° C (95° to 98.6° F), at the patient Y-tube, where the temperature is monitored. Decreased humidity will cause dried secretions and plugging. The humidifier should be checked for adequate water levels. The humidifier should not be overfilled as this may significantly increase circuit resistance and interfere with spontaneous breathing.

Flow patterns

The microprocessor ventilators can provide the same flow pattern breath-after-breath even against fairly high airway pressures. For example, on the Puritan-Bennett 7200 Microprocessor ventilator, square-wave, sine-wave, and decelerating flow patterns can be selected. Changing the flow pattern will affect inspiratory time, I:E ratio, and mean airway pressure. These changes should be considered before an adjustment to flow pattern.

Alarms
High pressure limit alarm

This alarm is triggered when the airway pressure is equal to or greater than the preset limit (see discussion on pressure limit).

Low inspiratory pressure or disconnect alarm

When airway pressure is below the preset minimum for one complete mandatory breath cycle, the disconnect alarm is triggered. In systems delivering PEEP or CPAP, this alarm should be set to trigger if baseline pressures fall either 5 cm H_2O or 20% below the set pressure level. This alarm will sound when the patient "over breathes" or draws in more air than the ventilator delivers. A leak or disconnection will also sound the alarm.

Low exhaled volume alarm

The low exhaled tidal volume or minute volume alarm should be set to trigger when either of those volumes fall 20% below established values. This alarm may be triggered by leaks in the humidifier, tubing connections, or artificial airway cuff or when a patient becomes disconnected. The alarm will also be activated when a patient on IMV stops spontaneous respirations.

High minute ventilation or tidal volume alarm

These alarms are set to warn of rise in minute ventilation by 20% of the established value.

I:E ratio alarm

For the A/C or control modes, an I:E ratio limit should be set to 1:1 to warn of changes in this parameter. Some ventilators allow this feature to be disabled to provide for unusual I:E ratios.

Low pressure oxygen or air inlet alarms

Most ventilators provide pressure sensor alarms to determine when pressure at the air or oxygen inlet falls below 35 psi.

Ventilatory failure alarm

Most ventilators have an alarm that will sound in the event of mechanical failure. Alarms are battery powered in the event of electrical failure.

Special Ventilatory Modifications
Sigh volume

The sigh mode delivers occasional larger breaths to patients, mimicking normal breathing patterns, to minimize or prevent atelectasis. Sigh breaths are usually limited to the control or A/C modes or when tidal volumes are set below the minimum of the specified range. The sigh volume is set to 1.5 to 2 times greater than the prescribed tidal volume. The sigh pressure limit is adjusted to 10 to 15 cm H_2O greater than the PIP during sigh mode. The sigh multiple should be set to 2, to deliver 2 consecutive sighs every 15 minutes. It is generally unnecessary to use sighs in the IMV mode where the mandatory breaths are usually delivered at higher tidal volumes, as compared to spontaneous breaths.

Inspiratory plateau or hold

With the hold modification, the volume or pressure is delivered and held for a period of time. This control may be set from 0 to 2 seconds (depending on the ventilator) and is used to help prevent airway closure and reduce microatelectasis. Setting an inspiratory hold may increase intrathoracic pressures and compromise cardiac output, so should be used only with a physician's order.

Expiratory retard

The expiratory retard setting slows the flow on expiration, mimicking pursed lip breathing. The resulting positive intraairway pressure prevents flaccid airways from collapsing in chronic obstructive disorders. A back pressure is generated in the thorax, increasing intrathoracic pressure and potentially decreasing cardiac output. This control is rarely used and should be applied only with a physician's order.

Negative end-expiratory pressure

Negative end-expiratory pressure (NEEP) is used to apply negative pressure to the breathing circuit on exhalation. The resulting subatmospheric pressure is applied to the patient's airways. This system was designed to counterbalance the increase in mean intrathoracic pressures caused by intermittent positive-pressure ventilation (IPPV). NEEP provides negative intrathoracic pressure, helping the venous blood to return to the right atrium.

Positive end-expiratory pressure

PEEP is used in mechanical ventilation to apply positive pressure during expiration. This modification prevents the airway pressure from reaching ambient pressure (defined as zero or atmospheric pressure) at end exhalation. The application of PEEP causes prevention of alveolar collapse during expiration, distension of patent alveoli, and recruitment of previously closed alveoli. There are many indications for PEEP,[18] but the most common use is for the management of hypoxemic respiratory failure, as seen in ARDS, hyaline membrane disease, and infant respiratory distress syndrome. When applied in ARDS, PEEP therapy is used to: (1) increase functional residual capacity, (2) reexpand collapsed and partially collapsed alveoli, (3) decrease right-to-left intrapulmonary shunting of blood, (4) improve ventilation/perfusion imbalances, and (5) improve oxygenation so that toxic concentrations of oxygen are no longer required. PEEP is generally instituted in the patient with a Pao_2 of <60 mm Hg on an Fio_2 of 60% or higher. The initial application of PEEP is in increments of 5 cm H_2O. Smaller patients or those

with impaired cardiac output may be initiated on 2.5 cm H_2O. Patients are evaluated at each PEEP level for 15 to 30 minutes before changes are made. The risk of complications of PEEP increases markedly above 25 cm H_2O.

The primary beneficial effect of PEEP is the improvement of Pao_2 because of an increased functional residual capacity (FRC). The increase in FRC occurs because exhalation does not return to the normal resting expiratory level. Because of the positive pressure left in the airways, the alveoli are kept slightly inflated, providing for optimal gas exchange. Airway closure is reduced and atelectatic lungs are reinflated. Pulmonary static compliance is also increased.

PEEP can cause numerous complications, including barotrauma, which can lead to pneumothorax, pneumoperitoneum, pneumomediastinum, and subcutaneous emphysema. An increase in intrathoracic pressure following expiration may also occur, impairing venous return. The reduction in left ventricular preload causes a decrease in cardiac output. The decreased venous return to the heart can also cause increased intracranial pressure, passive hepatic congestion, increased renal vein back pressure, decreased blood flow to the GI tract, and exacerbation of intracardiac shunts. One beneficial effect of the decreased venous return to the heart is that the reduction in preload may be helpful to the patient with ventricular failure. PEEP may also produce bulging of the ventricular septum into the left ventricle, reducing the left ventricular end-diastolic volume. Because of all of these complications, PEEP is contraindicated in patients with shock, intracardiac shunt, unilateral lung disease, bronchopleural fistula, pneumothorax, increased intracranial pressure, or COPD unless complicated by ARDS. A patient with a normal heart should tolerate 10 to 15 cm H_2O of PEEP without difficulty. A sick postoperative mitral valve patient, though, may do poorly even with 2.5 cm H_2O of PEEP.

A phenomenon called auto-PEEP, known as *gas trapping* or *breath stacking,* can occur when there is an unintentional development of positive pressure at the end of exhalation. Patients with airflow obstruction, as in COPD and asthma, tend to have auto-PEEP. The phenomenon is also seen in those patients with high minute ventilation requirements, such as with trauma, sepsis, and burns. Reduced expiratory time increases the probability of trapping gas during exhalation. The auto-PEEP phenomenon may have a detrimental effect on weaning from mechanical ventilation. In the spontaneously breathing ventilator patient, the inspiratory muscles have to develop an increased pressure to overcome the auto-PEEP before inspiratory flow will begin. To reduce auto-PEEP, the duration of inspiration must be reduced, thus maximizing expiratory time. The other option is to add PEEP to the auto-PEEP to improve the effective sensitivity as the pressure to trigger the machine rises to the end-expiratory alveolar pressure.[13]

Continuous-flow ventilation

Continuous-flow ventilation was designed as a weaning method and is able to use CPAP, IMV, and continuous gas flow near ambient pressure, all with one circuit for versatility. The design of the circuitry allows the patient's expired volumes to be monitored.[30]

Continuous positive airway pressure

CPAP is the application of positive-pressure during inspiration and expiration to the airway during spontaneous breathing. It is similar to PEEP with the same indications except that the patient is breathing spontaneously. CPAP is also used as a method for weaning from mechanical ventilation similar to T-tube weaning. CPAP can be administered through an ET tube, tracheostomy tube, mask, or nasal cannula. CPAP levels should be kept below 20 cm H_2O to avoid significant hemodynamic complications. The most accurate way to evaluate the optimal CPAP level required by a patient is to calculate the pulmonary venous admixture. Some researchers advocate increasing CPAP until the calculated venous admixture is decreased below 15% of cardiac output.

Expiratory positive airway pressure

Expiratory positive airway pressure (EPAP) is similar to CPAP in that the patient breathes spontaneously without controlled breaths; however, positive airway pressure is maintained during exhalation only. During a spontaneous inspiration the patient must lower the airway pressure to or below atmospheric pressure to inspire tidal air. This modification is thought to provide all the benefits of CPAP therapy while reducing the mean airway pressure. The work of breathing is significantly greater during EPAP therapy than during CPAP therapy.

Intermittent mandatory ventilation and positive end-expiratory pressure

IMV and PEEP are a combination of PEEP and CPAP. The patient receives controlled breaths intermittently between spontaneous breaths. Airway pressure never drops below atmospheric pressure.

ADJUSTING THE OXYGEN CONCENTRATION

The Pao_2 for most patients should be maintained between 60 and 100 mm Hg. Patients with COPD may be kept between a Pao_2 of 50 and 60 mm Hg if indicated. Consider patients' baseline Pao_2s and whether or not they are clinically symptomatic. A low Pao_2 of less than 55 mm Hg is more of a hazard than oxygen toxicity. The recommended practice is to start with a high Fio_2 (100%), check the Pao_2, and adjust the Fio_2 downward to achieve the Pao_2 goal. The steps in Skill 5-3 may be considered by some practitioners to be too cautious. A careful approach should be used, though, for an unstable patient with an unknown history.

THE PATIENT/VENTILATOR SYSTEM

The regular monitoring of the ventilator is usually the role of the respiratory therapist. The nurse needs to be familiar with the data being collected during routine ventilator checks, the modifications being made to the ventilator

---

Skill 5-3 Adjusting the Oxygen Concentration

EQUIPMENT AND SUPPLIES
- ABG kit
- Pulse oximeter
- Mechanical ventilator

NURSING INTERVENTIONS
1. Dial in initial Fio_2 to 100%.
2. Wait 20 minutes for a steady state to be reached.
3. Measure ABGs or pulse oximeter reading (see Chapter 4).
4. Adjust Fio_2 downward in the following steps to achieve a Pao_2 of 60 to 100 mm Hg.
   - If the Pao_2 is greater than 300 mm Hg, drop Fio_2 by steps of 20%.
   - If the Pao_2 is 150 to 300 mm Hg, drop Fio_2 by steps of 10%.
   - If the Pao_2 is 100 to 150 mm Hg, drop Fio_2 by steps of 5%.
5. Recheck the Pao_2 20 minutes after each downward adjustment.
6. If an Fio_2 greater than 50% is required to maintain the patient's Pao_2 at greater than 60 mm Hg, discuss with the physician the possibility of using PEEP.

---

system, the changes in the patient's condition, and the patient's response to ventilator settings. The ventilator should be checked at least every 1 to 2 hours or when a malfunction is suspected. In addition, specific patient measurements taken on and off the ventilator should be recorded every 1 to 4 hours. The measurements monitored will vary, depending on the ventilator flow chart used by the institution.

Settings and Patient Parameters to Monitor[43]
Ventilator settings
- Mode of ventilation
- Fio_2 ordered
- Tidal volume
- Rate (breaths/min)
- Inspiratory flow (L/min)
- I:E ratio
- Inspiratory hold/expiratory retard
- Sigh volume
- Sigh interval/sigh multiple
- Temperature
- Pressure limit
- Sensitivity
- PEEP/CPAP (cm H_2O)
- Alarm settings for apnea, pressure, volume, rate, and oxygen

Measurements taken with patient on ventilator
- Fio_2 delivered to patient—measure the Fio_2 delivered from the ventilator by analyzing the gas before it enters the humidifier. Adjust the control to the prescribed oxygen level. The oxygen percentage should be adjusted to within 2% of the ordered Fio_2.
- Minute volume (L).

Skill 5-4 Administration of Positive End-Expiratory Pressure

On ventilators, such as the Puritan-Bennett 7200 Microprocessor ventilator, PEEP is a feature incorporated into the design of the ventilator. On the less-sophisticated ventilators, PEEP can be added with external circuitry. Methods employed in the application of PEEP include underwater seal, Emerson water column, and Boeringer and Downs valves. Usually it will be the respiratory therapist's role to assemble the PEEP circuitry.

NURSING INTERVENTIONS

1. Verify that there is a written physician's order for PEEP.
2. Ensure that the equipment required to initiate PEEP is gathered and assembled. Test the equipment before initiating therapy.
3. Check charts for any indications of pneumothorax on recent chest x-rays or if any chest tubes were inserted.
4. If PEEP greater than 10 cm H_2O has been ordered, ensure that patient has a pulmonary artery catheter in place, as ordered.
5. Position the patient preferably in the semi-Fowler's position.
6. Auscultate the patient's chest and suction airways if needed. This will maximize air exchange and ventilation.
7. Obtain the following baseline physiological measurements:
   - Heart rate
   - Mean arterial pressure
   - Pulmonary artery systolic pressure (PASP)
   - Pulmonary artery diastolic pressure (PADP)
   - Pulmonary artery wedge pressure (PAWP)
   - Central venous pressure
   - Cardiac output
   - ABGs
   - Mixed venous oxygen saturation
   - Oxygen delivery = (arterial oxygen content) × (cardiac output) = $(O_2$ sat) × (Hemoglobin) × (1.34) × (CO) × (10)
   - Mechanics of ventilation (i.e., minute volume, TV, frequency, vital capacity, and maximal inspiratory force)
   - Total static lung compliance = (expired tidal volume) ÷ ([plateau inspiratory pressure] − [PEEP])
8. Follow these measurements to determine if PEEP therapy is improving arterial oxygenation (adequate Pao_2 at lower Fio_2) without having an adverse effect on oxygen delivery to the tissues. Total static lung compliance will provide an indication of when overdistension of the lungs and decreased compliance occurs.
9. Read PADP and PAWP at the end of expiration. During mechanical ventilation, measured filling pressures of PADP and PAWP increase during inspiration. Read the correct pressures as the lowest mean numbers that appear on the monitor.
10. Take into consideration that high values of PEEP can also affect cardiac pressure readings since one third of endobronchial pressure is distributed intrathoracically. To be more accurate, subtract one third of the PEEP value from the observed pressures. A patient on 15 cm H_2O PEEP with a PADP of 15 mm Hg has a real PADP of approximately 15 minus 5, equal to a PADP of 10 mm Hg.
11. Attach the patient to PEEP system and adjust to ordered pressure level. Adults are usually started on 5 cm H_2O, and children and neonates on 2 to 3 cm H_2O. Verify that the system is functioning properly.

12. Monitor the patient's cardiovascular measurements. Adverse effects will be noted first in the arterial and pulmonary artery pressures. The blood pressure may fall initially. If the values change significantly, notify physician immediately.
13. Continue to monitor cardiovascular measurements every 5 to 10 minutes until stable, then every 15 minutes.
14. Monitor all ventilator settings after initiation of PEEP, subtracting PEEP level from the measured value. For example, plateau pressure − PEEP pressure = adjusted plateau pressure.
15. Monitor urine output. The urine output may fall 40% with PEEP of 10 cm H_2O.
16. After 15 to 20 minutes and after each change in PEEP level, measure ABGs, hemoglobin, cardiac output, and total static lung compliance. If pulse oximetry is available, this continuous monitoring can replace the need for ABGs.
17. Perform a PEEP trial to determine the ideal or optimal level of PEEP. This is the level that provides the best arterial oxygenation and the greatest increase in pulmonary compliance with the least decrement in cardiac output.
18. Increase PEEP levels at increments of 2.5 to 5 cm H_2O at a time.
19. Continue to increase PEEP until the Pao_2 is 60 to 100 mm Hg with an $Fio_2 < 50\%$, without having a detrimental effect on cardiac output or pulmonary compliance. PEEP levels greater than 15 to 20 cm H_2O are rarely used. The risk of complications increases markedly at > 25 cm H_2O.
20. At PEEP levels of >20 cm H_2O, it may be necessary to augment cardiac output with dopamine or fluid challenges, as ordered.
21. Avoid periodical interruptions of PEEP, especially at levels of 15 cm H_2O or greater. Do not discontinue PEEP for transport, hemodynamic monitoring, or suctioning. The patient can be suctioned through a special PEEP valve.
22. Once patient has a Pao_2 of 80 to 100 mm Hg on an Fio_2 of $> 50\%$, wean from PEEP, as ordered.
23. Reduce PEEP by 2.5 to 5 cm H_2O. After 3 minutes, obtain ABGs or oximetry analysis. Restore the patient to the previous PEEP level.
24. Compare the 3 minute Pao_2 (or Sao_2) to baseline. If oxygenation drops to unacceptable level, reassess in 12 to 24 hours.[28]
25. When weaning from PEEP, observe the cardiac output carefully. A patient with ventricular failure who has benefitted from the reduced preload may not be able to compensate for the sudden increase in venous return to the heart.
26. Once a patient is weaned to 5 cm H_2O PEEP, pulmonary gas exchange is stable, and the underlying illness is stable, wean patient from the ventilator and extubate, as ordered.

- Rate (total breaths/min).
- Measured tidal volume—measure a minute volume using a portable respirometer or the ventilator spirometer. Divide the minute volume by the frequency to obtain an average machine tidal volume.
- Tubing compression volume—calculate by multiplying the PIP by the tubing compliance.
- Corrected tidal volume—calculate by subtracting the tubing compression volume from the measured tidal volume. The corrected tidal volume should be adjusted to within 50 ml of the ordered tidal volume.
- Sigh volume—volume of intermittent deep breaths administered to patient.
- Peak pressure—read as the highest pressure indicated by the manometer needle during inspiration. An increasing pressure reflects decreased pulmonary compliance from fluid accumulation by conditions such as pulmonary edema, interstitial edema, or secretion accumulation. Increased pressure may also indicate increased airway resistance, such as in bronchospasm.
- Plateau pressure—measure when there is no air flow in the patient/ventilator circuit. Measure plateau pressure by pinching the exhalation valve tubing during an inspiratory cycle, occluding the exhalation port momentarily after a breath is delivered. Observe the pressure manometer. It will indicate the PIP, then fall slightly (5 to 15 cm H_2O) and stabilize. Measure and note this later pressure on the flow sheet.
- Dynamic compliance—the compliance of the lungs, thorax, and the patient/ventilator circuit; measure by dividing the corrected tidal volume by PIP.
- Static compliance—an indicator of the compliance of the lungs and thorax; calculate by dividing the corrected tidal volume by the plateau pressure.

Skill 5-5   Monitoring the Patient/Ventilator System
▼ ....

NURSING INTERVENTIONS

1. Check for any changes in physician's orders.
2. Assess patient. Observe for patient comfort.
3. Check recent ABG and other physiological monitoring measurements.
4. Suction the patient as needed.
5. Check for proper ET tube position and cuff inflation pressure (see Chapter 4).
6. Always wash hands before and use aseptic technique when working with the ventilator.
7. Fill the humidifier to the proper level and drain the ventilator tubing of any condensate. Disconnect the tubing and drain into a water trap or a wastebasket with plastic bag lining. Never drain the condensate back into the humidifier.
8. Monitor ventilator settings, patient measurements on the ventilator, and patient measurements off the ventilator.
9. Adjust ventilator settings as required.
10. Record all ventilator settings and patient measurements on flow sheet.

- Circuit temperature—check the temperature of the air delivered to the patient with an in-line thermometer held as close to the patient connector as possible. Ensure that the delivered air temperature is close to body temperature.

Measurements taken with patient off ventilator
- Minute volume (L)
- Rate (breath/min)
- Tidal volume (L)
- Vital capacity (L)
- Maximum inspiratory force (Neg cm H_2O)
- Maximum voluntary ventilation (L/min)

TROUBLESHOOTING THE MECHANICAL VENTILATOR

When a patient on a mechanical ventilator develops a problem that has no immediate resolution, the patient should be immediately removed from the ventilator and provided with 100% oxygen through a manual resuscitator. A rapid assessment of the patient should be performed first, checking for bilateral breath sounds, chest movement, stable vital signs, improved respiratory function, and improved color. If the patient's condition improves, the problem could be attributed to the ventilator or the patient's response to the ventilator. The respiratory therapist will help troubleshoot the ventilator. If the condition (such as cyanosis or sudden hypotension) remains, then a patient problem (e.g., excessive administration of vasopressors or tension pneumothorax) will need to be diagnosed and corrected. Table 5-4 lists ventilator and patient problems with possible causes and corrections of these problems.[44] The corrections are not necessarily listed in order of priority, as the order will be determined by the situation. The alarms available will vary, depending on the ventilator being used; however, alarms may be classified into several different types, depending on their function.

ASSESSMENT

When caring for the patient receiving mechanical ventilation the nurse must continually assess the patient for problems and complications (Table 5-5). A nurse should always be within sight and sound of every patient being ventilated. A combination of data from the patient's physical assessment, the ventilator, and invasive and noninvasive monitoring devices should be evaluated at least every hour and can provide information on the patient's condition. The following measurements are a part of the nursing assessment.

- Observe and listen over the artificial airway. Assess for secure taping, proper position, and presence of cuff leak or heavy secretions.
- Auscultate the patient's chest for adventitious breath sounds: crackles (pulmonary edema and atelectasis) and rhonchi (may need suctioning).
- Compare breath sounds bilaterally (see Chapter 4).

Table 5-4   Troubleshooting the Mechanical Ventilator[44]

Problem	Causes	Interventions
Low exhaled TV	Altered settings; any condition that triggers high or low pressure alarm; patient stops spontaneous respirations; leak in system preventing TV from being delivered; cuff insufficiently inflated; leak through chest tube; airway secretions; decreased lung compliance; spirometer disconnected or malfunctioning.	Check settings; evaluate patient, check respiratory rate; check all connections for leaks; suction patient; check cuff pressure; calibrate spirometer.
Low inspiratory pressure	Altered settings; unattached tubing or leak around ET tube; ET tube displaced into pharynx or esophagus; poor cuff inflation or leak; tracheal-esophageal fistula; peak flows that are too low; low TVs; decreased airway resistance due to decreased secretions or relief of bronchospasm; increased lung compliance due to decreased atelectasis; reduction in pulmonary edema; resolution of ARDS; or change in position.	Reset alarm; reconnect tubing; modify cuff pressures; tighten humidifier; check chest tube; adjust peak flow to meet or exceed patient demand and correct for the patient's TV; reposition or change ET tube.
Low exhaled minute volume	Altered settings; leak in system; airway secretions; decreased lung compliance; malfunctioning spirometer; decreased patient-triggered respiratory rate due to drugs; sleep; hypocapnia; alkalosis; fatigue; and change in neurological status.	Check settings; assess patient's respiratory rate, mental status, and work of breathing; evaluate system for leaks; suction airway; assess patient for changes in disease state; calibrate spirometer.
Low PEEP/CPAP pressure	Altered settings; increased patient inspiratory flows; leak; decreased expiratory flows from ventilator.	Check settings and correct; observe for leaks in system; if unable to correct problem, increase PEEP setting.
High respiratory rate	Increased metabolic demand; drug administration; hypoxia; hypercapnia; acidosis; shock; pain; fear; anxiety.	Evaluate ABGs; assess patient; calm and reassure patient.
High pressure limit	Improper alarm setting; airway obstruction due to patient fighting ventilator (holding breath as ventilator delivers TV); patient circuit collapse; tubing kinked; ET tube in right mainstem bronchus or against carina; cuff herniation; increased airway resistance due to bronchospasm, airway secretions, plugs, and coughing; water from humidifier in ventilator tubing; decreased lung compliance due to tension pneumothorax; change in patient position; ARDS; pulmonary edema; atelectasis; pneumonia; or abdominal distension.	Reset alarms; clear obstruction from tubing; unkink and reposition patient off of tubing; empty water from tubing; check breath sounds; reassure patient and sedate if necessary; check ABGs for hypoxemia; observe for abdominal distension that would put pressure on the diaphragm; check cuff pressures; obtain chest X-ray and evaluate for ET tube position, pneumothorax, and pneumonia; reposition ET tube; give bronchodilator therapy.
Low pressure oxygen inlet	Improper oxygen alarm setting; oxygen not connected to ventilator; dirty oxygen intake filter.	Correct alarm setting; reconnect or connect oxygen line to a 50 psi source; clean or replace oxygen filter.
I:E ratio	Inspiratory time longer than expiratory time; use of an inspiratory phase that is too long with a fast rate; peak flow setting too low while rate too high; machine too sensitive.	Change inspiratory time or adjust peak flow; check inspiratory phase, or hold; check machine sensitivity.
Temperature	Sensor malfunction; overheating due to too low or no gas flow; sensor picking up outside air flow (from heaters, open doors or windows, air conditioners); improper water levels	Test or replace sensor; check gas flow; protect sensor from outside source that would interfere with readings; check water levels.

Table 5-5 Patient-related Complications of Intubation and Mechanical Ventilation[38,43]

Complication	Causes	Effects
Respiratory		
Barotrauma	High peak airway pressure (PAP), especially above 70 cm H_2O (includes high TVs and frequency); especially susceptible patients include those with necrotizing pneumonia, aspiration of gastric contents, and chronic lung disease.	Pressurized air may rupture alveoli of diseased or fragile lungs so that air enters thoracic cavity leading to tension pneumothorax, pneumomediastinum, pneumoperitoneum, pneumopericardium, subcutaneous emphysema, tracheal rupture, pulmonary interstitial emphysema (PIE), or vascualr air embolization.
Decreased respiratory drive	Hyperventilation causing decreased Pa_{CO_2} patient on hypoxic drive causing increased Pa_{O_2}; CO_2 narcosis causing increased Pa_{CO_2}.	Abnormal ABGs.
Air-trapping	High inspiratory flow rates, inverse I:E ratios, ball valve obstruction.	Inadequate alveolar ventilation.
Atelectasis	Secretion retention; decreased TV; constant TV; inappropriate sighing; decreased PEEP (with surfactant deficiently); inadequate chest physical therapy, turning, and postural drainage.	Ventilation/diffusion disturbances.
Hyperventilation	Increased minute ventilation ($\dot{V}E$), high amino acid or carbohydrate intake.	Hypocapnia (decreased (Pa_{CO_2}), respiratory alkalosis, and difficulty in weaning.
Hypoventilation	Decreased minute ventilation ($\dot{V}E$), cuff leak, displaced airway.	Hypercarbia (increased Pa_{CO_2}), respiratory acidosis, hypoxemia, and microatelectasis.
Nosocomial pulmonary infections	Contamination of high-output nebulizers and circuitry, unsterile suctioning technique, decreased resistance, aspiration of gastric contents.	High morbidity and mortality.
Oxygen toxicity	Exposure to >50% oxygen for prolonged period.	Syndromes of toxicity include absorption atelectasis, acute tracheobronchitis, acute lung injury resulting in ARDS and bronchopulmonary dysplasia.
Hypoxemia	Decreased Fi_{O_2}, decrease in PEEP level.	Decreased Pa_{O_2}.
Tracheal stenosis	Decrease in capillary circulation combined with irritation from the ET tube; high cuff pressure.	Narrowing of trachea by scar tissue.
Esophageal intubation	Difficult or rapid intubation without proper postintubation assessment.	Ventilation of the abdomen rather than the lungs with lethal effects if not corrected.
Intubation of right mainstem bronchus	Improper intubation technique and post-assessment.	Macroatelectasis secondary to obstruction of left mainstem bronchus.
Airway obstruction	Respiratory secretions, inadequate suctioning, tubing kinked or displaced, biting down on ET tube, bronchopasm, water in tubing, cuff herniation.	Hypoxemia and hypercarbia with lethal effects.
Cardiovascular		
Decreased venous return and stroke volume	Application of positive intrathoracic pressure (high TVs and PEEP levels and long inspiratory flow rates)	Decreased cardiac output, left ventricular afterload, blood pressure, Pa_{O_2}, and urinary output; increased heart rate, pulmonary artery pressure, and central venous pressure.
Cardiac dysrhythmias	Adverse reactions to intubation and sedation; rapid changes in O_2, CO_2, or pH levels.	Potential for cardiac arrest.
Neurological		
Increased intracranial pressure	Increased intrathoracic pressure due to high TVs and PEEP and prolonged inspiratory flow rates.	Decreased venous return to the heart, resulting in pooling of blood in the head.

Continued.

Table 5-5   Patient-Related Complications of Intubation and Mechanical Ventilation[38,43]—cont'd

Complication	Causes	Effects
Cerebral vasoconstriction	High Fio_2 or hyperventilation causing expiration of CO_2.	Low CO_2 levels cause vasoconstriction resulting in reduced blood supply to brain.
Renal, fluid, and electrolytes		
Fluid and sodium retention	Increased pressure on thoracic aorta baroreceptors causes increased production of antidiuretic hormone that stimulates renal system to retain water; excessive water in inspired gases; reduced insensible losses from respiratory tract.	Increased body weight and edema; electrolyte imbalances; increased intrathoracic water leading to pulmonary edema, decreased Pao_2, and increased $P(A-a)o_2$.
Decreased urine output	Decreased cardiac output, decreased in renal blood flow, increased in production of antidiuretic hormone.	Increased fluid volume.
Dehydration or mild hyperthermia	Inspired air improperly humidified or overheated.	Drying of pulmonary secretions and membranes; retention of secretions leading to infection.
Metabolic		
Acid-base disturbances	Use of control mode of ventilation, respiratory muscle fatigue, improper TV.	Electrolyte imbalances potentially leading to cardiac arrest.
Decrease in liver function	Downward pressure exerted by the diaphragm of the liver during inspiration, interfering with the portal blood flow.	Coagulation problems and decreased detoxification of drugs (especially depressants).
Increased work of breathing	Fighting the ventilator, small ET tube, hypoxia, decreased lung compliance, increased airway resistance.	Increased PAP, restlessness, intercostal muscle retractions, tachypnea.
Gastrointestinal		
Gastrointestinal (GI) ulcers	Stress, decreased nutrition, positive pressure interferes with perfusion to the spleen and GI tract.	Mucosal ischemia and increased susceptibility to acids in GI tract leading to ulceration and bleeding.
Gastric distention	Increased air swallowing in the presence of artificial airway.	Increased susceptibility for vomiting with pulmonary aspiration; restriction of diaphragmatic movement.
Paralytic ileus and fecal impaction	Positive pressure to abdomen, stress, decreased motility.	Decreased bowel movements, feeding difficulties.
Inadequate nutritional intake	Inaccurate estimation of caloric needs, presence of artificial airway, gastric distention, paralytic ileus.	Decreased respiratory muscle mass, altered surfactant production, pulmonary edema related to low serum albumin, respiratory muscle weakness, respiratory failure due to hypophosphatemia, increased susceptibility to infection, and difficulty in weaning.
Integumentary		
Damage to teeth, oral cavity, or upper airway	Rapid or careless intubation procedure.	Potential ulceration, abscesses, and infections.
Pressure sores, nasal necrosis, tracheal erosion, vocal cord damage	Friction from the ET tube, high cuff pressure.	Hoarseness for several hours after extubation, superficial infections.
Psychosocial		
Sensory overload	Lack of sleep, discomfort of artifical airway, manipulation of breathing pattern, noises from ventilator, suctioning, chest physical therapy, and turning.	Disorientation, anxiety, apprehension.
Inability to communicate verbally	Presence of artificial airway.	Frustration, anxiety, dependency, fear.
Psychological dependence on ventilator	Fear of being weaned and discharged.	Lack of cooperation, anxiety.

- Observe for asymmetry of chest movement indicating pneumothorax, splinting due to pain, and massive atelectasis. Assess for synchronization of chest movement with ventilator.
- Assess intercostal spaces for bulging, indicating tension pneumothorax.
- Observe for tachypnea.
- Assess for foul-smelling, tenacious sputum; elevated temperature; and tachycardia. Check any recent sputum cultures for the presence of pulmonary infection.
- Record results of most recent chest x-ray and pulse oximetry readings.
- Monitor ABGs with each ventilator change and with clinical changes. Determine if they are being maintained within acceptable limits for patient (see Chapter 4).
- Observe for dysrhythmias, tachycardia (>100), and increased blood pressure (>140/90), all early signs of acute respiratory failure.
- If the patient has a pulmonary artery catheter, evaluate the physiological variables (see Chapter 8).
- Monitor heart rate, blood pressure, and cardiac output after changes in PEEP level.
- Assess if the patient is fighting the ventilator; if so, evaluate for hypoxemia, hypercapnia, acidosis, pneumothorax, fear, anxiety, pain, or problems with ventilator, such as inadequate ventilatory mode, improper rate, or kinking of tubing. Assess need for paralysis/sedation.
- Determine Glasgow Coma Score. A decreased level of consciousness, confusion, and lethargy may indicate acute respiratory failure.
- Assess for signs of hypervolemia.
- Observe for a decreased urine output.
- Evaluate caloric and protein needs (see Chapter 16).
- Palpate abdomen for tautness and measure abdominal girth to evaluate for gastric distention.
- Assess gastric pH to determine effectiveness of stress ulcer therapy.
- Inspect mouth for need of better oral hygiene, to help prevent aspiration of oral bacteria.
- Assess bowel sounds for decreased motility that might lead to vomiting and aspiration. Evaluate for proper positioning (head of bed elevated 30 to 45 degrees) during continuous feedings.
- For patients assisting their own ventilation, observe for the use of accessory muscles. Palpate and observe the scalene muscles and parasternals at the second and third intercostal spaces. These accessory muscles are recruited when inspiratory work is increased.[4] Use of accessory muscles indicates an increased work of breathing. There may be an obstruction in the airway or circuit, the sensitivity may be set too high, or the patient may have developed fatigue.
- Assess for respiratory muscle fatigue by observing for paradoxical abdominal breathing.[19] When a patient breathes normally, the abdomen and the chest wall both move outward during inhalation. In paradoxical abdominal breathing, the abdominal wall moves inward on inhalation. When the diaphragm is exhausted, it weakens, and the abdomen flattens as the thoracic cage rises during inspiration.
- Assess for respiratory alternans, also indicating respiratory muscle fatigue.[19] In respiratory alternans, patients have periods of almost total use of the diaphragm and abdominal muscles for breathing interspersed with periods of almost total use of the chest wall muscles for breathing. This process is an innate attempt to rest the diaphragm.
- Assess patient for proper positioning for maximum lung expansion.
- Palpate patient's skin for subcutaneous emphysema, indicating a pneumothorax or dissection of air around tracheostomy.
- Observe for early indicators of acute respiratory failure, such as cool and dry skin, and late indicators, such as cyanosis and diaphoresis.
- Assess for skin ulceration at ET and tracheal tube sites.
- Assess patient's anxiety level by evaluating vital signs, body movements, and fighting of ventilator (frequent high pressure alarm).
- Determine need for assurance and assist with relaxation and diversion.
- Provide for patient and family teaching and explanation of ventilator.
- Determine if the patient can communicate (e.g., clipboard or alphabet board).

NURSING DIAGNOSIS

Possible nursing diagnoses for mechanically ventilated patients include the following:

- High risk for ineffective airway clearance related to copious secretions.
- High risk for infection related to compromise of normal defense mechanisms.
- Inability to sustain spontaneous ventilation related to neuromuscular defect.
- Decreased venous return related to positive intrathoracic pressure secondary to mechanical ventilation.
- Dysfunctional ventilatory weaning response related to history of malnutrition.
- High risk for impaired gastrointestinal tissue integrity related to stress and decreased perfusion secondary to mechanical ventilation.
- High risk for sensory overload related to continual manipulation secondary to mechanical ventilation.
- Impaired verbal communication related to presence of artificial airway.

PATIENT OUTCOMES

The following are examples of expected outcomes for mechanically ventilated patients. Patient evidences the following:

- Normal ABG values for patient with $Pao_2 > 60$ mm Hg, $Paco_2$ 35 to 45 mm Hg, pH 7.35 to 7.45, HCO_3^- 24 to 28 mEq/L, base excess (BE) + 2 mEq/L.
- Clear, well-secured, patent artificial airway.
- Bilateral clear, equal, and normal breath sounds with a rate of 12 to 20 breaths/min.
- Symmetrical chest movements, in synchronization with ventilator, without use of accessory muscles.
- Clear, white, odorless pulmonary secretions.
- Normal temperature 36° to 38° C (97° to 100.5° F), WBC count (<11,000 µl), and negative sputum cultures.
- Improved (increased) or normal static compliance (50 to 100 ml/cm H_2O).
- Tolerance to weaning from ventilator.
- Normal sinus rhythm of 60 to 100 and mean arterial pressure of 70 to 90 mm Hg.
- Normal physiological monitoring variables (see Chapter 8).
- Urine output > 30 ml/hr, urine specific gravity 1.003 to 1.030, and weight gain < 0.5 kg (1.0 lb) /24 hrs.
- Laboratory studies within normal limits.
- Clear, dry, warm, intact skin of normal color, especially around artificial airway entry sites.
- Moist tongue and mucous membranes and normal skin turgor.
- Relaxed, calm posture with heart rate <100 and restful sleep.
- Patient communicates well with staff using alphabet board or other device.
- Patient indicates feelings about being dependent on a ventilator.

WEANING FROM MECHANICAL VENTILATION

Weaning is the process whereby a patient is transferred from mechanical ventilatory support to spontaneous breathing. Most patients require a brief period of weaning. For those who require more gradual weaning, there are currently the following three methods[12,17,20]:

- Intermittent trials of spontaneous breathing on a T-piece alternated with mechanical ventilatory supported muscle rest. When a patient who is being ventilated with no more than 5 cm H_2O of PEEP needs to be weaned, spontaneous breathing trials can also be performed using a high-flow CPAP system rather than an ambient pressure T-piece. In the CPAP mode, though, the patient will still have to overcome the resistance of the demand valve. This increased workload may promote fatigue.
- IMV with a gradual reduction in the rate of mandatory breaths. Specialized forms of IMV available on some ventilators are extended mandatory minute volume (EMMV) and augmented minute ventilation (AMV). These modes guarantee a minimum minute volume that will be adjusted depending upon a patient's spontaneous efforts. If, during weaning, the pa-

Skill 5-6 Assessing Readiness for Weaning

NURSING INTERVENTIONS

1. Determine if the underlying disease process has been resolved or is in a stable state.
2. Ensure that the patient is alert and awake enough to protect the airway, has a normal drive to breathe, and is not in a state of sleep deprivation.
3. Assess the patient's psychological dependency on the machine.
4. Measure patient's vital signs to assess whether or not they are stable. Evaluate temperature for presence of fever.
5. Check the patient's laboratory values to determine the presence of anemia, infection, electrolyte imbalance (with a low potassium or phosphorus level), or a state of nutritional deprivation. These problems can cause muscle weakness.
6. Assess the stability of the patient's cardiovascular system and ensure that major inotropic support is not needed. Determine whether the patient is in shock or has a reduced cardiac output.
7. Determine that the patient is free of severe pain, especially in the thoracic area.
8. Assess that the patient has a normal amount and quality of airway secretions and a strong cough reflex.
9. Check the patient's ABGs to determine that they are within the patient's normal limits at an Fio_2 less than 40%. Ensure that there are no acid-base abnormalities, especially metabolic alkalosis and acidosis. The patient should evidence the following:
   - $Pao_2 > 60$ mm Hg on $Fio_2 < 40\%$ without PEEP
   - $Paco_2 < 45$ mm Hg
   - pH range 7.35 to 7.45
   The $Paco_2$ will probably be higher and the Pao_2 lower for a COPD patient.
10. Determine if the patient has sufficient respiratory muscle strength and reserve to maintain spontaneous ventilation. Perform bedside measurements of the following ventilatory parameters:[20,44]

Vital capacity	Greater than 10 ml/kg or 1½ to 2 times normal tidal volume
Respiratory rate	No greater than 25 breaths/min
Minute ventilation	Less than 10 L/min
Tidal volume	Greater than 5 ml/kg body weight
Inspiratory force	At least 20 cm H_2O

11. If these respiratory function variables are borderline, measure the maximal voluntary ventilation (MVV) to determine if it is more than twice the resting minute ventilation.
12. If desired, perform the following optional more-sophisticated tests of oxygenation and ventilation, keeping in mind that there is considerable risk in placing a patient on 100% oxygen therapy. Despite good respiratory muscle strength, the patient may be unable to achieve adequate blood oxygen levels because of significant lung injury.

$P(A-a)o_2$ breathing 100% oxygen	Less than 350 mm Hg
Shunt fraction breathing 100% oxygen	Less than 20%
Dead space/tidal volume ratio	Less than 0.6

tient's spontaneous breathing falls below the set minute volume level, mandatory breaths are delivered.

- Pressure-support ventilation (PSV) where the amount of pressure used to augment spontaneous ventilation is gradually reduced. PSV weaning can also be used in combination with either IMV or CPAP.[9] When used with IMV, the patient's spontaneous breaths are supported by a low level of pressure, and the patient is weaned by decreasing the number of ventilator breaths, as in standard IMV weaning. When PSV is used with CPAP, positive pressure is also maintained during expiration to reduce intrapulmonary shunting and to increase the Pao_2.

Readiness for Weaning

To determine if the patient is ready for weaning, an accurate assessment of the patient's condition is necessary (Skill 5-6). It is important to remember that many patients can be successfully weaned who do not meet all conventional weaning criteria. The weaning process may take anywhere from hours to days to complete, depending on the patient's condition. Nurses, physicians, and respiratory therapists will participate as a team in the weaning process.

INDEPENDENT LUNG VENTILATION

Occasionally, critical care patients will have unilateral lung disease where a pleural effusion, pulmonary contusion, or aspiration pneumonia, for example, is concentrated in one or more discrete areas of the lungs. When only one part of or only one lung is diseased and the patient is placed on mechanical ventilation, problems may occur. Because the healthy lung is more compliant, the gas flow will take the path of least resistance, causing hyperinflation and an increased chance of barotrauma to the healthy lung areas. The stiffer lung will receive less ventilation, resulting in increased alveolar collapse, causing ventilation-perfusion mismatching. An ideal solution to this problem would be to ventilate the two lungs independently using two synchronous mechanical ventilators.

Independent lung ventilation is performed using a double-lumen endobronchial tube. Each lung has its own ventilator so that volume, flow, Fio_2, PEEP, and alarm limits are independently adjustable for each lung. It is best to synchronize the two ventilators because asynchronous lung ventilation can cause changes in intrathoracic pressure, with adverse effects on the systemic and pulmonary circulations.[41] The Siemens Servo ventilator 900C and 900D have the capability for synchronous cycling with another machine. For other ventilators, a digital timer and relay driver can be attached across the terminals of the manual breath switches of two ventilators.[33]

Caring for a patient on two ventilators significantly increases the nurse's workload. Time periods when the nurse can receive help from other health care team members in turning and suctioning the patient will need to be carefully planned. The double-lumen endobronchial tube's lumens

Skill 5-7 Weaning with Intermittent Spontaneous Breathing (T-piece Trials)

▼ ....

An advantage of T-piece weaning is that theoretically it allows the respiratory muscles to work to the point of fatigue and then allows for complete rest when the patient is placed back on the ventilator. This alternation provides a training effect.

NURSING INTERVENTIONS

1. Check patient's chart for physician's weaning schedule.
2. Initially wean only during the day, preferably in the morning.
3. If patient receives bronchodilator treatments, postural drainage, chest physical therapy (CPT), suctioning, or procedures where energy is exerted, make sure that patient has rested on ventilator for 15 to 20 minutes afterwards.
4. Suction airway as needed.
5. Ensure that patient has not just received narcotics, other analgesics, or sedatives.
6. Talk to the patient and explain procedure. Allow patient to express fears and assure of close monitoring by staff.
7. Position patient in semi-Fowler's position to allow for good chest and lung expansion.
8. Set up high-flow humidified oxygen through a T-tube or tracheostomy collar at same or slightly higher Fio_2.
9. Turn off ventilator alarms, remove ventilator tubing, and attach T-tube or tracheostomy collar. Turn off ventilator.
10. Document date, time, and Fio_2.
11. Have the patient breathe spontaneously for approximately 5 to 10 min/hour initially. Gradually lengthen spontaneous breathing periods as tolerated.
12. Once patient is able to remain off ventilator for at least 15 minutes, obtain spontaneous ventilation measurements, vital signs, and ABGs just before the weaning period ends.
13. During the entire weaning process, continuously observe patient for the following adverse effects:[32]

Blood pressure	Rise or fall by 20 mm Hg
Heart rate	Increase by 20 beats/min
Respiratory rate	Increase by 10 breaths/min: > 25 or <8 breaths/min
Signs of respiratory muscle fatigue	Use of accessory muscles Asynchronous breathing Paradoxical breathing Respiratory alternans
ECG	Cardiac dysrhythmias
Oximeter	Decreasing oxygen saturation
ABGs	Rising Pco_2 that causes pH to drop below 7.35
Skin	Increased sweating
Mental status	Increased drowsiness or restlessness
Communications from patient	Panic, pain, fatigue, or dyspnea

14. Extubate the patient, as ordered, if no adverse effects have occurred and the following values are acceptable:

Pao_2	Acceptable (>80% of preweaning value)
pH	> 7.30 and stable

Skill 5-8   Weaning with Intermittent Mandatory Ventilation

Some of the advantages of weaning with IMV over T-piece weaning include a shortened mean ventilation time, decreased incidence of alkalosis, and lowered oxygen consumption during the transition to spontaneous ventilation. Also, if the patient suddenly becomes apneic, the ventilator will monitor the change.

NURSING INTERVENTIONS

1. Perform steps 1 to 7, Skill 5-7.
2. If necessary, change the ventilator mode to IMV or synchronized intermittent mandatory ventilation (SIMV).
3. Reduce "control" breath rate to level that will provide for desired Pa_{CO_2}.
4. Decrease IMV rate gradually in increments of 2 until a rate of 2 or zero is reached.
5. Perform a clinical evaluation of the patient with each rate reduction and obtain periodic ABG measurements.
6. When the IMV rate is reduced to as low as 2 to 3 breaths/ min, remove patient from the ventilator, as ordered, extubate, and place on a high humidity face mask or tracheostomy collar.

Skill 5-9   Weaning with Pressure-Support Ventilation

The advantages of PSV are that the amount of work of breathing by the patient can be regulated, and the patient may be more comfortable in this mode of ventilation. The patient has increased comfort because the pressure support decreases some of the inspiratory work of breathing imposed by the resistance of the demand valves and ET tube. Compared to T-piece weaning, PSV provides for more accurate oxygenation and humidity. The patient is also monitored continuously by the ventilator.

NURSING INTERVENTIONS

1. Perform steps 1 to 7, Skill 5-7.
2. Begin by providing a level of inspiratory PSV adequate to supply essentially all of the ventilatory demands of the patient. Some physicians begin with a level of pressure that produces a targeted tidal volume of approximately 8 to 10 ml/kg of ideal body weight.
3. Progressively decrease this level relatively rapidly so that the patient takes on more of the active work of breathing. Take care not to overwork the respiratory muscles too quickly.
4. Continuously evaluate whether the patient is clinically tolerating the level of spontaneous breathing work. Monitor the patient's spontaneous respiratory rate and ensure that it does not exceed 25 to 30 breaths/min.
5. If the respiratory rate is higher than desired, increase the PSV level until the targeted tidal volume is reached.
6. If the patient still has a high respiratory rate, help patient to relax. Patients will usually relax once the appropriate PSV level is found.
7. Extubate the patient at level of 5 cm H_2O pressure support, since the pressure is only overcoming the resistance of the ET tube at this point. Place on a high humidity face mask.

are narrower than a standard ET tube of the same size. Problems with prolonged endobronchial intubation include the following:

- Incorrect tube position.
- Kinking of tube at pharyngeal level.
- Frequent airway blockage because of retained secretions.
- Difficulty in suctioning narrow lumens.
- Cuff prolapse or abutment of the distal lumen against the airway wall.
- Mucosal erosion because of cuff pressure.

PEDIATRIC CONSIDERATIONS

Children are ventilated somewhat similarly to adults, but ventilation of the neonate differs radically because of the unique neonatal pulmonary physiology. The following physiological differences must be considered by nurses working with the neonate to provide appropriate care:

- Extremely compliant chest wall.
- Proportional decrease in the functional residual capacity.
- Reduced amount of pulmonary surfactant.
- Fewer developed alveoli and pulmonary capillaries.
- Less mature respiratory muscles.

Skill 5-10   Care of the Patient Receiving Independent Lung Volume Ventilation

NURSING INTERVENTIONS

1. Ensure that a large room is chosen for the patient, set up with extra electrical, suction, oxygen, and air outlets.
2. Position patient on side of healthy lung or as ordered. This helps blood to flow to the lung with better ventilation, improving the ventilation-perfusion ratio. It also allows for better inflation of the elevated, unhealthy lung.
3. Assess patient regularly for secure and proper tube placement. Auscultate for good bilateral air entry. Observe for adequate bilateral chest expansion. Check for a satisfactory airway pressure on the ventilator.
4. Monitor the cuff pressures regularly.
5. Constantly assess the amount and consistency of bronchial secretions.
6. Check the humidifier for proper functioning and provision of adequate airway humidification.
7. Suction when necessary. Suction through a PEEP valve if patient is on PEEP.
8. Maintain an adequate supply of narrow lumen suction catheters. A size 10 or 12 Fr suction catheter will be needed, depending on the size of the tube.[7]
9. Install a separate suction container and resuscitation bag for each lung to prevent cross-contamination.[7]
10. When providing manual inflation breaths before and after suctioning, carefully deliver a smaller tidal volume than when manually inflating two lungs. Excessive volumes can cause barotrauma and pneumothorax.
11. If the patient has been receiving PEEP, use a manual resuscitation bag with a PEEP valve.
12. Assess need for use of patient restraints or sedation, especially if the ventilators are not synchronized.

- Higher resistance to movement of air in the lungs secondary to smaller airway diameters.
- Increased oxygen use in the maintenance of body temperature.

The major indications for mechanical ventilation of neonates and pediatric patients are listed in the boxes on this page. Physical complications of mechanical ventilation are different in the neonate as compared to the adult patient (see box on bottom right). Retinopathy of prematurity or retrolental fibroplasia is caused by hyperoxygenation. Bronchopulmonary dysplasia is a consequence of lung injury and oxygen toxicity from positive-pressure ventilation.

Assessment of Respiratory Distress in the Infant

The most important and reliable tool for assessing the severity of respiratory impairment in the infant is ABG analysis. The following are key signs and symptoms of respiratory distress in the infant who is not yet on a mechanical ventilator:[16,22,36]

- Central cyanosis—may be absent in neonate with anemia or hyperbilirubinemia.
- Pallor.
- Decreased or absent inspiratory breath sounds.
- Tachypnea—respiratory rate greater than 60 breaths/min.
- Nasal flaring.
- Expiratory grunting—increases airway pressure during expiration, preventing airway closure and alveolar collapse.
- Stridor and prolonged inspiratory time if upper airway obstruction is present (such as subglottic stenosis).
- Prolonged expiratory time with wheezing if lower (or peripheral) airway obstruction is present.
- Retractions.

▼
Major Indications for Mechanical Ventilation of Pediatric Patients

RESPIRATORY FAILURE

$Pa_{CO_2} > 50\text{-}60$ mm Hg
$Pa_{O_2} < 70$ mm Hg

NEUROMUSCULAR DISORDERS

Muscular dystrophies
Guillain-Barré syndrome
Myasthenia gravis

INTRINSIC PULMONARY DISEASE

Viral pneumonia
Bacterial pneumonia
Aspiration pneumonia
Asthma
Cystic fibrosis

RESUSCITATION

Circulatory collapse
Postoperative cardiac surgery

INCREASED INTRACRANIAL PRESSURE

Direct trauma
Near drowning
Infection

From Betit P, Thompson JE: Mechanical ventilation. In Koff PB, Eitzman DV, Neu, J, editors: *Neonatal and pediatric respiratory care*, St Louis, 1988, Mosby–Year Book.

▼
Major Indications for Mechanical Ventilation of Neonates

RESPIRATORY FAILURE

$Pa_{CO_2} > 55$ mm Hg
$Pa_{O_2} < 50$ mm Hg

NEUROLOGICAL COMPROMISE

Apnea of prematurity
Intracranial hemorrhage
Drug depression

IMPAIRED PULMONARY FUNCTION

Respiratory distress syndrome
Meconium aspiration
Pneumonia

PROPHYLACTIC USE

Persistent pulmonary hypertension

From Betit P, Thompson JE: Mechanical ventilation. In Koff PB, Eitzman DV, Neu J, editors: *Neonatal and pediatric respiratory care*, St Louis, 1988, Mosby–Year Book.

▼
Neonatal Complications of Assisted Ventilation[24]

Extraneous air syndrome (airleaks)
Pulmonary interstitial emphysema
Subcutaneous emphysema
Perivascular emphysema
Retroperitoneal emphysema
Pseudocysts
Pneumothorax
Pneumopericardium
Pneumomediastinum
Pneumoperitoneum
Pneumoscrotum
Pneumatosis intestinalis
Air embolus
Retinopathy of prematurity
Bronchopulmonary dysplasia
Gastrointestinal complications
Central nervous system hemorrhage
Sepsis
Decrease in cardiac output

▼ **Danger Signs of Deterioration During Assisted-Ventilation of the Neonate**

RESPIRATORY

Color change: cyanotic, grey, mottled, pallid, or ruddy
Apnea associated with color change or bradycardia
Arterial: $Pao_2 < 50$, $Paco_2 > 60$
Capillary: $Po_2 < 40$, $Pco_2 > 60$
Diminished breath sounds
Sustained respiratory rate > 60 or < 25 breaths/min
Increased crackles and rhonchi
Pulmonary hemorrhage

CARDIOVASCULAR

pH < 7.25 or > 7.50
Systolic blood pressure < 40 or > 100
Pulse pressure > 30
Heart rate < 80 (bradycardia)
Heart murmur
Shift of point of maximum impulse
Diminished heart sounds
Loss of beat-to-beat variability
Hematocrit > 65 or < 40 (peripheral hematocrit can be 5 to 25% higher than central hematocrit)
Sudden drop in hematocrit
Failure to clot after punctures

NEUROLOGICAL

Full, tense fontanelle
Activity—seizures, jitteriness, flaccidity, hypertonia, or opisthotonos posturing

EXCRETORY

Urine output < 1 to 2 ml/kg/hour
Glycosuria $> 2+$
Proteinuria $> 2+$
Specific gravity < 1.004 or > 1.012
Projectile vomiting
Large residuals
Abdominal distention
Prominent bowel outline
Discoloration of abdomen
Occult blood in stools

MISCELLANEOUS

Excessive weight gain ($> 10\%$ of body weight/day)
Excessive total blood loss ($> 10\%$ of estimated blood volume)
Blood glucose < 40 mg % or > 150 mg %

From Katz K et al: Nursing care. In Goldsmith JP, Karotkin EH, editors: *Assisted ventilation of the neonate*, Philadelphia, 1988, WB Saunders.

• Paradoxical breathing—inward movement of chest wall on inspiration ranging to severe sign of "see-saw" motion whereby chest caves inward while abdomen moves outward.
• Hypotonia—decreased muscle tone.
• Acidemia—pH < 7.25.
• Hypercapnia—rising $Paco_2$.
• Hypoxemia—decreased Pao_2.
• Tachycardia—heart rate > 180 beats/min.

▼ **Neonatal Signs and Symptoms of Pneumothorax**

Small QRS complex
Bradycardia
Decreased breath sounds
Decreased heart sounds
Apnea
Cyanosis
Shifted point of maximum impulse
Hypotension
Sudden abdominal distention

From Katz K et al: Nursing Care. In Goldsmith JP, Karotkin EH, editors: *Assisted ventilation of the neonate*, Philadelphia, 1988, WB Saunders.

• Bradycardia—heart rate < 80 beats/min.

Problems may include a malpositioned ET tube, a malfunctioning ventilator, sepsis, a pneumothorax, central nervous system hemorrhage, and gastrointestinal complications. The critical care nurse should be able to recognize the danger signs of deterioration during assisted ventilation and the signs and symptoms of a pneumothorax (see the boxes on this page).

Ventilator Modes and Settings

Infants up to 10 kg (22 lbs) are predominantly ventilated using time-cycled, pressure-limited, continuous-flow IMV. In pressure-cycled ventilation a preset pressure is delivered, but the tidal volume may vary. This prevents high inflating pressures, decreasing the risk of barotrauma. If lung compliance is decreased or airway resistance is increased, less tidal volume will be delivered. Time cycling allows the ventilator to cycle from inspiration to expiration after a predetermined time has elapsed. This allows ease in changing the inspiratory time and I:E ratio. The following are general recommendations for initial neonatal ventilator settings:

• *Rate of breathing*—slow rate ventilation (20 to 40 breaths/min); rapid rate ventilation (60 to 80 breaths/min); rates above 80 breaths/min may be required to ventilate infants with pulmonary hypertension to decrease pulmonary artery pressure[11]; hyperventilation (100 to 150 breaths/min) used to lower the $Paco_2$; and high frequency ventilation (300 to 1800 breaths/min) used in bronchopleural fistulae, pulmonary barotrauma, and major airway disruption following surgery.
• *Inspiratory time*—0.3 to 0.5 seconds[36]; for small airway obstruction with hyperinflation (as in meconium aspiration), inspiratory time can be shortened to less than 0.3 seconds.
• *I:E ratio*—normally 1:2; inverse ratio of 2:1 or 3:1 has been used in early respiratory distress syndrome (RDS) without asphyxia.
• *PIP*—infants with normal lungs (12 to 18 cm H_2O); those with RDS (20 to 25 cm H_2O)[5]; and then adjusted so that the lowest possible PIP will still obtain satisfactory ventilation and oxygenation; an elevated

PIP increases the risk of barotrauma, causing air leaks, bronchopulmonary dysplasia, and impaired cardiac function.

- *Flow rate*—6 to 8 L/min.
- *Inspired oxygen concentration*—kept as low as tolerated to prevent risk of retinopathies, pulmonary oxygen toxicity, and bronchopulmonary dysplasia; an Fio_2 less than 60% is a safe level, contributing little to oxygen toxicity.
- *PEEP*—2 to 3 cm H_2O for infants with normal lungs; 4 to 5 cm H_2O for infants with RDS;[5] the use of high PEEP (> 5 to 6 cm H_2O) may decrease lung compliance; PEEP of 8 to 10 cm H_2O is used for markedly decreased lung compliance or lung volume but has many side effects.
- *Mean airway pressure (MAP)*—the mean pressure applied to the neonatal pulmonary system during a ventilatory cycle; incidence of barotrauma increases significantly with MAP greater than 12 cm H_2O;[2] in neonates with RDS, increases in MAP result in increases in oxygenation.
- *Waveform*—sine wave configuration most closely approximates the form of spontaneous breathing; square waveforms improve oxygenation when used with low rates and inverse I:E ratios. The longer time at peak pressure may improve distribution of ventilation.[11]

Larger children are supported with true volume-cycled ventilation, with or without IMV. Suggested initial ventilator settings for older children are listed in Table 5-6. Ventilatory parameters are set and adjusted according to individual needs and responses. Responses to check include breath sounds, adequacy of chest excursion, color, and perfusion status. Other assessment tools include ABG analysis, end tidal CO_2 monitoring, pulse oximetry, and transcutaneous O_2 and CO_2 monitoring (see Chapters 4 and 8).

New highly specialized ventilatory support modes used with children include high-frequency ventilation (HFV) and extra-corporeal membrane oxygenation (ECMO). HFV is used mainly in infants with pulmonary interstitial emphysema and other pulmonary air leak syndromes (see Table 5-2). In ECMO, venous blood is removed from the body and oxygenation and CO_2 removal occur during bypass through a membrane oxygenator before being returned to the body. The child's ventilatory support can then be decreased to less toxic settings and the lungs can rest while healing takes place. ECMO has been used for neonates in a variety of diseases, such as RDS, meconium aspiration syndrome, and congenital diaphragmatic hernia with coexistent pulmonary hypoplasia, sepsis, and primary persistent pulmonary hypertension of the neonate.[42] The most common pediatric application of ECMO has been for patients in severe cardiac failure, secondary to congenital or acquired problems. Pediatric respiratory diseases treated with ECMO include pneumonia, near drowning, trauma, pulmonary embolus, and pulmonary hemorrhage.[29]

PSYCHOSOCIAL CONSIDERATIONS

Being on a ventilator creates many adverse physical, psychological, and social experiences for patients in critical care units, on step-down units, and in the home. Patients' perceptions of these stressors and the nursing interventions helpful for improving the experience of mechanical ventilation are listed as follows:

Intubation

The act of being intubated is uncomfortable. Extubated patients have a fear of having to be reintubated and suffering through the discomfort again.

- Ensure that patient is not extubated or does not extubate prematurely.

Fear of Machine Failure and Human Error.[6]

- Inform patients that they will be constantly monitored. Briefly discuss purpose of alarms, other safety features, and backup systems.
- Exhibit a considerate, caring, and unhurried attitude.
- Establish a trusting relationship. Inform patient of procedures, provide explanations, and repeat information many times, checking for understanding.
- Provide for continuity of care by assigning the patient a primary nursing team.

Inability to Talk

One of the main outlets for stress is to be able to vocalize one's feelings and verify perceptions. Ventilator patients experience feelings of fear, anger, and frustration

Table 5-6 Suggested Ventilator Variables* for Initiation of Mechanical Ventilation

| Developmental Stage | Respiratory rate (breaths/min) | Tidal volume† (cc/kg) | Peak inspiratory pressure† | | I:E ratio |
			Normal lungs (cmH$_2$O)	Diseased lungs (cm H$_2$O)	
Newborn	30-40	10-20	15-20	20-30+	1:2 (1.5:1 or 1:1 may be
Infant	20-30	10-20	15-30	30-40+	needed if interstitial lung
Child	18-25	10-20	20-30	30-40+	disease is present)
Older child	12-22	10-15	25-35	30-40+	

*These variables should always be modified according to the patient's clinical condition. Once mechanical ventilation is begun, the nurse should continuously monitor the child's response to the ventilatory support.
†These variables should be adjusted after consideration of the resistance (or compliance) within the ventilator circuit (including tubing).
From Zander J, Hazinski MF: Pulmonary disorders. In Hazinski MF, editor: *Nursing care of the critically ill child*, ed 2, St Louis, 1992, Mosby–Year Book.

when attempts to communicate are not understood.[1]

- Prepare the patient adequately through preoperative instruction where possible.
- Maintain eye contact with the patient when possible. Anticipate needs and questions. Provide ample information and explanations, even if the patient does not seem to be alert and oriented.
- Provide patient with flash cards, language booklets, alphabet cards, alphabet boards, poster board, pen and paper, or magic slate for communication. Be aware that it is tiring for some patients to write.
- Have patient use hand gesturing and touch. Read the patient's lips if possible.
- Investigate the possibility of providing patient with an electronic or other talking device.

Suctioning

Shortness of breath and suction-induced coughing experienced during suctioning is reportedly very distressing. Patients also have difficulty readapting to the breathing pattern of the ventilator after suctioning, possibly because of an oxygen debt.[1]

- Hyperinflate the patient with 100% oxygen before and after each suction catheter pass, limiting the aspiration time to 10 seconds.
- Limit the suction catheter passes to three at a time or less.
- Assess the patient's breath sounds and suction only when necessary rather than at routine intervals.

Lack of Synchronization with Ventilator

The patient's breathing may be asynchronous with the mandatory timed breaths.[21]

- Ensure that the patient is not hypoxic.
- Help the patient to relax and breathe synchronous with the machine.
- Investigate the need to switch to a better-tolerated mode of ventilation.
- Evaluate the need for a neuromuscular blocking agent, administered with a tranquilizer or barbiturates.

Pain

ET tubes can cause a great deal of pain and discomfort; whereas tracheostomies are much more comfortable.[21] Other painful stimuli are tugging of ventilator tubing and ABG punctures.

- Anchor the ET tube securely.
- Draw ABG with as small a needle as possible. Assess the need for an arterial line for frequent ABGs.
- Use pulse oximetry if possible.

Dry Mouth and Throat

Intubated patients describe a feeling of thirst, dryness, and discomfort.[21]

- Provide good oral hygiene with toothbrush, toothpaste, water, mouthwash, and oral suction. This also prevents the aspiration of bacteria from the oral cavity.

- Provide ice chips if allowed.
- Keep area free of encrustations and lubricate lips with a petroleum jelly.

Noise

Ventilator patients are bothered by the noises of water in the circuit tubing, ventilator noise, alarms, noise from other patients, and loud talking by staff.[21]

- Establish alarm settings at appropriate levels, reset them promptly, and turn them off before changing ventilator circuits.
- Clear condensation from circuit tubing frequently.
- Calm and orient confused patients.

Inability to Sleep

Sleep disturbance can result in severe psychological impairment and complications.[21]

- Dim lights during nighttime hours. Bright lights make distinguishing between night and day a problem, contributing to the inability to keep track of time.
- Perform only essential procedures when patient should be sleeping. Coordinate rest periods with other staff members.
- Provide calendar and clock so that the patient can adapt to a routine sleep-wake schedule.
- Provide therapeutic touch, music, and other relaxation techniques to help patient relax and fall asleep.

Immobility

Ventilator patients may develop lower back pain if left in a supine position. The restriction of movement, wrist restraints, and the feeling of being "tied to a tube" is uncomfortable.[14]

- Provide for range of motion exercises.
- Release wrist restraints during periods of time when staff member is by bedside, observing patient.
- Provide position changes every 1 to 2 hours. Occasional complete 90 degree turns to the right or left lateral decubitus position will promote optimal lung drainage and improve ventilation-perfusion ratios.
- Assist patient out of bed to chair when stable. As patient becomes increasingly stable, assist to ambulate in ICU hallway, using manual resuscitator bag.

Social Isolation

Some ICU patients who have been on a ventilator for a prolonged time period express the need to see their family members more often. Others feel too ill or fatigued to have visitors. Those in the home find that they are more socially isolated unless they are able to obtain a portable unit that they can place on a wheelchair.

- Provide patient with access to a television and radio.
- Consider extending ICU visiting hours for long-term ventilator patients who desire more social interaction.
- Incorporate family into selected aspects of the physical care.
- Encourage patients in the home to make excursions

outside the home, accompanied by willing family members or friends.

Fear of Dying

Those on a ventilator for a prolonged period of time develop a feeling of doubtful recovery. They also feel that they will never be able to resume their normal activities. Patients who fail to be weaned off of the ventilator experience feelings of great despair, fearing an eternal ventilator dependence and the threat of imminent death.[1]

* Provide positive support and information. Keep the patient informed of progress.
* Discuss the options of returning home on assisted ventilation with a portable ventilator.

Weaning

During the weaning process many patients are afraid of being incapable of resuming spontaneous breathing.[1] Anxiety may precipitate shortness of breath, thus increasing the work of breathing and setting up a vicious cycle.

* Inform patient of improvement and documented readiness for weaning. Continue frequent positive feedback by all staff members for all patient and family improvements and progression.
* Warn that patient may experience dyspnea during the weaning.
* Ensure that call light is within reach of patient.
* Assure patient of being closely monitored.
* During initial weaning periods, remain at the patient's bedside and provide coaching, support, and encouragement.
* Provide consistency of care in all areas (i.e., nursing, medical, respiratory therapist, family, and others).
* Keep patient informed of progress.
* Investigate the need for a better-tolerated method of weaning, such as the pressure support mode.

HOME HEALTH CARE CONSIDERATIONS

Because of the shift in home health care in the 1980s, there has been a renewed interest and growth in home health care for ventilator-assisted patients. This growth was fueled by (1) cost restraints imposed on acute care hospitals, (2) the proliferation of home respiratory equipment companies, (3) the development of small liquid-oxygen systems and suitcase-sized oxygen concentrators, and (4) the arrival of easily operated, portable, compact home ventilators. To qualify for assisted ventilation in the home, a patient's cardiopulmonary status must be relatively stable.

Before the patient is discharged home, the patient and primary caregivers are instructed in each aspect of the patient's care and must be able to perform the procedures that follow. Often the manufacturers of particular home ventilators will provide a hospital training program. The patient or caregiver must also be able to do the following:[34]

* Perform appropriate handwashing technique.
* Clean ventilator circuit.

* Describe flow of air through tubing.
* Describe ventilator dials being used.
* Troubleshoot high and low alarms.
* Operate suctioning equipment.
* Operate manual resuscitator bag.
* Suction airway.
* Perform tracheostomy care, stoma care, and tracheostomy tube change.
* Perform cuff inflation procedure.
* Operate the nebulizer.
* Use a respirometer.
* Use an oxygen analyzer.
* Discuss how to prepare home environment, restricting visitors and smoking.
* Describe what to do if equipment failure occurs.
* Describe the signs of respiratory distress.
* Perform cardiopulmonary resuscitation.

Monitoring the Home Ventilator-Assisted Patient

Maintaining a home ventilator-assisted patient may at first seem overwhelming to the patient, family caregivers, and the home health nurse. It is helpful to establish a reg-

---

Skill 5-11   Cleaning Ventilator Equipment in the Home

▼ ....

Nondisposable ventilator circuits, aerosol tubing, suction catheters, nebulizers, and humidifiers can be reused in the home. They can be cleaned using clean rather than sterile technique. Ventilator circuitry may be changed every 3 days since the risk of infection in the home is less than in hospitals.[24] Suction equipment should be cleaned every day.

EQUIPMENT AND SUPPLIES

* Nonresidue-forming household detergent
* 2% vinegar and distilled water solution (1:3 dilution)
* Quatimine A or similar cleaner
* 70% ethyl alcohol solution
* Ventilator filter

NURSING INTERVENTIONS

1. Wash hands.
2. Change the ventilator circuitry.
3. Disassemble the dirty humidifier and tubing.
4. Wash the parts with a household detergent and warm water.
5. Thoroughly rinse and shake off excess water.
6. Disinfect by soaking for 10 minutes in a double-quaternary ammonium compound, such as Quatimine A, or a vinegar solution.[32]
7. Reuse the double-quaternary solution for 10 to 14 days. Replace the vinegar solution for each cleaning.[24]
8. Rinse the equipment well in water.
9. Shake off excess water and dry in a clean place.
10. Wipe off the exterior surfaces of the ventilator with a 70% ethyl alcohol solution or a commercially prepared broad spectrum germicide.
11. Change the ventilator filter as often as recommended by the manufacturer.

Table 5-7   Troubleshooting the Mechanical Ventilator in the Home[34]

Problem	Cause	Intervention
Green light or *on* light does not glow when ventilator is connected to 110-volt outlet. Green light or *on* light blinks slightly.	AC fuse is blown or circuit breaker is off. Power cord is not properly connected. This occurs when the batteries are fully charged and is a normal operation.	Check fuse or circuit breaker box. Check that power cord is plugged in.
Alarm sounds as soon as the ventilator is turned on.	The low pressure alarm will sound until the first breath that exceeds the low-pressure setting occurs.	
Alarm sounds as soon as the ventilator is turned on and the machine does not operate.	The DC fuse is blown.	Check fuse and replace. On units that have internal circuit breakers, push reset button.
Alarm sounds at peak pressure of each breath and increases as use continues.	Low-voltage alarm begins sounding when battery reaches low charge level.	Connect AC power cord.
Ventilator is operating but orange or red light does not glow.	Indicator lamp is defective.	Replace lamp. If green lamp is defective it will affect operation of red and orange lamps.
Ventilator is connected to external battery without AC power and ventilator operates with red lamp glowing.	Machine is not switching to external battery.	Check DC power cord connections.
External battery is connected without AC power; machine will not operate, red lamp glows brightly, and clicking sound is heard inside ventilator.	External battery is incorrectly connected.	Check wiring instructions.
Ventilator has been on external battery for extended time period. Orange and red lights both blink; there are clicking noises and erratic operation.	External battery is low. Machine is attempting to switch to internal battery.	Connect AC power cord.
Ventilator has been on external battery for extended time period. Unit is connected to AC power; green light blinks brightly, and clicking is heard.	Battery is at very low charge level. Clicking sound is produced by an automatic circuit breaker that opens when charge current is too high. As battery reaches higher charge level, circuit breaker will remain closed.	Recharge battery more often or use a stronger battery.

ular routine and checklist for assessing the patient and equipment for problems and hazards.

Troubleshooting the Home Mechanical Ventilator

Compact, portable, volume-preset positive pressure ventilators have been designed for home health care. These ventilators are easy to operate but have poor long-term performance records, so that a secondary backup ventilator must be on hand for ventilator dependent patients.[39] If the patient lives in an area where electrical power failures are common, a backup electrical generator must be available in the event of power outages. Power companies and local fire departments must be informed that the resident of that particular home is ventilator-assisted.

A home ventilator can be operated continuously on its own internal 12-volt DC battery for 1 to 2 hours or with an external 12-volt DC battery for 2 to 20 hours.[25] The home care patient's household electrical circuitry must be adequate to supply the necessary amperage for peak use periods. The electrical outlets used for medical devices should be placed on 15- to 20-amp-rated circuits with their own circuit breakers. Troubleshooting a home ventilator will be different from that of a hospital ventilator since home units are often connected to external batteries, and patients may occasionally have power failures with batteries or home electricity (Table 5-7).

REFERENCES

1. Bergbom-Engberg I, Haljamae H: Assessment of patients' experience of discomforts during respiratory therapy, *Crit Care Med* 17(10):1068, 1989.
2. Betit P, Thompson JE: *Mechanical ventilation*. In Koff PB, Eitzman DV, Neu J, editors: *Neonatal and pediatric respiratory care*, St Louis, 1988, Mosby–Year Book.
3. Blaufuss JA, Wallace CJ: Two negative pressure ventilators: current clinical application and nursing care, *Crit Care Nurs Q* 9(4):14, 1987.
4. Capps JS: Work of breathing: clinical monitoring and considerations in the critical care setting, *Crit Care Nurs Q* 11(3):1, 1988.
5. Carlo WA, Chatburn RL: *Assisted ventilation of the newborn*. In Carlo WA, Chatburn RL, editors: *Neonatal respiratory care*, St Louis, 1988, Mosby–Year Book.
6. Clark K: Psychosocial aspects of prolonged ventilator dependency, *Respir Care* 31(4):329, 1986.
7. Cooper KL, Burns K, Torsiello P: How do you use a double-lumen endobronchial tube? *Am J Nurs* 89(11):1503, 1989.
8. Dupuis Y: *Ventilators: theory and clinical application*, St. Louis, 1986, Mosby–Year Book.
9. Earl J: Should we support pressure support? *Resp Care* 34(2):125, 1989.
10. East TD: The ventilator of the 1990s, *Resp Care* 35(3):232, 1990.
11. Fox WW, Spitzer AR, Shutack JG: *Positive pressure ventilation: pressure- and time-cycled ventilators*. In Goldsmith JP, Karotkin EH, Barker S: *Assisted ventilation of the neonate*, Philadelphia, 1988, WB Saunders.
12. Geisman LK: Advances in weaning from mechanical ventilation, *Crit Care Nurs Clin NA* 1(4):697, 1989.
13. Geisman LK, Ahrens T: Auto-PEEP: an impediment to weaning in the chronically ventilated patient, *AACN Clin Issues Crit Care Nurs* 2(3):391, 1991.
14. Gries ML, Fernsler J: Patient perceptions of the mechanical ventilation experience, *Focus Crit Care* 15(2):52, 1988.
15. Gurevitch MJ: *Selection of the inspiratory:expiratory ratio*. In Kacmarek RM, Stoller JK, editors: *Current respiratory care*, Philadelphia, 1988, BC Decker.

16. Hazinski MF: Nursing care of the the critically ill child: a seven-point check, *Pediatr Nurs* 11:453, 1985.
17. Hess D: Perspectives on weaning from mechanical ventilation—with a note on extubation, *Respir Care* 32(3):167, 1987.
18. Hess D: The use of PEEP in clinical settings other than acute lung injury, *Respir Care* 33(7):581, 1988.
19. Hubmayr RD, Abel MD, Rehder K: Physiologic approach to mechanical ventilation, *Crit Care Med* 18(1):103, 1990.
20. Hudson LD: *Weaning techniques*. In Kacmarek RM, Stoller JK, editors: *Current respiratory care*, Philadelphia, 1988, BC Decker.
21. Johnson MM, Sexton DL: Distress during mechanical ventilation: patients' perceptions, *Crit Care Nurse* 10(7):48, 1990.
22. Katz K et al: *Nursing care*. In Goldsmith JP, Karotkin EH, Barker S: *Assisted ventilation of the neonate*, Philadelphia, 1988, WB Saunders.
23. Kirby RR: *Modes of mechanical ventilation*. In Kacmarek RM, Stoller JK, editors: *Current respiratory care*, Philadelphia, 1988, BC Decker.
24. Korones SB: *Complications*. In Goldsmith JP, Karotkin EH, Barker S: *Assisted ventilation of the neonate*, Philadelphia, 1988, WB Saunders.
25. Lucas J: *Ventilator care at home*. In Lucas J, Golish JA, Sleeper G et al, editors: *Home respiratory care*, Norwalk, Conn 1988, Appleton & Lange.
26. MacIntyre NR: *Pressure support: inspiratory assist*. In Kacmarek RM, Stoller JK, editors: *Current respiratory care*, Philadelphia, 1988, BC Decker.
27. Martin LM: *Pulmonary physiology in clinical practice. The essentials for patient care and evaluation*, St Louis, 1987, Mosby–Year Book.
28. Maunder RJ, Rice CL, Benson MS et al: Managing positive end-expiratory pressure (PEEP): the Harborview approach, *Respir Care* 31(11):1059, 1986.
29. McDermott BK, Curley MA: Extracorporeal membrane oxygenation: current use and future directions, *AACN Clin Issues Crit Care Nurs* 1(2):348, 1990.
30. McPherson SP, Spearman CB: *Respiratory therapy equipment*, St Louis, 1990, Mosby–Year Book.
31. McVan B et al: *Respiratory care handbook*, Springhouse, Pa, 1989, Springhouse.
32. Nett LM, Morganroth ML, Petty TL: Weaning protocols that work, *Am J Nurs* 87(9):1174, 1987.
33. Ray C: *Independent lung ventilation*. In Kacmarek RM, Stoller JK, editors: *Current respiratory care*, Philadelphia, 1988, BC Decker.
34. Riggs JH: *Respiratory facts*, Philadelphia, 1989, FA Davis.
35. Scanlan CL: *Selection and application of ventilatory support devices*. In Spearman CB et al, editors: *Eagan's fundamentals of respiratory care*, St. Louis, 1990, Mosby–Year Book.
36. Schussler NC, Scanlan CL: *Neonatal and pediatric intensive care*. In Spearman CB et al, editors: *Eagan's fundamentals of respiratory care*, St. Louis, 1990, Mosby–Year Book.
37. Deleted in proofs.
38. Swearingen PL, Sommers MS, Miller K: *Manual of critical care*, St Louis, 1988, Mosby–Year Book.
39. Thompson JE, O'Rourke PP: *Choosing a home care mechanical ventilator*. In Kacmarek RM, Stoller JK, editors: *Current respiratory care*, Philadelphia, 1988, BC Decker.
40. Toben BP, Lewandowski V: Nontraditional and new ventilatory techniques, *Crit Care Nurs Q* 11(3):12, 1988.
41. Weilitz PB: New modes of mechanical ventilation, *Crit Care Nurs Clin NA* 1(4):689, 1989.
42. White C, Richardson C, Raibstein L: High-frequency ventilation and extracorporeal membrane oxygenation, *AACN Clin Issues Crit Care Nurs* 1(2):427, 1990.
43. White GC: *Basic clinical lab competencies for respiratory care*, Albany, NY, 1988, Delmar Publishers.
44. Williams-Colon S, Thalken FR: *Management and monitoring of the patient in respiratory failure*. In Spearman CB et al, editors: *Eagan's fundamentals of respiratory care*, St Louis, 1990, Mosby–Year Book.

CHAPTER 6

ECG Interpretation

Objectives

After completing this chapter, the reader will be able to:

- Identify the parts of the conduction system of the heart and describe how the electrical impulse travels through the conduction network.
- Identify the five areas to auscultate heart sounds and describe how to assess heart sounds.
- Describe the elements of the normal ECG.
- Discuss cardiac monitoring.
- Describe how to perform a 12-lead ECG.
- Identify the major features of the sinus, atrial, junctional, and ventricular dysrhythmias.
- Describe and compare the three types of heart block: first, second, and third.
- Describe the effects of electrolytes and drugs on the ECG.
- Identify the changes produced on the ECG by a myocardial infarction.
- Contrast assessment findings of adults to findings of children.

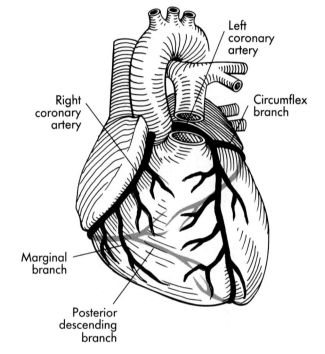

Fig. 6-1   Coronary arteries. (From Phipps WJ, Long BC, Woods NF, et al: *Medical-surgical nursing: concepts and clinical practice,* ed 4, St Louis, 1991, Mosby–Year Book.)

Cardiovascular diseases are the number one cause of mortality in Western society. The functional ability of the cardiovascular system is reflected in all other body systems. If the heart does not pump effectively, the function of the respiratory system, kidneys, and brain and the body fluid balance may quickly become impaired. Knowledge of the cardiovascular system and coronary arteries (Fig. 6-1) is very important to the nurse.

NORMAL HEART SOUNDS

Heart sounds arise from the acceleration and deceleration of blood in the cardiac chambers and from the closing of the heart valves. The first sounds to be identified are S_1 and S_2. Beginning at the aortic and pulmonic area, the loud, high-pitched S_2 sound is produced by the closing of the semilunar valves. The aortic and pulmonic valves do not close at the same time because of the difference in the

length of ventricular systole between the right and left ventricles. The right ventricle has a longer period of systole than the left ventricle. The aortic valve closure sound is more intense during inspiration because the decrease in intrathoracic pressure increases venous return to the right side of the heart and causes even more of a delay in right ventricular ejection and pulmonic valve closure. This phenomenon is referred to as *physiological splitting* (Fig. 6-2) and is best heard over the pulmonic area with the patient in the supine or sitting position, using the diaphragm of the stethoscope.

Reverse (paradoxical) splitting of S_2 occurs when left ventricular systole is delayed, resulting in pulmonic valve closure before aortic valve closure. Left bundle branch block, patent ductus arteriosus, aortic stenosis, uncontrolled hypertension, severe left ventricular disease, or

HEART SOUNDS   AREA HEARD BEST

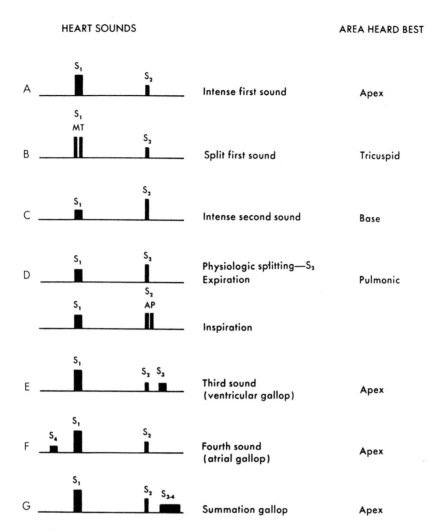

Fig. 6-2 The intensity and splitting of the first and second heart sounds, their relationships to the third and fourth heart sounds, and the auscultatory areas where these sounds are heard best. (From Andreoli KG, Zipes DP, Wallace AG, et al: *Comprehensive cardiac care,* ed 6, St Louis, 1987, Mosby–Year Book.)

atrial septal defects may be the cause of a reverse split in S_2.

Once the S_2 has been identified, the stethoscope is gradually moved towards the apex or mitral area of the heart. It is at the apex that the S_1 sound is the loudest. The S_1 sound is a result of the mitral and tricuspid valves closing. The occurrence of the S_1 can be correlated with the QRS complex on the ECG. It also occurs just before the carotid impulse and is approximately synchronous with the onset of the apical impulse. The S_1 sound can split the same as S_2, but it is not easily heard in the normal adult. It may be audible in children. It is referred to as splitting of the first heart sound. If the splitting of S_1 becomes more apparent, it can be a result of pulmonary hypertension (see Fig. 6-2).[1,3]

A third heart sound can be heard in children, adolescents and young adults, and is a normal finding under these circumstances. It is called a *physiological third heart sound.* It occurs during rapid ventricular filling following closure of the semilunar valves and opening of the AV valves. The third heart sound or S_3 is best heard with the

bell at the apex of the heart with the person supine or in a left semilateral lying position. S_3 is heard just after S_2.[1]

A low-pitched, fourth physiological heart sound may occur in normal adults over 50 years of age. The S_4 sound is heard just before S_1 and is a result of the atrial contraction adding to the ventricular filling. The S_4 sound may also be found in infants and children. The S_4 sound is often heard in patients with heart disease and hypertension. This sound is best heard at the point of maximum impulse (PMI) or slightly medial to the PMI with the bell of the stethoscope with the person in a supine or left semilateral position.[1]

ABNORMAL HEART SOUNDS

There are a number of abnormal heart sounds that can be auscultated. These include changes in the normal S_1 and S_2 sounds, as well as abnormal occurrences of the S_3 and S_4 heart sounds.

S_1, which occurs at the closure of the mitral and aortic valves, will change with any disease that affects these valves. Mitral or tricuspid stenosis can cause an increase in intensity of the S_1 sound. The S_1 sound will lose intensity if regurgitation in either of these valves occurs because of a decrease in velocity of the valve closing. In situations where ventricular systole occurs earlier in the cycle and the ventricles contract before the valves have had time to close, the intensity of S_1 will increase. If there is a lengthening of the time before ventricle systole occurs causing the mitral and tricuspid valves to be almost completely closed, then the S_1 sound will have less intensity. This can be seen by a shortening of the P-R interval in the first instance and a lengthening of the P-R interval in the second.

In situations where the force and velocity of ventricular contraction increases, this will increase the S_1 sound. This occurs in heart disease that produces a left-to-right shunt or with fever, hyperthyroidism, anemia, and tachycardia, which increases blood flow. Anything that would reduce the force and velocity of contraction of the ventricle, or reduce ventricular contractility, will produce a decrease in intensity of S_1. This will occur with myocardial infarction (MI), myocarditis, cardiac myopathy, and congestive heart failure. Dysrhythmias that produce a change in the P-R interval, such as first and second degree heart block, can produce a change in intensity of the S_1 sound. Also, with rhythms, such as atrial fibrillation and ventricular tachycardia, where the force and velocity of contractions change, the intensity of the S_1 and S_2 heart sounds will vary.

S_2 can change intensity and develop abnormal splitting. Changes in the arterial or pulmonary circulation can cause an increase in intensity that is associated with hypertensive states. The increase in the arterial system will increase the intensity of the aortic component of the S_2 sound. Increases in the pulmonary system will increase the pulmonic component of S_2. Situations that can cause an increase in the pulmonary arterial system include atrial or ventricular septal defects, patent ductus arteriosus, pulmonary emboli, mitral stenosis, or right ventricular failure. A decrease in intensity of S_2 is found with disease of both the aortic and pulmonic valves, such as stenosis.

Abnormal splitting of the S_2 sound will occur with situations that accentuate the difference in the closing of the pulmonic and aortic valves. This can occur when right ventricular ejection is prolonged due to delayed closure of the pulmonic valve, such as with pulmonic stenosis or with bundle branch block.

Widening of the S_2 split can occur with congestive heart failure, ventricular septal defect, and pulmonary hypertension because of early closure of the aortic valve and a delayed closing of the pulmonic valve.

Paradoxical splitting of S_2 occurs when there is a prolonging of left ventricular systole. Conditions, such as left bundle branch block and overload of the left ventricle, are associated with paradoxical splitting. In these situations, respirations will affect the splitting with the sounds becoming more noticeable during expiration and less noticeable during inspiration.

The S_3 sound is called a gallop rhythm because its rhythm resembles that of a galloping horse. Both the abnormal S_3 and S_4 sounds occur during diastole. If the sound is heard after S_2, it is called an S_3 or *ventricular gallop* (S_{3g}). When the sound occurs immediately before S_1, it is termed an S_4 gallop (S_{4g}).

The S_{3g}, when heard, resembles the word "Kentucky" (Ken-tuck-y) and is best heard with the bell of the stethoscope. It is a dull, low-pitched sound. It is frequently heard in normal children and young adults, disappearing by ages 25 to 30 years. It is also heard in older individuals and often is associated with myocardial failure or incompetence of the mitral or tricuspid valve. An S_{3g}, unlike the S_3, will not disappear when the person stands and will increase in intensity when the person assumes a left lateral position or exercises.

The S_{4g} or *atrial gallop* resembles the word "Tennessee" (Ten-nes-see). The S_{4g} is a low-pitched sound best heard with the bell of the stethoscope. It is usually heard over the apex or just medial to the apex but can also be heard at the base of the heart. Situations that increase resistance to ventricular filling will produce an S_{4g} sound. These include hypertensive cardiovascular disease, coronary artery disease, myocardiopathy, or aortic stenosis. The sound can be intensified with forced inspiration or following exercise. It will disappear if the patient performs the Valsalva maneuver, is sitting, or is using rotating tourniquets.

Quadruple rhythms are those that follow the cadence of the S_1 and S_2 plus S_3 and S_4. When the heart rate is not abnormally fast, all four sounds can be heard.

A *summation gallop* is a triple gallop produced by a delayed AV conduction time or by the presence of tachycardia. In this rhythm, S_3 and S_4 fuse to form a single sound during mid-diastole.

Heart murmurs are vibratory sounds of increased duration resulting from turbulent blood flow through the heart valves. Heart murmurs are categorized according to their timing within the cardiac cycle (i.e., systolic or diastolic).

Systolic murmurs are the most common type of murmur. They are generally ejection (crescendo-decrescendo) murmurs or regurgitant (pansystolic) murmurs. Ejection murmurs follow S_1, increasing and then decreasing in intensity. They terminate before S_2. *Regurgitant murmurs* are loud, long, and are heard in the mitral or tricuspid areas. *Functional or innocent murmurs* are frequently heard in

▼ ....

Rating Scale for Heart Murmurs

GRADE	DESCRIPTION
1	Very soft, almost inaudible.
2	Soft but can be heard easily.
3	Moderately loud, but unaccompanied by thrill.
4	Loud and thrill is present.
5	Very loud, thrill present.
6	So loud that it can be heard with the stethoscope slightly off of the chest, thrill present.

young people and need to be differentiated from those murmurs that indicate heart disease. Functional murmurs are short ejection murmurs. They may become inaudible when the patient rises from a supine to a sitting position. Functional murmurs are heard best in the aortic and pulmonary areas.

Diastolic murmurs can be classified into two types: high-pitched decrescendo murmurs of aortic and pulmonic regurgitation and low-pitched murmurs of mitral and tricuspid stenosis.

Murmurs are usually characterized by timing in the cardiac cycle, intensity, quality, pitch, location, and radiation (see the box on p. 102).

Other heart sounds can be heard, including snaps, clicks, and rubs.

ASSESSMENT

Cardiac assessment is important for all patients and crucial for those patients experiencing cardiac symptoms or with a history of cardiovascular disease. The assessment of the cardiovascular system should be performed quickly while evaluating the patient's general condition. If the patient is severely compromised, life-threatening situations must be corrected before proceeding with the assessment. The techniques of assessment of the cardiovascular system are inspection, palpation, percussion, and auscultation.

▼ **Pain Assessment**

Onset	When was pain first noticed?
Manner of onset	Was the pain sudden or gradual?
Duration	How long did (does) the pain last?
Location	Where did (does) the pain originate? Does it radiate? If so, where?
Quality	What does the pain feel like? (Allow the patient to describe in own words.)
Intensity	How severe or intense is the pain? (On a scale of 1 to 10, 1 being almost no pain and 10 being severe pain, where would you place your pain?) Has pain interfered with activities?
Chronology	Has this pain occurred before? If so, how often?
Associated symptoms	Are there any other signs or symptoms that occur at the same time, before, or after the pain episode?
Precipitating factors	What causes the pain to start (e.g., anxiety, emotions, exercise)?
Aggregating symptoms	What makes the pain worse?
Relieving factors	What makes the pain ease or go away?

Skill 6-1   Conducting the Cardiac Assessment

EQUIPMENT AND SUPPLIES

- Stethoscope with bell and diaphragm
- Sphygmomanometer and cuff
- Adequate lighting
- Pen light
- Watch with second hand

NURSING INTERVENTIONS

1. See Chapter 8 for additional cardiac assessment.
2. Conduct a patient interview.
   a. Chief complaint
      - Determine the chief cardiac complaint.
      - Ask how long the problem existed, how it started, and what are the precipitating factors.
      - Determine the symptoms: location, radiation, intensity, duration, associated symptoms, aggravating, and alleviating factors.
      - List treatments and medications.
   b. Pain history
      Chest pain or discomfort is one of the cardinal symptoms of cardiac disorders. It is essential to make a careful assessment of chest pain (see the boxes on Pain Assessment [above] and Characteristics of Angina Pectoris [p. 104]).
   c. Personal health history
      - General health and past illnesses.
      - Weight.
      - Determine previous cardiac problems, including heart enlargement, congestive heart failure, congenital heart disease, rheumatic fever, coronary artery disease, MI, murmurs, hypertension, intermittent claudication, elevated cholesterol, and triglycerides. Obtain chronology.

   - Determine previous cardiac surgeries or invasive diagnostic procedures, such as cardiac catheterization.
   - Determine previous thrombolytic therapy.
   d. Family history
      - Determine family history of heart disease, high blood pressure, coronary artery disease, stroke, kidney disease, and diabetes.
   e. Social history
      - Determine what medications the patient is taking, including over-the-counter drugs.
      - Determine alcohol intake, recreational drug use, and smoking.
      - Ask patient to describe his or her personality type, for example, striving, rushing, achieving or relaxed, calm, resting.
      - Determine activity level.
      - Determine type of diet (e.g., high in fats and carbohydrates).
      - Inquire about educational background, occupation, family support system, daily routine, and recreational activities.
3. Observe the patient's general affect. Determine if the patient is calm, anxious, energetic, tired, or in acute distress.
4. Inspect the skin. Determine color and temperature. Observe for cyanosis or cold areas. Observe for dry areas, clubbing of fingers (indicating chronic hypoxia from various conditions, such as chronic obstructive pulmonary disease (COPD), right-to-left shunting, thickened nails, edema, loss of hair on skin and extremities, or splinterlike hemorrhages, which might indicate bacterial endocarditis).

Continued.

Skill 6-1   Conducting the Cardiac Assessment—cont'd

Characteristics of Angina Pectoris

LOCATION

Beneath sternum, radiating to neck and jaw
Upper chest
Beneath sternum, radiating down left arm
Epigastric
Epigastric, radiating to neck, jaw, and arms
Neck and jaw
Left shoulder, inner aspect of both arms
Intrascapular

DURATION

30 seconds to 30 minutes

QUALITY

Sensation of pressure or heavy weight on the chest
Feeling of tightness, like a vise
Visceral quality (deep, heavy, squeezing, aching)
Burning sensation
Shortness of breath, with feeling of suffocation
Most severe pain ever experienced

RADIATION

Medial aspect of left arm
Jaw
Left shoulder
Right arm

PRECIPITATING FACTORS

Exertion/exercise
Cold weather
Exercising after a large, heavy meal
Walking against the wind
Emotional upset
Fright, anger
Coitus

NITROGLYCERIN RELIEF

Usually within 45 seconds to 5 minutes of administration

From Thelan LA, Davie JK, Urden LD: *Textbook of critical care nursing: diagnosis and management,* St Louis, 1990, Mosby–Year Book.

5. Inspect the eyes. Yellow lipid lesions are associated with hyperlipidemia. Petechiae may indicate bacterial endocarditis or fat embolus.
6. Adjust lighting to shine on neck area. Inspect the neck bilaterally. Observe the jugular veins for pulse waves and pressure levels. In the normal person in the sitting position, no jugular venous pulsations can be seen. When the person is lying at a 45-degree angle, the jugular pulse does not rise more than 1 to 2 cm above the level of the manubrium. When the person is lying down, the venous pressure is evident. In right-sided heart failure, the neck veins will be distended more than 2 cm above the sternal angle when the patient is reclining at a 45-degree angle.
7. If mild right ventricular failure is present, assess the jugular vein for the hepatojugular reflex. Place the hand over the patient's liver and exert mild pressure for at least 1 minute. Observe the neck veins. An elevation in the jugular pressure during and immediately following liver compression indicates that

the right ventricular pressure is persistently elevated. This indicates an inability of the right ventricle to sufficiently pump an increased venous return.

8. Measure the height of the venous pulsation by measuring the distance that the veins are distended above the manubrium of the sternum (see Chapter 8). NOTE: The patient should be sitting with the thorax elevated to a 45 degree angle from the horizontal to begin this assessment.
9. Observe the jugular vein pulsation using the right internal jugular vein. Jugular vein pulsations are evaluated for contour. The contour of this pulse reflects alterations in pressure related to changes in the cardiac cycle. The normal jugular venous pulse consists of a, v and c waves and two negative slopes, the x and y descents. Normally only the a and v waves are visible (see Chapter 8).
10. Observe the carotid arteries for contour or pulses, unusually large or bounding pulsations.
11. Expose the thoracic area. Cover the abdominal area with the sheet or gown. Cover the breasts of female patients with a drape or towel until inspection is carried out.
12. Begin inspection of the chest by noting its contour. Compare the anterior-posterior diameter to the transverse diameter. The normal ratio is 1:2 and 5:7. An increase in this ratio may indicate COPD. Also, observe for skeletal deformities.
13. Inspect for intercostal retractions or bulging.
14. Place patient in a supine position, if the patient can tolerate this position.
15. Adjust lighting so that subtle movements can be observed and inspect the chest area for pulsations in the following areas:
    • Sternoclavicular area: directly over the upper portion of the sternum where the clavicles join.
    • Aortic area: second intercostal space to the right of the sternum.
    • Pulmonic area: second intercostal space to the left of the sternum.
    • Right ventricular area: lower half of the left sternal border.
    • Apical area: fifth intercostal space along midclavicular line. This is the PMI. It is visible in approximately 50% of normal adults. When visible, it helps to establish cardiac size.
    • Epigastric area: near the xiphoid process. Observe for pulsations, retractions, heaves, or lifts. Pulsations are normal over the apical area; retractions are normal on the chest wall medial to the midclavicular line in the fifth intercostal space; and heaves or lifts are not normal findings and indicate that the work of the right ventricle is increased.
16. Palpate the cardiac area carefully beginning at the apex, moving to the left sternal border, and then to the base of the heart. Use palmar surfaces of the fingers and base of the hand. Palpate for the apical impulse, abnormal heaves, and abnormal retractions. Audible murmurs may result in a palpatory sensation known as *thrill.* It is important to describe pulsations in relation to their timing in the cardiac cycle. Simultaneously, palpate the carotid artery with the left hand, while palpating the heart with the right.
17. Continue to palpate until all of the areas listed in step 14 have been assessed methodically.
18. Palpate the skin for temperature and moisture. Determine warmth of the extremities.
19. Assess for edema or dehydration.
20. Determine if edema is present especially in the feet, ankles, sacrum and abdomen. This may indicate right-sided heart failure or other cardiac diseases. If edema is present, assess severity by pressing a finger or thumb carefully into the area to determine the amount of edema present. See Table 6-1 for pitting edema scale.

Skill 6-1   Conducting the Cardiac Assessment—cont'd

Table 6-1   Edema Scale

Depth	Edema
0-5 mm (0-¼ inch)	+1 pitting
6-9 mm (¼-½ inch)	+2 pitting
10-25 mm (½-1 inch)	+3 pitting
26 mm and greater (1 inch and greater)	+4 pitting

21. Locate the carotid artery by placing the fingers lightly over the patient's trachea, then slide fingers into the trough between the trachea and the sternocleidomastoid muscle. Palpate only the lower half to prevent too much pressure on the carotid sinus. Undue pressure can stimulate carotid sinus baroreceptors, causing a slowing of the heart, dropping blood pressure, and potentially a syncopal episode. Palpate each carotid artery. Palpate only one carotid artery at a time to avoid excessive carotid sinus massage.
22. Palpate each peripheral artery for elasticity of vessel wall, rate and rhythm, strength, equality, and type of pulse:
    - Radial pulse.
    - Brachial pulse.
    - Femoral pulse (place patient in supine position).
    - Popliteal pulse (flex knee or turn patient).
    - Posterior tibial pulse.
    - Dorsalis pedis pulse.
23. Percuss the heart to determine heart size. Percuss the left cardiac border for dullness. Begin at the fifth intercostal space, anterior axillary line. Move the fingers along the intercostal space at about 1-cm intervals, tapping lightly, until the sternal border is reached or dullness is heard. Repeat at the fourth and third intercostal spaces. When the change in the sound is heard, the left sternal border has been reached. In the adult, this will usually be 10 to 12 cm from the midsternal line and always within the midclavicular line.
24. Auscultate the heart using a stethoscope with both a bell and diaphragm. The diaphragm is used for high-pitched sounds while the bell is used for low-pitched sounds. It is important for the nurse to concentrate on one component of the cardiac cycle at a time. Using the bell of the stethoscope, auscultate the carotid arteries for bruits. *Bruits* are produced by turbulent blood flow through narrowed vessels caused by vascular obstructions, such as arteriosclerotic plaques. Normally, no bruits are heard, although at times they are heard in the absence of pathology. Bruits of long duration, especially those that are continuous, may indicate obstructions, fistulas, high-output states, or aortic valve stenosis.
25. If the initial auscultation was performed while the patient was lying in a supine position, move or ask the patient to move onto the left side, then auscultate the apex again using the bell, listening for the presence or absence of low-frequency diastolic sounds, such as filling sounds or a mitral valve murmur.[1,3] Continue auscultating with the diaphragm while the patient is in a sitting position. Auscultate during the normal respiratory cycle and while the patient holds his/her breath.
26. Auscultate the following:
    - Aortic area.
    - Pulmonic area.
    - Third intercostal space left sternal border, Erb's point.
    - Tricuspid area.
    - Mitral (apical) area (Fig. 6-3)

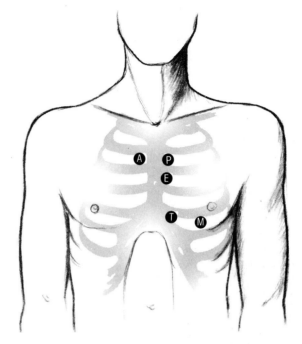

Fig. 6-3   Anatomical locations for auscultation of the cardiac sounds. *A,* Aortic area; *P,* pulmonary area; *E,* Erb's point; *T,* tricuspid area; *M,* Mitral area. (From Guzzetta CE, Dossey BM: *Cardiovascular nursing: holistic practice,* St Louis, ed 2, 1992, Mosby–Year Book.)

27. Listen at each of these areas for the S_1 and S_2 heart sounds.
28. Identify each of the sounds (S_1 and S_2). Auscultate each area with the diaphragm. Repeat the same process with the bell.
29. Repeat the assessment using both the diaphragm and bell with the patient in the left lateral and sitting positions.
30. If an abnormal sound is heard, listen to the surrounding chest surface to determine its distribution and radiation. Describe the following:
    a. *Timing.* When in the cardiac cycle does the sound occur? Systole? Diastole? Both?
    b. *Intensity.* How loud is the sound?
    c. *Location.* Where is the sound heard best? The mitral, tricuspid, aortic, or pulmonary areas?
    d. *Radiation.* Does the sound radiate in a specific direction? For example, mitral murmurs appear to radiate to the axilla or left, whereas ventricular murmurs project to the carotid arteries and the base of the heart.
    e. *Quality.* What is the tonal character of the sound? Harsh? Blowing? Rumbling? Musical? Whooping?
    f. *Configuration.* What is the shape of the sound? Crescendo (increasing), decrescendo (decreasing), crescendo-decrescendo (diamond shaped)?
    g. *Pitch.* What is sound frequency? High? Medium? Low? If it is best heard with the diaphragm, it is high pitched. If best heard with bell, it is low pitched. If it is heard equally with either bell or diaphragm, it is medium pitched.
31. Auscultate the apical pulse while palpating the radial pulse.
32. Monitor serum enzymes, CBC, and electrolyte laboratory studies.
33. Monitor 12-lead ECG (see ECG section); evaluate rhythm strips.

NURSING DIAGNOSIS

Sample nursing diagnoses for the patient who has undergone cardiovascular assessment include the following:

- Decreased cardiac output related to decreased myocardial contractility secondary to cor pulmonale.
- Decreased arterial blood pressure related to hypovolemia secondary to blood loss in cardiac surgery.
- Decreased peripheral tissue perfusion related to decreased afterload secondary to congestive heart failure.
- Disturbance in cardiac conduction related to atrial flutter.
- Alteration in sinus conduction related to sinoatrial exit block.
- Decreased atrial-ventricular conduction related to premature junctional systole.
- High risk for injury related to dysrhythmias secondary to MI.
- High risk ineffective coping related to chest pain secondary to MI.
- Impaired adjustment related to change in role function secondary to MI.
- Anxiety related to impending heart surgery.
- Pain related to myocardial ischemia.
- High risk for infection related to multiple intravenous catheters.
- Knowledge deficit associated with rehabilitation after MI.

PATIENT OUTCOMES

Possible outcomes for patients with cardiovascular alterations include evidence of the following:

- Pulse within normal limits (60 to 100 beats/min.).
- Respirations (12 to 20/minute).
- Bilateral clear and equal breath sounds.
- Temperature 36° to 38° C (97° to 100.5° F).
- Mean blood pressure within normal limits for patient. Blood pressure between 90/60 to 140/90, unless patient is hypertensive.
- Alertness, wakefulness, orientation to time, person, and place.
- Strong palpable pulses in all extremities.
- Capillary refill in less than 3 seconds (immediate); more than 3 seconds (delayed).
- Expresses fears and anxieties.
- Skin intact, warm, dry, of normal sensation, temperature, and turgor.
- Normal ECG:
  —P wave 0.06 to 0.12 second and not over 3 mm.
  —PR interval from 0.12 to 0.20 second.
  —QRS complex between 0.06 to 0.10 second.
  —QT interval of 0.31 to 0.38 second at a heart rate of 72 (depends on pulse rate).
  —T waves not above 5 mm in limb leads and not above 10 mm in precordial leads.
- Provides self-care within limits of prescribed activities.

THE HEART'S CONDUCTION SYSTEM

The conduction system of the heart consists of highly specialized tissue that keeps the heart working uniformly (Fig. 6-4). The electrical activity that causes normal depolarization in the cardiac tissue occurs in the sinoatrial (SA) node located in the upper portion of the right atrium. The SA node dominates the conduction system and usually determines the rate of contraction and the intrinsic heart rhythm. From the SA node, the impulse travels through the atria via internodal tracts to the atrial muscle fibers reaching the AV node. The AV node acts as a relay station to pass the impulse from the atria to the ventricles and serves as a second pacemaker should the SA node falter or stop functioning. It also controls how rapidly the impulse is passed to the ventricles to provide for maximum filling before contraction occurs. From the AV node, the impulse passes through the bundle of His and then to the right and left bundle branches. After the bundle branches, the impulse goes to the Purkinje fibers producing ventricular muscle depolarization.

All of this activity is generated by the movement of sodium ions ($Na+$) and potassium ions ($K+$) across the cell membranes. Fig. 6-5 illustrates the process of electrical activity, or action potential, in a single cell.

Phase 0: Depolarization

Depolarization, or phase 0, occurs when an electrical stimulus causes the resting cell to move towards 0 mV or become less negative. Sodium rushes into the cell through pathways called *fast channels,* changing the polarity of the cell (Fig. 6-6). This sudden movement of $Na+$ into the cell changes the intracellular potential to nearly $+20$ mV.

Phase 1: Rapid Repolarization

Following depolarization, the cell begins to move toward repolarization. After the upstroke of the action potential, there is a brief period of rapid repolarization when the membrane potential returns to 0 mV. This is stimulated by the electrical gradient created across the cell membrane during phase 0. Potassium begins its exodus from the cell and a small amount of chloride enters the cell.

Phase 2: Plateau

During phase 2 of the action potential, or the plateau, calcium enters the cell through the *slow channels* that have remained open after depolarization. Potassium continues to leave the cell. Calcium-mediated mechanical contraction (or systole) occurs.

Phase 3: Repolarization

In phase 3, repolarization accelerates until the resting potential is regained. Potassium rapidly exits from the cell.

Phase 4: Diastole

The resting state is then achieved and is seen in phase 4. At this point, the cell is repolarized and ready for another stimulus and the cycle will begin again. Two im-

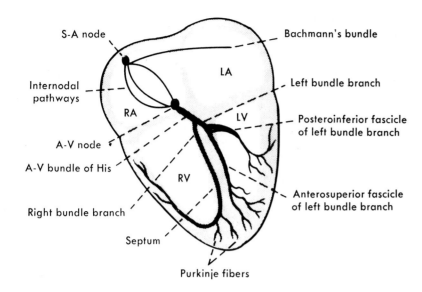

Fig. 6-4 Conduction system of th heart, showing rates of the potential pacemakers. (Adapted from Kinney MR, Packa DR, Andreoli KG, et al: *Comprehensive cardiac care,* ed 7, St Louis, 1991, Mosby–Year Book.

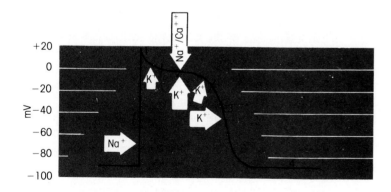

Fig. 6-5 Process of depolarization and repolarization. **A,** Resting (polarized) cell. Impulse is received at **B,** which begins the process of depolarization. Arrow above cell B illustrates direction of current flow. **C,** Totally depolarized cell. **D,** Process of repolarization. **E,** Return to resting (polarized) state. (From The Methodist Hospital: *Basic electrocardiography: a modular approach,* 1986, St Louis, Mosby–Year Book.)

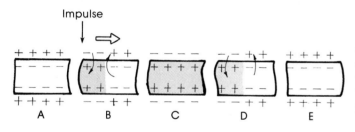

Fig. 6-6 Action potential phases 0 to 4 with arrow indicating the direction of ion flow. (From Guzzetta CE, Dossey BM: *Cardiovascular nursing: holistic practice,* St. Louis, ed 2, 1992, Mosby–Year Book.)

portant events occur in phase 4:

- Restoration of an electronegative chemical state across the cell membrane, as the sodium-potassium pump actively pumps potassium into the cell and sodium out of the cell.
- Initiation of spontaneous diastolic depolarization, or automaticity, the fundamental property of pacemaker cells in the SA node, lower portion of the AV node, bundle of His, and Purkinje's system.

Pacemaker cells have the highest degree of automaticity; they depolarize spontaneously (without an external stimulus). The SA node does this more rapidly than the other pacemaker cells and is the main force for cardiac depolarization. Once the pacemaker cells provide the stimulus, the flow is passed from cell-to-cell along the conduction pathway until the cardiac muscle cells are stimulated to contract. The inherent rate of impulse formation in the SA node is 60 to 100 beats/minute. The AV junction has much the same action potential as the SA node, but its inherent rate is slower (40 to 60 beats/minute). As long as the SA node is functional, it will control the heart rate, because of its action potential. If the SA node is suppressed, then the AV junction takes over but at a slower rate of 40 to 60 beats/minute. The bundle of His and Purkinje fibers can also control depolarization when the higher order pacemaker cells can no longer control heart rate. These cells have the lowest rate and will drive the heart at 20 to 40 beats/minute.[1,2]

The main regulator of this activity is found in three primary electrolytes: sodium, potassium, and calcium. In the beginning of depolarization or phase 0, the Na+ enters the cell rapidly by the fast channels in the cell membrane. Potassium then leaves the cell thus changing the homeostasis of the cell. During the plateau or phase 2 of the potential, a second inward current develops. This second current is primarily controlled by Ca++ and uses the slower channels. As the Na+ level within the cell rises and K+ falls, the normal homeostasis mechanism takes over, removing Na+ from the cell and taking up K+. This continues to occur until the cell has returned to its resting membrane potential. One of the unique features of cardiac cells that separates them from skeletal muscle cells is their action potential. Skeletal muscle cells respond to a repeated stimulus applied to the cells and tetany occurs. The cardiac muscle cells have a protective mechanism that prohibits depolarization from occurring during certain phases of the action potential no matter the strength of the electrical stimulus. During phase 2 and the early portion of phase 3, the cardiac cells are in the absolute refractory period. This protects the heart from being overstimulated and causing tetany. During the later portion of phase 3, the cardiac cells move into what is called the relative refractory period. Here the cells will respond to an electrical stimulus of sufficient strength. The stimulus must be stronger than the normal stimulus that would cause depolarization in the resting phase, or Phase 4. As the resting potential is regained, the cell is no longer refractory and enters what is referred to as the super-normal period during which a mild electrical stimulus can produce another action potential. This is thought to occur because of the availability of fast Na+ channels for depolarization.[1,18]

THE ELECTROCARDIOGRAM (ECG)

Electrical energy produced by charged ions as they move across myocardial cell membranes during depolarization and repolarization causes flow of electric current in the body. This current creates electrical potential that extends to the surface of the body. The surface ECG is a graphic recording of the electrical activity within the segments of the heart muscle. The ECG can be obtained at rest, or with exercise, and is a valuable diagnostic tool. Two electrodes applied to the body and the voltage between them measured on the ECG machine is called a lead. The placement of electrodes has been standardized. The routine ECG is composed of 12 different leads (Figs. 6-7 to 6-9). Each lead has a positive and a negative pole (electrode).

Standard Limb Leads (I, II, III)

The standard limb leads use the limbs to measure the electrical activity between a positive and negative pole (Fig. 6-7). Since there are always two active measurement points, a positive (+) and a negative (−), the standard limb leads are often termed the *bipolar limb leads*. The electrodes are placed in the area of the right arm, left arm, and left leg. The right leg serves as the ground. It makes no difference if the electrode is attached to the end of a limb or very close to the body, such as the shoulder. These three electrodes can be thought of as a triangle of electrical activity with the heart at the center. This is known as *Einthoven's triangle*. Since the left arm in this lead is positive, when the heart directs a voltage toward the left, one will record a positive or upward deflection on the ECG. If the heart directs a voltage toward the right, one will record a negative or downward deflection. Since lead II parallels the wave of depolarization, from right to left, in the heart, its complexes are taller than those of the other two standard limb leads. Lead II most clearly depicts the heart's rhythm, so it is most frequently used to obtain a rhythm strip (Fig. 6-8).

Augmented Limb Leads (aV$_R$, aV$_L$, aV$_F$)

Another set of leads in the 12-lead ECG are the augmented or unipolar leads (Fig. 6-9). They are obtained by connecting the positive electrode to one of the apices of Einthoven's triangle, and the negative electrode to the two remaining points on the triangle. Since there is only one active electrode, the positive one, which one is comparing to electrical zero, these leads are termed *unipolar*. The designation V signifies a unipolar system that has a zero reference point. Because of their low amplitude, the ECG augments the deflections 1½ times, as denoted by the prefix *a* in the name of the leads. The R, L, and F represent the position of the active or positive electrode on the right arm, left arm, and left foot, respectively. The QRS complex will have a negative deflection in lead aV$_R$ because the wave of depolarization in the heart travels away from that lead. The standard and augmented limb leads are called the frontal plane leads because they represent the electrical activity of the heart in specific directions in one plane, as if the patient were a flat cardboard cutout.

Precordial, Chest, or V Leads (V$_1$ through V$_6$)

The remaining leads completing the 12-lead ECG are the V leads. Again, the designation V signifies a unipolar system that has a zero reference point. The positive electrode will be placed at specific well-defined points on the chest (see Fig. 6-7). In this system the electrical activity directed from the electrical center of the heart toward or away from the positive electrodes located on the chest can be measured. This measures the forces directed anteriorly, posteriorly, right, and left, termed the *cross-sectional plane*. Combining the information from all 12 of the leads enables one to form a three-dimensional picture of the

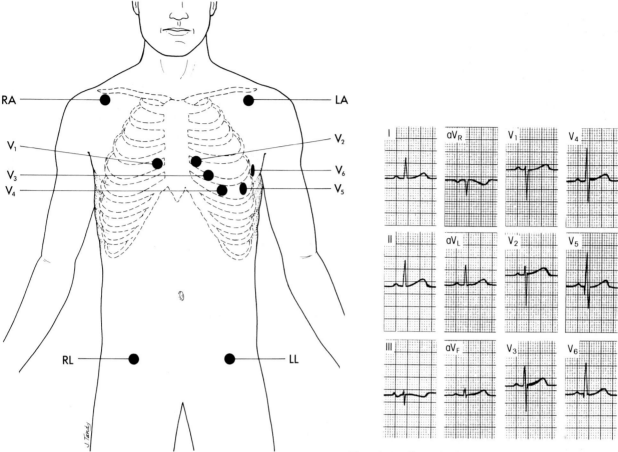

Fig. 6-7   ECG leads, showing placement of the limb electrodes (LL, RL, RA, LA) and the chest electrodes (V₁-V₆).

Fig. 6-8   Normal 12-lead ECG. (From Guzzetta CE, Dossey BM: *Cardiovascular nursing bodymind tapestry,* St Louis, 1984, Mosby–Year Book.)

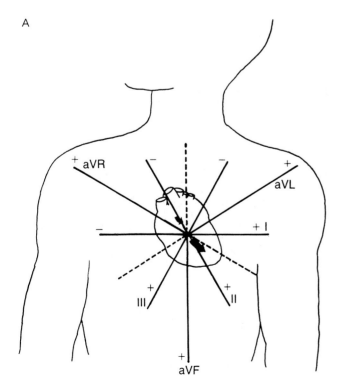

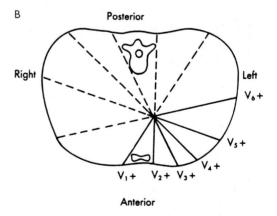

Fig. 6-9   **A,** All leads of the frontal plane, including augmented leads aVR, aVL, and aVF. **B,** The precordial reference figure. Leads V₁ and V₂ are called right-sided precordial leads; leads V₃ and V₄, mid-precordial leads; and leads V₅ and V₆, left-sided precordial leads. **A** from Lounsbury P, Frye SJ: *Cardiac rhythm disorders: a nursing process approach,* ed 2, St Louis, 1992, Mosby–Year Book.) **B** from Andreoli KG, Zipes DP, Wallace AG, et al: *Comprehensive cardiac care,* ed 6, St Louis, 1987, Mosby–Year Book.)

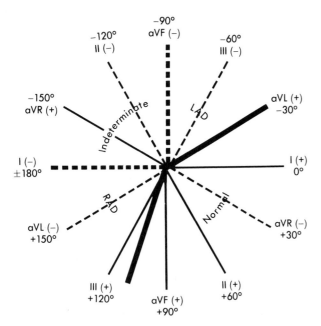

Fig. 6-10   The hexaxial reference system. (From Thelan LA, Davie JK, Urden LD: *Textbook of critical care nursing,* St Louis, 1990, Mosby–Year Book.)

heart's electrical activity. Electrical forces traveling toward one of the chest leads produces a positive deflection, while those traveling away from it produce a negative deflection. Thus it becomes possible to identify beats originating in the left or right ventricle, helping to detect left and right bundle branch block, and to differentiate ventricular ectopic from aberrant conduction.

Hexaxial Reference System

The hexaxial reference system is used to calculate the electrical axis of the heart, which indicates the general direction of the wave of depolarization (Fig. 6-10). Each pole of any lead has a value of 30 degrees. All poles below lead I are positive and those above lead I are negative in value. The normal axis is from −30 degrees to +110 degrees. Left axis deviation runs from −30 to −90 degrees; right axis deviation is from +100 to +180 degrees.[9] The axis is normal when the QRS complexes are positive in leads I and aV_F. Changes in the electrical axis will occur with an alteration in the conduction of the impulse through the ventricles. These alterations may be due to fibrosis, ischemia, injury of the conduction system, or changes in ventricular muscle mass. In the diagnosis of intraventricular conduction defects, determination of axis is especially important.

ECG Paper

The ECG paper is composed of a series of horizontal and vertical lines. The horizontal lines are 1 mm apart and are used to measure amplitude. The vertical lines are also 1 mm apart and measure time or duration. Every fifth line both vertically and horizontally is darker than the preced-

ing lines, forming a large square with five smaller squares within it. The usual speed of the paper is 25 mm/sec, making each small box 0.04 second long and 0.1 mV high.

Normal Deflections

Amplitude is recorded in millimeters or millivolts, and duration of deflection is recorded in seconds or milliseconds. The deflections seen on the ECG are positive when they go above the baseline and negative when below the baseline. If a deflection is partly above the baseline and partly below it, it is referred to as biphasic or diphasic. Positive deflections show that the electrical current is flowing toward the positive electrode. Likewise, negative deflections show that the electrical current is flowing away from the positive electrode. Normally, leads aV_R, V_1, V_2, and V_3 show strong negative deflections.

WAVES AND COMPLEXES

The major complexes seen on the ECG are identified by letters. These are P, Q, R, S, T, and U respectively (Fig. 6-11).

P Wave

The first wave seen is the P wave, which represents atrial depolarization. It begins in the SA node and then travels through the atria. The duration of the P wave is normally between 0.06 to 0.12 second in the normal heart and indicates the time it takes the impulse to travel through the atria muscle. The height of the P wave is normally not over 3 mm. The P wave is upright or positive in leads I, II, aV_F, and V_4 to V_6; inverted in aV_R; and biphasic in III and V1. The normal contour is rounded not pointed or notched.

PR Interval

Following the P wave is a flat line. The duration of the P wave and this flat line constitute the PR interval. The PR interval starts with the beginning of the P wave and goes to the beginning of the QRS complex. It represents the time it takes the impulse to travel from the atria to the AV node. The time interval is normally from 0.12 to 0.20 second duration. The impulse is then delayed in the AV node for about 0.01 second before traveling into the ventricles and the remainder of the conduction system. The AV node is the area of the heart with the slowest conduction time. This allows for atrial contraction and for adequate filling time for the ventricles. The PR interval includes all atrial and nodal activity for each beat.

The QRS Complex

The QRS complex represents ventricular depolarization. The QRS complex is comprised of three waves: Q, R, and S. The Q wave is the first negative deflection, the R wave is the first positive, and the S wave is the second negative deflection. Small letters are used to describe subsequent negative or positive deflections. The impulse travels through the ventricles rapidly, and the complex normally measures between 0.06 to 0.10 (but less than 0.12) second in duration.

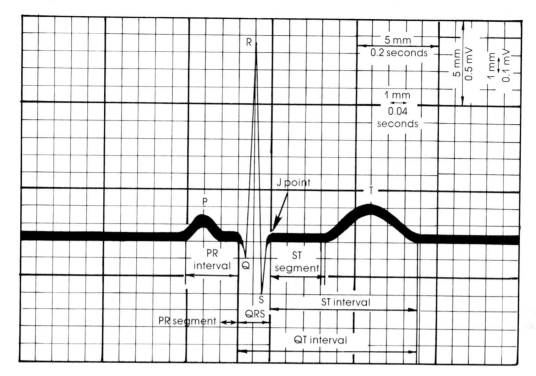

Fig. 6-11   Deflections and intervals in a normal ECG. (From The Methodist Hospital, Basic electrocardiography: a modular approach, 1986, St Louis, Mosby–Year Book.)

RP Interval

The RP interval is measured from the beginning of the QRS complex to the beginning of the next conducted P wave. Ordinarily the length of any PR interval is dependent on the length of the preceding RP interval. This inverse relationship between RP and PR intervals is called RP-PR reciprocity.

ST Segment

The ST segment extends from the QRS complex to the beginning of the T wave. The ST segment represents the time during which the ventricles have completely depolarized and the beginning of repolarization. Deviation of the ST segment is normal, if not elevated above the baseline more than 1 mm or below the baseline by 0.5 mm.

J Point

The J point is the angle at which the QRS complex ends and the ST segment begins. If the ST segment is depressed or elevated, the J point will deviate from the isoelectric line.

The QT Interval

Following the ST segment is the QT interval. This is measured from the beginning of the QRS complex to the beginning of the T wave. It represents the time it take for ventricular depolarization to occur and for ventricular repolarization to begin. The time interval of a QT segment is 0.34 to 0.43 second and varies with heart rate, sex, and age. In normal sinus rhythm, the QT interval is less than half the preceding R-to-R interval.

The T Wave

The T wave represents ventricular repolarization. At this time in the cardiac cycle, the ventricles are refractory. The peak of the T wave is when the relative refractory period of the action potential occurs and a larger number of fast Na+ channels are available. This period in the cycle is referred to as the vulnerable period when a stimulus can produce ventricular tachycardia or fibrillation.[5] The T wave is slightly rounded and slightly asymmetrical. A sharply pointed symmetrical T wave may indicate MI. The T wave is normally positive in leads I, II, aV_L, aV_F, and V_3 to V_6; inverted in aV_R; and inverted or upright in V_1. In leads III and V_2, the T wave may vary. The T wave normally is not above 5 mm in height in the standard limb leads and not above 10 mm in the precordial leads.[1,2]

The U Wave

The U wave is a small wave of low voltage that follows the T wave and occurs in the same direction as the T wave. Many times it is not seen on the ECG because of its low electrical voltage. The U wave may be elevated in hypokalemia and inverted in heart disease.[1,2,18]

Determining the Heart Rate

The heart rate can be determined in the following ways:
- Count the number of QRS complexes in a 1-minute strip.
- Count the number of small boxes between two R waves and divide that number into 1500.
- Count the number of large boxes between two R waves and divide that number into 300.

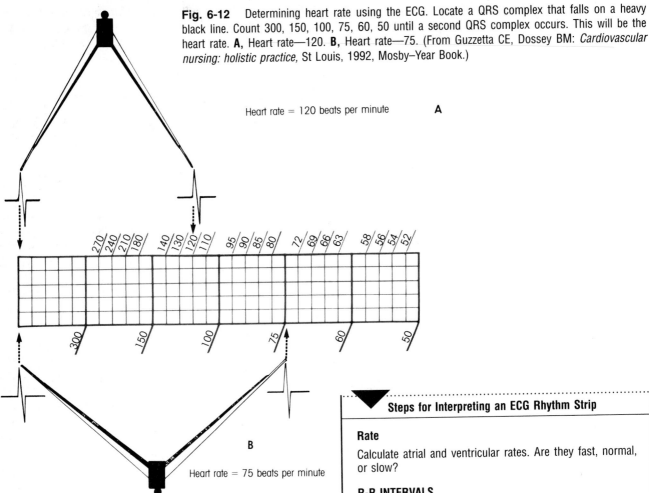

Fig. 6-12 Determining heart rate using the ECG. Locate a QRS complex that falls on a heavy black line. Count 300, 150, 100, 75, 60, 50 until a second QRS complex occurs. This will be the heart rate. **A,** Heart rate—120. **B,** Heart rate—75. (From Guzzetta CE, Dossey BM: *Cardiovascular nursing: holistic practice,* St Louis, 1992, Mosby–Year Book.)

Heart rate = 120 beats per minute **A**

Heart rate = 75 beats per minute

- Run a 6-second strip and count the number of R waves, then multiply that number by 10.
- Find a QRS complex that falls on a heavy black line (Fig. 6-12). Then count off the heavy lines as follows: 300, 150, 100, 75, 60, 50 until the next QRS complex occurs. The resulting number will be the heart rate.

Regularity

The rhythm on the ECG strip is examined for regularity by observing the intervals between the P waves and R waves for uniformity of length. If the rhythm is irregular, these intervals will be represented on the ECG strip by a pattern of varying distances. Each P wave should be clearly related to a QRS complex, and the PR interval should be normal and constant. In some dysrhythmias, the P wave may follow the QRS complex. When this occurs, the RP interval is measured. Finally, all P waves and QRS complexes should be determined identical and normal in contour and intervals should fall within normal limits (see box on Interpreting an ECG Rhythm Strip on the right).

THE 12-LEAD ECG

The 12-lead ECG gives a complete picture of the heart since it examines the heart's electrical potential from 12

▼ **Steps for Interpreting an ECG Rhythm Strip**

Rate

Calculate atrial and ventricular rates. Are they fast, normal, or slow?

R-R INTERVALS

Are they regular or irregular?

P WAVES

Are they present or absent? Are they before, buried in, or after the QRS? Normal in shape (no more than 3 small blocks high or wide) and position (upright)?

PR INTERVALS

Are they present? Normal (0.12-0.20 sec), short, or prolonged? In a regular pattern (before each QRS)?

QRS COMPLEXES

Are they present? Narrow or wide (no greater than 0.12 sec)? Normal, upright, and regular pattern?

ST SEGMENTS

Are they normal, depressed, or elevated?

T WAVES

Are they in an upright position? Normal height (no more than 10 small blocks in chest leads and 5 small blocks in others)?

ECTOPIC BEATS

Are they present or absent? Atrial, junctional, or ventricular?

SYMPTOMS

Is the patient tolerating the rate and rhythm?

different views at once. The recording of a 12-lead ECG is useful in identifying the following:

- Bundle branch blocks
- Hypertrophy
- Cardiac electrical axis
- Pacemaker electrode position
- Progress, extent, and location of acute MI
- Dysrhythmias
- Effects of drug therapy
- Myocardial disease

Signals from the 12 leads can be recorded sequentially on a single-channel ECG with manual or automatic switching or recorded simultaneously on a multichannel recorder. Three-channel ECGs are now commonly used. Many of the 12-lead ECG machines are computerized and have ECG interpretation programs. They use 10 seconds of ECG data to identify the QRS complex and waves, perform morphology measurements, and analyze the rhythm.

SIGNAL-AVERAGED ELECTROCARDIOGRAPHY[15]

Signal averaging is a computer-based technique that generates a high-quality, noise-free ECG. Noise is generated from muscle, power lines, and electronic noise from electrodes. The computer combines hundreds of QRS complexes. Because noise is random, the computer cancels extraneous signals, leaving a high-resolution, noise-free signal that can be amplified to identify the late potentials that usually occur with supraventricular tachycardia (SVT) (since SVT usually originates from a reentry circuit). The signal-averaged ECG requires 10 to 20 minutes to perform.

CONTINUOUS ECG MONITORING

When performing continuous monitoring, lead placement will be determined by the number of monitor leads available and the area of the heart to be monitored. Leads are placed on the chest rather than on the extremities (Fig. 6-13). *Text continued on p. 116.*

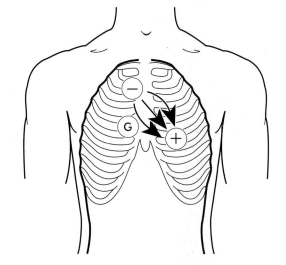

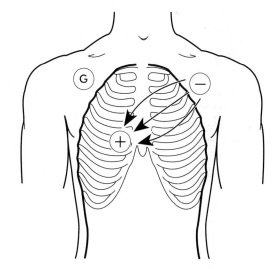

Three-lead system:
(A) Lead II
    (1) Apply negative electrode to first intercostal space, right sternal border.
    (2) Apply positive electrode to fourth intercostal space, left midclavicular line.
    (3) Apply ground electrode at fourth intercostal space, right sternal border.

(B) MCI$_1$ (modified chest lead V$_1$)
    (1) Apply negative electrode just inferior to left clavicle, midclavicular line.
    (2) Apply positive electrode to fourth intercostal space, right sternal border.
    (3) Apply ground electrode just inferior to right clavicle, midclavicular line.

Fig. 6-13 Electrode placement for continuous monitoring. **A,** Lead II provides clear P wave and tall, distinct R wave. **B,** MCI$_1$ (modified chest V$_1$) identifies bundle branch blocks, atrial and ventricular dysrhythmias, and ventricular conduction.

Continued.

C

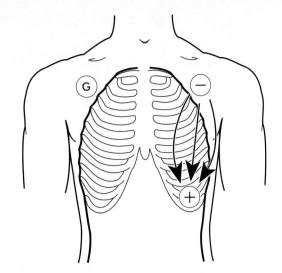

D

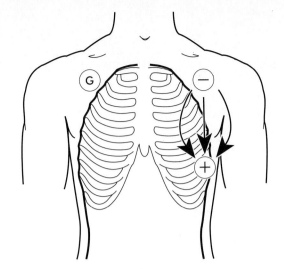

(3)   MCL₃ (modified chest lead III)
   (1)   Apply negative electrode just inferior to left clavicle, midclavicular line.
   (2)   Apply positive electrode on last left intercostal space, midclavicular line.
   (3)   Apply ground electrode inferior to right clavicle, midclavicular line.

(D)   MCL₆ (modified chest lead V₆)
   (1)   Apply negative electrode inferior to left clavicle, midclavicular line.
   (2)   Apply positive electrode to fifth intercostal space, midclavicular line.
   (3)   Apply ground electrode inferior to right clavicle, midclavicular line.

E

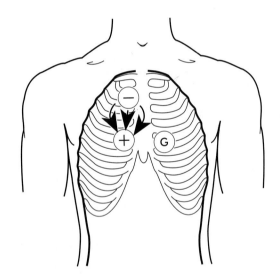

F

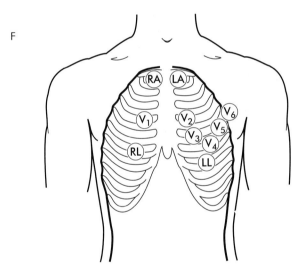

(E)   Lewis lead
   (1)   Apply negative electrode at first intercostal space, right sternal border.
   (2)   Apply positive electrode at fourth intercostal space, right sternal border.
   (3)   Apply ground electrode at the fourth intercostal space, left sternal border.

(F)   Five-lead system
   (1)   Apply RA electrode inferior to right clavicle, midclavicular line.
   (2)   Apply LA electrode inferior to left clavicle, midclavicular line.
   (3)   Apply RL electrode on sixth intercostal space, right midclavicular line.
   (4)   Apply LL electrode on sixth intercostal space, left midclavicular line.
   (5)   Apply chest lead electrode on selected chest sites V₁, V₂, V₃, V₄, V₅, or V₆ position.

Fig. 6-13, cont'd.   C, MCL₃ (modified chest lead III) offers another lead for a positive R wave. **D,** MCL₆ (modified chest lead V₆) is used for patients with median sternotomy incisions and for telemetry monitoring and provides a good R wave and identifies ventricular dysrhythmias and bundle branch block. **E,** Lewis lead. Good P waves for atrial dysrhythmia identification. **F,** Five-lead system. The fifth V lead electrode can be applied to a selected chest site; obtains a precise, multiplaned view of heart's activity; detects hemiblocks. (From Millar S et al: *AACN procedure manual for critical care,* Philadelphia, 1985, WB Saunders.)

Skill 6-2 Recording a 12-Lead ECG

EQUIPMENT AND SUPPLIES

- ECG machine with leads
- Electrode gel, alcohol pads, or disposable electrodes
- Tissues or gauze sponges
- Razor, soap, and water

NURSING INTERVENTIONS

1. Obtain patient's name, identification number, age, sex, approximate weight and height, presence of pacemaker, chest pain, and cardiac or thyroid medications.
2. Introduce self, identify patient, and explain procedure. Discuss briefly the function of an ECG and the fact that the procedure will not cause pain.
3. Position patient in a reclining position with the head of the bed slightly raised only if necessary. Ensure that no parts of the patient's body are touching any metal parts.
4. Ensure that the patient is comfortable and relaxed because muscle tensing and contracting will distort the tracing. The patient should not talk during the recording.
5. Bring the ECG machine to the patient's left side if possible, since it is easier to place the patient's precordial leads from this side. Plug machine to the wall electrical outlet and turn it on to let it warm up.
6. Drape patient to provide for privacy. Take patient's left arm out of hospital gown and pull back gown to observe for electrode placement sites. If necessary, remove perspiration and oil from skin with alcohol wipes. This will prevent distortion of ECG.
7. Select sites with a minimum of hair; shave excessively hairy areas if necessary so that better skin contact can be obtained.
8. Place disposable electrodes or conductive gel on electrode sites. Use alcohol pads for limb ECG. If using gel, apply to skin and rub in with electrode to reduce skin resistance.
9. Place limb electrodes as follows (see Fig. 6-7):
   RA: Place below right clavicle near, not on, shoulder.
   LA: Place below left clavicle near, not on, shoulder.
   RL: Place on torso below rib cage position in line with outside of right ankle.
   LL: Place on torso below rib cage position in line with outside of left ankle.
10. For ECG leads that use rubber straps rather than clips, place as follows:
    RA and LA: Place on inside of patient's forearms.
    RL and LL: Place on inside of patient's ankles.
11. Prepare to place chest electrodes or electrode gel. Placement must vary less than 5 mm from the proper location with each recording. Locate the angle of Louis, which is a bony ridge about 2 inches below the suprasternal notch. Just below the angle of Louis is the second intercostal space or count down from the clavicle to the fourth intercostal space and begin placement as follows:
    V_1: Just to the right of the sternal border, fourth intercostal space.
    V_2: Just to the left of the sternum, fourth intercostal space.
    V_3: Midway on a straight line between V_2 and V_4.
    V_4: The midclavicular line, fifth intercostal space. The midclavicular line is a vertical projection from a point halfway between the midline of the body and the upper-outer point of the shoulder. It usually passes through the nipple, but the nipple line is variable.
    V_5: On a horizontal line from V_4 in the anterior axillary line, which is a vertical projection from the band of pectoral muscles that can be felt joining the upper chest to the anterior surface of the shoulder.

V_6: On the same horizontal line from V_4 in the midaxillary line, which is a vertical projection from the midpoint of the armpit. Leads V_5 and V_6 are on a horizontal line running around the chest from V_4 and therefore will not usually be in the fifth intercostal space, which curves up and back.

12. Center the electrode cable on the patient's abdomen and connect the proper wires of the cable to the correct electrodes. Be sure to position the lead wires without bending or kinking them. The cables will be marked for the appropriate location and will be color coded as follows:

RA—white	LL—red
LA—black	Chest—brown
RL—green	

13. Ensure that the machine has paper. Press calibration button to check for standardization of tracing. The ECG is usually standardized to ensure that at 1 mV the deflection will be 10 mm. One-half standardization is occasionally required when the ECG complexes are unusually tall.[8]
14. Set paper speed to 25 mm/second.
15. Provide patient information, such as name, weight, and medications, as required by the machine's computer.
16. Press auto-run button. Inspect tracing critically for presence of *lethal dysrhythmia.* If patient requires immediate defibrillation, never place defibrillator paddles on ECG electrodes. Place the paddles so that some skin (and thus impedance) exists between the electrodes and the paddles.
17. Observe tracing for presence of *muscle tremor.* If present, help patient to relax and repeat tracing. Choose an electrode position where movement is at a minimum, such as where the limb joins the trunk.
18. Check tracing for *reversed limb leads* (RA for LA). In the normal ECG the T wave is always positive in lead I and negative in lead aVR.
19. Observe for *irregular baseline,* identified by bizarre, inconstant, and irregular deflections of the baseline. This is usually caused by broken lead wires, poor electrical contact, or metallic particles between the electrode and the patient's skin. Consider shaving patient's body hair to maintain better electrode contact.
20. Observe for *wandering baseline,* identified by a rhythmic up and down motion of the entire ECG. This is caused by motion of the patient, motion of the electrode, or by high skin resistance. It may be necessary to have the patient stop breathing briefly in midinspiration when recording leads V_5 and V_6 to eliminate a wandering baseline.
21. Check for signs of *alternating current interference,* identified by a fuzzy baseline that is completely regular like the teeth of a saw, showing 60 cycles/second. Check for proper grounding. Check for good electrode contact. Ensure that the cable tips are clean and bright. Check the electrical connections. Move the patient away from metal or from the wall, since there may be wiring that is causing the interference.
22. Make copies, as necessary. Remove electrodes from patient and cleanse sites with tissues or soap and water. Clean limb lead electrodes using alcohol wipes. Disconnect suction cup chest electrodes (if used) and hold under running water.

Continuous monitoring of patients in the ICU is a routine practice. Patients are continuously monitored for changes in cardiac rhythm; to document cardiac dysrhythmias or changes in cardiac axis; to select an appropriate ECG lead to enhance cardiac diagnosis; and to provide clean ECG tracings free of artifacts. Modifications of the standard 12-lead ECGs are used for routine cardiac monitoring at the bedside.

There are many types of cardiac monitors. Common to all, however, are certain components and capabilities. One of the basic components of a cardiac monitor is the oscilloscope, which is a television-like screen upon which the patient's ECG appears. As the heart beats, the ECG tracings move across the oscilloscope. The pulse meter registers the heart rate/minute and registers each cardiac cycle with an audible beep and a flash of light. The beep and light correspond to each QRS complex. The beep can become disturbing to the patient. In this event, the volume can be turned down.

Every monitor has alarms for the heart rate. These can be set individually for a maximum high pulse rate and a minimum low pulse rate. If the heart rate exceeds or drops below the set rates, an alarm will go off. Other factors may also cause the rate alarm to sound. The high rate alarm may go off because of skeletal muscle activity, loose electrodes, damaged or broken wires or cables, or improper connection of cables. The low alarm may go off if there is insufficient contact between the skin and electrodes. When this occurs, the tracing may resemble asystole. Alarms should never be set on stand-by and when sounding should always be investigated.

There may be several other dials on the monitor. The gain dial controls the size of the tracing. The position dial controls the position of the tracing on the oscilloscope. If other monitoring systems, such as arterial pressure monitoring or pulmonary artery pressure catheter monitoring, are hooked into the monitor, it may be necessary to reposition the ECG tracing to provide space and prevent superimposing tracings. The alarm silencer can be used to turn off the alarm briefly while mechanical problems are being dealt with or a disconnected lead or cable is being connected.

Skill 6-3   Continuous Bedside Monitoring

EQUIPMENT AND SUPPLIES

- Bedside hard-wire monitor
- 3- to 5-lead ECG cable (as indicated)
- Chest leads (3 to 5)
- Electrode pads
- Electrode gel
- Alcohol wipes
- Razor, soap, water
- Towel, washcloth
- 4 × 4 gauze pads

NURSING INTERVENTIONS

1. Turn on monitor to warm up before patient admission so that it is ready when needed.
2. Connect electrode wires to ECG cable and attach cable to monitor. Assess the condition of the wires and ensure that the connections are secure.
3. Ensure that the switches are on their standard settings as follows:
   - The sweep speed switch, controlling the rate that the light beam crosses the screen, is usually set at 25 mm/second.
   - The filter switch, controlling the amount of external interference with tracing, is usually set on "monitor," since this switch filters out most of the muscle artifact.
4. Introduce yourself, identify the patient, and explain what is to be done.
5. Wash hands.
6. Expose the chest area. Assess skin condition.
7. Mark the electrode placement on stationary areas of the chest, usually over ribs. Placement will depend on the purpose of the monitoring. Avoid the clavicle, ribs, neck, shoulder, breast tissue, areas with dressings, and hairy areas. Hair may have to be clipped if the patient has a great deal of it on the chest. Shaving may nick the skin and may lead to infection.[5]
8. Clean skin completely with alcohol to remove any residue on the skin that might interfere with monitoring.
9. If the skin is particularly smooth, abrade slightly by rubbing the sites with a gauze pad to ensure conduction.[5]
10. Peel disposable electrode pads from backing, or place electrode gel on nondisposable electrodes.
11. Attach the electrode pads to the areas marked. Press down firmly.
12. Attach leads to the pads.
13. Determine what lead is being used and calibrate the monitor according to the manufacturer's instructions.
14. Change pads whenever they become nonadhering or every 24 to 48 hours. Change the sites slightly at this time and observe skin under pads for irritation and blistering. Wipe away remaining paste from previous electrode sites.
15. After placing the electrodes and adjusting the monitor, observe the ECG on the screen.
16. Adjust the position of the baseline with the position knob. If the complexes are not tall enough to be counted by the monitor's rate meter, increase size by adjusting the sensitivity knob.
17. Set the millimeter/second control, which regulates the speed of the waveform as it moves across the screen at 25 mm/sec for routine monitoring. A speed of 50 mm/sec may be needed to identify some dysrhythmias, such as supraventricular tachycardia.
18. Note rate on rate meter. Periodically monitor pulse as well. Set rate alarms, depending on the rate that would indicate danger for the patient. This rate needs to be individualized depending on the patient's status and heart rate. For patients within normal range, this interval is usually ±20 beats/min. For patients with very slow or very high cardiac rates, this interval may be shortened to ±10 beats/min.
19. Allow patient to hear the alarm so he or she will not be startled if it sounds.
20. Leave alarm on at all times. Check patient immediately if it sounds.
21. Run a printout strip by pressing the appropriate button.

Accurate continuous monitoring requires the nurse to troubleshoot possible sources of interference. Improper grounding may cause electrical interference to appear on the monitor.[14] It is important to ensure that both the bed and the monitor are grounded. A very weak signal may also reflect an interruption or interference with the electrical transmission. The nurse should check for poor electrical contact between the skin and electrodes and for improper cable connections. If the electrodes move when the patient moves or breathes, a wandering baseline may result.

Telemetry Monitoring

Continuous measurement of the cardiac activity of a patient with dysfunction that requires prompt detection and treatment can be performed by telemetry. The patient is attached to a telemetry transmitter via two lead wires. The transmitter sends ECG data to the central console of a telemetry unit located at the nurses' station. Telemetry is generally used in the patient who does not need to be continuously attached to a bedside monitor and can ambulate further and move with less restriction. The electrodes are placed as shown in Fig. 6-13. Lead II is used for monitoring. The areas for electrode placement should be free of hair and oil. The two lead wires are attached to a small transmitter; the patient can carry it around the neck or waist in a pouch. The patient is instructed not to leave the range of the telemetry unit; get the telemetry unit wet; use electric appliances, e.g., a hair dryer or razor; and to notify the nurse if the electrodes become disconnected.

DYSRHYTHMIAS ORIGINATING FROM THE SINUS NODE
Normal Sinus Rhythm

The sinus impulse originates in the SA node. The normal heart rate is between 60 to 100 beats/min in adults, 80 to 110 beats/min in children, and 120 to 180 beats/min in

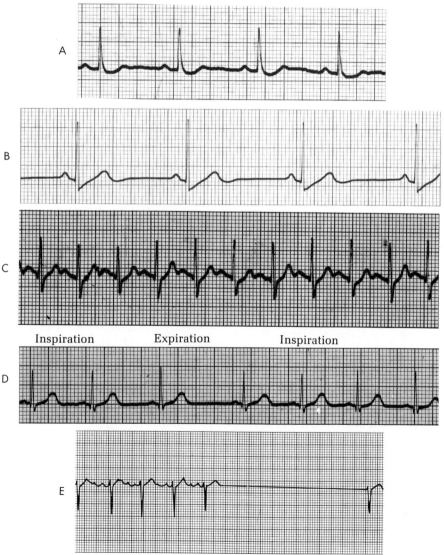

Fig. 6-14 Dysrhythmias originating from the sinus node: **A,** Normal sinus rhythm. **B,** Sinus bradycardia. **C,** Sinus tachycardia. **D,** Sinus dysrhythmia. **E,** Sinus arrest (sinoatrial block). (**A** and **B** from Guzzetta CE, Dossey BM: *Cardiovascular nursing: holistic practice,* St Louis, ed 2, 1992, Mosby–Year Book. **C, D,** and **E** from Conover MB: *Understanding electrocardiography: arrhythmias and the 12-lead ECG,* ed 6, St Louis, 1992, Mosby–Year Book.)

infants. Each QRS complex is preceded by a P wave and both atrial and ventricular rhythms are regular. All complexes appear the same. The PR interval in the adult is 0.12 to 0.20 second. The QRS complex measures between 0.06 to 0.10 second (Fig. 6-14, *A*).

Sinus Bradycardia

In sinus bradycardia the SA node is the pacemaker, but it discharges at a rate slower than 60 beats/min in adults, at less than 80 beats/min in children, and below 100 beats/min in infants. Both atrial and ventricular rhythms are regular and each QRS complex is preceded by a P wave. All P waves and QRS complexes appear the same, and the PR interval is between 0.12 to 0.20 second in duration. The QRS complex is normal in appearance and measures between 0.06 to 0.10 second in duration. This rhythm can occur with good cardiac reserve, such as seen in an athlete. It can be caused by pathological conditions of the heart, increased intracranial pressure, and hypothyroidism. Treatment is not needed unless the patient is symptomatic (Fig. 6-14, *B*).

Sinus Tachycardia

Sinus tachycardia occurs when the SA node in an adult has a rate of 100 to 180 beats/min. The rhythm is regular and a P wave appears before each QRS complex. The QRS complex is normal and each complex appears the same. If the rate is rapid enough, the P wave may be superimposed on the preceding T wave. The PR interval in the adult is within normal range, 0.12 to 0.20. This rhythm can be related to physiological factors, such as stress, exercise, fever, and increased consumption of tobacco or coffee. Pathological heart conditions, such as pulmonary emboli, myocardial ischemia, congestive heart failure, or shock may also cause sinus tachycardia. Treatment of this dysrhythmia is not necessary unless the patient is symptomatic, then the underlying cause is treated (Fig. 6-14, *C*).

Sinus Dysrhythmia

In sinus dysrhythmia, the pacemaker is the sinus node and conduction is normal. The rhythm speeds and slows alternately. The rate varies with respiration, increasing with inspiration and slowing with expiration. The irregularity disappears when the individual holds his or her breath. P waves, the QRS complex, and the PR interval are normal and all complexes appear the same. There is no treatment for this type of dysrhythmia and many times the rhythm will disappear when adulthood is reached (Fig. 6-14, *D*).

Sinus Arrest (Sinoatrial Block)

Sinus arrest occurs when the SA node fails to initiate an impulse and ventricular asystole occurs. There is usually more than one complete complex dropped. The rate is slow due to the dropped complexes, and the rhythm is irregular because of the lack of electrical activity. This type of rhythm is also labeled as sinus block, if the normal rhythm resumes as if nothing had occurred. The P waves, when present, appear normal but are absent during periods of asystole. The PR interval is normal where the P waves are present. The QRS complexes are normal when present, but the normal complexes could be replaced by a junctional or ventricular rhythm if the higher pacemakers fail to fire. This rhythm can occur as a result of the normal aging process or with hypoxia of the SA node. It can also occur with increased vagal tone or in response to drug use. Treatment occurs if the patient becomes symptomatic as a result of the slow heart rate (Fig. 6-14, *E*).

DYSRHYTHMIAS ORIGINATING FROM THE ATRIA

The atria have the next to the highest pacing rate, so if the SA node quits or if a location in the atria becomes irritable, the atria take over the pacemaker function. Rhythms that arise from the atria are known as *atrial dysrhythmias.* Atrial dysrhythmias are caused when the atrial rate becomes faster than the sinus rate, either by escape or by irritability. The only difference in conduction is that it is slower and rougher than in normal sinus rhythm.

Wandering Atrial Pacemaker

The wandering atrial pacemaker involves the passive transfer of the dominant pacemaker focus from the sinus node to latent pacemakers within the atria or the AV junctional tissue. Only one pacemaker dominates at a time, but passing the pacemaker role from the node to the irritable site occurs. The rate varies from slow as the pacemaker approaches the AV node to faster as the focus moves back to the SA node. The rhythm is slightly irregular due to the shifting pacemaker. Each QRS complex is preceded by a P wave but the P waves change in appearance because of the change in pacemaker site. The P waves from atrial beats are not the normal round waves but are pointed, flattened, notched, or diphasic. If the pacemaker moves into the junctional tissue, the P wave may become lost in the QRS complex or could follow the QRS complex. The PR interval will vary, depending on where the pacemaker is located in relation to the AV node. The closer the pacemaker is to the SA node, the more normal the PR interval will be. The QRS will appear normal and will measure within normal limits of 0.06 to 0.10 second. This type of dysrhythmia can occur with heart disease, such as SA node ischemia, atrial inflammation, or chronic lung disease. If the patient is asymptomatic, therapeutic intervention is not needed (Fig. 6-15).

Premature Atrial Contraction

A premature atrial contraction (PAC) is a beat that occurs in the right or left atria before the next SA node impulse (Fig. 6-16, *A*). When measuring the P-to-P interval, the P wave will occur early in the cycle. PACs can be unifocal or multifocal, meaning they occur in only one site of the atria or in many sites. They may also occur in a bigem-

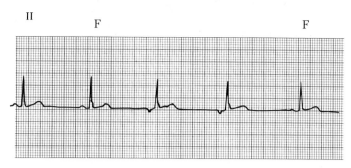

Fig. 6-15   Wandering atrial pacemaker. (From Conover MB: *Pocket guide to electrocardiography,* St Louis, 1990, Mosby–Year Book.)

iny, trigeminy, or quadrigeminy pattern. *Bigeminy* is a normal beat followed by a premature contraction; *trigeminy* is two normal beats followed by a premature contraction; and *quadrigeminy* is three normal beats to a premature contraction. The P waves of the premature beats do not appear the same as the normal P waves. The rate will vary, depending on the number of premature beats; the rhythm will be irregular but can have a regular pattern to it. The PR interval is within normal limits but will vary for the premature beats. The QRS complexes are typically normal and measure within normal limits. The PAC can on occasions be conducted through the ventricular tissue in an abnormal pathway. When this occurs, the QRS will appear abnormal. This is referred to as *aberrancy.* If the premature beat occurs during the refractory period of the ventricles, the impulse will not be transmitted through the ventricles. In this instance the P wave will appear on the ECG strip but will not be followed by a QRS complex. Causes of PACs include atrial hypoxia and irritability, fatigue, anxiety, and medications or stimulants, such as tobacco or coffee. PACs are not usually life threatening in patients without a history of cardiac disease.[16] Treatment includes monitoring the dysrhythmia and removing the underlying cause if possible. This type of dysrhythmia can result in a sustained atrial tachycardia, fibrillation, or flutter.

Paroxysmal Atrial Tachycardia

In paroxysmal atrial tachycardia (PAT) (Fig. 6-16, *B*), a single focus in the atria becomes so irritable that it begins to fire regularly and therefore overrides the SA node for the entire rhythm. All of the P waves in PAT have the atrial configuration. PAT is characterized by a regular rhythm. It is usually quite rapid with a rate of between 150 and 250 beats/minute. Because of the rapid rate, P waves may be hidden in the preceding T waves.

Patients with PAT have an excessive number of stimuli traveling through the AV junction. Increasing vagal tone may suppress this. The patient can perform a Valsalva maneuver or the physician may attempt carotid massage. Drugs, such as verapamil, are highly effective, as are digitalis and propranolol.

Atrial Flutter

Atrial flutter occurs when the atria become so irritable that they fire at a rate between 250 to 300 beats/min. The AV node does not permit all the impulses to reach the ventricles. It controls the ventricular response through the number of impulses it transmits, from two to eight. The rhythm of the atria and the ventricles is regular in pure flutter, but if the block varies, then ventricular response varies. The P waves are absent and replaced by sawtoothed F waves. PR intervals are not measurable. The QRS complexes are normal and measure between 0.06 to 0.10 second but may be difficult to measure because of the flutter waves. Atrial flutter almost always indicates the presence of organic heart disease. It can also occur during fetal life or within the first week of life and is referred to as congenital atrial flutter. Paroxysmal atrial flutter can also occur after 3 weeks of age and is more common in males. Treatment usually requires some type of medical intervention either with drug therapy or synchronized electrical countershock (Fig. 6-16, *C*).

Atrial Fibrillation

Atrial fibrillation occurs when the atria become so irritable that they are no longer beating but are quivering as a result of multiple irritable foci in the atria. The rate of the atria is greater than 300 beats/min. The AV node controls the number of impulses that reach the ventricles. The ventricular rate varies depending on the number of impulses that are transmitted, but the rhythm is irregular. P waves are not present. The atrial activity is displayed as a wavy undulating line on the ECG and is referred to as *F waves* or fibrillatory waves. The F waves are conducted in an extremely chaotic pattern, producing a grossly irregular RR interval. PR intervals are not measurable. The QRS complexes will vary in electrical voltage but usually appear normal and may measure within normal limits. Atrial fibrillation only occurs in the presence of organic heart disease. It is a relatively uncommon occurrence in infancy and early childhood. Treatment usually requires medical intervention to keep the ventricular rate within sinus limits of 60 to 100 beats/min (Fig. 6-16, *D*).

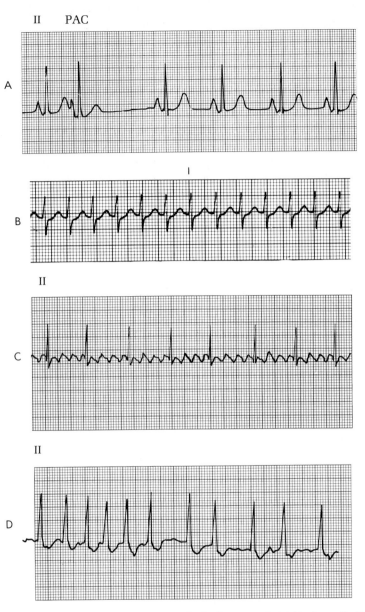

Fig. 6-16   **A,** Premature atrial contraction (PAC). **B,** Paroxysmal atrial tachycardia (PAT). **C,** Atrial flutter. **D,** Atrial fibrillation. (**A, C,** and **D** from Conover MB: *Pocket guide to electrocardiography,* ed 2, St Louis, 1990, Mosby–Year Book. **B** from Goldberger AL, Goldberger E: *Clinical electrocardiography: a simplified approach,* ed 4, St Louis, 1990, Mosby–Year Book.)

JUNCTIONAL RHYTHMS

In junctional rhythms, the SA node loses the ability to be the pacemaker of the heart. When this occurs, the next highest order pacemaker, the AV junctional tissue, takes over as the pacemaker. The rate is between 40 to 60 beats/min. The rhythm is regular for both the atria and ventricles.

Electrical impulses that arise from the AV junction cause the heart to be depolarized in an unusual manner. Since the AV junction is located in the middle of the heart, junctionally generated electrical impulses spread in two di-

rections simultaneously. When this occurs, the atria and ventricles depolarize at about the same time. The method by which the atria are depolarized is known as *retrograde conduction.* The electrical pattern on the ECG will show an inverted P wave.

In junctional rhythms, the P wave does not always precede a QRS complex, since it is possible for the ventricles to depolarize before the atria. If this occurs, the QRS complex will precede the P wave. If both atria and ventricles depolarize at the same time, the P wave will be hidden in the QRS complex.

PR intervals in junctional rhythms are short, since the impulse occurs lower in the heart than the SA node and does not have as far to travel. The QRS complex is generally normal in appearance. The rhythm can be a normal phenomenon owing to the effects of vagal tone on higher pacemakers or it may occur during pathological slow sinus discharge and heart block as a safety mechanism. Treatment will depend on the cause of the rhythm, but usually none is necessary. If the patient becomes symptomatic because of a slow heart rate, then medication that will increase heart rate will be used.

Premature Junctional Contraction

In premature junctional contraction (PJC), an irritable focus in the junction stimulates an early cardiac cycle (Fig. 6-17, *A*). A PJC is generally a single beat and interrupts the underlying cardiac rhythm. The RR interval may be regular or irregular, depending on the underlying rhythm, but the PJC will come earlier than expected.

In healthy individuals, PJCs may result from a variety of sources, for example, emotion, tobacco, or caffeine. PJCs are commonly seen in patients in digitalis toxicity and are the result of enhanced automaticity.

Junctional Escape Rhythm

Junctional escape occurs when there is an undue time lapse in the conduction of the electrical impulse from the SA node to the AV node. The junction senses the failure of the SA node to fire and the junction pacer cells reach threshold, discharge, and assume the pacemaker function. The RR interval will be regular. The P wave may appear before or after the QRS or it may be hidden within the QRS. The junctional escape rhythm is a normal failsafe mechanism rather than an irritable dysrhythmia (Fig. 6-17, *B*).

AV junctional escape rhythms may be seen in patients experiencing digitalis toxicity, toxic reaction to beta-blockers or calcium channel blockers, acute myocardial infarction (AMI), hypoxemia, or hyperkalemia.

Accelerated Idiojunctional Rhythm

An accelerated idiojunctional rhythm occurs because of enhanced automacity within the AV junction. The rate is between 40 and 100 beats/min (Fig. 6-17, *C*). Accelerated idiojunctional rhythm is commonly seen in patients with digitalis toxicity.

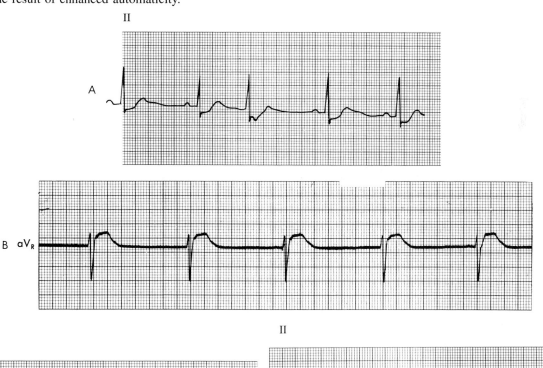

Fig. 6-17 **A,** Premature junctional contraction. **B,** Junctional escape rhythm. **C,** Accelerated junctional rhythm. **D,** Junctional tachycardia. (**A, C,** and **D** from Conover MB: *Pocket guide to electrocardiography,* ed 2, St Louis, 1990, Mosby–Year Book. B from Goldberger AL, Goldberger E; *Clinical electrocardiography: a simplified approach,* ed 4, St Louis, 1990, Mosby–Year Book.)

AV Junctional Tachycardia

Junctional tachycardia is an irritable dysrhythmia. Since the rate of the junction is slower than the sinus node, the rate of the rhythm can exceed 100 beats/min. Both the atrial and ventricular rhythms are regular. This type of dysrhythmia usually occurs with some heart diseases or following open heart surgery. It can also be a result of digitalis toxicity (Fig. 6-17, D).

SUPRAVENTRICULAR TACHYCARDIA (SVT)

SVT is not a specific dysrhythmia but is a term to describe a family of regular tachydysrhythmias that originate above the ventricles. They have indistinguishable P waves and fall within a common rate range. The RR intervals are constant and the rhythm is regular. The rate is usually between 100 and 250 beats/min.

The P waves in SVT precede, are imbedded in, or follow the QRS complex. If visible, the P wave is inverted. If the P wave precedes the QRS complex, the PR interval will be less than 0.12 second. If it falls in the QRS complex or follows it, there will be no PR interval. SVTS would include sinus tachycardia, PAT (including AV junctional tachycardia, atrial fibrillation, atrial flutter, and multifocal atrial tachycardia.

Paroxysmal Supraventricular Tachycardia

The exact mechanism causing paroxysmal supraventricular tachycardia (PSVT) is not known but it is thought to be AV nodal reentry or reentry over an accessory pathway. *AV nodal reentry* is the return of an impulse through the AV node to activate a pathway within the AV node for the second time. The impulse travels down the bundle tissue causing ventricular depolarization but also travels backward through the AV node producing another AV node depolarization (Fig. 6-18). The rate is rapid, usually between 170 to 250 beats/min. In children, the rate can be faster than 250 beats/min. The causes of this type of dysrhythmia are related to factors, such as overexertion, emotional stimuli, caffeine, and smoking. The occurrence of paroxysmal supraventricular tachycardia does not indicate heart disease. The person experiencing the attack may have symptoms ranging from palpitations, nervousness, or anxiety to angina, frank heart failure, or shock, depending on the duration of the tachycardia and the presence of an existing heart disease. Treatment depends on the clinical situation and how well the patient tolerates the rhythm. Treatment can include the simple intervention of rest and sedation to more complex medical intervention.

HEART BLOCK

There are several different dysrhythmias that do not originate in the SA node or in the AV junction but are a result of an abnormal delay or failure of impulse conduction within the AV node, bundle of His, or the surrounding tissue. This family of dysrhythmias is known as heart block.

Heart block can be permanent or transient, anatomical, or functional. It is classified according to degrees, such as first-degree, second-degree (type I and type II), and third-degree complete heart block.

First Degree AV Heart Block

First degree AV heart block is prolonged conduction from the SA node to the AV node, displayed by a PR interval greater than 0.20 seconds in adults; greater than 0.18 seconds in children; and greater than 0.15 seconds in infants. First degree AV heart block indicates that a conduction problem at the AV node is present but not complete. All impulses are conducted but each undergoes a delay before being conducted. The rhythm is regular and the rate is generally between 60 to 100 beats/min but will depend on the underlying cardiac rhythm. Each QRS complex is preceded by a P wave, and the QRS is within normal limits of 0.06 to 0.10 second. First degree AV heart block does not have to occur with heart disease. It can accompany viral infections, drug toxicity, or occur during heart surgery and cardiac catherization (Fig. 6-19, A). First degree AV heart block generally produces no symptoms and requires no treatment.

Second Degree AV Heart Block

Second degree heart block is more serious than first degree block because some impulses are actually blocked, while others are conducted. A key feature of second degree heart block is that not every P wave is followed by a QRS complex. Second degree heart block is divided into type I and type II. Type I, also referred to as *Wenckebach* or *Mobitz I,* has a rate within normal limits (60 to 100 beats/min). The ventricular rate is slightly lower because of dropped beats. The rhythm of the atria is regular while the ventricles have a cyclically irregular rhythm. The P waves are normal in shape and appearance. In type I heart block, each impulse from the atria to the ventricles seems to have increasingly more difficulty being conducted. The P-to-P and R-to-R intervals get progressively shorter. The PR interval gradually increases until a beat is dropped (the P wave is not followed by a QRS complex). The Wenckebach cycle then repeats itself. The ECG pattern for this

V_1

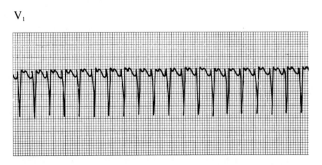

Fig. 6-18 Paroxysmal supraventricular tachycardia. (From Conover MB: Pocket guide to electrocardiography, ed 2, St Louis, 1990, Mosby–Year Book.)

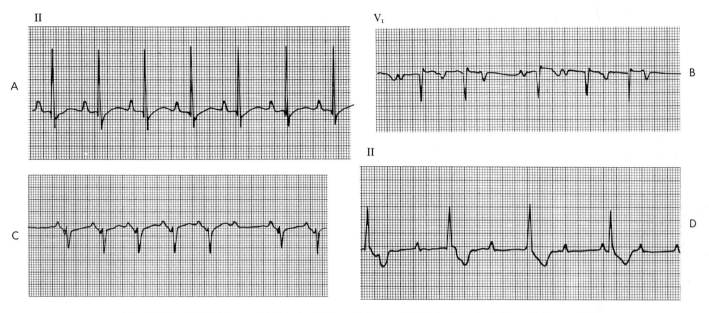

Fig. 6-19   **A,** First-degree AV block. **B,** Second-degree AV block, Type I. **C,** Second-degree AV block, Type II. **D,** Third-degree (complete) AV block. (From Conover MB: *Pocket guide to electrocardiography:* ed 2, St Louis, 1990, Mosby–Year Book.)

type of conduction disturbance is characterized by a clustering of QRS complexes followed by a longer pause that represents the dropped beat. The QRS complex is normal, measuring between 0.06 to 0.10 second. Although type I degree heart block is usually a benign type of dysrhythmia associated with reversible conditions, such as inferior myocardial ischemia, rheumatic fever, digitalis toxicity, or the postoperative period of open heart surgery, it does have some limited potential to progress to higher degree heart blocks[4] (Fig. 6-19, *B*).

Type II second degree heart block (*classical* or *Mobitz II* heart block) has a more serious prognosis than type I (Wenckebach). The difference between Wenckebach and classical second degree heart block is that with the type II condition fewer P waves are conducted. This results in a pattern of more P waves than QRS complexes.

The atrial heart rate for type II is between 60 to 100 beats/min, while the ventricular rate is less due to dropped ventricular beats. The ventricular rate may be in the brachycardic range. The rhythm is regular for the atria and irregular for the ventricles. The P waves all appear the same and are normal in shape. The PR interval may be normal or it may be prolonged; however, it is constant for every conducted beat to the ventricles. The QRS complex in type II is often associated with a bundle branch block (BBB) pattern, so the QRS complex can be greater than 0.10 seconds. The risk with this type of block is it can progress to complete heart block and transvenous pacing will be necessary (Fig. 6-19, *C*).

Third Degree Heart Block

Third degree heart block (complete heart block) occurs when all impulses from the SA node are blocked at the AV node; no impulses get through to the ventricles. The atria and the ventricles beat independently, therefore complete heart block is one form of complete AV dissociation. The atrial rate is usually in the normal rate, while the ventricular rate is slower. If a junctional focus is controlling the ventricles, the rate will be 40 to 60 beats/min, and if the focus is ventricular, the rate will be 20 to 40 beats/min.

The rhythm of the atria and the ventricles is regular. The P waves will appear normal, but there will be no PR interval to measure, since the atria are not controlling the ventricles. The QRS complex can be normal in appearance or it may be prolonged, depending on where the pacemaker for the ventricles is located, but there is no relationship between the P wave and the QRS complex (Fig. 6-19, *D*). If the junctional tissue takes over and becomes the pacemaker, the complex can appear normal, but if the ventricles themselves become the pacemaker, the QRS complex will be greater than 0.10 second. The R-to-R interval is regular. The causes of third degree heart block can be many and include drug toxicity, degenerative diseases, or electrolyte imbalances, as well as cardiac disorders. Risks associated with the slow ventricular rate include the following:

- Lethal ectopic rhythms.
- Ventricle asystole.
- Stokes-Adams syncope.
- Severe bradycardia.
- Ventricular tachydysrhythmias.

VENTRICULAR RHYTHMS

Ventricular rhythms originate in the ventricles below the branching of the bundle of His. They are serious dysrhythmias since the efficiency of the heart is greatly reduced.

Further, since the inherent escape mechanism of the ventricles is the last, there is no further mechanism to keep the heart pumping if it fails.

Premature Ventricular Contractions

Premature ventricular contractions (PVC), the most common of all dysrhythmias, originate in the ventricles and occur early in the cardiac cycle. With PVCs, an etopic electric impulse in one of the ventricles (usually the left) triggers a contraction before the SA node fires. The rate will depend on what the pacemaker is for the heart. The P waves will appear normal for the sinus beats, but the PVC will not have a P wave preceding the QRS complex. The QRS complex for the premature beat will be wide and abnormal in appearance. The T wave that follows the QRS complex will be in the opposite direction from the QRS complex. Because the ventricle beat occurs early, it disrupts the regular rhythm and produces a *compensatory pause,* equal to two normal cycles, following the premature beat (Fig. 6-20, *A*). In some situations a P wave may follow the early ventricle beat and be conducted to the ventricles with a long PR interval. This is called an *interpolated beat* and no compensatory pause occurs following the premature beat. Also, two foci can cause ventricle depolarization to occur simultaneously and the complex will be a blend of the premature beat and the normal beat. This is called a fusion beat. The ventricular fusion complex will often be narrower and of lesser amplitude than the ectopic beat alone. If the patient has

had an acute MI ventricular fusion beats may warn of congestive heart failure.

Ventricular premature beats, like atrial premature beats, can occur in pairs or groups. This pattern indicates increasing cardiac irritability. When there are two PVCs in a row, it is referred to as a couplet (Fig. 6-20, *B*). There can also be a grouping of three or more PVCs, called a run of PVCs (Fig. 6-20, *C*). Premature beats may have different contours. When this occurs, it is referred to as *multiform premature ventricular contraction.* If PVCs are occurring from more than one ectopic focus, they are referred to as *multifocal premature ventricular contractions.*

Occasionally, frequently occurring PVCs fall into a pattern surrounding the normal beats. This phenomenon is referred to as grouped beating. For example, when one normal beat precedes a PVC and this pattern continues, it is called *bigeminy* (Fig. 6-20, *D*). A group of two sinus beats followed by a PVC in a repeated pattern is known as *trigeminy* (Fig. 6-20, *E*). *Quadrigeminy* refers to a repeated pattern of three normal beats and one PVC (Fig. 6-20, *F*). The presence of premature beats in individuals without heart disease may be of no significance; however, the development of premature ventricular systoles following an MI, adds a risk factor for subsequent death.

The individual experiencing premature ventricular contractions complains of symptoms of palpitations or discomfort in the chest or neck. Premature ventricular contractions can also produce angina or hypotension in patients with heart disease.

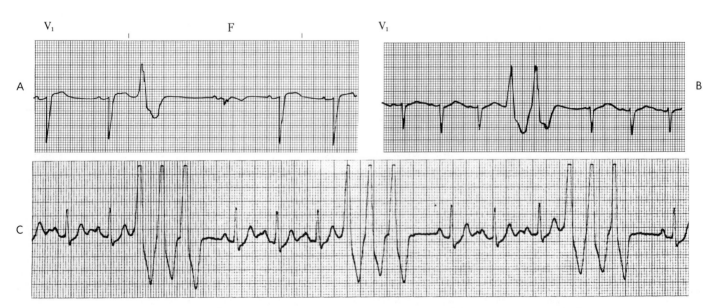

Fig. 6-20   A, Ventricular fusion complex. **B,** Paired PVCs (couplet). **C,** A run, or salvo, of PVCs.

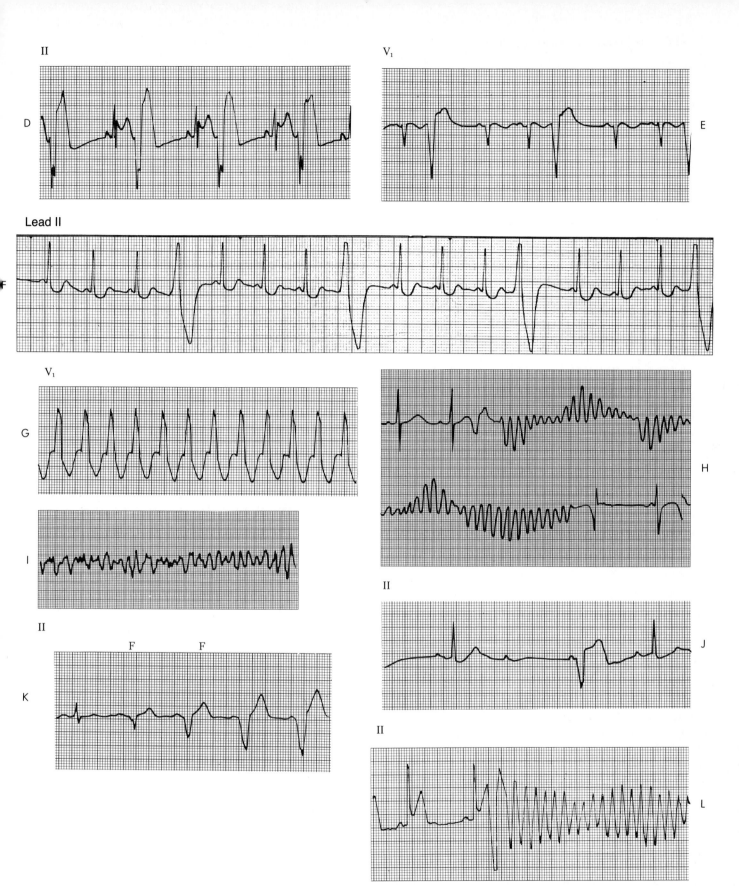

Fig. 6-20 cont'd **D,** Ventricular bigeminy **E,** Ventricular trigeminy. **F,** Ventricular quadrigeminy. **G,** Ventricular tachycardia. **H,** Torsades de pointes. **I,** Ventricular fibrillation. **J,** Idioventricular rhythm. **K,** Accelerated idioventricular rhythm. **L,** R-on-T phenomenon. PVC patterns that are dangerous and require special attention include: 1) more than 6 PVCs per minute, 2) R-on-T phenomenon, 3) bigeminy, 4) 2 or more PVCs in a row, and 5) multifocal PVCs. (**A, B, D, E, G, J, K,** and **L** from Conover MB: *Pocket guide to electrocardiography,* ed 2, St Louis, 1990, Mosby–Year Book. **C** and **F** from Lounsbury P, Frye SJ: *Cardiac rhythm disorders: a nursing process approach,* ed 2, St Louis, 1992, Mosby–Year Book. **H** and **I** from Beare PG, Myers JL: *Principles and practice of adult health nursing,* St Louis, 1990, Mosby–Year Book.)

Ventricular Tachycardia

If the myocardium becomes extremely irritable, the ventricles' focus could speed up and override the higher pacemaker sites. Ventricular tachycardia presents with a sustained run of premature ventricular beats. The atrial rate cannot be measured because P waves are hidden within the QRS complex. The ventricular rate is between 100 to 250 beats/min. The rhythm is regular or slightly irregular for both the atria and the ventricles. PR intervals cannot be measured because the P waves cannot be seen. The QRS complex is wide, greater than 0.10 second, and abnormal in appearance. The T wave is usually in the opposite direction of the QRS complex. The presence of tachycardia is indicative of some heart disease and is another form of AV dissociation. If the dysrhythmia is left untreated, ventricular fibrillation may result (Fig. 6-20, *G*).

Torsades de Pointes

Torsades de pointes (twist around points) is an atypical polymorphic ventricular tachycardia characterized by QRS complexes of changing amplitudes that seem to twist around the isoelectric line at a rate of 150 to 250 beats/min (Fig. 6-20, *H*).[12] Torsades de pointes is a potentially lethal syndrome characterized by prolonged ventricular repolarization and therefore a prolonged QT interval. Torsades de pointes may be indicated by a late diastolic PVC that occurs during a prolonged TU wave or by a long-short ventricular cycle but it may terminate spontaneously or degenerate into ventricular fibrillation.

An incorrect ECG diagnosis of Torsades de pointes may cause harm to the patient because Torsades de pointes may not be treated by class I antidysrhythmics (lidocaine, procainamide, or quinidine).

Ventricular Flutter

Ventricular flutter is a dysrhythmia similar to VT, but the ventricular rate is greater than 300. The ventricles depolarize at such a fast rate that the ECG pattern becomes very uniform. The pattern resembles a side view of a coiled spring. There is little difference between VT and ventricular flutter, except the rate.

Ventricular Fibrillation

Ventricular fibrillation occurs when the ventricles become extremely irritable, and many foci fire in a chaotic, ineffective manner. The rate cannot be measured and the rhythm is completely irregular. P waves are not visible, thus PR intervals cannot be measured. The QRS complex is bizarre with no consistent pattern. This type of dysrhythmia is lethal. Death results if immediate interventions are not initiated to halt the rhythm and restore a normal heart rate. Cardiac output is reduced and the patient loses consciousness, the pulse is absent and within 3 minutes, brain death will occur (Fig. 6-20, *I*).

Idioventricular Rhythm (Ventricular Escape)

Idioventricular rhythm is a ventricular escape rhythm where the ventricles take over the role of the heart's pacemaker because of failure of the higher pacemakers. The inherent rate of the ventricles is 20 to 40 beats/min. The rhythm is usually regular, although it can slow as the heart dies. There are no P waves in this dysrhythmia. The QRS complex is wide and bizarre, measuring at least 0.12 seconds (Fig. 6-20, *J*).

When this rhythm is in its terminal phases as the patient is dying, the QRS complexes lose some of their form and become irregular. This rhythm of the dying heart is known as *agonal,* especially if the rate drops below 20 beats/min.

Accelerated Idioventricular Rhythm

Accelerated idioventricular rhythms occur when an area of increased automaticity within the ventricles paces the heart at a rate greater than the inherent rate of the ventricles but less than 100 beats/min. The rate is generally within 10 beats of the SA node so that control of the cardiac rhythm is exchanged back and forth as the two pacemaker sites compete. As a result, fusion beats can be seen on the ECG as the sites exchange. The rhythm can be regular or irregular (Fig. 6-20, *K*). P waves generally present but may be lost in fusion beats. This dysrhythmia is often seen with acute MI or as a result of digitalis intoxication.

R-on-T Phenomenon

The R-on-T phenomenon refers to PVCs in which the R wave hits the T wave of the preceding normal beat. This is important to note because the T wave has a vulnerable phase, or relative refractory period, located on its downslope where an electrical impulse could generate an aberrant depolarization of the heart. An R-on-T therefore has the potential of throwing the heart into an uncontrolled repetitive pattern (Fig. 6-20, *L*).

BUNDLE BRANCH BLOCK

Bundle branch blocks (BBB) result in intraventricular conduction defects. BBB causes the heart to be activated in a lopsided fashion, i.e., one ventricle and then the other, instead of simultaneously. BBBs are frequently associated with acute MI and may be temporary or permanent. Other factors that contribute to BBB include congenital abnormalities, valvular disorders, cardiac disease, atherosclerotic disease of the conduction system, and some cardiac drugs.

Some prolongation of the QRS complex is seen. In incomplete BBB, it may be between 0.01 and 0.12 seconds and longer than 0.12 seconds in complete BBB.

Right Bundle Branch Block

The right bundle branch (RBB) is considerably smaller than the left bundle branch (LBB). RBB block (RBBB) does not interfere with the initial left-to-right depolarization of the ventricles. In RBBB, the two ventricles are activated one after the other. The left ventricular depolarization remains normal with the right ventricle taking slightly longer.

RBBB is frequently seen in both normal and diseased tissue and because of the extensive conduction remaining, is not viewed as life-threatening.

In uncomplicated complete RBBB, the QRS complex is 0.11 seconds or wider. The asynchronous activation of the ventricles produces a secondary component to the ventricular complex in the right precordial leads. Called an R′ wave, the QRS complexes may take a variety of shapes, such as rsr′, rSR′, rR′, or an M-shaped pattern that is frequently seen in the V_1 and V_2 leads. Small Q waves and wide S waves are seen in leads I, aV_L and V_6 (Fig. 6-21). Incomplete RBBB is demonstrated on the ECG by a QRS complex of less than 0.12 seconds in addition to the indications described above.

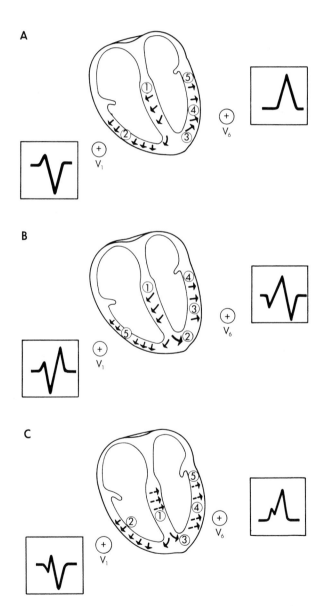

Fig. 6-21 **A,** Sequence of ventricular depolarization. **B,** Sequence of ventricular depolarization when right bundle branch block is present. **C,** Sequence of ventricular depolarization when left bundle branch block is present. (From Thelan LA, Davie JK, Urden LD: *Textbook of critical care nursing: diagnosis and management,* St Louis, 1990, Mosby–Year Book.)

Left Bundle Branch Block

Since the LBB conducts impulses to the left ventricle, a disturbance in its conduction reflects serious underlying cardiac disease. LBB block (LBBB) results in disruption of the normal life-to-right activation pattern of the ventricles. When the LBB is blocked, the RBB receives the impulse first. The impulse then travels across the septum to the left ventricle.

LBBB is most easily diagnosed using the left precordial leads of V_5 and V_6. The initial Q waves are absent, the QRS complex is wide (more than 0.12 seconds), and notched with a late intrinsicoid deflection. In the right precordial leads, the S wave is widened and R waves are small or absent. The ST segment and T wave shift are 180 degrees opposite the major QRS deflection (see Fig. 6-21). LBBB can mask the ECG signs of an acute MI.

Hemiblocks

A hemiblock occurs when conduction to half of the left ventricle is hampered. Involvement of the anterosuperior fascicle is known as left anterior hemiblock (LAH) and a block in the posteroinferior fascicle is known as left posterior hemiblock (LPH).

ECG diagnosis of LAH depends on the identification of a marked left axis deviation (greater than a −45 degree angle or beyond) in the frontal plane. The QRS width is less than 0.12 seconds. The S wave in lead aV_F equals or exceeds the R wave in lead I.

LPH produces a QRS angle in the frontal plane of approximately +120 degree angle or more, an initial Q wave in lead III, and a terminal S wave in lead III. The QRS width is less than 0.12 seconds.

Hemiblocks may result from coronary artery disease after an anteroseptal MI that involves the RBB and one of the divisions of the LBB. Treatment in the presence of MI requires the use of a temporary transvenous pacemaker because more advanced AV block may follow. Pacemaker implantation without MI is not usually necessary.

Artificial Pacemaker Rhythms

Artificial pacemakers are electronic devices that deliver an electrical stimulus to the heart through electrodes placed in contact with the endocardium. The electrodes are attached to a battery box, which delivers an electrical stimulus that will stimulate the cardiac cells to depolarize, causing ventricle depolarization. The use of pacemakers can be either temporary or permanent. What is seen on the ECG when an individual has a pacemaker is a pacer spike appearing before the QRS complex. P waves may be seen but they have no relationship to the QRS complexes. As a result, PR intervals cannot be measured. Because depolarization begins in the right ventricle, the QRS complex becomes wide and abnormal in appearance. If any beats are produced by the sinus node, the P wave will precede the beat, the QRS will be normal and measure between 0.05 to 0.10 second, and the PR interval will be within normal limits of 0.12 to 0.20 seconds. In studying this rhythm, it is important to identify the pacer spikes and know the type of pacemaker being used. Bipolar pacemakers have two electrodes in contact with the heart muscle; unipolar pacemakers have one. The unipolar pacemaker has a pulse generator that senses the cardiac impulses. It produces a large, easy to see artifact. See Chapter 7 for more information on this topic and on the ECG strips.

ECG CHANGES RESULTING FROM ELECTROLYTE IMBALANCES

Potassium and calcium both have an effect on the heart and the ability of the heart to depolarize and repolarize. These effects will become more prominent with changes in the levels of these electrolytes and can produce distinct changes on the ECG.

Hyperkalemia

Potassium imbalances produce characteristic changes. *Hyperkalemia* (serum K+ levels greater than 5.5 mEq/L) will produce wide P waves and R waves (Fig. 6-22, *A*). The T waves will be tall, narrow and symmetrical. The QT interval will be shortened. As the K+ level rises, intraven-

tricular block may develop, shown by prolongation of the PR interval. As the K+ level continues to increase, QRS complexes will become wide and bizarre, P waves will disappear, and the ST segment will become depressed. As the myocardial activity becomes depressed, changes in the heart rhythm will occur, such as sinus bradycardia, AV blocks, intraventricular conduction defects, escape rhythms, ventricular tachycardia or fibrillation, or asystole.

Hypokalemia

Hypokalemia (below 3.6 mEq/L) will produce changes in the ECG. These are evidenced by a flattened or depressed ST segment and T waves. The U wave will appear, if not present before, or become more prominent, if already present (Fig. 6-22, *B*). The QT interval will become prolonged, and the P waves will become peaked. The lowered potassium levels result in electrical instability associated with supraventricular tachydysrhythmias and frequent premature ventricular beats. Hypokalemia enhances the cardiovascular effects of digitalis on the heart and may produce symptoms of digitalis toxicity. Treatment of this imbalance involves increasing the potassium level in the patient, generally by adding potassium to the IV solution.

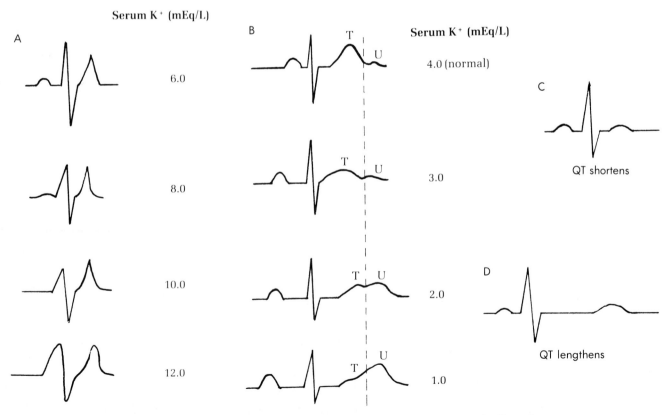

Fig. 6-22   A, Hyperkalemia. **B,** Hypokalemia. **C,** Hypercalcemia. **D,** Hypocalcemia. (From Conover MB: *Pocket guide to electrocardiography,* ed 2, St Louis, 1990, Mosby–Year Book.)

Hypercalcemia

The main function of calcium is to enhance cardiac contractility. *Hypercalcemia* (serum levels greater than 11 mg%) increases myocardial contractility. The ECG changes include shortening of the ST segment or shortening of the QT intervals. The QRS complex will prolong during severe hypercalcemia and AV block may develop (Fig. 6-22, *C*). One important aspect is that high calcium levels oppose the effects of high potassium, and low calcium levels oppose the effects of low potassium. If the calcium varies in direct opposition to the potassium, the effect of the potassium level can be enhanced.

Hypocalcemia

Hypocalcemia (serum levels below 9 mg%) reduces myocardial contractility. As the ECG changes, this produces lengthening or prolongation of the ST segment or QT interval without changing the QRS or T waves, although the T wave may change polarity (Fig 6-22, *D*). Treatment requires returning the calcium level to normal range.

ECG CHANGES WITH MEDICATIONS

Many drugs can effect the ECG. Usually changes are nonspecific, but several commonly used drugs do produce distinct changes. Digitalis and quinidine are two of these drugs.

Since one of the effects of the cardiac drug digitalis is to shorten the repolarization time intervals of the ventricles, the QT interval on the ECG is shortened. Digitalis can also prolong the PR interval because of its effect on the AV node. Digitalis preparations often produce a characteristic scooping of the ST-T complex. This is known as the digitalis effect (Fig. 6-23, *A*). When this occurs, the ST segment and the T wave fuse.

Quinidine, procainamide, and disopyramide are drugs that also effect ECG tracings. These drugs prolong ventricular repolarization. Hence, the QT interval is prolonged and the T wave is flattened (Fig. 6-23, *B*). U waves may also be seen.

ECG CHANGES RESULTING FROM PERICARDITIS AND PERICARDIAL EFFUSION

In response to pericarditis, the ECG reflects an elevated ST segment (Fig. 6-24). Changes can be seen on all leads. This differs from ST segment changes seen with MI that are limited to either the anterior or the inferior leads because of the localized damage. The ECG changes that accompany pericarditis mirror the more generalized involvement of the heart. Pericarditis also affects repolarization of the atria, as seen by depression of the PR segment in limb leads and left chest leads (V_5 and V_6). In acute pericarditis, the PR segment and the ST segment point in different directions.

The ECG change seen most commonly with pericardial effusion is low voltage of the QRS complex. This is probably due to the fluid surrounding the heart.

ECG CHANGES WITH MYOCARDIAL ISCHEMIA

Myocardial ischemia results when the cardiac muscle does not receive as much blood as it needs to function. The major symptom expressed by the patient is pain. Myocardial ischemia (with or without infarction) may be limited to the subendocardial layer of the ventricle. This is because this area is most removed from the blood supply provided by the coronary arteries. The most common ECG change seen with myocardial ischemia is ST segment depression (Fig. 6-25).

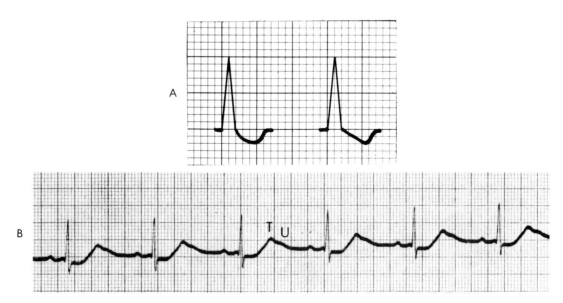

Fig. 6-23 ECG changes with medications. **A,** Digitalis. Note scooping of ST-T changes. **B,** Quinidine. (From Goldberger AL, Goldberger E: *Clinical electrocardiography,* ed 4, St Louis, 1990, Mosby–Year Book.)

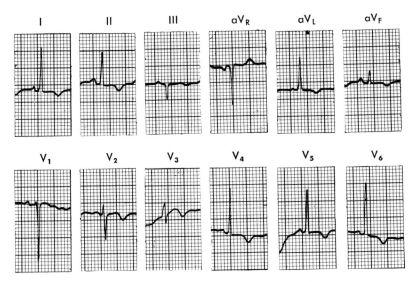

Fig. 6-24 ECG changes resulting from pericarditis. Note changes on all leads. (From Goldberger AL, Goldberger E: *Clinical electrocardiography,* ed 4, St Louis, 1990, Mosby–Year Book.)

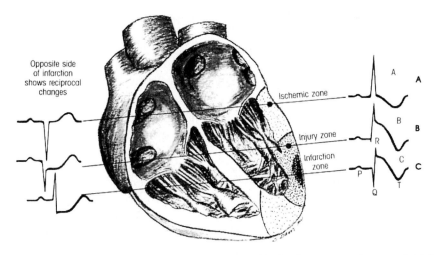

Fig. 6-25 Electrocardiographic alterations associated with the three zones of myocardial infarction. Changes occur in the leads whose positive electrodes face the damaged area. Ischemia results in T wave inversion (from altered tissue repolarization). Injury results in S-T segment elevation (from abnormal repolarization). Infarction/necrosis results in pathologic Q wave (from abnormal depolarization or from scar tissue that cannot depolarize). (From Guzzetta CE, Dossey BM: *Cardiovascular nursing: body-mind tapestry,* St Louis, 1984, Mosby–Year Book.)

ECG CHANGES WITH ANGINA PECTORIS

Angina pectoris is a clinical syndrome of ischemic heart disease. It is manifested by transient attacks of pain in the chest and adjacent areas. Angina is commonly caused by atherosclerosis. The classic attack of angina is characterized by complaints of a dull, boring, burning, pressing, heavy, crushing, or squeezing substernal or retrosternal pressure or pain. Angina is classically precipitated by stress, exertion, exposure to cold, strong emotion, and other such events. It is relieved by nitroglycerin. Anginal pain may radiate to the neck, jaw, teeth, back, both shoulders, arms, elbows, and wrists. Anginal pain tends to radiate to the left, but it may radiate to the right. Patients who develop anginal pain may also show symptoms, such as nausea, vomiting, anxiety, diaphoresis, and shortness of breath. Many (but not all) patients who develop angina may show ECG tracings similar to those of subendocardial ischemia with characteristic ST segment depressions during an attack. Interestingly, when the pain subsides, the ECG returns to the pattern previously demonstrated by the patient (Fig. 6-26).

Many patients with coronary artery disease (CAD) present with a normal ECG at rest. When CAD is suspected, an exercise ECG is frequently performed to confirm or rule out this disease. The stress ECG is recorded while the patient walks a treadmill or pedals a stationary bicycle. This test is anxiety producing for patients who have experienced chest pain on exercise. The stress ECG is stopped when the patient develops angina, fatigue, produces ST changes, or when the patient's heart rate reaches

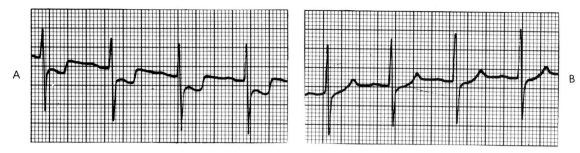

Fig. 6-26 Angina. **A,** During anginal pain episode. Note the ST depression. **B,** 5 minutes after nitroglycerin. Note ST segments have returned to normal. (From Goldberger AL, Goldberger E: *Clinical electrocardiography,* ed 4, St. Louis, 1990, Mosby–Year Book.)

Fig. 6-27 Location of infarction in the ventricular wall. (From Guzzetta CE, Dossey BM: *Cardiovascular nursing: holistic practice,* ed 2, St Louis, 1992, Mosby–Year Book.)

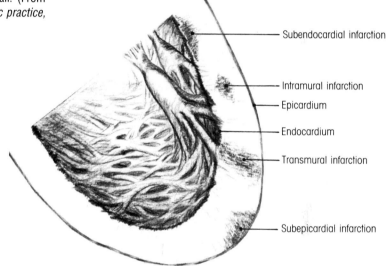

Subendocardial infarction

Intramural infarction

Epicardium

Endocardium

Transmural infarction

Subepicardial infarction

85% to 90% of maximum pulse rate value for the patient's age. The appearance of an ST depression constitutes an abnormal test.

A small group of patients do show ST elevations when experiencing angina. The ST elevations are transient. This atypical angina is known as *Prinzmetal's angina.* It can also be differentiated because anginal pain symptoms frequently occur at night or when the patient is at rest.

MYOCARDIAL INFARCTION

ECG changes that occur with MIs are caused by alterations in ventricular depolarization and repolarization that result from ischemia, injury, or infarction. Each of these events produces different levels of myocardial damage and creates different alterations on the ECG. The infarction zone produces abnormal Q or QS waves. This is because electrical activity cannot occur, since the cells are dead. The zone of injury (see Fig. 6-25) produces ST segments, which are displaced. The ischemic zone produces ECG patterns with symmetrical T-wave inversion.

Types of Infarctions

Myocardial infarctions are classified by the layers of the myocardium that are involved and by the location of the myocardial damage (Fig. 6-27).

Classification by layer

In a *subendocardial infarction* (non Q-wave infarction), the area of necrosis is confined to the subendocardial layer of the heart[12] (see Fig. 6-27). This area of the myocardium is most distant from the blood supply of the coronary arteries. It is also closest to the high pressure of the ventricular cavity. For these reasons, it is especially vulnerable to ischemia. A subendocardial infarction is caused by insufficient coronary blood flow that lasts long enough for necrosis to develop. Tissue damage can be localized, occurring in the area supplied by one coronary artery, or it can be diffuse. When actual subendocardial infarctions occur, several changes can be seen on the ECG (Table 6-2). It generally affects ventricular repolarization (ST-T complex). Fig. 6-28 illustrates an ECG of a subendocardial infarction.

Table 6-2 Classification of MI and ECG Changes

Classification	ECG changes
By layer	
Subendocardial MI (Non-Q-wave infarction)	Q waves do not generally occur. ST segment depressed. T-wave inversion without a QRS complex alteration.
Transmural MI (Q-wave infarction)	Acute phase. ST segment elevations; Tall T waves in some leads sometimes. Evolving phase (occurring in hours or days). Deep T-wave inversions in leads that previously showed ST elevations and pathologic Q waves.
By location	
Anterior wall MI	Q waves seen in V_1, V_2, V_3, possibly V_4, I, and aV_L. ST segment elevation and T wave inversion in leads V_1 to V_4. Reciprocal changes may occur in leads II, III, and aV_F.
Inferior (diaphragmatic) wall MI	Abnormal Q waves, ST segment elevation and T wave inversion can be seen in leads II, III, and aV_F. Reciprocal changes occur in leads V_1 through V_3.
Posterior wall MI	Reciprocal changes are seen in leads V_1 and V_2; these include tall R waves and depressed ST segments. This is because the MI is posterior. T waves are seen in the evolving phase, since the deep T waves appear at the back of the heart.
Lateral wall MI	ST-T changes in leads V_5 and V_6.
Right ventricle MI	Q wave and ST segment elevations in leads II, III, and aV_F. ST elevations in right precordial leads (V_{4R} and V_{6R}). ST-T changes in V_5 and V_6 if lateral infarction present.

An MI that destroys a full thickness of the myocardium is known as a *transmural MI* (see Fig. 6-27). This type of infarction results in changes in both depolarization (an abnormal Q wave lasting 0.04 seconds or one that is deep) and repolarization (ST-T complex). Abnormal Q waves are characteristic markers of transmural myocardial infarctions.

Classification by location

Myocardial infarctions are further described in terms of their location on the left ventricular wall: anterior, inferior, posterior, lateral, apical, anterolateral, and anteroseptal. Presently, right ventricular infarctions are being diagnosed and are felt to be more common than previously expected.

An acute anterior MI involves the anterior wall of the left ventricle (Fig. 6-29, *A*). Anterior MIs account for approximately 25% of all MIs and have a mortality rate of 25%. Patients who experience an anterior MI have more myocardial damage, significantly higher mortality rates, and greater prevalence of congestive heart failure and cardiogenic shock than patients who have MIs located in other areas of the left ventricle. ECG changes for anterior MIs are listed in Table 6-2 and can be seen in Fig. 6-29, *B*.

An inferior MI involves the inferior (diaphragmatic) wall of the left ventricle (Fig. 6-30, *A*). Approximately 17% of all MIs are inferior MIs. The mortality rate is 10%. (See Fig. 6-30, *B* for ECG changes.)

A posterior MI occurs on the back surface of the left ventricle (Fig. 6-31, *A*). True posterior infarctions are relatively rare, occurring only in about 2% of all MIs. Most posterior infarctions occur in conjunction with lateral or inferior infarctions of the left ventricle. The posterior MI may be difficult to diagnose, since the characteristic abnormal ST elevations may not be evident in any of the leads. Instead, a tall R wave and ST segment depression may be seen on leads V_1 and V_2 (reciprocal to the Q wave and ST segment elevations that would be seen at the back of the heart). See Fig. 6-31, *B* for an ECG of a posterior MI. When the posterior MI extends to the lateral wall of the left ventricle, changes can be seen in lead V_6. If the posterior MI extends to the inferior wall, changes will also be seen in leads II, III, and a V_F. When there appears to be an overlap between inferior and posterior infarctions, the more general term, *inferoposterior,* can be used.

Lateral MIs are confined to the lateral wall of the left ventricle. As with the posterior MI, this type is rare, occurring in about 3% of MIs.

An apical MI occurs in the apex of the heart. An anterolateral infarction affects the heart's front lateral side. An anteroseptal MI involves the septum of the heart.

A right ventricular infarction occurs in the right ventricle. About 3% to 8% of all MIs are right ventricular infarctions and occur more often in patients with an inferoposterior infarction. Clinically, patients with right ventricular infarctions present with neck vein distension and elevated central venous pressure. This is because of the abnormally high diastolic filling pressures in the right side of the heart. If damage to the right ventricle is severe, the patient may develop hypotension, bradycardia, and cardiogenic shock. When these clinical findings are present in a patient with an acute inferoposterior MI, one should suspect right ventricular infarction as well. Recognition of a right ventricular infarction is very important, since volume expansion may be necessary in hypotensive patients who have low or normal pulmonary artery wedge pressures in spite of elevated systemic venous pressure (see Fig. 6-32 for ECG changes). *Text continued on p. 135.*

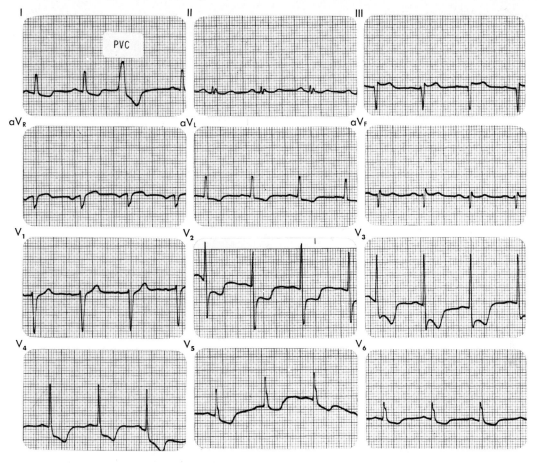

Fig. 6-28 Subendocardial infarction. ST depressions can best be seen in leads V_2 to V_5. A PVC can be seen in lead 1. (From Goldberger AL, Goldberger E: *Clinical electrocardiography,* ed 4, St Louis, 1990, Mosby–Year Book.)

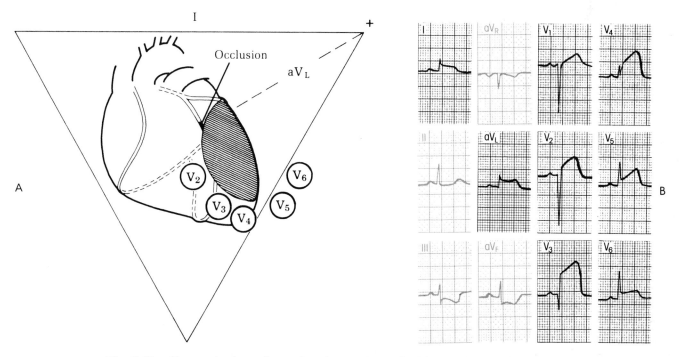

Fig. 6-29 Hyperacute phase of anterolateral acute myocardial infarction. **A,** Darkened area indicates extensive anterior-wall infarct (anterolateral). **B,** Elevated ST segment in 1, aV_L, V_2 to V_6 with diagnostic Q waves in V_1, V_2, and V_3. Reciprocal changes are seen in leads III and aV_F. (Figure from Conover MB: *Understanding electrocardiography,* St Louis, 1984, Mosby–Year Book. ECG from Guzetta CE, Dossey BM: *Cardiovascular nursing: bodymind tapestry,* St Louis, 1984, Mosby–Year Book.)

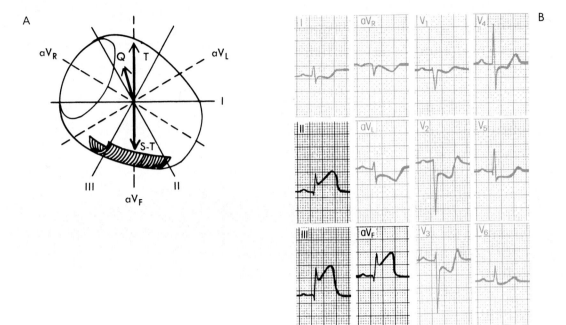

Fig. 6-30 Hyperacute phase of inferior acute myocardial infarction. **A,** Vectors of a diaphragmatic myocardial infarction. The ST vector indicates the injured zone. **B,** ST segment is elevated in leads II, III, and aV$_F$ with Q waves in II, III, and aV$_F$. Reciprocal changes are seen in I, aVL, and V$_1$ to V$_5$. (**A** from Kinney MR, Packa DR, Andreoli KG, et al: *Comprehensive cardiac care,* ed 7, St Louis, 1991, Mosby–Year Book. **B** from Guzzetta CE, Dossey BM: *Cardiovascular nursing: holistic practice,* St Louis, 1992, Mosby–Year Book.)

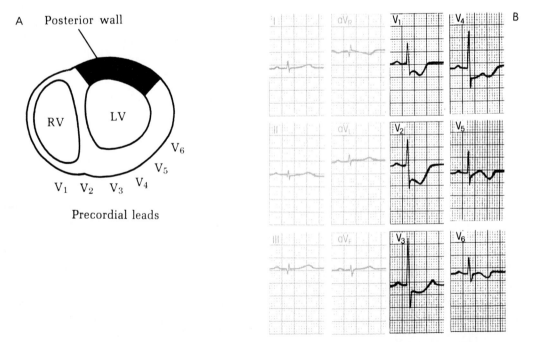

Fig. 6-31 Hyperacute phase of posterolateral acute myocardial infarction, **A,** Darkened area indicates damage to posterior wall. **B,** Increased R waves are seen in V$_1$ and V$_2$ with wider T waves in V$_1$, V$_2$, and V$_3$. (**A** from Conover MB: *Understanding electrocardiography,* ed 4, St Louis, 1984, Mosby–Year Book. **B** from Guzzetta CE, Dossey BM: *Cardiovascular nursing: holistic practice,* St Louis, 1992, Mosby–Year Book.)

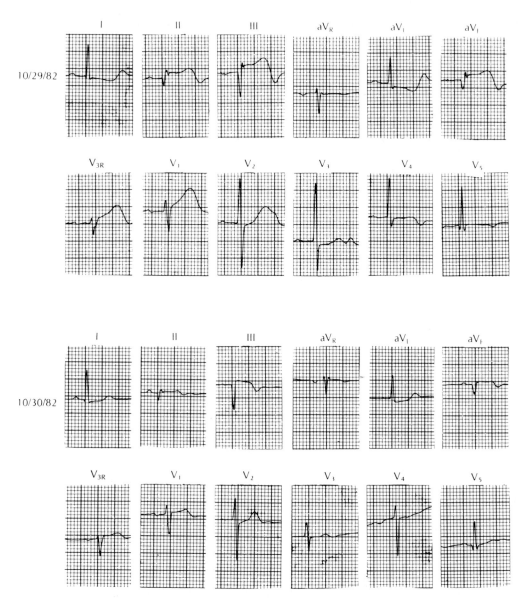

Fig. 6-32   Acute right ventricular infarction. Note Q waves and ST segment elevations in leads II, III and aV$_F$. ST elevations in right precordial leads V$_{3R}$ and V$_I$. ST-T changes in V$_5$ and V$_6$ indicate lateral wall ischemia. (From Goldberger AL, Goldberger E: *Clinical electrocardiography,* ed 4, St Louis, 1990, Mosby–Year Book.)

ECG Changes with Myocardial Infarction

The ECG can be a useful tool in confirming the diagnosis of an MI. The ECG will not always show changes, but if changes are present, it will support the diagnosis. The following three changes occur when the heart is damaged:

* ST segment changes, indicating ischemia.
* T wave changes, indicating an area of injury.
* Q wave changes, indicating necrosis.

The ECG helps to locate the MI area. The heart is divided into topographic regions where infarctions occur. The regions are anterior, producing changes in leads V$_1$, V$_2$, V$_3$; diaphragmatic or inferior, producing changes in leads II, III, aV$_F$; and lateral, producing changes in I, aV$_L$, V$_5$, and V$_6$.

Location of the positive pole when placed over the area of infarction assists in the diagnosis. The posterior position has no positive leads directly over it. Changes in depolarization occur and produce ECG changes on the point anteriorly, away from the site of the infarct.[1] The ECG changes produced in a pure posterior infarct are best seen in leads V$_1$ and V$_2$. The changes will be tall, broad R waves, ST segment depression, and tall, upright T waves.

The changes that occur following an acute myocardial injury include ST segment elevation, reflecting ischemia; greater than 1 mm in the leads over the site of injury; and depression in leads opposite the damaged area. The depression of the ST segment should be greater than 0.5 mm.

These changes are not permanent and will last only about 1 week.

Changes reflecting injury produce T wave inversions over the area of damage and peaks in leads opposite the damaged area. Early in the infarction, the T waves may be peaked over the area of damage. The ischemic changes may be permanent or transient.

The change on the ECG that is most important and the one that will be permanent is that of Q waves. Q waves can normally appear on the ECG and in those leads the Q waves will become more prominent (i.e., V_5, V_6, aV_L, and I; small waves may be present in leads II, III and aV_F; and deep wide Q waves in aV_R and V_1). Normally, the Q wave will be one third the height of the QRS complex and will be one box in width or 0.04 seconds and greater than 4 mm in depth. The appearance of the Q wave in leads where Q waves are not normally present indicates necrosis. Leads that do not usually have Q waves are aV_R, V_1, and V_2. Q waves may appear at the time of damage or within the first several days.

The evolution of an MI occurs in a specific sequence and length of time. Within the first few hours, or *hyperacute state,* ST segment elevation and tall, upright T waves appear in leads over the area of damage. Q waves may appear early or not for several days. The ST segment begins to return to the baseline within several days, but the T wave will progress to inversion. After weeks or months to years, the T wave will become shallow and may return to normal. The Q wave is the one change that will remain as a permanent record of the infarction. Persistent ST segment elevation beyond 6 weeks may be a result of a ventricular aneurysm.[1,2]

PEDIATRIC CONSIDERATIONS
Assessment

The history of infants and children is obtained from the parents. Older children should be consulted and asked to add information. In addition to the child's health history, the mother should be interviewed regarding her prenatal, natal, and postnatal history; health; and family history.

The cardiac assessment is performed while the child is quiet. This may be at the beginning of the assessment or later, depending on the child's level of agitation. The assessment of the infant or scared child can be performed while the child sits on a parent's lap, if the child's condition permits.

The size and growth pattern are probably the most useful indicators of the adequacy of cardiovascular function. The child with heart disease will tend to be undersized and undernourished in appearance. The examiner observes the child's activity pattern for any signs of distress, especially while playing, noting cyanosis, squatting, or sweating.

Much of the assessment of the cardiovascular system described in this chapter is relevant for the assessment of infants and children. There are some cardiac differences that are normal in children, however, that are not normal in adults.

Table 6-3 Variations in Pulse Rate by Age

Age	Average pulse rate (beats/min)
Birth	140
First 30 days	130
1 month to 6 months	130
6 months to 1 year	115
1 to 2 years	110
2 to 4 years	105
5 to 10 years	95
10 to 14 years	85
14 to 18 years	82

The pulse rate varies with age. It is high at birth and slowly decreases in rate until adulthood. See Table 6-3 for average pulse rates. Assessment of all pulses is important, particularly those of the lower extremities. Absence of the femoral pulse may indicate coarctation of the aorta.

During infancy the heart has a larger diameter in relation to the chest than in the adult. The apex is one or two intercostal spaces above that which is considered normal for the adult. The apex is located at the third or fourth intercostal space, just left of the midclavicular line. This changes rapidly as the child grows and is found at the fifth intercostal space by 7 years of age. The PMI will depend on the child's age.

Palpation of the child's chest wall can give the examiner more information than palpation of an adult's chest wall because of the thinner chest structure. The blood vessels of the child are soft and pliable when palpated.

Auscultation of the heart should be performed using both the bell and the diaphragm of the stethoscope while the child is sitting up and lying down. The first (S_1) and second (S_2) heart sounds should be clearly audible. S_1 is usually heard best over the fifth intercostal space and S_2 at the second intercostal space. The S_2 is frequently split during inspiration. Transient murmurs may be heard in neonates during the first 48 hours after birth from late closure of the foramen ovale or the ductus arteriosus. The third heart sound (S_3) may be heard in the preschool and school-aged child. This is normal in children and can be heard best at the apex of the heart. Innocent murmurs are usually located in the pulmonic area and can recur in as many as 50% of normal children. Innocent murmurs are characteristically systolic in timing, are grade 1 or 2 in intensity, and are not transmitted to other areas. They are loudest when the child is reclining and may not be audible when the child sits up. It is difficult to determine if a murmur is innocent or not, but a murmur of grade 3 or louder generally indicates pathology.

A venous hum is commonly heard in children. It is characterized by a continuous, high-pitched sound that originates in the internal jugular vein. It is auscultated either above or below the clavicles. It is more pronounced when the child is sitting and disappears when the child reclines.

ECG

The normal ECG of the newborn and the infant resembles a pattern of right ventricular hypertrophy.[17] The PR interval is 0.10 to 0.25 second in infants and 0.13 to 0.18 in children. Tall R waves can be seen in the right chest leads and the right axis deviation. Notching of the T wave is common. Until the child is about 10 years old, T waves in the right to middle chest leads are normally inverted.[17] If this continues throughout the teen years and into adulthood, this is called the juvenile T wave variant. Another normal variant that can be seen is the tall voltage in the chest leads.

Monitoring

Most monitoring systems for children use only three leads with no lead selection. Therefore leads should be placed to record maximal potential changes originating in the heart. Electrodes should be placed at the right upper lateral chest wall below the clavicle and the left lower chest wall in the anterior axillary line below the PMI. The ground electrode is placed on the upper left chest wall.

Many infants and children are monitored using a cardiorespiratory monitor. The tracing is displayed on a visual screen with the child's respiratory pattern as well.

PSYCHOSOCIAL CONSIDERATIONS

Patients with conduction disturbances may experience a flood of emotions related to fears about their health status and its implications for future role performance. A life-threatening event, such as a MI, requires a major emotional adjustment towards the goal of regaining control. That process can be divided into the following four stages:
1) Defending oneself/denial by minimizing the seriousness of the situation.
2) Acknowledgement of the event, characterized by an effort to understand and come to terms with it.
3) Learning to live, during which the patients attempt to establish guidelines for living and to regain a sense of trust in their abilities.
4) Living again, the stage in which patients place the MI event behind them and allow other aspects of their lives to take precedence.

Patients must be allowed to verbalize their concerns and should be helped by the nurse to identify and fully use their coping resources. Patients in the early stages of adjustment will often hide their fears and anxieties, so the nurse must display qualities of compassion, competency, and caring.

PATIENT AND FAMILY TEACHING

Patient teaching for ECG enables the patient to understand what is happening and to cooperate with the procedure. The patient needs to know that the ECG reflects the activity of the heart and will not hurt them. Teaching should also address fears of electrocution. The patient must be instructed to remain at rest during the ECG and not to talk, since body movement may result in an erratic ECG tracing.

HOME HEALTH CARE CONSIDERATIONS

The Holter monitor is an ECG recorder that records a continuous ECG over a 24-hour (or longer) period of time. The recorder is about the size of a small tape player, weighing about 19 ounces (532 gm). Leads are attached using a 5-chest lead system. The patient wears the recorder as he or she maintains usual activities of daily living. This type of recording is useful to evaluate cardiac dysrhythmias that occur intermittently and that have not been assessed.

The patient is asked to maintain a log to record times, medications, activities (e.g., walking, stair climbing, sleeping, urinating, sexual activities, emotional upset, or physical symptoms), and related cardiac symptoms so that these events can be integrated and correlated with the tape from the Holter monitor.

The Holter monitor can be used to track the effectiveness of a pacemaker, to monitor the patient on cardiac drugs, to monitor the patient with an MI, or to track chest pain.

REFERENCES

1. Abels L: *Critical care nursing,* St. Louis, 1986, Mosby–Year Book.
2. Andreoli KG, Zipes DP, Wallace AG, et al: *Comprehensive cardiac care,* ed 6, St. Louis, 1987, Mosby–Year Book.
3. Bates B: *A guide to physical assessment,* Philadelphia, 1987, JB Lippincott.
4. Catalano T: SA Wenckebach, *Crit Care Nurse* 10(10):16-21, 1990.
5. Conover MA: *Understanding electrocardiography: arrhythmias and the 12-lead ECG,* ed 6, St. Louis, 1992, Mosby–Year Book.
6. DeAngelis R: Hypocalcemia, *Crit Care Nurse* 11(7):71, 1991.
7. Drew BJ: Using cardiac leads the right way, *Nurs '92* 22(5):50, 1992.
8. Elder AN: Setting up and using a cardiac monitor, *Nurs '91* 21(3):58-63, 1991.
9. Goldberger AL, Goldberger E: *Clinical electrocardiography: a simplified approach,* ed 4, St. Louis, 1990, Mosby–Year Book.
10. Johnson JL: Morse JM: Regaining control: the process of adjustment after acute myocardial infarction, *Heart Lung* 19(2):126, 1990.
11. Knapik ML: Determination of electrical axis deviation, *Crit Care Nurse* 10(6):57-63, 1990.
12. Lefor N, Cardello FP, Felicetta JV: Recognizing and treating Torsade des Pointes, *Crit Care Nurse* 12(5):23, 1992.
13. McMillan JV, Little-Longeway CD: Right ventricular infarction, *Focus Crit Care* 18(2):158, 1991.
14. Scalzo T: Managing the patient on remote telemetry, *Nurs '92* 22(3):57, 1992.
15. Schactman M, Greene JS: Signal-averaged electrocardiography: A technique for determining which patients may be at risk for sudden cardiac death, *Focus Crit Care* 18(3):202, 1992.
16. Snowberger P: Premature atrial contractions, *RN* 54(6):38, 1991.
17. Snowberger P: Wandering atrial pacemaker, *RN* 54(9):37, 1991.
18. Thelan LA, Davie JK, Urden LD: *Textbook of critical care nursing,* St Louis, Mosby–Year Book, 1990.

CHAPTER 7

Pacemakers

Objectives

After completing this chapter, the reader will be able to:

- Identify components of the conduction system.
- Describe the relationship of heart rate and stroke volume.
- Describe the hemodynamic benefits of dual-chamber pacing.
- Identify the primary indications for pacing.
- Define pacemaker functions—pacing, sensing, and capture.
- Discuss three contraindications for temporary external pacing.
- Explain the significance of pacing thresholds.
- Identify the complications of pacing.
- Discuss pediatric considerations.
- Describe the telephone pacemaker check.

Cardiac pacing is the delivery of an electrical stimulus to the heart to initiate a contraction. In 1906, Einthoven recorded the first tracing of complete heart block. From this and other early investigations, the concept of cardiac pacing to treat heart block evolved. Today pacing technology has been incorporated as a standard treatment for patients with conduction defects requiring short-term temporary pacing or long-term permanent pacing (see Chapters 6 and 8 for discussion of the conduction system and cardiac hemodynamics).

THE ARTIFICIAL PACEMAKER SYSTEM

A pacemaker system works using the principles of electricity. To function, a power source (generator or pacemaker), a means of delivery (leads), a recipient of the current (patient's heart), and an intact circuit are required. The lead is an insulated conductive wire with two electrodes, one positive (the anode) and one negative (the cathode). The lead makes a conductive pathway from the generator to the heart and back to the generator completing the circuit.

Temporary and permanent pacemaker systems work in the same way, but there are two major differences—duration of use and access to the controls. Temporary systems use an external device to control pacing; with permanent pacing the controls are implanted under the skin and an external device is required to change settings. The device that changes pacemaker parameters is called a *programmer.*

The generator houses the battery and controls for regulation. The power from the battery is referred to as *current.*

The second part of the system is the lead wire, constructed to transmit the current. There are two ways to describe a lead—by the method of insertion and the configuration of the lead. The method of insertion indicates if the lead is passed through a vein (transvenous or endocardial) or transcutaneously (transthoracic or epicardial). A transvenous insertion threads the lead through a vein (usually the cephalic), until it rests against the endocardial wall of the heart. It is passed into the heart until it reaches the apex of the right ventricle. A transthoracic lead is passed through the skin or an incision in the chest wall until it is secured to the outer surface of the left ventricle. The method of insertion is determined by the patient's condition, contraindications to one of the approaches, and the choice of the physician.

Configuration of the lead refers to the placement of the electrodes. There are two types of leads—bipolar and unipolar. A bipolar lead has both the positive and negative electrode at the tip of the wire inside the heart. The positive electrode is a few centimeters back from the tip of the lead and is referred to as a *ring electrode,* and the negative electrode is at the tip of the lead. The unipolar lead has the generator as the positive electrode located outside the heart, and the negative electrode is at the tip of the wire inside the heart. Choice of lead depends on the physician's preference. The system is completed when the lead interfaces with the endocardial surface of the heart to deliver the stimulus.

The Intersociety Commission on Heart Disease (ICHD) (now referred to as [NBG]) had previously developed a coding system for temporary and permanent pacing. It is now referred to as the North American Society of Pacing and Electrophysiology code. By using the code, one can differentiate a single-chamber (Table 7-1) versus a dual-chamber (Table 7-2) pacemaker and identify what chambers of the heart will be affected by the pacemaker. The first letter of the code refers to the cardiac chamber that is paced. The second letter designates which chamber is sensed. The third letter indicates the response to the sensed event. For example, the code VVI on Table 7-1 signifies the following:

1. Electrical current is being delivered to the ventricle (i.e., the ventricle is being paced).
2. The intrinsic activity of the ventricle is being sensed by the pacemaker.
3. The pacemaker response is inhibited by the patient's natural heartbeats.

A single-chamber (SC) pacemaker has only one lead inserted into the heart. The lead may be either in the atrium or the ventricle to pace that chamber. SC pacemakers are simple in design and easy to assess for proper function. Single-atrial chamber pacing depends on an intact AV nodal system to assure ventricular depolarization after a pacing stimulus. Single-ventricular chamber devices pace the ventricles but cannot coordinate pacing with the patient's intrinsic atrial rate. The result is AV asynchrony. A dual-chamber (DC) pacemaker has a two-lead system. One lead is placed in the atrium, and the other is placed in the

Table 7-1 NBG Pacing Codes–Single-Chamber

Code	Chambers paced*	Chambers sensed	Pacemaker response mode
AAI	A	A	Inhibited
VVI	V	V	Inhibited
VVT	V IHR/PHR	V	Triggered
AOO/VOO	A	None	Asynchronous

*IHR, Intrinsic heart rate; PHR, pacing heart rate.

Table 7-2 NBG Pacing Codes–Dual Chamber

Code*	Chambers paced	Chambers sensed	Pacemaker response mode
VVD	V	A and V	A triggered/V inhibited
DVI	A and A/V	V	Inhibited
DDD	A, V, and A/V	A and V	A triggered/V inhibited
DOO	A/V	None	Asynchronous

*D, double; O, none.

Table 7-3 Cardiac Pacing Identified by Duration, Method, and Chamber Paced

Duration	Method	Chamber
Short-term (1-18 hrs)	Transcutaneous	Atrium/ventricle
Short-term (3-7 days)	Transvenous	Atrium
		Ventricle
		Atrium/ventricle
Short-term (3-7 days)	Transthoracic	Atrium
		Ventricle
		Atrium/ventricle
Long-term (lifetime)	Single chamber (transvenous or epicaridal	Atrium
		Ventricle
Long-term (lifetime)	Dual chamber (transvenous or epicaridal)	Atrium/ventricle

ventricle to maintain AV synchrony (synchronous contraction of the atrium and then the ventricle). This is also known as *physiological pacing.*

If the pacemaker is an SC device, the pacing occurs immediately and a pacemaker spike is seen on the ECG. The DC system is different. In DC pacing, a triggered mode senses atrial activity but paces the ventricle after a predetermined period of time. The time period is called the *AV delay* and represents the same time interval as the PR interval. Another name for this is *tracking.*

The code is helpful in learning how the paced ECG with each system looks. It provides an organized approach to analysis of the paced ECG. Another use of the code is in teaching patients about their system. If patients do not have their identification cards or know much about their pacemakers, they can at least provide the code information to health care providers. Table 7-3 summarizes the pacing methods discussed by duration of pacing, method of pacing, and the chambers paced.

Indications for Artificial Cardiac Pacing

The indications for temporary external pacing (TEP) and for the temporary transvenous pacemaker (TPM) can be found in the upper box on p. 140. Presently, the external method of pacing is most often used for pacing less than 18 hours, in emergency situations, and when the need for pacing occurs because of a medical procedure. Regardless of the rhythm or method of initiating pacing, the final determinants in selecting pacing include the following:

- Prevention of a catastrophic event.
- Stability of the patient.
- Access to the technology.
- Location of the event.
- Physician's preference.

The indications for permanent pacing include the persistence of the problem, the affect on hemodynamics, and the probability of increasing severity of the problem. If doubt exists, an electrophysiology study (EPS) permits an indepth analysis of the patient's conduction system and aids in determining the need for long-term pacing. An EPS is performed by inserting specialized catheters for multiple-site pacing and recording electroconduction from inside the heart. The standard 12-lead ECG recording and symptoms provide additional information.

Indications for permanent pacemaker implantation can be divided into three classes. The Class I indications are the most significant and most often seen. Class II indications require extensive documentation. Class III are usually not indications for implantation of a pacemaker. Class I indications for permanent pacing include seven groups of patients. Each group has been subdivided into categories to correspond to a more specific final diagnosis (see box on p. 140).

ELECTRICAL SAFETY

An electrical accident is an event that occurs in the clinical environment involving electrical current creating a negative patient outcome; (e.g., the application of suffi-

▼ **Indications for Temporary Pacemakers**

TEMPORARY EXTERNAL PACING

Asystolic arrest
Bradycardia
Ventricular asystole
Support for insertion of a temporary wire
Management of high-risk patients (e.g., cardiac catheterization)
Emergency transport
Support during insertion of permanent pacemaker
Standby for loss of capture with a temporary system or during administration of cardioactive drugs

TEMPORARY TRANSVENOUS PACING

Acute myocardial infarction (MI) (Mobitz II AV block, complete heart block [CHB], bilateral bundle branch block)
Cardiac arrest
Bradydysrhythmias with decreased cardiac output (CO) or syncope
Second-and third-degree AV block
Hemiblocks with symptoms (right bundle branch block [RBBB] with left anterior hemiblock [LAH], RBBB with left posterior hemiblock [LPH], left bundle branch block [LBBB] with first-degree AV block, and alternating BBB)
Control ectopy with bradydysrhythmias
Overdrive suppression of tachydysrhythmias
Inhibition of a permanent pacemaker (PPM)
Maintain heart rate in presence of failing PPM
Diagnostic testing (e.g., stress test, sinus node recovery time, electrophysiology)
Cardiac surgery
Cardiac catheterization or pressure monitoring
Congestive heart failure (CHF)
Trial with cerebral insufficiency to improve blood flow
Standby during treatment of tachydysrhythmias

▼ **Class I Indications for Permanent Pacing[9,11]**

GROUP I—ACQUIRED AV BLOCK IN ADULTS

- Permanent or intermittent complete heart block (CHB).
- Permanent or intermittent second-degree atrioventricular (AV) block.
- AV block with atrial fibrillation, flutter, or supraventricular tachycardia (SVT).

GROUP II—AV BLOCK WITH MYOCARDIAL INFARCTION

- Persistent or advanced AV block or CHB (decision made before discharge).

GROUP III—BIFASCICULAR AND TRIFASCICULAR BLOCK (CHRONIC)

- Bifascicular with intermittent CHB (associated with symptomatic bradycardia).
- Bifascicular with intermittent second-degree AV block (with symptoms).

GROUP IV—SINUS NODE DYSFUNCTION (SYMPTOMS CORRELATE WITH DYSRHYTHMIA)

- Sick sinus syndrome.
- Sinus bradycardia with symptoms.
- Bradycardia-tachycardia syndrome.

GROUP V—HYPERSENSITIVE CAROTID SINUS SYNDROME

- Recurrent syncope associated with carotid sinus stimulation (> 3 sec pause).

GROUP VI—PACEMAKERS IN CHILDREN

GROUP VII—PACING FOR TACHYDYSRHYTHMIAS

- Symptomatic SVT.
- Symptomatic ventricular tachycardia

cient electrical current directly to the heart, resulting in ventricular fibrillation). Normally, the patient and personnel in the hospital have the skin as natural protection from electrical accidents. Intact skin acts as a high-resistance barrier to conduction of electrical currents to the vital organs of the body.[16,24] The insertion of pacing wires breaks the protective skin barrier and creates a low resistance pathway directly to the heart causing the patient to be electrically sensitive.

Placement of various types of electrical equipment in the clinical environment is another source of concern. During operation of equipment, electrical current is being drawn from a power source, through an electrical pathway, and back to the source or through a ground.[15] The *ground* in a system is a means of providing a planned, low-resistance path for current to be safely directed back to the earth. Electricity always takes the path of least resistance to the earth. However, the system does not recover all of the current, creating leakage current. Nurses may inadvertently place themselves in the circuit by simultaneously touching the electrical equipment and the pacing wire, thereby acting as an alternate path for the current and directing it down the pacing wire.

The degree of electrical hazard is determined by the amount of leakage current conducted to the patient. The current delivered directly to the heart is called a *microshock*. Ventricular fibrillation occurs with the delivery of less than 1 mA (1000 microamperes) directly to the heart. In contrast, 1 mA delivered to the skin results in a tingling sensation because it is at the threshold of pain perception.[24] The magnitude of a possible electrical accident makes electrical safety a primary responsibility of the nurse during care of the pacemaker patient (see box on p. 141).

▼ **Electrical Safety Precautions**

PACEMAKER

Insert a new battery before each use of the pacemaker.
Maintain a log of generator use.
Keep the faceplate cover over the generator controls.
Do not change the battery with the unit in operation.
Wear rubber gloves when handling the pacing wire.
Discharge stray current on a metal surface before approaching the patient.
Do not allow contact of both extensions of the pacing wire.
Cover all exposed parts of the pacing wire with a rubber glove.
Use a battery-operated ECG machine to record intracardiac electrograms (ICEs) and ECGs.
Do not simultaneously touch electrical equipment and the pacing wire.

ENVIRONMENT

Minimize use of additional line-powered equipment.
Disconnect electric beds.
Turn line-operated equipment off before disconnecting from an outlet.
Disconnect the patient cable from monitor before turning it on or off.
Do not use remote outlets to service equipment on the patient.
Keep the patient and area dry.
Do not touch electrical equipment with wet hands.
Monitor room humidity. Keep at 50% to 60% to decrease static electricity.
Minimize use of patient-owned equipment. Develop a patient handout about the use of home equipment.
Report sockets that do not hold plugs securely.
Know source of emergency power.
Do not use cheaters or extension cords.
Do not permit temporary or makeshift equipment repairs.

EQUIPMENT

Test all new equipment before use.
Check inspection tags on equipment in use.
Use only properly grounded equipment—three-prong plugs.
Use only hospital-grade power cords.
Inspect strain relief on equipment power cords.
Do not step on plugs or line cores.
Do not unplug equipment by pulling the cord from the outlet.
Do not use damaged equipment.
Report all complaints of shocks or tingling sensations from equipment.
Unplug equipment giving off warning signs.
Report all equipment that has been dropped.
Do not tolerate any deviations from the expected performance of the equipment (e.g., poor tracing on the screen).

PATIENT[14]

Remove excess gel.
Keep bed linens dry.
Monitor tracing on-screen for quality.
Maintain equipment.

The electrical safety consideration for TEP and TPM vary. The noninvasive TEP eliminates a direct electrical pathway to the heart because the procedure requires the application of electrodes to the chest. A conductive gel is used to decrease the amount of resistance between the electrodes and the skin. If excessive gel is used, the potential for skin burns is increased. The risk for burns also increases if it is necessary to defibrillate the patient during an episode of pacing.

ASSESSMENT

The patient who has been admitted to the hospital with a conduction disturbance requires a thorough assessment. The assessment data defines the physical and psychosocial status of the patient and the response to the dysrhythmia. This information helps identify the factors contributing to the conduction problem and helps determine the effect of the dysrhythmia on hemodynamic measurements (Skill 7-1).

NURSING DIAGNOSIS

Sample nursing diagnoses for the patient who requires artificial pacing include the following:

- Ineffective breathing pattern related to chest contractions with temporary external pacing (TEP).
- High risk for injury related to pacemaker malfunction.
- Noncompliance related to impaired ability to comprehend instructions.
- Noncompliance related to previous unsatisfactory responses to treatment.
- Ineffective coping associated with knowledge deficit secondary to pacemaker implantation.
- Anxiety related to a perceived threat of requiring a pacemaker.
- Activity intolerance related to decreased CO secondary to bradydysrhythmia.
- Powerlessness related to dependency on a permanent pacemaker.
- Depression related to perceived inability to work secondary to permanent pacemaker.
- Disturbance in self-concept related to body image changes secondary to pacemaker implant.

PATIENT OUTCOMES

Possible outcomes for patients requiring artificial pacing include the following:

Before discharge the pacemaker patient:

- Evidences the following:

    Heart rate greater than or equal to the lowest rate set for pacing; the usual rate is 50 to 70 beats/min in either the SC or DC system.

    Regular heart sounds when in sinus rhythm and reversed or paradoxical split S_2 when ventricular paced. The split sound occurs because with right ventricular pacing conduction is the same as with a left bundle branch block (LBBB). The heart sounds must also be easily heard to rule out tamponade.

Skill 7-1 Assessing the Patient with Conduction Disturbance

EQUIPMENT AND SUPPLIES

- Stethoscope
- Watch
- Chart
- ECG
- Monitor

NURSING INTERVENTIONS

1. Obtain a family and medical history (see Chapter 6).
2. Obtain chief complaint and ask the following questions to establish cardiac function:
   - What are your recent physical complaints?
   - Do you experience fainting, dizziness, memory loss, palpitations, chest pain, fatigue, or difficulties in breathing?
   - What are your symptoms? When do they occur? Location? Duration? Cause and relief?
   - Can you participate in self-care and normal daily activities?
   - Describe alterations in activities of daily living that occurred as a result of your health problems.
   - How do you cope with your problem?
   - How do you manage your leisure time, job responsibilities, family activities, and family role?
3. Obtain a hemodynamic history by asking the following questions:
   - What is your response to your dysrhythmia? (Use words patient can understand.)
   - How does the dysrhythmia affect normal ability?
   - How are you compensating for the deficiency?
4. Assess pulse for rate and rhythm. Monitor blood pressure.
5. Compare the patient's heart rate and blood pressure with available baseline measures.
6. Obtain pulse pressure and mean blood pressure. (Determine the pulse pressure by subtracting the diastolic blood pressure from the systolic blood pressure.) The pulse pressure is indicative of stroke volume. Wide pulse pressure indicates increased stroke volume. The mean pressure, indicative of afterload or the resistance the heart must overcome to pump the blood, is obtained by taking one third the pulse pressure plus the diastolic pressure. When the mean pressure is above normal, the heart has an increased workload, further decompensating the cardiovascular system.
7. Obtain other baseline data (e.g., ECG, arterial blood gases [ABGs], electrolytes, coagulation studies, drug levels, and complete blood count [CBC]).
8. Auscultate the heart sounds. Deviations from normal with the various degrees of heart block and BBBs can be found in Table 7-4.
9. Determine whether coexisting problems are present that may have a potential to affect the patient once the pacemaker is implanted. CHF, preexisting BBBs, structural heart defects, hypertension (HTN), and neurological defects are of particular importance.
10. Complete the general assessment of the remaining systems.
11. Record data.

Table 7-4 Heart Sounds with Heart Blocks

Degree of block	Heart sound
First	Decreased intensity in the S_1
Mobitz I	Cyclic decrease in the S_1 intensity
Mobitz II	S_1 uniform
CHB	Marked variation in the S_1 intensity
	Explosive S_1 with short PR interval (bruit de canon)
	S_2 according to escape pacemaker
LBBB	Paradoxical split in the S_2
RBBB	Wide split in the S_2

ECG or Holter monitor recording of normal pacemaker function.

Stable blood pressure between 90/60 and 140/90, unless the patient is usually hypertensive.

Temperature between 36° and 38° C (97° and 100.5° F) for 24 hours.

Bilateral clear and equal breath sounds.

Respiratory rate between 12 to 20 breaths/min.

Normal chest x-ray with no evidence of congestion; the lungs are fully expanded and heart within normal size for the individual patient. (Previous enlargement may be present.)

- Displays a clean, dry pacemaker incision site of minimal swelling, slight ecchymosis, and normal warmth.
- Performs range of motion in extremity nearest pacemaker site, limited to elevation of the arm to shoulder height in front and lateral motion to the side. The patient is not to extend the arm over the head or complete any backward motion. This limited range of motion protects the implant site, prevents bleeding, and prevents a frozen shoulder related to prolonged immobility and prevents lead displacement.
- Operates the transtelephonic monitoring equipment correctly, if appropriate.
- Reports signs and symptoms of complications to the physician.
- Identifies potentially hazardous situations in the environment that might affect the pacemaker.
- Expresses confidence in ability to perform role-related responsibilities.
- States date of the first pacemaker clinic visit.

TEMPORARY PACING MODES

Temporary pacing supports and enhances cardiac output by increasing heart rate and in some cases maintaining synchrony between the atrial and ventricular contractions. Temporary pacing can be accomplished using a fixed rate (pacing at the set rate regardless of patient's own rhythm), inhibited mode (pacing is suppressed by the patient's own rhythm), or triggered mode (an event [sensed] by the pacemaker controls the pacing).

▼ Guidelines for Care of the Patient with a Temporary Pacemaker[3,6]

After insertion of the temporary pacemaker, the nurse should do the following:

- Provide emotional support for the patient and family members to include patient teaching, stress-management techniques, and listening.
- Monitor the patient's hemodynamic status, response to the pacemaker, status of the underlying rhythm from monitor tracings, insertion site, vital signs including temperature, and symptoms.
- Assess heart sounds after insertion for complications. Changes in heart sounds occurring after insertion of a pacing wire include presystolic clicks related to diaphragmatic or intercostal muscle stimulation, systolic clicks and murmurs related to movement of the catheter in the ventricle, tricuspid insufficiency related to the catheter, and friction rubs related to contact of the catheter with the wall of the ventricle or with perforations.[17] Also, during the pacing episodes, there is the paradoxical splitting of S_2.
- Monitor function of the pacemaker. Select a monitor lead to detect the QRS and pacing spike (see ECG chapter), record 12-lead ECGs as ordered by the physician, check pacemaker settings each shift, note new ectopy that may be caused by the pacemaker lead in the heart, use the status indicator on the generator, check connections each shift, and record thresholds daily. Ordinarily it is the physician's responsibility to check daily thresholds.
- Initiate safety measures to prevent complications and system malfunctions. Document preinsertion safety checks and post safety signs by the patient's room to notify other health care staff of the temporary pacemaker in operation, perform the shift and daily connection checks, keep side rails up, secure position of the arm to prevent lead displacement, and transport patient only if absolutely necessary. (ECG monitoring is mandatory when transporting the patient.)
- In case of defibrillation, turn off the generator and disconnect the lead from the generator if time permits, place the paddles so the current vector from the defibrillator is perpendicular to the sensing vector of the pacemaker, use as low a current as possible (start with 200 J), and monitor closely after defibrillation for 100% capture. Recheck thresholds 24 hours after defibrillation.
- Identify and intervene in pacing complications.
- Prepare a plan of care for the patient using the nursing process identified earlier in the chapter.
- Prepare the patient for insertion of a permanent pacemaker, if required.

Temporary Transcutaneous Pacing

Transcutaneous pacing is a noninvasive pacing technique that functions by placing electrodes on the patient's chest and delivering sufficient current (mA) through the skin to initiate cardiac contraction. This form of pacing is also referred to as *noninvasive pacing* or *temporary external pacing (TEP)*. TEP is the first line of defense for a patient in hemodynamic distress from a bradydysrhythmia.

TEP simultaneously activates the atrium and ventricle, resulting in a significant decrease in mean arterial pressure and systemic vascular resistance. The hemodynamic response is better cardiac perfusion and a decrease in workload.

Contraindications for TEP include the following:
- Chest trauma.
- Flail chest.
- Cervical spine injury.
- Weight < 30 kg (66 lbs) unless a pediatric application is available.
- Heart rate > 40 beats/min unless the cardiac output is severely depressed.

Complications with TEP are usually limited to inability to capture, interference with sensing because of muscle contractions or patient agitation, sharp pain or burning sensation with pacing, skin burns or electrical microshock, and coughing.[25,29]

Conditions exist that affect the current requirements for pacing (pacing threshold). Patients with dilated cardiomyopathy, chronic obstructive lung disease, obesity, hypoxia, or metabolic acidosis may not achieve pacing because of the extremely high current thresholds required.[25] This occurs when the amount of current required exceeds the capabilities of the device (maximum 200 mA) or levels that will not be tolerated by the patient. The desired current level is less than 40 mA. A range of 40 to 90 mA produces chest discomfort. Current levels greater than 90 mA result in pain and chest contractions interfering with respirations. A few patients can tolerate up to 120 mA. See Table 7-5 for patient responses to the amount of electrical current used.[14,23] It is important to differentiate between the current required to pace and the amount of current that results in pain.

Temporary Transvenous and Transthoracic Pacing

In temporary transvenous pacing, the pacing wire is passed through a vein to the apex of the right ventricle or atrium (Fig. 7-1). Insertion sites include the antecubital, brachial, subclavian, internal jugular, or femoral vein. Access to the vein is obtained by venous cutdown or percutaneous puncture. A guide, referred to as an introducer, is inserted into the puncture site to facilitate passage.

The transthoracic approach is more direct but has a higher complication rate. A needle is directed to the right ventricle using the subxiphoid or parasternal approach. In the subxiphoid approach a puncture is made in the space between the left xiphoid edge and the left costal margin. The parasternal approach consists of a puncture in the fourth or fifth intercostal space above the lower rib and near the sternum.[21] Caution must be used to avoid puncture of the internal mammary artery or the lung. The transthoracic approach is not the method of choice except in an extreme emergency. This is most often seen in a surgical ICU for patients undergoing heart surgery.[4]

Before insertion of the temporary pacemaker, the pa-

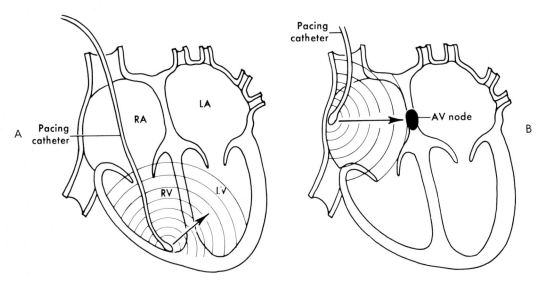

Fig. 7-1 **A,** Ventricular pacing. Impulses are initiated in ventricle. **B,** Atrial pacing. Impulses are initiated in atrium and travel to ventricles by normal conduction system. (From Phipps WJ, Long BC, Woods NF, et al: *Medical-surgical nursing: concepts and clinical practice,* ed 4, St Louis, 1991, Mosby–Year Book.)

tient must sign an informed consent. If the patient is unable to do so, permission may be obtained from a member of the family. During the insertion procedure, the nurse must be prepared to assist with changing the access approach from percutaneous to cutdown. This may be necessary if complications occur.

Complications related to temporary cardiac pacing are relatively low. The complications of temporary cardiac pacing are divided into electrical accidents, patient problems, and system problems. Electrical accidents require preventive measures and compliance with the recommendations for electrical management of the pacemaker patient. Patient problems include the following:

- Extracardiac stimulation (e.g., chest wall and diaphragm).
- Right ventricular perforation with or without tamponade.
- Bleeding.
- Bacteremia.
- Insertion site hematoma.
- Infections at insertion site or systemic infections.
- Thrombophlebitis.
- Dysrhythmias.
- Pneumothorax.
- Twidler's syndrome.
- Emboli.

System problems usually involve the generator, the lead, or the lead/patient interface. The nurse must assess the rhythm strips to identify system problems. Table 7-6 gives tips for troubleshooting. *Failure to pace* is noted when the pacemaker spike is not evident on the ECG.

Capture is the response of the heart to pacing stimuli, an atrial contraction, a ventricular contraction, or both. *Failure to capture* is the inability of the stimulus to depolarize the heart; either the P wave with the atrial spike or the QRS complex with the ventricular spike is not recorded. This problem may also be intermittent or continuous and is life threatening to a patient with minimal or no underlying heart rhythm when occurring with the ventricular output. Failure to capture warrants immediate attention.

Sensing variations are *failure to sense* (the pacemaker does not identify the patient's intrinsic rhythm) or *oversensing* (the pacemaker responds to signals other than the patient's intrinsic rhythm). The sensing variations may be intermittent or continuous. Some interventions require the physician. Under those circumstances, the nurse is to prepare the patient and equipment (see box on p. 143 for Guidelines for Care of the Patient with a Temporary Pacemaker).

Table 7-5 Patient Responses to Current with Transcutaneous Pacing

Output mA*	Response
20	Prickly sensation on skin
30	Slight thump on chest
40	Definite thump on chest
50	Coughing
60	Diaphragm pacing and coughing
70	Coughing and knock on chest
80	More uncomfortable than 70 mA
90	Strong, painful knock on chest
100	Leaves bed because of pain

*Responses noted with the Z011-NTP unit.

<u>**Skill 7-2**</u>   **Application of a Transcutaneous Pacemaker**

EQUIPMENT AND SUPPLIES

- Cardiac monitor
- Noninvasive pacemaker
- External adhesive pacing electrodes
- External pacing cable
- ECG electrodes
- Pulse sensor
- ECG recording paper
- Skin preparation
- Code cart
- Defibrillator
- Pain medication, as ordered
- Respiratory support (oxygen and ventilator)
- Pulse oximeter
  (Variations in equipment and supplies occur, depending on the device in use.)

NURSING INTERVENTIONS[4,6,25,36]

1. Obtain written informed consent. Permit nothing by mouth. Remove artificial devices, such as glasses, teeth, or contact lenses for patient safety.
2. Inform patient of procedure. Advise the patient of muscle twitching and a thumping sensation in the chest when the device is pacing. During sensing, the device does not cause discomfort.
3. Have code cart available.
4. Assess the patient's respiratory status. The patient may be intubated to maintain adequate ventilation, because chest wall contractions can interfere with the patient's breathing.
5. Administer supplemental oxygen, if needed, to facilitate oxygenation during pacing.
6. Start IV line, if appropriate.
7. Prepare the designated equipment, as delineated by the operator's manual.
8. Connect patient to cardiac monitor and obtain a clear ECG pattern. The standard monitor will be overloaded by the pacing signal. The alternative is to initiate monitoring through the pacing device. This will also be necessary for the device to sense cardiac activity and function in the demand mode.
9. Obtain a baseline ECG and vital signs. Include a pulse oximetry reading, if available, to obtain a baseline value and to monitor for adequate oxygenation.
10. Prepare the skin for electrodes. Do not use alcohol or benzoin on the skin because burns may result. Clean and dry the skin. Trim the chest hair with scissors to avoid cuts. Skin cuts increase the pain during pacing.
11. Check functioning of generator. Apply the electrodes (Fig. 7-2). The electrodes are applied by the nurse following the physician's order to initiate TEP. The electrode configuration minimizes pectoral muscle stimulation and facilitates low pacing thresholds. It may be necessary to move the electrodes to achieve a low pacing threshold.
    a. Apply the posterior or negative electrode first. Place it on the back between the left scapula and spine at heart level.
    b. Apply the anterior or positive electrode over the precordium below the left pectoral muscle between the V_2 and V_5 position.
12. Once the electrodes are securely in place, press firmly around the outer edge of the electrode, press on the center of the electrode for good skin contact, and connect them to the pacing cable and to the pacing generator.

13. Inform the patient when pacing will be started.
14. Start pacing. Set the device to 0 mA, heart rate 10 beats/min above the patient's rate. Turn the unit on. Steadily increase the mA until capture is observed, usually less than 90 mA and preferably less than 40 mA to have minimal chest contraction.
15. Evaluate for 100% capture. Every pacing spike will be followed by a QRS complex greater than 0.14 milliseconds, a T wave, and suppression or competition with the patient's intrinsic heart rhythm (Figs. 7-3 and 7-4).
16. Set the device for demand pacing. Decrease the heart rate to 10 beats/min less than the patient's rate. The muscle contractions of an agitated patient causes the unit to falsely sense the muscle activity as cardiac activity and to not pace the patient. Observe for competition between the patient's rhythm and the pacemaker.
17. Reposition electrodes for noncapture, high current requirements, or excessively painful stimuli (mA requirements > 90).
18. Medicate the patient for discomfort according to the physician's order. Take caution with administration of pain medication before the procedure. Assess patient's hemodynamic status: blood pressure, heart rate, and respirations. Pain medication during the pacing interval is given to control chest discomfort resulting from TEP. Chest pain of cardiac origin demands further evaluation by the nurse and physician.
19. Monitor vital signs to verify effectiveness of pacing. Calculate the mean blood pressure as described in the assessment section. Effective pacing is evidenced by the expected decrease in mean pressure as the heart rate increases. Check the radial or pedal pulses to be sure that true pulse is present and not just chest muscle contraction with stimulation.
20. Observe rhythm for return of an adequate intrinsic rate (Fig. 7-5).
21. Disconnect the pacing electrodes from the generator, if defibrillation is required, to avoid damage to the generator. Check operator's manual because this may not be required by the device in use.
22. Discontinue pacing according to physician's order. (Check hospital policy to determine if the nurse or the physician will turn off the device.) The physician monitors the patient's intrinsic rhythm and determines when pacing can be stopped. Termination of pacing is gradual. Begin by turning down the rate. The patient's own rhythm should take over as the pacing rate is decreased. Once the patient's own rhythm is sustained, the device can be turned off or left at the low backup rate until one is certain the patient will maintain an adequate rate (Fig. 7-6). An alternate method of taking the patient off the pacemaker is to slowly decrease the mA output until a subthreshold current level is reached (Fig. 7-7). Observe the patient closely for asystole in the event that the intrinsic rhythm does not take over.
23. Assess the skin for irritation from the electrodes and treat accordingly. Cleanse the skin thoroughly with soap and warm water. Apply topical burn cream, if appropriate.
24. Keep TEP unit on standby for 24 hours after discontinuation of pacing and removal of electrodes in the event that bradycardia or block return.

A

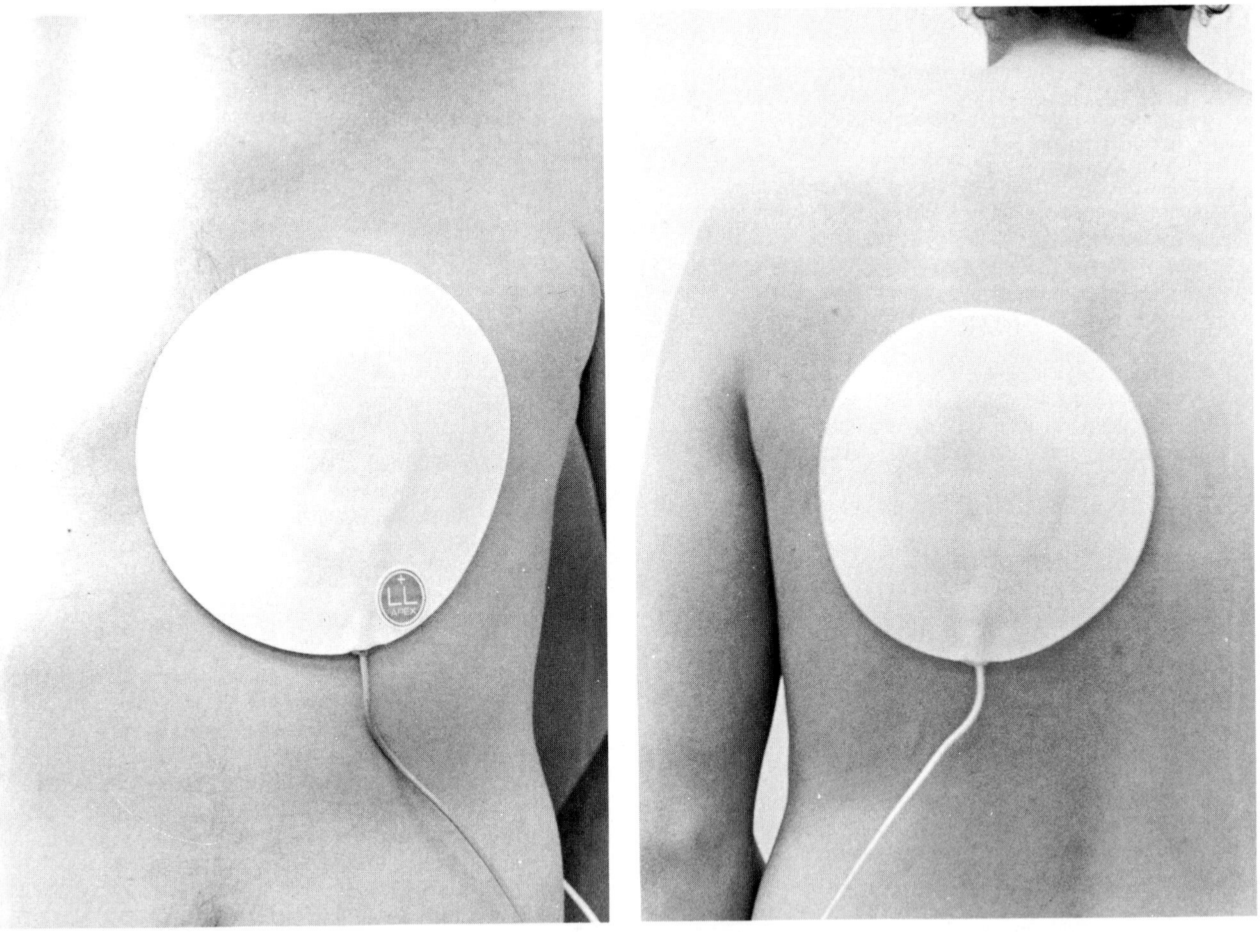

B

Fig. 7-2 Electrode placement for temporary external pacing. **A,** Anterior. **B,** Posterior. (From Persons CB: *Critical care procedures and protocols: a nursing approach,* Philadelphia, 1987, JB Lippincott.)

Table 7-6   Troubleshooting a Temporary Pacemaker

Complication	Cause	Intervention	Complication	Cause	Intervention
Failure to pace	Battery depletion	Change battery		Perforation	Notify doctor
	Generator failure	Change unit			Obtain chest x-ray
	Loose connection	Secure connections			Obtain ICE
	Sensitivity high	Decrease sensitivity			Reposition lead
	Spike not visible	Change monitor lead			Treat tamponade
		Increase monitor gain		Complexes not	Change monitor lead
		Check on/off control		visible	Increase monitor gain
	Lead fracture	Notify docto			
		Change lead	Failure to sense	Lead displacement	Notify doctor
		Unipolarize lead			Obtain chest x-ray
		Reverse electrodes			Obtain ICE
	Electromagnetic	Perform electrical			Reposition lead
	interference (EMI)	check		Inadequate signals	Check insertion thresholds
	Lead displacement	Notify doctor		(competition)	Obtain ICE
		Obtain chest x ray			Reverse electrodes
		Obtain ICE (intracardi-		Sensitivity high	Decrease sensitivity
		ac electrogram)		EMI	Perform electrical check
		Reposition lead		Concealed	Administer antidysrhythmic
	Crosstalk	Decrease atrial output		conduction	therapy
	(No V pace)	Decrease ventricular		Fusion beats	No intervention
		sensitivity		Crosstalk	Decrease atrial output
		Increase ventricular		(oversensing)	Decrease ventricular sensitivity
		blanking period			Increase ventricular blanking
	Incorrect	Reverse lead			period
	chamber paced	connections			Other interventions:
					Turn off pacer with an
Failure to capture	Low mA	Increase mA			adequate rate
	Acute threshold rise	Increase mA			Overdrive intrinsic heart rate
		Administer steroids			(IHR)
	Lead fracture	Notify doctor			Unipolarize lead
		Change lead			Stabilize patient in
		Unipolarize lead			ventricular fibrillation (VF)
		Reverse electrodes			or ventricular tachycardia
	Lead displacement	Reposition patient			(VT)
		Limit patient activity		Generator failure	Replace pulse generator
		Notify doctor			Submit defective unit for repair
		Obtain chest x ray		Pacemaker mediated	Check retrograde conduction
		Obtain ICE		tachycardia (PMT)	Evaluate settings
		Reposition lead			
	Loose connection	Secure connections			
	Battery failure	Change battery			

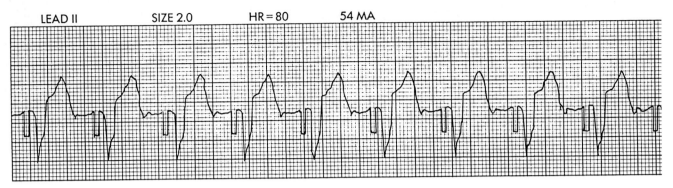

Fig. 7-3   Pacing capture with a transcutaneous pacemaker.

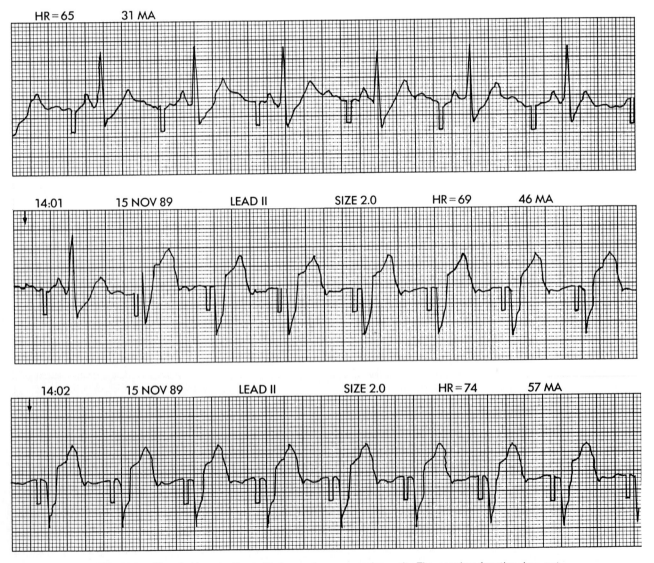

Fig. 7-4   Threshold evaluation with transcutaneous pacing unit. The sensing function has not been adjusted.

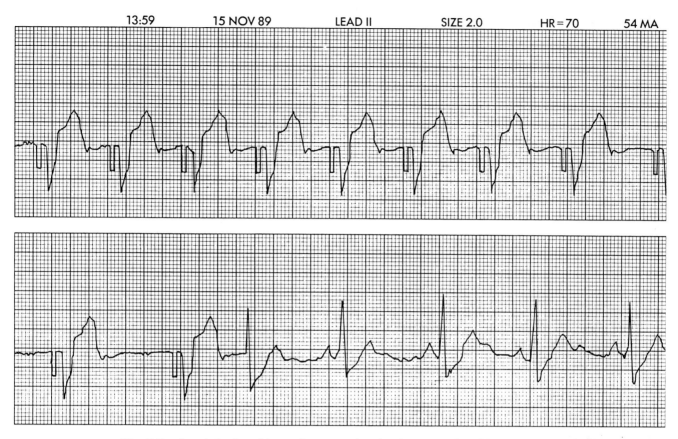

Fig. 7-5   Sample tracing of transcutaneous pacing showing resumption of intrinsic rhythm.

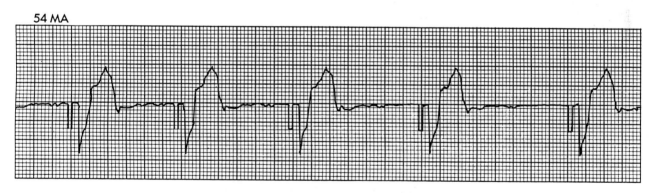

Fig. 7-6   Back-up rate setting with transcutaneous pacing.

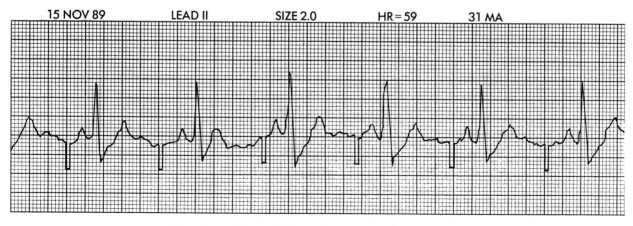

Fig. 7-7   Subthreshold stimuli with transcutaneous pacing.

PACEMAKER THRESHOLDS

Pacemaker thresholds are an important component for the initiation of effective pacing and maintenance of the pacing system. There are two types of thresholds, a pacing or stimulation threshold and a sensing threshold. The *stimulation threshold* is the minimal amount of current delivered by the pacemaker that will consistently cause the heart to contract. The contraction of the heart is referred to as capture. The threshold is measured in milliamperes (mA) or volts (V). The *sensing threshold* refers to the pacemaker's ability to sense intrinsic rhythm. The threshold is the minimal cardiac signal sensed by the pacemaker's circuit. It is measured in millivolts (mV).

Threshold testing is performed during insertion of a pacemaker by the physician with the assistance of the nurse. Thresholds provide a degree of familiarity with the system to determine the pacing needs of the patient. Pacemaker threshold should be checked as soon as possible after insertion. Events that affect pacing thresholds are (1) the addition of antidysrhythmics to the treatment protocol (e.g., flecainide, quinidine, and procainamide), (2) disturbance in acid-base status, (3) electrolyte imbalances (primarily potassium), (4) administration of β-blockers (e.g., propranolol), (5) administration of calcium channel-blockers (e.g., verapamil), (6) ischemic events, or (7) defibrillation. They are the same for temporary and permanent pacing. Per-

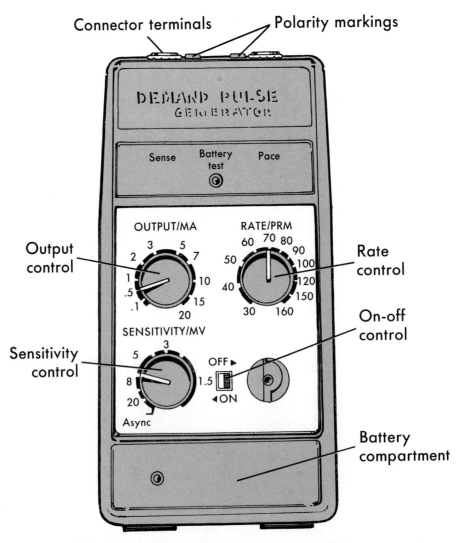

Fig. 7-8   Temporary pulse generator. (Example shown is a Medtronic Demand Pulse Generator.) (From Beare PG, Myer JC: *Adult Health Nursing,* St Louis, 1990, Mosby–Year Book.)

manent thresholds are recorded with a pacing system analyzer (PSA) available from the pacing manufacturer. A PSA can be used on a temporary system, but the practice is rare.

It is recommended that the sensing threshold be tested first. Once the patient has been paced, intrinsic rhythm may be suppressed. This is one of the inherent dangers in pacing. The suppression of the intrinsic heart rate (IHR) is not permanent. By testing the sensing threshold, the position of the lead in the heart is verified, and time is saved for the final hookup to the generator.

TROUBLESHOOTING WITH TEMPORARY PACING

Frequent checks of the system may prevent crises with temporary pacing. When making rounds, the nurse should note the following (see Fig. 7-8):

- Device is turned on or off.
- Settings are correct for the patient (mA, rate, AV interval, and sensitivity).

- All connections are secure.
- Patient is maintaining correct arm positions.
- Patient is moving around amount that is safe.
- Monitoring lead correct.
- Patient had an x-ray or other test done.
- How long patient has had the pacemaker for threshold considerations.

TERMINATION OF SHORT-TERM PACING

The precise method of termination is determined by the physician and is guided by the patient's condition. The potential methods are to: (1) turn off the device and remove the lead at that time; (2) turn off the device, disconnect from the lead, and remove the lead after 24 hours observation; or (3) set the device to a backup rate for 24 hours and then discontinue. The patient's underlying rhythm, rate, and stability are all considered when terminating the pacing procedure.

Skill 7-3 **Threshold Evaluation for Temporary Pacing**

EQUIPMENT AND SUPPLIES

- Intact pacing system
- ECG machine (battery-operated preferred)
- V lead connection from the ECG machine
- Sterile connector cable with alligator clips
- Rubber gloves
- Indifferent pacing electrode

NURSING INTERVENTIONS

1. Observe electrical safety precautions. Wear rubber gloves to handle the pacing wire.
2. Set up the ECG machine for recording if not done during the insertion process. Check the status of the paper to be sure of recording the entire sequence.
3. Check attachment of the distal tip of the pacing wire to the V lead of the machine. NOTE: This is the only lead on the standard ECG machine that is isolated. It has a built-in high resistance to prevent conduction of stray current down the pacing lead.
4. Record a tracing from the distal tip of the pacing wire (Fig. 7-9). The ICE verifies: (1) the quality of the signal the pacemaker will use to sense the overall amplitude of the P wave or QRS complex; (2) the position of the lead in the apex of the right ventricle described by the small R wave and deep S wave; and (3) the ST-segment elevation, showing good contact with the endocardial wall of the ventricle, at least 5 mm in amplitude.
5. Attach the pacing wire to the gray cable and generator. Observe polarity of the connections. Again verify position of the lead before initiating stimulation threshold measurements to avoid triggering a lethal dysrhythmia.
6. Set the generator approximately 10 beats/min above the IHR, the mA at 3, and the sensitivity at asynchronous.

7. Turn the generator on.
8. Observe for capture.
9. Gradually decrease the output while observing for continuous capture. Stop at each value on the dial and state the current value so the physician is aware of the setting.
10. Continue to decrease the output in this manner until consistent capture is lost. The lowest current setting with consistent capture is the *stimulation threshold*. The process is repeated for the atrium and ventricle, if both are to be paced (DVI or DDD pacing).
11. Verify threshold by slightly decreasing the current. Observe for continued capture. Table 7-7 gives the acceptable thresholds. If the thresholds are too high, the lead will have to be repositioned by the physician. Initial values should be low. Over a period of several days, the thresholds can rise 5 to 10 times the initial values, and exceed the capabilities of the pacemaker. CAUTION: Once the patient has been 100% paced to check thresholds, intrinsic rhythm may be suppressed. Do not abruptly turn off the generator. Once thresholds are obtained, the physician may ask the patient to deep breathe, cough, or change position to evaluate the stability of the lead position.[17]
12. Monitor the patient's vital signs and response to the procedure.
13. Set the generator for the final pacing settings based on the thresholds obtained, output, sensitivity, and rate. It is recommended that the current be set 3 times higher than the stimulation threshold for a safety margin. The sensitivity setting is adjusted for demand pacing.
14. Monitor the ECG for normal pacemaker operation, that is appropriate pacing, sensing, and capture.
15. Document the ICE recording, thresholds, and final settings.

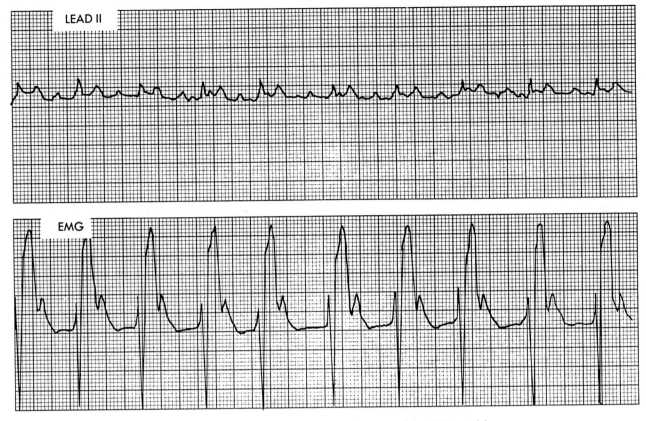

Fig. 7-9   Intracardiac electrogram from the apex of the right ventricle.

Table 7-7   Pacing and Sensing Thresholds

	Pulse width	Volts	Max V	mA	Ohms*
Stimulation					
Atrial	1 ms	1	2	3	< 1000
Ventricular	0.5 ms	0.5-1	1	1-1.5	< 1000
	mV				
					Slow rate
Atrial	1.5				.5 V/sec
Ventricular	4				.5 V/sec

*Ohms are resistance on the lead.

Selection of the Pacemaker System

The selection of a permanent pacemaker is determined by the underlying problem. If it is an irreversible problem, a permanent pacemaker is required. The hemodynamic assessment is needed to evaluate the patient's response to the disturbance. The degree of hemodynamic embarrassment is then quantified. The remaining task is to select the correct system for the patient.

Selection of the system is complex. The main factor is the interaction between the indication for pacing and the response of the patient. The pacemaker must provide the patient with optimal CO. Therefore the physician matches the capability of the individual with a system that will meet the demands. This evaluation includes the following:

- Physical and mental status of the patient.
- Associated medical problems that may affect the long-term prognosis.
- Presence of an underlying cardiac disease adversely affected by the dysrhythmia.
- Physical activity level.
- Access to medical care.
- Need for medication that has depressant effects on the heart.

Skill 7-4 Troubleshooting for Nonpacing/Noncapture

EQUIPMENT AND SUPPLIES

- Transcutaneous pacing system, if available
- Replacement generator
- Replacement lead
- 9-volt battery
- Skin electrode to unipolarize the system
- Rubber gloves
- Defibrillator
- Code cart
- Atropine and/or Isuprel
- Insertion kit

NURSING INTERVENTIONS

1. Detect the problem (Fig. 7-10 shows ECG examples).
2. Categorize the problem: (a) spike present without capture—look to the patient or lead; (b) spike absent—look to the generator.
3. Assess the patient: (a) stable with own rhythm—attend to the system; (b) unstable with an inadequate rhythm or asystole—attend to the patient.
4. Institute transcutaneous pacing, if available, until temporary pacing is established.
5. Increase the mA setting on the generator to 3 to 5 times the threshold, 10 mA with a ventricular lead, or 20 mA with an atrial lead.
6. Check all connections. Start close to the patient and work toward the unit.
7. Position the patient to last known effective pacing position, usually the left lateral decubitus position. This will reposition the lead against the endocardium.
8. Consider full CPR status, if pacing has not been established, and the patient is unstable. Elapsed time to this point should be less than 2 minutes.
9. Prepare for drug administration—Atropine 0.5 mg IV push or isoproterenol 1 mg in 250 D_5W at an infusion rate of 4 μg/min (1 ml/min) are the drugs of choice. Precautions with isoproterenol include not to run as the main infusion, observe the patient for VT, and discontinue the infusion for a heart rate greater than 90 beats/min or if premature ventricular contractions occur.
10. With asystole, first attempt pacing. Position forearm along the axis of the sternum with a clenched fist approximately 20 to 25 cm (8 to 10 inches) above the sternum. Deliver blows to the middle third of the sternum at a rate of 1/sec. Avoid fracturing the sternum. Check carotid pulses during the procedure to determine the efficiency of the blows.
11. Initiate full CPR if pacing has not been established.
12. Document all events occurring during the crisis.
13. Investigate the cause of the problem and initiate corrective action once the crisis event has been resolved.
14. Prepare for unipolarization of the system or lead change if determined as the cause of the problem. Unipolarization is done by inserting the skin electrode into the positive terminal of the generator. The electrodes of the pacing wire are tested for integrity. Whichever electrode is intact is inserted into the negative terminal of the generator to establish pacing.
15. Change the generator battery, if required.
16. Decrease the mA setting of the device. A continuous requirement for > 10 mA current settings on a ventricular lead indicates a problem. The 10 mA setting with ventricular pacing increases the potential for VT should competition develop. This is not a safe setting.
17. Obtain a chest x-ray after the interventions.
18. Record an ICE to confirm position and establish thresholds.
19. Assess the patient for response to the event and corrective actions taken.
20. Document final resolution of the problem and patient status.

Skill 7-5 Termination of Short-Term Pacing

EQUIPMENT AND SUPPLIES

- Defibrillator
- Code cart
- Sterile gloves
- Suture removal kit
- Site dressing
- ECG monitor
- Culturette
- Povidone-iodine solution

NURSING INTERVENTIONS

1. Explain the procedure and the reason for termination of pacing to the patient.
2. Prepare the insertion site by removing the dressing and cleaning the area with a povidone-iodine solution.
3. Turn the pacing rate down slowly until the intrinsic heart rate (IHR) takes over. The device should never be abruptly turned off.
4. Continuously monitor the cardiac rhythm as the physician removes the pacing wire, since dysrhythmias may occur as the lead is removed.
5. Continue monitoring during removal.
6. Inspect the site for signs of infection or abnormal swelling. Apply the dressing.
7. Send the pacing wire tip for culture, if ordered. Periodical cultures are a component of a quality assurance program to evaluate patient care.
8. Obtain a chest x-ray for cardiac silhouette and lung status, if ordered.
9. Maintain cardiac monitoring for 24 hours, since dysrhythmias may occur during that time.
10. Provide emotional support. The patient may express a fear of activity related to a potential for return of symptoms.
11. Monitor the patient for internal or external bleeding after removal of temporary epicardial wires, heart sounds, blood pressure, and heart rate.
12. Cover ends of the pacing wires separately with rubber gloves if only the generator is removed.
13. Have transcutaneous pacing available in the event that it will be required.
14. Assess the physical status of the patient for return of previous symptoms and hemodynamic stability.
15. Document procedure.

Strip #1 = Normal pacemaker function - pace, sense, capture.

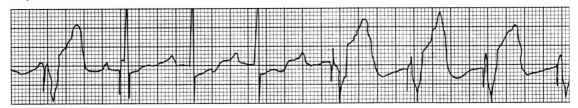

Strip #2 = Complete cessation of pacemaker function with no underlying rhythm.

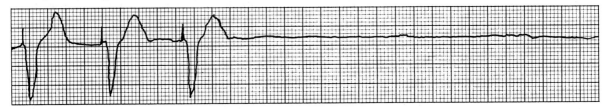

Strip #3 = Complete loss of capture but pacing spikes are visible. There are P waves visible without QRS responses.

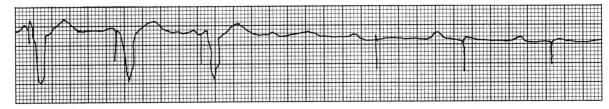

Strip #4 = Pacemaker spikes only. The return of the stylus to baseline (spike decay) gives the appearance of a possible complex.

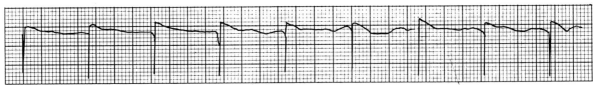

Strip #5 = Pacemaker spikes are present, no capture. Underlying rhythm is CHB, rate 30. Sensing preserved.

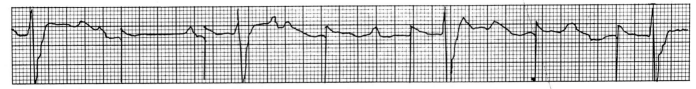

Fig. 7-10   ECG recognition of problems for crisis management.

- Susceptibility to a cardiovascular accident if perfusion is diminished for any reason.
- Input received from patient's family or caregivers.
- Symptoms attributed to bradycardia (e.g., transient dizziness, light-headedness, near syncope, or frank syncope as manifestations of transient cerebral ischemia, marked exercise intolerance, or CHF.)[12]
- Intraventricular conduction disturbances with an MI.

The pacemaker will be either a SC system or a DC system. The SC system does not truly optimize cardiac performance. The augmentation of CO is of short duration and in some cases the function may deteriorate.[8,34] The main advantage of the SC system is demand rate pacing. Bradycardia is prevented, but the rate cannot adapt to the needs of a changing environment. For some patients, this is an appropriate selection. Another option is an SC rate-adaptive system. These units provide the rate mechanism for improved exercise endurance. If the patient's needs extend beyond the rate component, the DC system is the device of choice. The DC, or physiological, system is close to the normally functioning heart. It provides the rate adaptation and restores AV synchrony. Sensors have been added to the dual chamber systems as well. Should the sinus mechanism default, the sensor will take over rate adaption.

Implantation of a Permanent Pacemaker

Once the hardware is selected, the system is implanted. The method of implantation depends on the preference of the physician and available resources in the hospital. It is critical to prepare the patient for pacemaker insertion.

The preferred method of implantation is the endocardial or transvenous technique. The patient remains awake for the procedure, recovers more quickly, and has fewer side effects from the anesthetic agent.

Complications of Permanent Pacing

Complications of permanent pacing are similar to temporary pacing. One would have a difficult time differentiating a temporary from a permanent pacing system by looking at a tracing. Interventions are also similar but are performed by magnet application to check pacing, test the device, and elicit end of service (EOS). Capture may be accomplished by programming the output to a higher level or widening the pulse width. Sensing problems can also be corrected by using the programmer to change settings or refractory periods (see Table 7-7).

In addition to the normal events in permanent pacing, the nurse should be alert for alteration in function caused by the effects of electromagnetic interference (EMI). EMI occurs when electrical emissions from equipment operating in the vicinity of the patient alter functions of a pacemaker.[27] Causes of EMI can include the following:
- Uninsulated wires.
- Electrocautery.
- Cardioversion/defibrillation.
- Small electrical appliances.
- Radio stations.
- Arc welding.
- Myopotentials from muscle tremors.
- Other devices, such as implanted defibrillators, transcutaneous electrical nerve stimulation (TENS) units, and crosstalk between atrial and ventricular channels in the same unit.
- Magnetic resonance imaging (MRI).
- Some telemetry power packs with telemetry monitoring.
- Lithotripsy.

EMI interferes with the pacer signal. The pacer may respond to the EMI by triggering, inhibiting, converting to a fixed rate, reprogramming, reverting to a backup mode, or not responding.

EMI is recognized on the tracing or ECG by the following:
- Baseline artifact (e.g., distorted or rapid, spiky undulations).
- Inappropriate pauses that are not a multiple of the basic rate.
- Inappropriate rate increases greater than the pacing rate, greater than the upper rate limit, greater than the rate protection limit in the device (120 to 300 beats/min), or rates not possible in the device.
- Intermittent abnormal pacing and sensing operations.
- Backup pacing modes.
- Tingling sensations on the skin.
- Syncopal episodes.
- Event analysis.

Outside of the manufacturers' interventions, programming is the principle method to alter the effects of EMI. For example, making the pacemaker less sensitive, changing the mode, changing the level of responsiveness to the sensor, programming the rate, and using magnet mode.

Another complication of the permanent pacemaker to troubleshoot is the potential for premature or expected EOS in the device. Manufacturer variations will include life expectancy of the device, how it functions as the battery voltage decreases, access to the information, and warranty. Generally the life expectancy is about 8 to 10 years, depending on how the pacemaker is programmed. High-energy settings deplete the battery at a higher rate. Factors that may indicate EOS for the pacemaker include the following:
- Pulse width widening.
- Voltage decrease.
- Increased cell (battery) impedance.
- Mode changes.
- Backup pacing.
- Telemetry information stating EOS.
- Pacing and sensing alterations.
- Magnet rate variations.
- Threshold test variations.
- Pacing rate decrease.
- Dim battery light indicator.
- Antitachycardia and rate adaptive responses inactivated.

The patient-related complications to permanent pacing vary from those of temporary pacing because of the duration of pacing. The long-term complications include the following:

- Perforation with or without tamponade.
- Poor wound healing.
- Dysrhythmia interference with the pacemaker.
- Pacemaker-induced dysrhythmias.
- Battery migration.
- Externalization of the generator.
- Infection.
- Emboli.
- Endocarditis.
- Congestive heart failure (CHF).
- Hematoma/bleeding.

Additional complications may occur with implantation during the first 24 hours. These complications include the following:

- Pneumothorax.
- Extracardiac stimulation.
- Perforations.
- Bleeding.
- Air in the pocket.
- Dysrhythmias.

Analysis of Normal Pacemaker Function

The pacemaker is a constant component in the care plan once it has been implanted. Assessment of the pacemaker requires evaluation of pacing, sensing, and capture.

PEDIATRIC CONSIDERATIONS

Indications for pacing in children are similar to those for adults. There are specific considerations in pediatric pacing. Pediatric indications for cardiac pacing include the following[10,13]:

- Second- or third-degree AV block with symptomatic bradycardia.
- Advanced second- or third-degree AV block with moderate-to-marked exercise intolerance.
- External ophthalmoplegia with bifascicular block.
- Sinus node dysfunction with symptomatic bradycardia.
- Supraventricular tachycardia (SVT).
- Bradycardia-tachycardia syndrome with the need for antidysrhythmics (not digitalis).
- Congestive heart failure (CHF).
- Congenital AV block with wide QRS escape rhythm.
- Congenital heart failure.
- Asymptomatic patient after cardiac surgery with advanced second- or third-degree AV block persisting 10 to 14 days after surgery.

Several factors have lead to a greater incidence in permanent pacing in children. Improved and simplified techniques for implantation have made the procedure more realistic. Advanced technology, such as rate programmability, can better meet the needs of children, from neonate to adolescent. Capability and longevity of the pacing system may be sacrificed, however, for size. A final factor in the increased use of pacing with children has been its achievement of better cardiovascular performance in AV block in comparison to the strict use of chronotropic agents to increase rate.[5]

Problems that must be overcome with pediatric pacing include the following[2,18,30,31]:

- Taut leads from growth of the child, necessitating surgery to release the tension.
- Erosions through the skin, if a small generator is not used.
- Retromammary placement of the generator for cosmetic reasons in the adolescent female.
- Rate management in children requiring a wide range of programmable rates since as the child matures, the normal heart rate slows. Therefore the pacemaker can be programmed to fire at a slower rate. For example:
  Less than 2 years, 100 to 110 beats/min.
  2 to 10 years, 90 to 100 beats/min.
  More than 10 years, 75 to 80 beats/min.
  Later adolescent, 70 beats/min.
- Consideration given to the activity of the child. Extremely violent type of play and sports should be discouraged.
- Electronic toys available for children that interfere with the implanted device.
- Early teaching of the patient and parents to avoid overprotection of the child (more critical when the child is pacemaker-dependent).

Temporary external pacing (TEP) is also available for pediatric application. Four of the following indications have been identified for beneficial application of TEP:[2]

- Sick sinus syndrome requiring cardioversion for children with atrial tachydysrhythmias who may be bradycardiac after conversion.
- Complete heart block (CHB) after a surgical procedure resulting in severe bradycardia from general anesthesia.
- Patients with permanent pacemakers who are at risk during pacemaker reprogramming or replacement.
- Patients with drug-induced bradycardia.

PSYCHOSOCIAL CONSIDERATIONS

Patients who require artificial pacing may have difficulty adjusting emotionally to feelings of loss, altered body image, and fear of dependency on the pacing device. Additional concerns that the nurse must consider in planning care for these patients involve the following[32,33]:

- Patient's need for long-term follow-up and replacement of the device.
- Possibility of life-style changes.
- Cost of ongoing care.
- Potential effect on employment.
- Perceived benefits of the pacemaker.
- General state of the patient's health.

The patient's ability to communicate these concerns and the previous experience with emergency events determines

Skill 7-6 Analysis of Pacemaker Function

EQUIPMENT AND SUPPLIES

- Monitor tracing recorded for 1 minute
- ECG with and without magnet
- Pacemaker magnet
- Calipers
- Mini-clinic
- Implant record on pacemaker, if available
- Pacemaker identification card
- Pacemaker specifications manual
- ICHD code chart (see Tables 7-1 and 7-2)

NURSING INTERVENTIONS

1. Obtain an ECG with and without magnet or a monitor tracing recorded for 1 minute to evaluate pacemaker function.
2. Obtain the supporting data to interpret the tracing. This includes an event history from the patient, indication for pacemaker implant, implant date, implant thresholds (if available), the name of implanting or monitoring physician, pacemaker manufacturer, and magnet function.
3. Identify the implanted device (not all implanted devices are pacemakers). Know the model, type of device (SC, DC, and rate adaptive), pacemaker settings, and idiosyncrasies of the device.
4. Obtain an electronic analysis using the mini-clinic. Place the mini-clinic on the patient's bare skin (usually the chest), turn on, and record the parameters displayed in the window at the top of the device. The pacing interval or automatic interval is first, then pacing rate, atrial/ventricular pulse width interval, and the AV interval with a DC pacemaker. The patient must be pacing at the time the readings are taken. Repeat the values in the magnet mode.
5. Identify the patient's underlying rhythm, if apparent on the tracing. Observe for rate, rhythm, site of origin, and ectopy. DC devices require P waves to track during normal operation.
6. Determine system configuration: bipolar showing a small pacing spike and unipolar showing a large pacing spike.
7. Determine chamber placement of the lead (Fig. 7-11). Lead placement can be recognized on the ECG by the bundle branch block (BBB) configuration. Use the monitor lead, modified chest lead V_1 (MCL$_1$). Pacing from the right ventricle results in a LBBB. Pacing from the left ventricle results in a RBBB. The BBB configuration should not change. Changes indicate perforation of the opposite ventricle. The P wave after the spike indicates atrial pacing. Both responses are indicative of a DC system.
8. Determine pacing operation. Identify the spikes on the tracing. Measure the automatic interval (time from one spike to the next). This evaluates the timing cycle and defines the pacing rate. Evaluate the spike for visibility when no intrinsic events are evident, appropriate spike-to-spike intervals for the device, spikes within the range of the device settings (lower rate and upper rate limits), that polarity of the spike is consistent, and consistent size of the spike.

9. Determine sensing operation. Evaluate the tracing for the opportunity to sense. The SC system looks for QRS complexes, and the DC system looks for P waves and QRS complexes. Measure the escape interval to determine what is being sensed. The escape interval in SC is the same as the automatic interval and in DC it is the ventriculoatrial (VA) interval. (Subtract the duration of the AV interval from the automatic interval to obtain the VA interval.) Sensing in the SC results in demand operation. Sensing in the DC results in tracking or inhibition of the device. Cardiac events occurring in the pacemaker's refractory period will not recycle the device and appear to be nonsensed events.
10. Assess the response to pacemaker operation, atrial and/or ventricular capture. SC pacing evokes a broad QRS complex in response to each pacemaker spike or a P wave if it is an atrial system. DC pacing evokes a paced QRS complex (similar to SC pacing) after each sensed P wave after timing out the AV interval. If both spikes are emitted, each should be followed by the appropriate response—P wave after the atrial spike and QRS complex after the ventricular spike. Capture will not occur if the spike is in the heart's absolute refractory period.
11. Rule out pseudomalfunctions in the evaluation such as magnet operation, programming errors, programming not documented, hysteresis (a programmed longer escape interval that mimics failure to pace), refractory periods, dysrhythmias, pseudofusion/fusion beats, idiosyncrasies of the device, iatrogenic artifacts such as the recording of the IVAC artifact, or interpretation errors. Rule out the responses of the pacemaker to electrical interference (see section on complications on pp. 155-156).
12. Use additional options for pacemaker assessment, such as the following:
    - Programmer interrogation of the device.
    - ICEs from the implanted pacemaker through the programmer.
    - Marker channels built into the device and accessed through the programmer. (Marker channels label each ECG event as paced or sensed.)
    - Magnet activation.
    - Threshold testing.
    - X-rays.
    - Patient's response to activity maneuvers (e.g., isometric exercises).
13. Evaluate length of time from implant to detect battery end of life (EOS). (See EOS characteristics in pacemakers on pp. 155-156).
14. Summarize the findings as normal functions, pseudomalfunction, malfunction, or a combination.
15. Determine appropriate interventions.

the rate and degree to which adjustment is achieved. Between 15% to 29% of patients may not adapt successfully.[29] The nurse's knowledge and use of the patient's support system along with the provision of counseling and education help facilitate a maximal adjustment.

PATIENT AND FAMILY TEACHING

The education program for the pacemaker patient must begin at the time the need for a pacemaker is determined. There is a great deal of information to be given to the patient in a short period of time. In some cases as few as 3 days are available from the decision point to discharge with the pacemaker.

Planning in advance minimizes the risks of incomplete discharge teaching and patient complications. The content of a pacemaker education program depends on the technology in use, the skills of the educator, available time, patient motivation, family support, and hospital resources. A pacemaker education program should cover the following information[22,25,32,34]:

- General pacemaker information to be provided for the patient and family including the following:
    Indication for pacemaker specific to the patient.
    Diagram of the heart and vessels used for pacemaker insertion.
    Purpose of the pacemaker—rate management, rate adaptation, and AV synchrony.
    Realistic benefits of the pacemaker, both short-term and long-term.
    Available support system for the patient and family.
    Importance of expressing feelings and asking questions.
    Cardiac monitoring with selected pacing method.
    Pacing duration expected with pacing method.
    Preparation for the procedure (i.e., skin preparation, IV infusion, and medications).
    Insertion or implant procedure.
- Temporary external pacemaker (TEP) including the following:
    Purpose of the electrodes.
    Sensations experienced during episodes of pacing.
- Temporary transvenous pacemaker (TPM) including the following:
    Purpose and placement of the pacing wire.
    Mild sedation and small incision on the upper chest for implant.
    Range of motion to avoid complications.
    Electrical safety measures.
- Permanent pacing including the following:
    How the system implanted operates to achieve its purpose (i.e., SC, DC, or SC or DC rate responsiveness.
- Health behaviors for patient including the following:
    Take and record the pulse. Patients are told the rate limits of their devices. SC have a minimum rate. DC have both a minimum pacing rate and an upper limit pacing rate. Rate adaptive devices also have rate ranges.

Carry the pacemaker identification card; obtain and wear a Medic-Alert necklace or bracelet.
Report recurrence of previous or new symptoms.
Continue to take prescribed medications, as ordered by physician.
Continue diet, as indicated by physician.
Notify physician regarding travel plans. In addition, security personnel at the airport should be notified of the pacemaker before the patient goes through the metal detector. If available, a telephone monitor should be taken along with the patient.
Notify physicians seen for other procedures, of the pacemaker and type of pacemaker (e.g., dentists and surgeons). Sensors in the rate adaptive pacemaker react to stimuli other than those generated by the patient. The pacemaker should have the rate adaptive mode programmed off.
Safely maintain small appliances in the home, including microwave ovens. Electrical appliances should be kept 10 to 15 cm (4 to 6 inches) away from the pacemaker. Do not pass electric razors directly over the pacemaker. Maintain a safe distance from open ignition systems, such as in a car or lawn mower. Hospital equipment, such as diathermy, cautery, therapeutic radiation, or MRI can affect the pacemaker.
Do not manipulate the pacemaker (Twidler's syndrome).
Perform proper wound care after implantation and long term. Check for swelling, redness, irritation, pain, drainage, or migration of the device. Avoid restrictive or irritating clothing over the pacemaker site. Shower for the first week to 10 days. Obtain shower chair if needed.
Maintain pacemaker follow-up by way of physician's office, hospital-based pacemaker clinic, or telephone monitoring.
Resume sexual activity, as recommended by physician.
Resume work, as directed by the physician.
Adhere to the treatment programs for new or existing medical problems. The physician evaluates interactions with the pacemaker during the decision-making process.

HOME HEALTH CARE CONSIDERATIONS

The initial 2 months after implant are the most critical. The incision and pocket are healing. The pacemaker stimulation threshold is also going through its evolution to chronic levels. Consequently, during this time, full range of arm motion, heavy lifting, or active sports could result in bleeding in the pacemaker pocket, lead dislodgement or disruption in the integrity of the incision. (Active fixation leads can also be pulled out of place.) After 2 months, the patient can perform any activities not contraindicated by the patient's state of well-being. Limits are usually im-

Right Ventricular Pacing	Left Ventricular Pacing
ECG: Left Bundle Branch Block pattern	ECG: Right Bundle Branch Block pattern

— Positive QRS lead I
      Negative QRS lead II
	— Negative QRS lead I
	      Positive QRS lead II

The ECG pattern may vary with placement of the lead in the chamber or placement of the ECG electrodes for recording the ECG.	The ECG pattern may vary with placement of the lead in chamber or placement of the ECG electrodes for recorc the ECG.

Lead placement: Transvenous approach
                  Right ventricle - apex or outflow tract
	Lead placement: Epicardial approach
	                  Surface left ventricle - apex or lateral wal

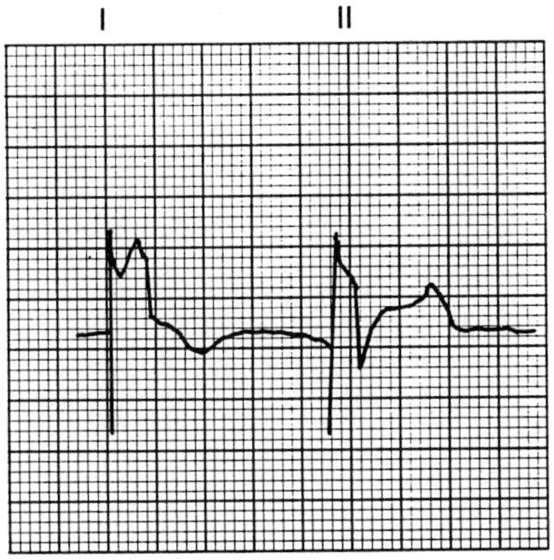

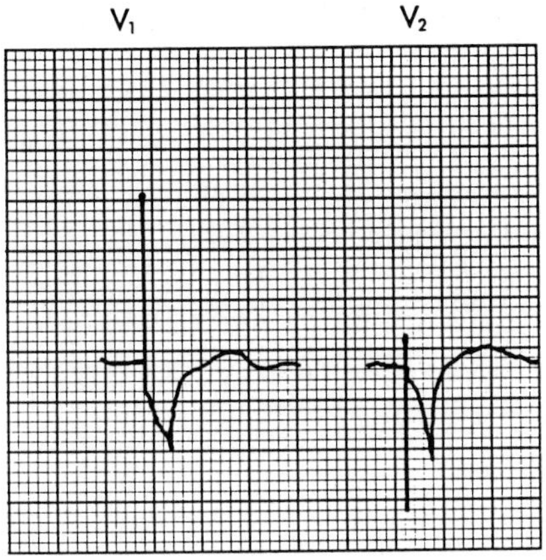

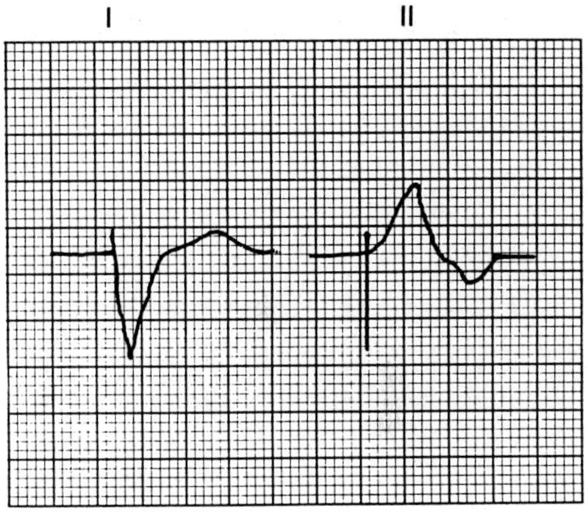

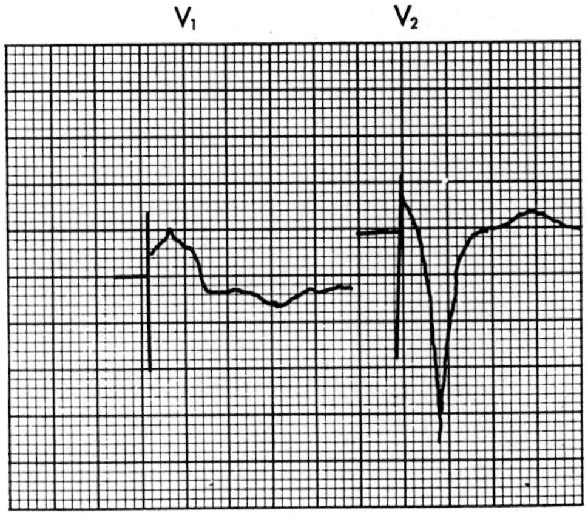

Fig. 7-11   Recognition of pacemaker lead placement by ECG.

posed by the patient's overall cardiovascular status.

In the home, patients take responsibility for themselves based on the teaching performed by the nurse and the physician. The nurse monitors, assesses, and evaluates the plan of care that was established in the hospital to determine if the patient understands it and can carry out self-care. Patients and family members can troubleshoot pacemaker function in the home by monitoring for infection and pain and monitoring the environment for safety hazards.

At home, the pacemaker patient can safely turn on light switches, lamps, televisions, radios, and may sleep under an electric blanket. The patient can use electrical tools, tooth brushes, and hair dryers, but they should not be held right next to the pacemaker. These appliances, if held directly over the insertion site, could produce electric signals that interfere with the pacemaker.

If the patients are in doubt about the safety of a microwave oven, caution them to stand at least 6 feet away from the oven when it is in use.[35]

When traveling, advise the patient to identify self to airport personnel before going through the metal detector and show the pacemaker identification card. Patients who work near electric arc welders, steel furnaces, or radio or telephone transmitters should be advised to discuss this with their physician. Rarely will a change in occupation be necessary.

The Telephone Pacemaker Check

A resource available to the pacemaker patient is the transtelephonic monitor, which the patient takes home. The receiver is in the hospital or physician's office. The physician may have the patient call at predetermined intervals to evaluate pacer function, or more frequently, if the patient suspects a problem.

Patients who are monitored at home by telephone can buy or rent a device about the size of a phone modem to transmit a single-lead ECG by telephone. The heart sounds are converted to electronic signals and are then transmitted by phone. The cost varies and some insurance companies cover these charges. Even with telephone monitoring, the patient should be evaluated in the office at least once a year for SC and twice a year for DC and rate adaptive.

REFERENCES

1. Beland MJ, Hesslein PS, Finlay CD et al: Noninvasive transcutaneous cardiac pacing in children, *PACE* 10:1262, 1987.
2. Branyon M, Schuch C: *Care of the cardiac patient.* In Andreoli K, Zipes E, Wallace A et al, editors: *Comprehensive cardiac care,* St Louis, 1987, Mosby–Year Book.
3. Braun AE: Transthoracic pacing in the emergency department, *J Emerg Nurs* 12(6):354, 1986.
4. Casta A, Mehta AV: Evaluating pediatric arrhythmias, *Fam Pract Recertification* 10(2):25, 1988.
5. Dugan L: What you need to know about permanent pacemakers, *Nursing '91* 21(6):46, 1991.
6. Fisch C (Task Force Chairman): Guidelines for implantation of cardiac pacemakers and antiarrhythmia devices, *J Am Coll Cardiol* 18(1):1-13, 1991.
7. Frye RI, Collins JJ, De Sanctis RW et al: Guidelines for permanent cardiac implantation, *Circulation* 70:331a, 1984.
8. Furman S, Schwedel JB: An intracardiac pacemaker for Stokes-Adams seizures, *New Engl J Med* 261(19):943, 1959.
9. Furman S, Hayes DL, Holmes DR: *A practice of cardiac pacing,* Mt Kisco, New York, 1986, Futura.
10. Guillette PC: Advances in treatment of supraventricular tachydysrhythmias in children, *Mod Concepts Cardiovasc Dis* 58(7):37, 1989.
11. Horrow JC: Electrical safety, *Curr Rev Respir Crit Care* 9:35, 1986.
12. Kaye GC, Butrous GS, Allen A et al: The effect of 50 Hz external electrical interference on implanted cardiac pacemakers, *PACE* 11:999, 1988.
13. Kaye W: Invasive therapeutic techniques: emergency cardiac pacing, pericardiocentesis, intracardiac injections and emergency treatment of tension pneumothorax, *Heart Lung* 12(3):300, 1983.
14. Lawrence PA: Cardiac pacing in children, *AACN Clinical Issues* 2(1):150, 1991.
15. Martinez R: *Emergency cardiac pacing.* In Sternbach G, editor: *Topics in emergency medicine,* Gaithersburg, Md, 1988, Aspen.
16. Means B, Taplett L: *Cardiac pacemakers.* In: *Quick reference to critical care nursing,* Gaithersburg, Md, 1986, Aspen.
17. Meibom J, Vilhelmsen R, Madsen JK: *A new noninvasive temporary pacemaker (Zoll-NTP),* University Hospital, 1986, Copenhagen, Denmark.
18. Miller K: *Electrical safety for patients and medical device operators.* In Miller S, Sampson L, Soukup M, editors: *AACN procedure manual for critical care,* Philadelphia, 1985, WB Saunders.
19. Pearsons CB: External cardiac pacing in the emergency department, *J Emerg Nursing* 12(6):348, 1986.
20. Reiffel JA, Coromilas J, Zimmerman JM et al: Drug device interactions: clinical considerations, *PACE* 8:369, 1985.
21. Sager DP: Current facts on pacemaker electromagnetic interference and their application to clinical care, *Heart Lung* 16(2):211, 1987.
22. Strathmore N, Mond H: Noninvasive monitoring and testing of pacemaker function, *PACE* 10:1359, 1987.
23. Walsh CA, McAlister HF, Andrews CA et al: Pacemaker implantation in children: a 21-year experience, *PACE* 11:1940, 1988.
24. Walsh J, Pearsons CB, Wieck L: *Manual of home health care nursing,* Philadelphia, 1987, JB Lippincott.
25. Wilson JG, Macgregor DC, Goldman BS et al: Factors affecting patient recovery following pacemaker implantation, *Clin Prog Pacing Electrophysiology* 2(6):554, 1984.
26. Wingate S: Levels of pacemaker acceptance by patients, *Heart Lung* 15(1):93, 1986.
27. Wirtzfeld A, Schmidt G, Himmler FC et al: Physiological pacing: present status and future developments, *PACE* 10:41, 1987.
28. Witherell CL: Questions nurses ask about pacemakers, *Am J Nurs* 90(12):20, 1990.
29. Zoll PM: Resuscitation of the heart in ventricular standstill by external electrical stimulation, *New Engl J Med* 247:768, 1952.

CHAPTER 8

Hemodynamic and Respiratory Monitoring

Objectives

After completing this chapter, the reader will be able to:

- Discuss the concept and measurement of central venous pressure.
- Describe the setting up, balancing, calibration, and validation of a pressure monitoring system.
- Discuss the concept of arterial pressure monitoring and variations in the arterial pulse.
- Discuss principles and monitoring of pulmonary artery and wedge pressures.
- Analyze pulmonary artery pressure values and waveforms in common disease states.
- Describe principles and monitoring of left atrial pressure.
- Describe the concept and measurement of cardiac output, including the different injectate methods.
- Apply the principles of hemodynamic monitoring to preload, afterload, and contractility manipulation.
- Describe the principles of respiratory monitoring, including the use of respiratory formulas, capnography, compliance measurements, and continuous monitoring of mixed venous oxygen saturation.
- Formulate nursing diagnoses and patient outcomes for patients requiring hemodynamic and respiratory monitoring.
- Specify the nursing interventions helpful for the patient and family experiencing the need for psychosocial support and teaching.
- Differentiate between pediatric and adult hemodynamic monitoring.

Hemodynamic monitoring is the measurement of hemodynamic status. *Hemodynamic status* is an index of the pressure and the flow within the pulmonary and systemic circulations. Patients with heart failure, fluid overload, shock, pulmonary hypertension, and other such problems have altered hemodynamic status. Invasive hemodynamic moni-

toring requires cardiac catheterization and arterial pressure monitoring. The advent of the Swan-Ganz catheter, first introduced in 1970, made bedside catheterization feasible and revolutionized hemodynamic evaluation. The critical care nurse must be able to competently operate hemodynamic monitoring equipment, assess and interpret trends in values, and formulate a nursing care plan.

CENTRAL VENOUS PRESSURE MONITORING

Central venous pressure (CVP) is measured in the superior vena cava, or right atrium, and is a direct measurement of right atrial (RA) pressure. The CVP reflects the preload of the right ventricle or right ventricular end-diastolic pressure (RVEDP), thereby providing information about the patient's blood volume, right ventricular (RV) performance, and venous capacitance. Cardiac events that produce the CVP waveform are shown in Fig. 8-1.

Indications for Monitoring

Monitoring of CVP is indicated for patients who have disturbances in circulating blood volume but in whom cardiopulmonary function is relatively normal. CVP measurements are most useful during early resuscitation from acute injury when there is little time to set up a pulmonary artery pressure (PAP) monitoring system. The CVP may be used to guide fluid therapy after hemorrhage, accidental and surgical trauma, sepsis, and emergency conditions associated with blood volume deficits. Valuable information can be obtained from the CVP concerning a patient's tolerance to a volume load or fluid challenge over a prescribed period of time. The CVP can indicate the reserve capacity of the heart and vascular tree.

Significance of Values

The CVP may be measured by a pressure transducer in millimeters of mercury (mm Hg) or by a water manometer in centimeters of water (cm H_2O). To convert mercury to water, the mercury value is multiplied by 1.36 (mm Hg $\times$ 1.36). To convert water to mercury, the water value is divided by 1.36 (cm $H_2O \div 1.36$). Fluid overload produces an elevated CVP, indicating that fluids have been overad-

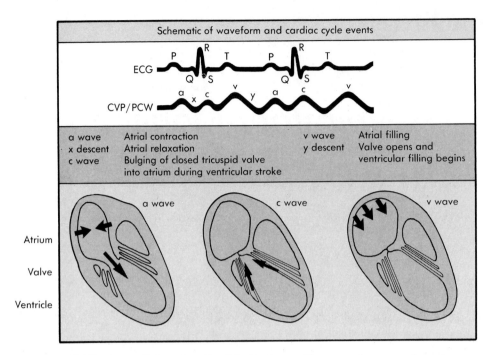

Fig. 8-1   Cardiac events that produce the CVP waveform with a, c, and v waves. A wave represents atrial contraction; x descent represents atrial relaxation; c wave represents the bulging of the closed tricuspid valve into the right atrium during ventricular systole; v wave represents atrial filling; y descent represents opening of the tricuspid valve and filling of the ventricle. (From Thelan LA, Davie JK, Urden LD: *Textbook of critical care nursing: diagnosis and management*, St Louis, 1990 Mosby–Year Book.)

ministered or administered too rapidly. A hypovolemic patient has a low CVP, indicating that there is insufficient blood volume in the ventricle at end diastole to produce an adequate stroke volume. CVP valves are as follows:

0-8 cm H_2O	Healthy ambulatory person lying down.
10-12 cm H_2O	Upper limit of normal for acutely ill patients.
15-18 cm H_2O	Upper limit of acceptable CVP values before a pulmonary artery catheter should be used to obtain pulmonary artery wedge pressures (PAWPs) for more precise titration of fluid administration.
20-25 cm H_2O	Values seen in critically ill patients on mechanical ventilation with positive end-expiratory pressure (PEEP), who require fluid volume to maintain arterial pressure.

Limitations

The CVP is not a reliable indicator of left-ventricular (LV) dysfunction or preload of the left side of the heart. A patient can have severe deterioration of LV function that will not be reflected in changes in RA or vena cava pressures. CVP measurements are not as accurate at reflecting hypovolemia as they are at indicating fluid overload. In the hypervolemic state and in right heart failure, blood accumulates behind the right ventricle, and the venous tree becomes distended. While this venous engorgement in-

creases, the CVP also increases so that high peripheral pressures reflect high CVP values. It is incorrect, however, to assess blood volume status from CVP values because there are many factors that influence CVP values, including vasopressor therapy, intrinsic venous tone, increased intraabdominal or intrathoracic pressures, cardiac performance, and blood volume. Wide variations in the CVP may also occur in cases of tricuspid insufficiency, when the central line slips into the right ventricle, and with severe right heart failure and dilation of the atrioventricular ring.

Complications

Some of the complications associated with central vein catheter placement include hemothorax, pneumothorax, nerve injury, arterial puncture, and thoracic-duct perforation. Once the catheter is placed the following problems may occur: systemic or local infection, perforation or erosion of vascular structures, thrombosis, and catheter or air embolism. When an open vein under negative pressure is exposed to atmospheric air, the potential for air emboli exists. Simple interventions that minimize the risk of air emboli include using heparin caps, avoiding cracks or defects in the tubing, and securing connections with Luer-Loks.

The most important consideration in measuring the CVP is to establish a consistent "zero" point so that changes may be followed by different individuals on different shifts. The reference point on the patient's chest should be marked with an X at the level of the right atrium so that it may be used consistently. The right atrium is located at the midaxillary line in the sixth intercostal space. Another way to determine the level of the right atrium is to use the phlebostatic axis and the phlebostatic level (Fig. 8-2). If the phlebostatic axis is used, any head-of-bed position up to 45 degrees may be accurately used for CVP readings.

EQUIPMENT AND SUPPLIES

- Stationary or portable CVP manometer with three-way stopcock
- Intravenous (IV) fluid container, IV tubing, and pole
- CVP catheter connected to IV tubing

NURSING INTERVENTIONS

1. Connect the IV tubing. Turn the stopcock off to the manometer by turning the flat side toward the manometer (Fig. 8-3, *B*). Spike the IV bottle, and run the fluid through the tubing, expelling all air bubbles.
2. After the physician inserts the central vein catheter, connect the catheter to the IV tubing, and flush the tubing to ensure patency. Order a chest x-ray to ensure proper placement, and observe for signs of complications of insertion.
3. Mark an X on the patient's chest at the phlebostatic axis (see Fig. 8-2).
4. Ensure that the patient is lying supine. The head of the bed may be elevated. Hold the manometer next to the patient so that the zero level of the manometer is at the phlebostatic level (see Fig. 8-3). Be careful not to touch the patient's skin with the manometer, since this leads to skin breakdown.

5. Turn the stopcock so that the flat side faces the CVP catheter. Allow fluid to flow into the manometer up to about the 20- or 25-cm level (Fig. 8-3,*C*).
6. Turn the stopcock so that the flat side is toward the IV fluid container line (Fig. 8-3,*D*). The fluid will flow out of the manometer into the CVP catheter and will fluctuate slightly with the patient's respirations.
7. Measure the CVP from the base of the meniscus of water at the end of expiration. End expiration is associated with a relatively constant intrapleural pressure. Do not disconnect a patient using a ventilator for a CVP reading.
8. If the manometer fluid does not fluctuate, there may be an obstruction of flow. Place the IV container below the level of the catheter, and check for a blood return. If blood does not return, the catheter is not patent. Check the tubing and catheter for kinks, and have the patient change position.
9. There may be a clot at the tip of the catheter, requiring aspiration with a syringe. After aspirating, discard the aspirated blood, and then gently flush the tubing to clear it of all blood. When irrigating, never force the solution in against great resistance. If the catheter is obstructed by a large clot, it will need to be irrigated with declotting agents according to a protocol (see Chapter 15).

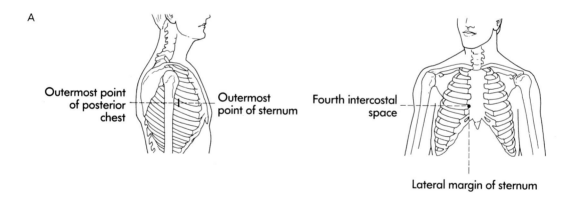

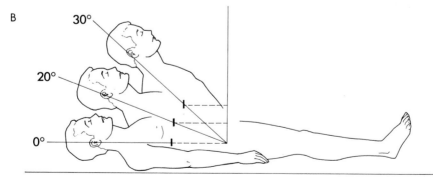

Fig. 8-2 The phlebostatic axis and the phlebostatic level. **A,** The phlebostatic axis is the intersection of two imaginary reference lines: one drawn halfway between the anterior and posterior surfaces of the chest, and another drawn from the point where the fourth intercostal space joins the sternum to the side of the body under the axilla. **B,** The phlebostatic level is a horizontal line through the phlebostatic axis. The line must be level with the zero mark on the manometer or the air-fluid interface of the transducer balancing port stopcock. As the patient moves from the supine to the semi-Fowler's position, the level stays horizontal through the same reference point.

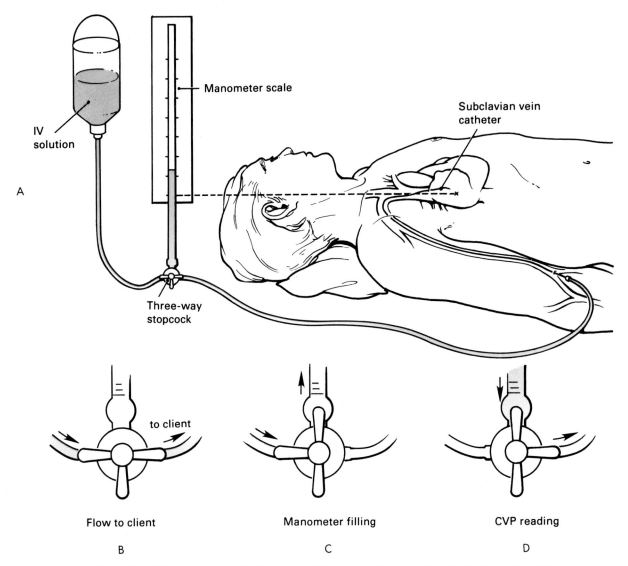

Manometer scale

IV solution

Subclavian vein catheter

A

Three-way stopcock

to client

Flow to client

Manometer filling

CVP reading

B   C   D

Fig. 8-3 CVP measurement. **A,** Placement of the manometer in relationship to the patient. The zero level of the manometer is at the phlebostatic axis. **B,** Stopcock is turned for intravenous flow to the patient. **C,** Stopcock is turned so that manometer fills with fluid. **D,** Stopcock is turned so that fluid in manometer flows to the patient. A CVP reading is obtained when the fluid level stabilizes. (From Lewis SM, Collier IC: *Medical-surgical nursing: assessment and management of clinical problems,* St Louis, 1992, Mosby–Year Book.)

COMPONENTS OF INVASIVE BLOOD PRESSURE MONITORING SYSTEMS

The basic components of an invasive blood pressure (BP) monitoring system found in an intensive care unit (ICU) are shown in Figs. 8-4 through 8-6. They consist of the following:
- Catheter entering patient's blood vessel.
- IV flush solution in pressure bag. Counterpressure from the pressure bag prevents backflow of blood into the monitoring system.
- Macrodrip IV infusion set.
- Pressure tubing kept as short as possible.
- Continuous-flush device with a manual fast-flush system.

- One or two stopcocks.
- T connector used to withdraw blood.
- Pressure transducer, converts movement into electrical signal.
- Transducer dome.
- Transducer arms.
- Balancing port stopcock.
- Amplifier system that provides output voltage.
- Oscilloscope. The pressure waveforms are displayed on a calibrated oscilloscope.
- *Digital displays.* The digital displays present quantitative data from the pressure waveforms.
- *Strip chart recorder.* Recorders print out dynamic response characteristics.

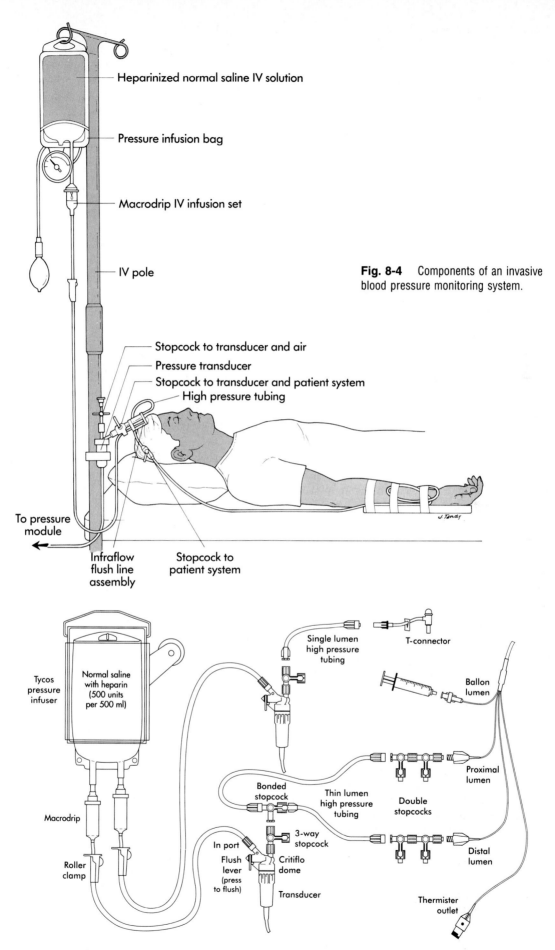

Heparinized normal saline IV solution

Pressure infusion bag

Macrodrip IV infusion set

IV pole

Fig. 8-4   Components of an invasive blood pressure monitoring system.

Stopcock to transducer and air
Pressure transducer
Stopcock to transducer and patient system
High pressure tubing

To pressure module

Infraflow flush line assembly

Stopcock to patient system

Tycos pressure infuser

Normal saline with heparin (500 units per 500 ml)

Single lumen high pressure tubing

T-connector

Ballon lumen

Proximal lumen

Macrodrip

Roller clamp

Bonded stopcock

Thin lumen high pressure tubing

Double stopcocks

Distal lumen

In port

Flush lever (press to flush)

3-way stopcock

Critiflo dome

Transducer

Thermister outlet

Fig. 8-5   Invasive blood pressure monitoring system used for monitoring systemic arterial pressure, right atrial pressure (CVP), and pulmonary artery pressure.

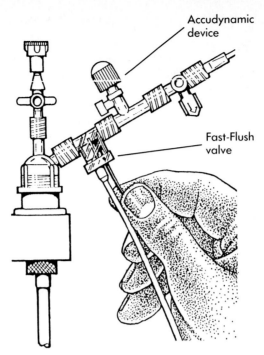

Fig. 8-6   Pull the pigtail to prime the tubing. Accudynamic device can be added to the monitoring system to absorb the unwanted frequency vibration. (Courtesy of Sorenson Research, Division of Abbott Laboratories, Salt Lake City, Utah.)

Skill 8-2   Setting Up a Pressure Monitoring System with a Disposable Pressure Transducer

EQUIPMENT AND SUPPLIES

- IV pole with a transducer holder
- IV pressure bag
- Heparinized flush solution with label
- Cardiac patients: 500 ml 5% dextrose in water (D_5W) with 500 units heparin
  Other patients: 500 ml NS with 500 units heparin
- Macrodrip IV infusion set (produces fewer bubbles)
- Stopcocks
- Disposable pressure transducer kit with pressure tubing
- Monitor and monitor cable

NURSING INTERVENTIONS

1. Turn on monitor and plug in the transducer cable. Allow the monitor several minutes to warm up.
2. Open the disposable transducer kit, and aseptically remove contents from the package. Add additional components as needed, but keep lines as short as possible. The longer the tubing, the more compromised the frequency response.
3. Tighten all connections. The components may have loosened during sterilization and shipping.
4. Slide the transducer into the pole mount, and connect the transducer to the monitor cable. This connection should be made before filling the system with fluid to avoid inadvertent fluid drippage into the transducer-monitor cable connection. Moisture within the connector may cause malfunction of the monitor cable or inaccurate pressure readings.
5. Remove all air from the IV bag by inserting a 22-gauge needle into the medication port and withdrawing the air. This minimizes the possibility of air emboli as the fluid level in the bag decreases or if the bag is placed in a horizontal position for transport.
6. Obtain an IV infusion set and move the roller clamp up near the drip chamber. Close the roller clamp and spike the IV bag with the IV macrodrip set. This eliminates entrapped air during initial priming. When monitoring two

pressure lines, a second IV tubing can be inserted into the medication port of the infusion bag (see Fig. 8-5).
7. Hang the IV bag about 60 cm (2 feet) above the patient. This generates approximately 45 mm Hg of pressure to prime the system through gravity.
8. Squeeze the drip chamber and fill at least halfway with flush solution. Open roller clamp.
9. Locate fast flush device, and either pull the pigtail or press the device (depending on manufacturer) to prime the kit in fast-flush mode. Flush the tubing slowly to prevent the formation of air bubbles (Fig. 8-6).
10. Turn the stopcock on the side that will lead to the patient's catheter to OFF position. Hold the transducer at an upward angle to prime the transducer. This allows the air to rise and leave the transducer more easily.
11. Replace the vented cap at the transducer vent port with a nonvented cap. Vented caps are used during sterilization to allow gas to reach all inner lumens.
12. Turn stopcock off to the transducer vent port, and fill remaining lines. All vented caps should be replaced with nonvented caps.
13. Pump up the IV pressure bag to no more than 300 mm Hg. The pressure gradient should be 200 mm Hg more than the pressure being measured to obtain flow through the flush device.
14. Flush the system. Aseptically connect the tubing to the catheter and begin monitoring. Always ensure that all air bubbles are eliminated from the system before connecting to the patient's catheter. Proceed with the balancing, calibration, and validation of system's dynamic response (the square-wave test).
15. Change flush solution and tubing every 48 hours, based on institutional policies.
16. Repressurize IV bag occasionally, since air may gradually escape from the pressure bag.
17. Ensure that no air bubbles are ever between the flush device and the patient catheter.

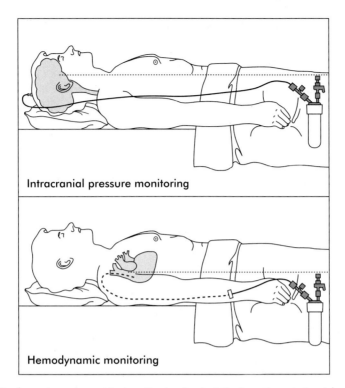

Intracranial pressure monitoring

Hemodynamic monitoring

Fig. 8-7   For hemodynamic monitoring, the top level of the transducer balancing port stopcock (air-fluid interface) should correspond to the phlebostatic axis, located at the patient's right atrium. In intracranial pressure monitoring the pressure source is the foramen of Monroe.

Skill 8-3   Balancing (Zeroing) a Pressure Transducer

Monitoring equipment is not always stable and has a tendency to drift, similar to a weight scale that drifts away from zero when the scale is empty. A pressure transducer should be balanced (or zeroed) every 8 hours and when dramatic variances in the waveform or readings are observed. To zero a transducer, the transducer will need to be opened to air, since atmospheric pressure is read as zero. By balancing, atmospheric pressure is established as the baseline for the patient's pressure readings. This prevents atmospheric pressure from affecting the patient's pressure readings.

EQUIPMENT AND SUPPLIES

• Carpenter's level or closed-loop water leveler

NURSING INTERVENTIONS

1. Adjust the level of the transducer balancing port stopcock (air-fluid interface) to correspond to the phlebostatic level

(see Figs. 8-2 and 8-7). This can be done with a carpenter's level, a closed-loop water leveler, or by sighting (eyeballing) the correct level.
2. Remove and save the vented cap, and adjust transducer stopcock so that it is turned off to the patient and the transducer balancing port stopcock is open to the atmosphere.
3. Depress the ZERO button on the monitor or adjust the ZERO knob to read 0 mm Hg.
4. Observe the oscilloscope screen. You will see a flat wave at zero.
5. Turn the stopcock, closing the transducer balancing port to atmosphere and resume patient monitoring. Replace vented cap.
6. Calibrate the monitor with the transducer (Skill 8-4).
7. Maintain the transducer balancing port at the proper level throughout monitoring. For each inch off the proper level, one can expect a 2 mm Hg error in the pressure reading.

Skill 8-4   Calibrating the Monitor to the Transducer Using a Mercury Manometer

Before monitoring a patient's pressure, ensure that the monitor will interpret the transducer's signal correctly. For a monitoring system to be accurate, the equipment must be calibrated to known standards. A known quantity of pressure will need to be applied to the transducer with either a mercury column, electronic calibrator, or water manometer calibration scale. The monitor will then need to be adjusted to reflect that known pressure. The monitor should be calibrated to the transducer every 8 hours and with any noted change in pressure measurements that might require a major change in therapy.

EQUIPMENT AND SUPPLIES

- Mercury sphygmomanometer
- Plastic Y connector
- Three pieces of rubber tubing
- Stopcock

NURSING INTERVENTIONS

1. Begin by balancing the transducer (see Skill 8-3).
2. Check the calibration of the monitor, which will be determined by a built-in electronic calibration factor.
3. Depress the CALIBRATE button on the monitor system. A known pressure will be applied internally (e.g., 200 mm Hg).
4. After the readout stabilizes, adjust the control knob to obtain the appropriate readout value of 200 mm Hg.
5. Ensure that the transducer balancing port stopcock is at the phlebostatic level.
6. Attach rubber tubing adaptor pieces to three ends of Y-connector (Fig. 8-8).
7. Remove the cuff from the mercury sphygmomanometer.
8. Attach the rubber tubing to one arm of the Y-connector.
9. Attach the sphygmomanometer's bulb to the other arm of the Y-connector.
10. Connect the foot of the Y-connector to the transducer balancing port stopcock.
11. Ensure that the stopcock on the patient's side of the transducer is off to the patient to prevent air embolism.
12. Open the stopcock between the Y-connector and the dome.
13. Check the monitor to ensure that a zero reading on the mercury manometer produces a zero reading on the pressure module. If there is a discrepancy, adjust the monitor to read zero.

14. Pump up the sphygmomanometer until the column reaches 200 mm Hg. This applies 200 mm Hg to the transducer's diaphragm. Adjust monitor's CALIBRATION control knob to display 200 mm Hg at the digital readout and wave tracing on the oscilloscope.
15. Lower mercury level to zero again.
16. Close the stopcock on the transducer to the air and re-open the stopcock to patient monitoring.

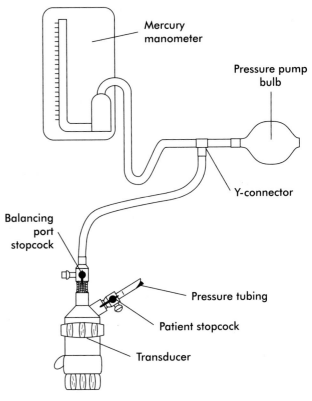

Fig. 8-8   Setup for calibrating the monitor with the transducer using a mercury manometer.

Skill 8-5   Calibrating the Monitor to the Transducer Using a Water Manometer Calibration Scale

When a transducer is calibrated with pressurized air while it is connected to a patient, the patient may be exposed to an air embolism. A safer method is to connect a piece of sterile IV extension tubing to a position vertical to the transducer's balancing port stopcock, and then use the fast flush device to fill the tubing with a column of fluid.

EQUIPMENT AND SUPPLIES

- Water manometer calibration scale

NURSING INTERVENTIONS

1. Insert water manometer calibration scale into transducer holder (Fig. 8-9).
2. Remove nonvented cap from tubing set.
3. Turn transducer vent port stopcock off to patient, and remove nonvented cap. Zero monitor.
4. Replace nonvented cap, and turn vent port stopcock on to patient. Hold open end of patient line at 30 mm Hg. Mark and adjust monitor to 30 mm Hg if needed. Calibration at this pressure will ensure proper system accuracy for entire operating range.

Skill 8-6   Removing Bubbles from Transducer

EQUIPMENT AND SUPPLIES

- 10-ml syringe

NURSING INTERVENTIONS

1. Attach a 10-ml syringe to transducer vent port.
2. Turn transducer vent port stopcock off to patient, and pull a slight vacuum (0.3 to 0.5 ml) inside syringe.
3. Activate flush device and slight vacuum will instantaneously empty old fluid with air bubble. Keep activating flush device and pulling back on syringe plunger until transducer is filled with bubble-free solution.
4. Remove syringe and rezero monitor.
5. Turn stopcock on to patient and replace nonvented cap. Resume monitoring.

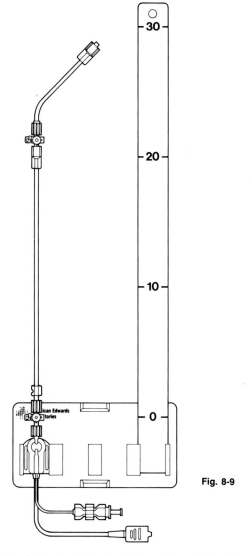

Fig. 8-9

Fig. 8-9   Setup for calibrating the monitor with the transducer using a water manometer calibration scale. *(Courtesy of Baxter Healthcare Corporation, Edwards Critical-Care Division, Santa Ana, Calif.)*

Skill 8-7   Performance of the Square-Wave Test to Validate the Pressure Monitoring System's Dynamic Response

A patient pressure monitoring system must be able to respond to changing blood pressures. This is referred to as a *dynamic response*. The catheter-tubing-transducer system used in ICUs has a measurable natural frequency and a measurable damping coefficient, which indicate how quickly a system comes to rest after being excited. An underdamped system will produce a waveform that is artificially spiked and exaggerated. An overdamped system will produce a waveform that is artificially rounded and blunted.[7] The dynamic response of a pressure monitoring system can be assessed by performing a square-wave test.

NURSING INTERVENTIONS

1. Validate the dynamic response of the pressure monitoring system whenever the pressure waveform appears to be damped or otherwise distorted, at least once each shift, and after each opening of the system, such as for drawing blood, changing the tubing, or balancing the transducer.
2. Turn on the strip chart recorder of the monitor.
3. Open the valve of the continuous flush device by pulling and quickly releasing the pigtail or pressing the lever (depending on the manufacturer). The rapid closure generates a square wave. Check that the square wave exceeds 200 mm Hg.
4. Observe for the oscillation of the pressure wave directly after the square wave. An optimal dynamic response would consist of two or three rapid oscillations extending sharply below the baseline and then displaying a rapid recovery to the original pressure waveform (Fig. 8-10, *A*).
5. Observe for a possible overdamped system in which the end of the square wave does not oscillate below the baseline. The pressure tracing that follows appears unnaturally smooth, and the waveform has an absent or diminished dicrotic notch (Fig. 8-10, *B*). Observe for false low-systolic and high-diastolic pressure readings.
6. To optimize the dynamic response of the system:[9]
   - Remove any air bubbles.
   - Ensure that there is no soft, compliant tubing in use.
   - Shorten the tubing to less than 4 feet.
   - Reduce the number of stopcocks to fewer than three.
   - Ensure that the pressure bag is pumped up to 300 mm Hg.
   - Eliminate kinks in the system.
   - Flush the tubing free of clotted blood.
   - Ensure that the catheter tip is not against a vessel wall.
   - Aspirate clots from the catheter tip if necessary.
7. Observe for a possible underdamped system (low damping coefficient) characterized by too many oscillations or vibrations in the waveform following the square wave (see Fig. 8-10, *C*). This indicates excessive "noise" in the system. Observe for false high-systolic and low-diastolic pressures on the monitor.
8. To induce damping, make the following changes to the system:
   - Add a device (Accudynamic or Rose) to the monitoring system to absorb the unwanted frequency vibration (see Fig. 8-6).
   - Add a 8-cm (3-inch) extension tubing to the monitoring system.
   - Turn a stopcock slightly.

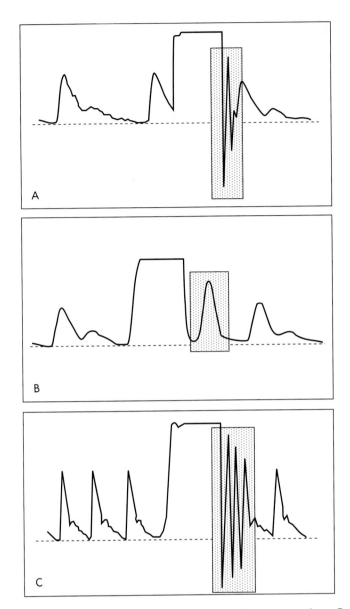

Fig. 8-10   Square wave testing using the fast-flush valve. **A,** Accurate waveform. **B,** Overdamped. **C,** Underdamped. *(Courtesy of Baxter Healthcare, Irvine, Calif.)*

ARTERIAL PRESSURE MONITORING

The continuous invasive monitoring of arterial pressure is used in the following situations:
- When cuff blood pressures are not audible.
- If there is a need for frequent, accurate BP.
- When patients need to be undisturbed while BP is observed.
- During intraaortic balloon counterpulsation.
- When there is a need for frequent arterial blood gas (ABG) measurements.

Systolic pressure is the maximal pressure with which the blood is expelled from the left ventricle during systole. Roughly, the upper limit of normal for systolic pressures is 100 plus the patient's age (Table 8-1). The *diastolic pressure* reflects both the vessel's elasticity and the rapidity of flow of the ejected blood through the arterial system. The mean arterial pressure (MAP) is most frequently used to assess perfusion because MAP represents perfusion pressure throughout the cardiac cycle. The MAP is calculated as shown in Table 8-1. It is important to ensure that a pa-

Table 8-1   Hemodynamic Pressures and Calculated Hemodynamic Values

Hemodynamic pressure or value	Abbreviation	Definition and explanation	Normal range	Formula
Mean arterial pressure	MAP	Average perfusion pressure created by arterial blood pressure during the complete cardiac cycle. The normal cardiac cycle is ⅓ systole and ⅔ diastole. These three components are divided by 3 to obtain the average perfusion pressure for the whole cardiac cycle.	70-90 mm Hg	$$\frac{(\text{Diastolic} \times 2) + (\text{Systolic} \times 1)}{3}$$
Central venous pressure	CVP	Pressure created by volume in the right side of the heart. When the tricuspid valve is open, the CVP reflects filling pressures in the right ventricle. Clinically, the CVP is often used as a guide to overall fluid balance.	0-8 cm water (H_2O) 0-6 mm Hg	$$\frac{(\text{CVP diastolic} \times 2) + (\text{CVP systolic} \times 1)}{3}$$
Left atrial pressure	LAP	Pressure created by volume in the left side of the heart. When the mitral valve is open, the LAP reflects filling pressures in the left ventricle. Clinically, the LAP is used after cardiac surgery to determine how well the left ventricle is ejecting its volume. In general the higher the LAP, the lower is the ejection fraction from the left ventricle.	5-10 mm Hg	$$\frac{(\text{LAP diastolic} \times 2) + (\text{LAP systolic} \times 1)}{3}$$
Pulmonary artery pressure (systolic, diastolic, mean)	PAP, PA systolic (PAS), PA diastolic (PAD), PAP mean (PAP$_M$)	Pulsatile pressure in the pulmonary artery, measured by an indwelling catheter.	PAS 20-30 mm Hg PAD 6-12 mm Hg PAM 10-15 mm Hg	$$\frac{(\text{PAD} \times 2) + (\text{PAS} \times 1)}{3}$$
Pulmonary capillary wedge pressure or pulmonary artery wedge pressure	PCW or PCWP or PAWP	Pressure created by volume in the left side of the heart. When the mitral valve is open, the PAWP reflects filling pressures in the pulmonary vasculature, and pressures in the left side of the heart are transmitted back to the catheter "wedged" into a small pulmonary arteriole.	PAWP 6-15 mm Hg	
Cardiac output	CO	The amount of blood pumped out by a ventricle. Clinically, it can be measured using the thermodilution CO method, which calculates CO in liters per minute (L/min).	5-6 L/min (at rest)	Heart rate × Stroke volume

Adapted from Thelan LA, Davie JK, Urden LD: *Textbook of critical care nursing: diagnosis and management,* St Louis, 1990, Mosby–Year Book.

Continued.

Table 8-1   Hemodynamic Pressures and Calculated Hemodynamic Values—cont'd

Hemodynamic pressure or value	Abbreviation	Definition and explanation	Normal range	Formula
Cardiac index	CI	Cardiac output divided by body surface area (BSA), tailoring the CO to individual body size. A BSA conversion chart is necessary to calculate CI, which is considered more accurate than CO because it is individualized to height and weight. CI is measured in liters per minute per square meter BSA ($L/min/m^2$).	2.5-4.0 $L/min/m^2$	$\dfrac{CO}{BSA}$
Stroke volume	SV	Amount of blood ejected by the ventricle with each heart beat. Hemodynamic monitoring systems calculate SV by dividing cardiac output (CO in L/min) by the heart rate (HR) then multiplying the answer by 1000 to change liters to milliliters (ml).	60-130 ml	$\dfrac{CO}{HR} \times 1000$
Stroke volume index	SI	SV indexed to BSA.	40-50 ml/m^2	$\dfrac{SV}{BSA}$
Systemic vascular resistance	SVR	Mean pressure difference across the systemic vascular bed, divided by blood flow. Clinically, SVR represents the resistance against which the left ventricle must pump to eject its volume. This resistance is created by the systemic arteries and arterioles. As SVR increases, cardiac output falls. SVR is measured in either units or $dynes/sec/cm^{-5}$. If the number of units is multiplied by 80, the value is converted to $dynes/sec/cm^{-5}$.	900-1200 $dynes/sec/cm^{-5}$	$\dfrac{MAP - CVP}{CO} = units$ $\dfrac{MAP - CVP}{CO} \times 80 = dynes/sec/cm^{-5}$
Systemic vascular resistance index	SVRI	SVR indexed to BSA.	2000-2400 $dynes/sec/cm^{-5}/m^2$	$\dfrac{MAP - CVP}{CI} \times 80 = dynes/sec/cm^{-5}/m^2$

Table 8-1 Hemodynamic Pressures and Calculated Hemodynamic Values—cont'd

Hemodynamic pressure or value	Abbreviation	Definition and explanation	Normal range	Formula
Pulmonary vascular resistance	PVR	Mean pressure difference across pulmonary vascular bed, divided by blood flow. Clinically, PVR represents the resistance against which the right ventricle must pump to eject its volume. This resistance is created by the pulmonary arteries and arterioles. As PVR increases, the output from the right ventricle decreases. PVR is measured in either units or dynes/sec/cm^{-5}. PVR is normally ⅙ of SVR.	1.2-3.0 units or 150-250 dynes/sec/cm^{-5}	$$\frac{PAP\ mean - PAWP}{CO} = units$$
Pulmonary vascular resistance index	PVRI	PVR indexed to BSA.	225-315 dynes/sec/cm^{-5}/m^2	$$\frac{PAP\ mean - PAWP}{CI} \times 80 =$$ dynes/sec/cm^{-5}/m^2
Left cardiac work index	LCWI	Amount of work the left ventricle does *each minute* when ejecting blood. The hemodynamic formula represents pressure generated (MAP) multiplied by volume pumped (CO); 0.0136 is a conversion factor to change mm Hg to kilogram-meter (kg-m). LCWI is always represented as an indexed volume (BSA chart). LCWI increases or decreases because of changes in either pressure (MAP) or volume pumped (CO).	3.4-4.2 kg-m/m^2	1. MAP × CO × 0.0136 = LCW 2. $\dfrac{LCW}{BSA}$ = LCWI
Left ventricular stroke work index	LVSWI	Amount of work the left ventricle performs with *each heartbeat*. The hemodynamic formula represents pressure generated (MAP) multiplied by volume pumped (SV); 0.0136 is a conversion factor to change ml/mmHg to gram-meter (g-m). LVSWI is always represented as an indexed volume. LVSWI increases or decreases because of changes in either pressure (MAP) or volume pumped (SV).	50-62 g-m/m^2	1. MAP × SV × 0.0136 = LVSW 2. $\dfrac{LVSW}{BSA}$ = LVSWI

Continued.

Table 8-1 Hemodynamic Pressures and Calculated Hemodynamic Values—cont'd

Hemodynamic pressure or value	Abbreviation	Definition and explanation	Normal range	Formula
Right cardiac work index	RCWI	Amount of work the right ventricle performs *each minute* when ejecting blood. The hemodynamic formula represents pressure generated (PAP mean) multiplied by volume pumped (CO); 0.0136 is a conversion factor to change mm Hg to kilogram-meter (kg-m). RCWI is always represented as an indexed value (BSA chart). Similar to LCWI, the RCWI increases or decreases because of changes in either pressure (PAP mean) or volume pumped (CO).	0.54-0.66 kg-m/m²	1. PAP mean $\times$ CO $\times$ 0.0136 = RCW 2. $\dfrac{RCW}{BSA}$ = RCWI
Right ventricular stroke work index	RVSWI	Amount of work the right ventricle does *each heart beat*. The hemodynamic formula represents pressure generated (PAP mean) multiplied by volume pumped (SV); 0.0136 is a conversion factor to change mm Hg to grammeter (g-m). RVSWI is always represented as an indexed value (BSA chart). Similar to LVSWI, the RVSWI increases or decreases because of changes in either pressure (PAP mean) or volume pumped (CO).	7.9-9.7 g-m/m²	1. PAP mean $\times$ SV $\times$ 0.0136 = RVSW 2. $\dfrac{RVSW}{BSA}$ = RVSWI

tient's MAP does not drop below 60 mm Hg, since this pressure is necessary to perfuse the brain, coronary arteries, and kidneys. Arterial pressure reflects a patient's overall circulatory status and does not directly measure reductions of blood flow and volume but rather the failure of circulatory compensations. When deficits in blood volume or cardiac function exist, such as in shock and trauma states, the body has compensatory neurovascular mechanisms that will sustain arterial pressures. Therefore arterial pressures are useful only for screening and for rapid assessment of trends in emergency conditions, especially gastrointestinal (GI) bleeding and trauma. It is important to know a patient's baseline pre-illness arterial pressure, since there is such a wide range of normal pressures. The critical care nurse should assess and treat the clinical situation and BP trends rather than absolute numbers.

INTERPRETATION OF THE ARTERIAL PRESSURE WAVEFORM

The normal arterial pressure waveform begins with a sharp upstoke as blood is rapidly ejected from the left ventricle through the aortic valve (Fig. 8-11). The highest point is the systolic pressure. After peak ejection, there is a decrease in pressure as blood flows into the periphery. As the pressure falls the aortic valve closes, producing a characteristic dicrotic notch on the downstroke of the waveform. The dicrotic notch signifies the onset of diastole. The remainder of the descending waveform represents runoff of blood flow into the arterial system. The lowest point recorded is diastole. Variations from the normal arterial pulse can occur because of many physiological conditions as shown in the box on p. 117 and Fig. 8-12.

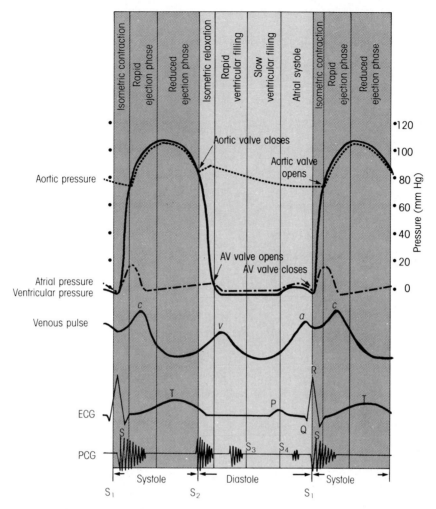

Fig. 8-11 Cardiac cycle, showing events of systole and diastole, venous pressure waves, ECG, and heart sounds. (From Guzzetta CE, Dossey BM: *Cardiovascular nursing: holistic practice,* St Louis, 1992, Mosby–Year Book.)

Comparisons of Indirect versus Direct Blood Pressure Monitoring

Direct BP monitoring is an invasive method of measuring arterial pressure. The tip of a hollow catheter is inserted into an artery to the selected point of measurement. The vascular pressure is then transmitted through fluid (usually saline) to a pressure transducer. Pressure transducers contain a diaphragm and convert pressure against this diaphragm into an electrical signal. Electrical elements alter the electrical signal by an amount proportional to the applied pressure. The electrical signal is then amplified, processed, and displayed by a monitor as a numerical value or pressure waveform. The most common site for in-traarterial catheterization is the radial artery, since the collateral circulation of the hand is distal to the site of cannulation. This minimizes the risk of vascular complications. Before inserting the arterial line into the radial artery, the Allen's test can be performed to determine the adequacy of blood supply to the hand.

Indirect BP monitoring is a noninvasive method of measuring arterial pressure. Various techniques for obtaining BP are through auscultation, palpation, automatic blood pressure machines, and dopplers. There may be inconsistencies between direct and indirect BP values. In normal conditions, pressures obtained from intraarterial catheters are approximately 2 to 8 mm Hg higher than cuff pres-

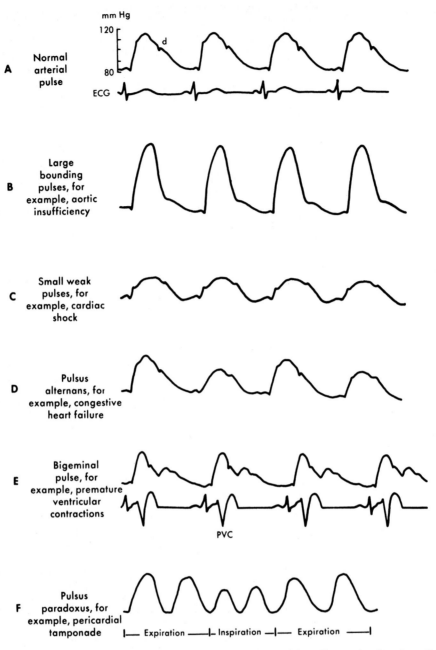

mm Hg

120

A Normal arterial pulse

80

ECG

B Large bounding pulses, for example, aortic insufficiency

C Small weak pulses, for example, cardiac shock

D Pulsus alternans, for example, congestive heart failure

E Bigeminal pulse, for example, premature ventricular contractions

PVC

F Pulsus paradoxus, for example, pericardial tamponade

|— Expiration —|— Inspiration —|— Expiration —|

Fig. 8-12 Variations in contour of the arterial pulse with selected cardiovascular disorders. (From Andreoli KG et al: *Comprehensive cardiac care*, ed 6, St Louis, 1987, Mosby–Year Book.)

sures. In critically ill patients, intraarterial pressures have been found to be 10 to 30 mm Hg higher than cuff pressures. When there is severe vasoconstriction with low stroke volume, cuff pressures are often inaccurate. Some monitoring systems produce artificially high readings during amplification of incoming signals. This increases the discrepancy between directly and indirectly obtained values.[13] Rather than waste precious time attempting to correlate cuff and arterial line pressures, nurses should accept that a disparity of 5 to 20 mm Hg is within an acceptable

range. It is more important to monitor BP trends and evaluate other indices, such as mentation, cardiac index, and pulmonary artery pressures.

In some cases in which there is a discrepancy in the BP measurements, the monitoring system may be underdamped. The systolic pressure obtained by intraarterial catheter is higher than that obtained by cuff, whereas the diastolic pressure is lower. The pressure monitoring system's dynamic response can be tested as in Skill 8-7 or evaluated with the monitored occlusion technique (Skill 8-8).

▼
Variations in the Arterial Pulse

Pulsus magnus—large, bounding pulse consisting of a large, rapid upstroke, a brief peak, and a fast downstroke; seen in association with exercise, anxiety, fear, hyperthyroidism, anemia, patent ductus arteriosis, aortic regurgitation, complete heart block with bradycardia, and hypertension; it is also found in elderly persons who have arteriosclerosis and rigidity of the arterial system.

Pulsus parvus—small, weak pulse characterized by diminished pulse pressure. The pulse contour shows a slow gradual upstroke, a delayed peak, and a prolonged downstroke; it is found in severe left ventricular failure as a result of decreased stroke volume and in moderate-to-severe cases of aortic stenosis as a result of slow ejection of blood through the valve.

Pulsus alternans—heart beats with a regular rhythm but with alternating strong and weak beats; seen in left-sided heart failure. When the heart contracts, some damaged cells take longer to recover. These recovering cells do not contribute to contraction with the subsequent beat. Therefore every other contraction ejects more volume.

Bigeminal pulse—one that alternates in amplitude from beat to beat, usually when every other contraction of the heart is premature. The stroke volume of the premature beat is less than that of the normal beat.

Pulsus paradoxus—the pulse diminishes significantly in amplitude (more than 10 mm Hg in the systolic blood pressure) during inspiration, because of a diminished stroke volume; it is seen in cardiac tamponade, severe emphysema, constrictive pericardial disease, congestive heart failure caused by chronic myocardial disease, restrictive cardiomyopathy, and hypovolemic shock.

Pulse deficit—the heart rate counted at the apex is higher than that of the pulse counted by palpation at a peripheral artery. Not every cardiac contraction is strong enough to reach the periphery because of the presence of dysrhythmias, such as atrial fibrillation and premature contractions.

Decreased pulse pressure—when the difference between the systolic and diastolic pressures decreases because of falling stroke volume; this often precedes decreases in diastolic pressure in patients developing hypovolemic shock and is one of the first clinical signs of blood volume loss; this also occurs in cardiac tamponade when fluid in the pericardial sac limits the venous inflow and diastolic filling of the heart.

Increased pulse pressure—an early sign of volume restoration; this is also associated with systemic arteriovenous fistulas and aortic valve insufficiency; it may be a sign of increased intracranial pressure, especially in presence of an increase in systolic pressure without a diastolic rise.

Skill 8-8 Monitored Occlusion Technique[4]
▼
NURSING INTERVENTIONS

1. Position one observer near the BP manometer and the second observer in sight of the oscilloscope screen.
2. The first observer places the BP cuff around the extremity above the intraarterial catheter and inflates the cuff until the pressure wave on the oscilloscope screen disappears.
3. The first observer deflates the BP cuff while observing the mercury manometer.
4. The second observer signals when the first "blip" appears in the flat line on the oscilloscope screen as the pressure wave reappears.
5. The first observer notes the value on the mercury manometer when the blip occurs, representing the true systolic pressure.
6. If there is a large discrepancy in the value obtained and that displayed by the monitor, corrections can be made as in step 8, Skill 8-7.

Skill 8-9 Obtaining a Blood Sample from an Arterial Line
▼
EQUIPMENT AND SUPPLIES

- Blood tubes
- Needle
- 10-ml syringe
- 10- or 20-ml syringe
- Sterile 4 × 4 sponges in packets

NURSING INTERVENTIONS

1. Turn off arterial pressure alarm.
2. Open sterile 4 × 4 sponge packet, leaving packet intact, and rest sampling stopcock on sponges.
3. Remove stopcock port cap and place on sterile field.
4. Insert 10-ml syringe into sampling port, and turn stopcock off to flush solution bag.
5. Aspirate flush solution from arterial line into syringe until blood is obtained. Close stopcock to the halfway position, remove syringe, and discard.
6. Attach new syringe to stopcock port, close stopcock to flush solution bag line, and aspirate blood gently, allowing arterial pressure to fill syringe.
7. Turn stopcock off to arterial line, and remove syringe. Attach needle to syringe, and inject blood into blood tubes.
8. Point sampling port down over 4 × 4 sponges, and clear stopcock of blood using fast-flush valve. Replace cap over port.
9. Turn stopcock off to sampling port, and flush arterial line until all traces of blood are removed.
10. Reset arterial pressure alarm, and check monitor for reappearance of normal arterial waveform.

PULMONARY ARTERY PRESSURE MONITORING
Indications

The development of the balloon-tipped, flow-directed pulmonary artery (PA) catheter by Swan and Ganz in 1970 represented a major advance in hemodynamic monitoring. Made of pliable, radiopaque polyvinyl chloride, the catheter most commonly has four lumens (Fig. 8-13). The clinical advantages of using PA catheters include their ability to (1) measure intracardiac pressures and waveforms, (2) obtain mixed venous blood samples, (3) determine cardiac output, (4) monitor mixed venous oxygen saturation, (5) act as a temporary pacemaker of the atrium or ventricles, and (6) administer drugs directly into the central circulation. The information obtained from the PA catheter can be used to assess fluid volume status, ventricular performance, and tissue oxygen supply and demand. The information can also be used to calculate the derived hemodynamic and respiratory indexes and to diagnose cardiopulmonary pathologies.

One of the most important clinical applications of a PA catheter is to assess left ventricular (LV) performance. Besides providing information about the cardiac output, the PA catheter can provide an estimate of the preload of the left ventricle, also known as the *left ventricular end-diastolic pressure (LVEDP)*. The LVEDP conveys the "state of fullness" of the left ventricle before its contraction begins. Measuring the LVEDP enables one to assess the fluid volume status of the patient and the function of the left ventricle. Most normal hearts show a LVEDP of 5 to 15 mm Hg. A ventricle that requires a filling pressure greater than 20 mm Hg to pump is severely dysfunctional. Once the LVEDP is known, it can be manipulated to improve LV performance.

Direct bedside monitoring of the pressures in the left side of the heart is not commonly performed in ICUs. The right side of the heart, however, is easily accessible by cannulating the great veins (subclavian and jugular) that lead directly to the right heart. The PA catheter, inserted into the right heart, can be used to measure pressures on the left side of the heart through the pulmonary artery wedge pressure (PAWP) and the pulmonary artery diastolic pressure (PADP) (Figs. 8-14 and 8-15). At the tip of the PA catheter is a balloon that, when inflated, is carried up the bloodstream until it "wedges" in a branch of the pulmonary artery. With the catheter wedged, the tip is no longer exposed to pressure from the right heart. During ventricular diastole when the mitral valve is open, there is a clear pathway between the tip of the catheter and the left ventricle. Therefore the PAWP is identical to the LVEDP. The PAWP cannot reflect LV preload in the presence of mitral regurgitation or stenosis, left atrial myxoma, pulmonary hypertension, reduced or increased LV compliance, thoracic tumors pressing on pulmonary veins, or when the catheter tip is in lung zone 1 or 2 (Fig. 8-16).

Pulmonary Artery Pressure Waveforms

The PAP waveform looks very similar to an arterial line tracing except that the pressures are generally lower (Fig. 8-17). RV systole causes opening of the pulmonic valve and a rush of blood into the PA. This causes the initial positive upstroke in the PA pressure tracing. The dicrotic notch occurs on the downstroke when the pulmonary valve closes.

The PAWP waveform reflects events in the left atrium, so it will have a, c, and v waves that have physiological origins similar to those of the RA pressure waveform. The a wave represents LA contraction, and the c wave is produced by closure of the mitral valve. The v wave reflects LA filling and posterior bulging of the mitral valve during LV systole (Fig. 8-18).

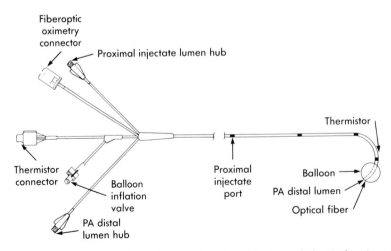

Fig. 8-13   Pulmonary artery catheter. The proximal injectate lumen hub attaches to a pressure line to measure right atrial CVP. This is also the hub where the solution will be injected to measure CO. The injectate solution will exit at the proximal injectate port, located in the right atrium.

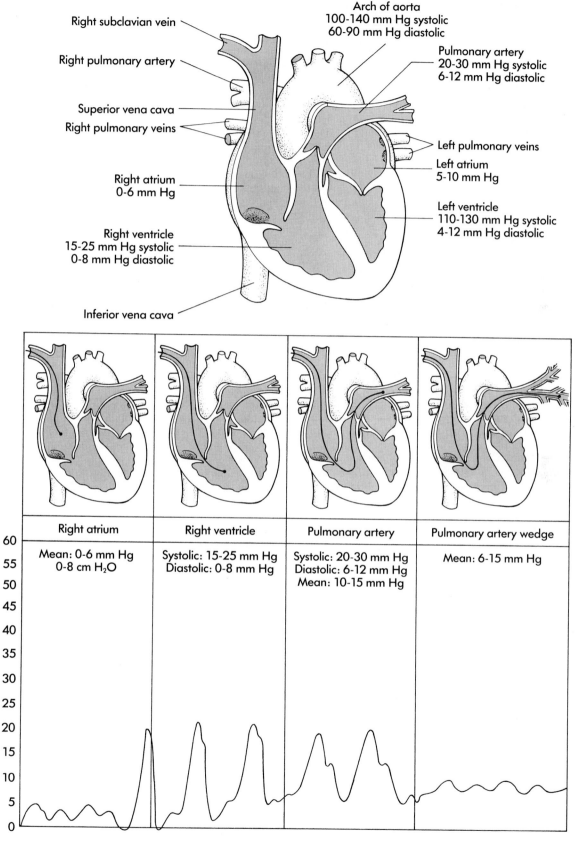

Fig. 8-14 *Above,* Representation of the heart showing all four chambers and valves visible in the anterior view. *Below,* PA catheter insertion with corresponding waveforms and pressures.

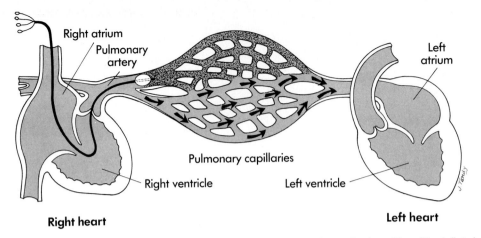

Fig. 8-15 Representation of the pulmonary artery catheter in the wedged position. The inflated balloon floats into a segment of the pulmonary artery. No blood flows distally to the balloon-occluded segment. This creates a nonmoving column of blood that allows the electronic monitoring equipment to "look through" a nonactive segment of the pulmonary circulation to the left atrium.

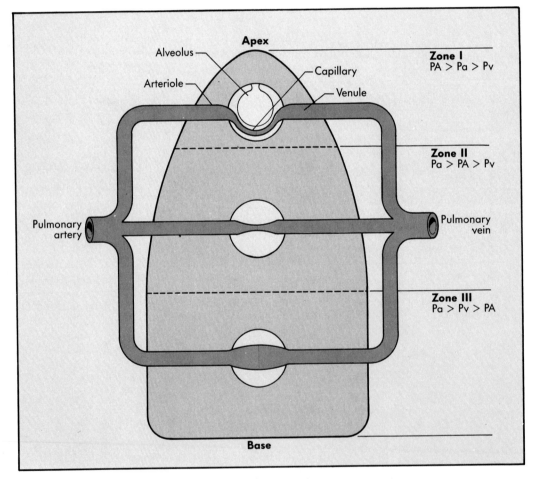

Fig. 8-16 West lung zones. The upright lung can be separated into three zones. In *zone 1,* or the upper third of the lung, alveolar pressure exceeds pulmonary venous and pulmonary artery pressure (PAP). In *zone 2,* the middle third, PAP is greater than alveolar pressure, which is greater than pulmonary venous pressure. In *zone 3,* the lowest third of the lung, PAP is greater than pulmonary venous pressure, which is greater than alveolar pressure. Because of these pressure differentials, if a PA catheter is placed in the upper zone of the lung, it might erroneously be measuring alveolar or pleural pressure rather than the pressure of the pulmonary artery. The best place to measure the PAWP is in zone 3 because the diameter of the capillary lumen in this area is unaffected by alveolar pressure. One might suspect that the catheter is malpositioned outside of zone 3 if the PAWP is greater than the PADP, especially when PEEP artificially raises alveolar pressure. (From McCance KL, Huether SE: *Pathophysiology: the biologic basis for disease in adults and children,* St Louis, 1990, Mosby–Year Book.)

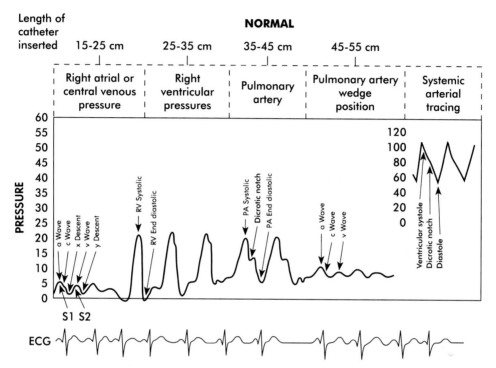

Fig. 8-17 Normal PA catheter and systemic arterial pressure tracings. (From Victor LD: *Manual of critical care procedures,* Rockville, Md, 1989, Aspen.)

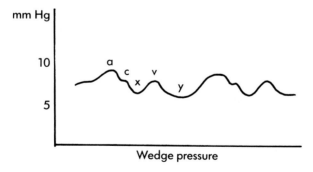

Fig. 8-18 PAWP waveform. The *a wave* = atrial contraction; the *c wave* = bulging of the valve into the atrium, resulting from ventricular contraction; the *x descent* = a drop in pressure in response to further atrial volume changes during ventricular contraction; the *v wave* = a rise in pressure during the remainder of systole resulting from continuous venous inflow; the *y descent* = a pressure drop in the atrium that accompanies the transfer of blood from the atria into the ventricles.

Variable Pulmonary Artery Pressure Values

The normal PAP mean is 10 to 15 mm Hg, and the normal PAWP is 6 to 15 mm Hg (see Table 8-2). Since the PAWP equals the pulmonary capillary pressure, it is a critical measurement of the movement of fluid from the vascular bed to the interstitial and alveolar spaces of the lungs. The nurse should be aware that once the PAWP is elevated to 18 to 20 mm Hg, mild pulmonary congestion is usually evident and should be reported. Once the PAWP is above 30 mm Hg, acute pulmonary edema occurs. Likewise, if a patient has a PAWP of 0 to 5 mm Hg, the nurse should be alert for septic or hypovolemic shock (Table 8-2). Rather than evaluate isolated measurements, though, the nurse should observe trends in values, especially since certain chronic disease states will have an elevated PAWP. Patients with slow-onset, chronic elevations in LA pressure, such as mitral insufficiency or mitral stenosis, may tolerate a very high PAWP. Even with PAWPs as high as

35 mm Hg, these patients are protected from the development of pulmonary edema because of the mechanisms of diminished permeability of the pulmonary capillary membrane, supernormal pulmonary lymph flow, and reactive constriction of the pulmonary arterioles, causing a reduction in pulmonary blood flow (see box on p. 183 for causes of intracardiac pressure changes).

Waveform Analysis in Common Disease States

Through critical analysis of systemic and intracardiac pressures and waveforms, the nurse can evaluate mechanical events in the heart to obtain valuable diagnostic and therapeutic infomation in a wide variety of cardiopulmonary pathologies. Figs. 8-19 to 8-25 illustrate the various pressure waveforms that can be expected in hypovolemic shock, cardiac tamponade, pericardial constriction, mitral regurgitation, mitral stenosis, aortic stenosis, and aortic insufficiency.

Table 8-2   Summary of Hemodynamic Data

Diagnosis	CVP/RA	RV (mm Hg)	PA (mm Hg)	PA Mean	PAWP (mm Hg)	Systemic arterial pressure (mm Hg)
Normal	0-6	20-30/0-6	20-30/6-12	10-15	6-15	100-140/60-90 70-90M
Hypovolemic or hemorrhagic shock	0-2	15-20/0-2	15-20/2-6		0-5	85-100/50-80
Septic shock early, "warm"	0-2	15-20/0-2	15-20/2-6		0-5	85-100/50-80
Septic shock late,"cold"	0-2	15-20/0-2	15-20/2-6		0-5	60-80/40-60
Acute LV failure	4-6	45/4-8	45/>18-20		>18-20	100-140/90-100
Chronic LV failure	0-10	NL or >	60/25-35	>35	>18	100-140/60-90
LV failure, severe cardiogenic shock	0-6		30-45/>20	20-30	>20	<100/50
Massive pulmonary embolism	10-20	50-60/12	50-60/8-12		<12-14	90-100/50-60
RV infarction	10-20	15-30/10-20	15-30/10-20		<15	90-100/50-60
Cardiac tamponade	12-20	25/12-16	25/12-16		12-20 = CVP	90/60
Acute mitral regurgitation	2-6	25-35/2-6	>25/6-12		Large v wave	
Severe mitral stenosis	15-20	40-120/20-30	40-120/20-30			
Primary pulmonary hypertension	0-6	80-100/0-6	80-100/6-12		<12	
Secondary pulmonary hypertension	>6	80/>6	80/25-35		<12	100-140/60-90

Adapted from Victor LD: *Manual of critical care procedures*, Rockville, Maryland, 1989, Aspen.

Causes of Intracardiac Pressure Changes

CENTRAL VENOUS (RA) PRESSURE
Causes of increased values
Volume overload
RV failure caused by RV infarction or cardiomyopathies
RV failure caused by pulmonary embolism, chronic obstructive pulmonary disease (COPD), sepsis, or adult respiratory distress syndrome (ARDS)
RV failure caused by left heart dysfunction, such as left ventricular (LV) failure or mitral stenosis/insufficiency
Tricuspid stenosis and regurgitation
Constrictive pericarditis
Cardiac tamponade/effusion
Pulmonary hypertension or embolism
Positive pressure breathing/PEEP or increased airway resistance
Pneumothorax
Ascites or abdominal distention
Systemic hypertension
Causes of decreased values
Hypovolemia
Shock
PULMONARY ARTERY PRESSURE
Causes of increased values
Volume overload
Pulmonary hypertension or embolism
Ventricular septal defect
Left heart dysfunction, such as mitral stenosis/insufficiency, decreased LV compliance, or LV failure
Cardiac tamponade/effusion
Left-to-right cardiac shunt

Constrictive pericarditis
Pulmonary parenchymal disease
Positive pressure breathing/PEEP
Causes of decreased values
Hypovolemia
RV failure
Pulmonic stenosis
Shock
PULMONARY ARTERY WEDGE PRESSURE
Causes of increased values
Volume overload
Pulmonary edema
Left heart dysfunction
LV faliure
Mitral stenosis/insufficieny
Decreased LV compliance
Increased pulmonary vascular resistance (PVR) caused by pulmonary embolism, COPD, ARDS, hypoxemia, sepsis, or shock
Cardiac tamponade/effusion
Constrictive pericarditis
Positive pressure breathing/PEEP
Causes of decreased values
Hypovolemia
Shock
RV failure
Pulmonic stenosis
Pulmonary embolism

CO L/min	CI L/m²	Stroke volume mL/beat	Svo2 %*	A/Vo2 diff. volume %	Systemic vascular resistance dyne/sec/cm⁵	Pulmonary vascular resistance dyne/sec/cm⁵	Heart rate
5-6	2.5-4	60-130	60-80	3-5	900-1200	150-250	60-100
<5	<2.5-4	NL or <	NL or <	NL or <	NL or >	NL	NL or >
>5	High				<900		>80-100
<5	<2.5				>1200		>80-100
<5	<2.5-4	<	NL ≤ 60	NL or >	>1500	NL or<250	Variable
<5	<2.5					>250	
<5	<2.1		<60	>	>1500	<160	>90
					>1500	>400	>90
					>1500	>250	>90
<5	<2	Low	<60		>1500	<160	>90
<5	<2	NL or >					
<5						>1500	
					>1500	>500	
	<2				>1500	>400	

*Svo2, Venous oxygen saturation.

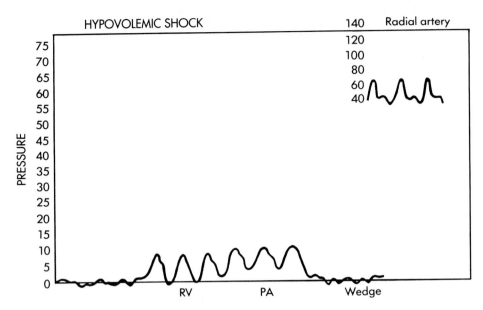

Fig. 8-19   PA catheter and systemic arterial pressure tracing showing hypovolemic shock. All cardiac chambers and the systemic arterial pressure show abnormally low pressures. PA catheter pressures may even dip below zero. The tracing has a "damped" appearance. There is little distinctness of waveforms between heart chambers. (From Victor LD: *Manual of critical care procedures,* Rockville, Maryland, 1989, Aspen.)

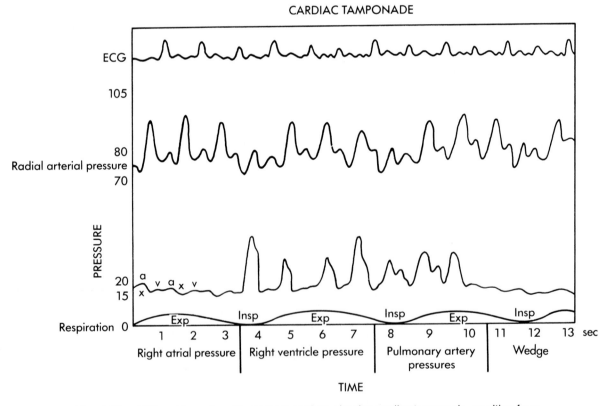

Fig. 8-20   ECG and hemodynamic pressure tracings showing cardiac tamponade, resulting from a rapid accumulation of fluid in the pericardial sac and characterized by global impairment of ventricular function during diastole. As can be seen, there is equalization of all diastolic pressures and respiratory variation. There is usually an inspiratory decrease in RA, RV, PA, and PAW pressures, although not consistently. The systemic arterial pressure shows pulsus paradoxus. The RV waveform loses its diastolic dip. The ECG shows electrical alternans. (From Victor LD: *Manual of critical care procedures,* Rockville, Maryland, 1989, Aspen.)

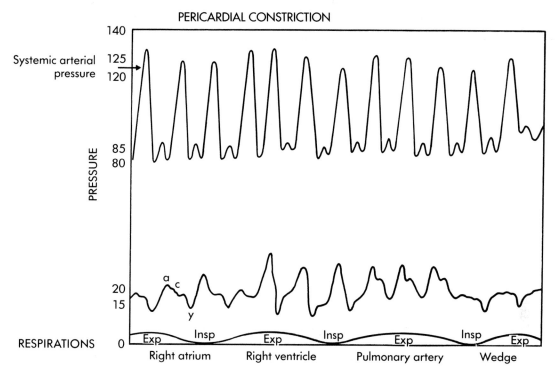

Fig. 8-21 Hemodynamic pressure tracing showing pericardial constriction (constrictive pericarditis), resulting from an abnormally rigid pericardial sac, causing impairment of diastolic filling. There is equalization of diastolic pressures in all chambers. Respiratory variation occurs with an inspiratory increase in RA pressure. RA waveform has dramatic y descent. Systemic arterial waveform shows only mild decrease in systolic pressure with inspiration. (From Victor LD: *Manual of critical care procedures,* Rockville, Maryland, 1989, Aspen.)

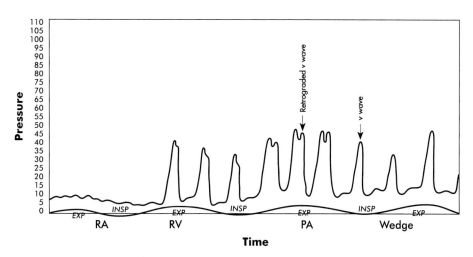

Fig. 8-22 PA pressure tracing showing mitral regurgitation where the left atrium must accommodate large volumes of regurgitant blood. This causes dramatic increases in pulmonary venous pressure and pulmonary edema. Respiratory variation occurs. The PA waveform shows a bifid peak in the systolic pressure, reflecting the retrograde v wave from the LA. The wedge pressure is elevated and has a very large v wave. (From Victor LD: *Manual of critical care procedures,* Rockville, Md, 1989, Aspen.)

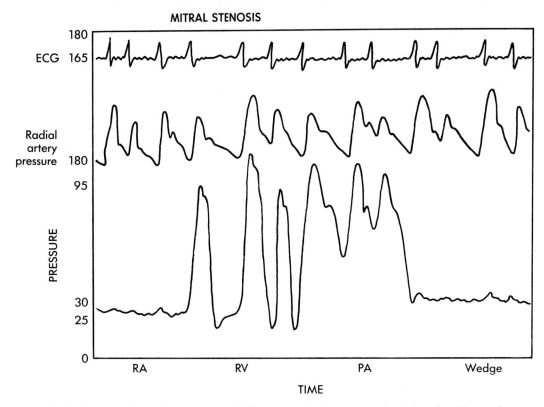

Fig. 8-23 Hemodynamic pressure and ECG tracing showing severe mitral stenosis with associated tricuspid stenosis and atrial fibrillation. With narrowing of the mitral valve, there is increasing compromise to diastolic ventricular filling, resulting in elevated LA pressures. Retrograde transmission of this elevated pressure causes secondary pulmonary hypertension. The RA waveform has a very elevated pressure. The RV waveform shows dramatic RV hypertension. The PA waveform shows severe pulmonary hypertension with varying systolic peak pressures secondary to the atrial fibrillation. The wedge waveform is massively elevated with indistinct a waves and x descents. (From Victor LD: *Manual of critical care procedures,* Rockville, Maryland, 1989, Aspen.)

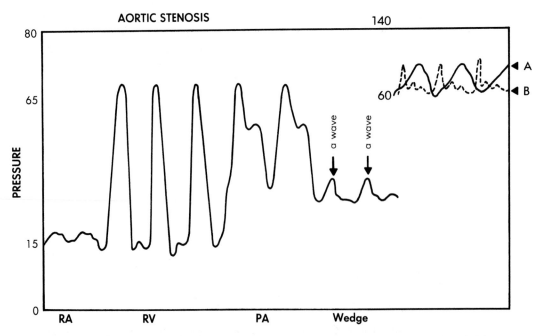

Fig. 8-24 Hemodynamic pressure tracing showing advanced aortic stenosis with chronic biventricular failure. This results in overloading of the LV during systole because of the presence of outflow obstruction and results in LV hypertrophy. The RA, ventricular, and PA systolic and diastolic pressures are elevated. The wedge tracing demonstrates a prominent a wave. (Adapted from Victor LD: *Manual of critical care procedures,* Rockville, Maryland, 1989, Aspen.)

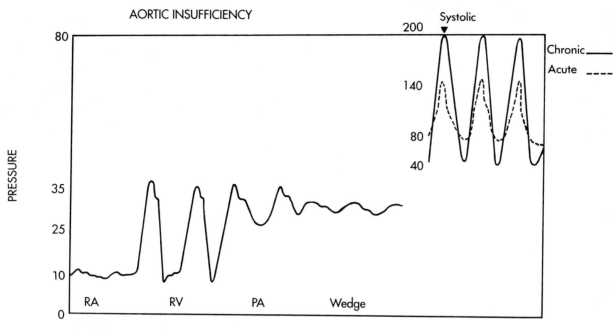

Fig. 8-25   Hemodynamic pressure tracing showing acute and chronic aortic insufficiency with acute LV failure. In acute aortic insufficiency, there is regurgitation of blood into the LV during diastole. This results in a precipitous rise in the LVEDP, LAP, and PAWP. A severe reduction in CO can occur resulting in acute pulmonary edema. As shown, the PA pressures are elevated and the wedge pressure is extremely elevated. The systemic arterial pressure waveform is more elevated in chronic aortic insufficiency and neither of these waveforms shows a dicrotic notch. (Adapted from Victor LD: *Manual of critical care procedures,* Rockville, Maryland, 1989, Aspen.)

Skill 8-10   Insertion of Pulmonary Artery Catheter

EQUIPMENT AND SUPPLIES

- Defibrillator
- Syringe of 100-mg bolus dose of xylocaine (Lidocaine)
- PA catheter
- Percutaneous sheath introducer kit
- Two prepared transducer/pressure-monitoring setups on IV pole
- Two 2-foot pressure-monitoring extension lines
- Pressurized heparin-flush monitoring system
- Pressure monitor with switch turned on
- Cardiac output module
- IV fluid and tubing
- Small sterile cup of sterile saline to test balloon integrity
- Vial of xylocaine 1%
- Povidone-iodine solution (optional)
- 4 × 4 gauze sponges
- Sterile gloves, gowns, and drapes
- Surgical masks and caps
- Razor and soap
- Dressing for the site
- Black silk skin suture
- Clean sheets to make a sheet roll

NURSING INTERVENTIONS

1. Calibrate the pressure transducer system (see Skill 8-4).
2. Ensure that patient has an IV line and obtain baseline vital signs. Inform patient about procedure and that some transient local discomfort may be felt.
3. Place head of bed flat and insert sheet roll between the shoulders.
4. Ensure that all personnel are wearing caps and masks.
5. Shave insertion site if necessary, and prepare skin with povidone-iodine solution.
6. Assist physician with donning surgical gown, opening sterile equipment, and placing on sterile field. Hold vial of xylocaine so that physician can withdraw solution and apply local anesthetic.
7. Assist physician in testing balloon for integrity. Catheter tip will be submerged in sterile saline and inflated to test for leaks. Test thermistor port by plugging it into the cardiac output module.
8. Connect the multipressure monitoring system to the distal or PA port and the proximal or RA port.
9. Connect the IV fluid to the extension line on the RA port.
10. Prime all lumens of the PA catheter.
11. Observe waveforms on electrocardiogram (ECG) and pressure monitor as physician inserts PA catheter and threads through introducer (see Fig. 8-14). When the RA tracing is seen, the physician will inflate balloon with 1.5 ml of air, depending on manufacturer's recommended inflation volume.
12. Observe monitor for ventricular ectopy when catheter tip is in the RV position. The physician will advance the catheter until a PAWP waveform is noted on the monitor and then deflate the balloon.
13. On deflation of balloon, ensure that PA waveform has returned. The physician will remove the introducer, coil the excess external catheter, and suture the catheter to the skin.
14. Apply sterile dressing, and order chest x-ray to verify placement and rule out pneumothorax.
15. Balance and recalibrate transducer, and record PAP and PAWP.
16. Set monitor alarms 20 mm Hg above and below patient's range.

Skill 8-11   Measurement of Pulmonary Artery Pressures

EQUIPMENT AND SUPPLIES

- PA catheter
- Pressure monitor with strip chart recorder
- Transducer setup

NURSING INTERVENTIONS

1. Ensure that transducer balancing port stopcock is level with the phlebostatic axis at the RA during pressure readings each time the level of the head of the bed is changed (see Figs. 8-2 and 8-7). To get the most accurate PAP measurements, keep the patient's backrest position within a range of 0 to 20 degrees.
2. For patients with significant respiratory variation of the PAP waveforms, record pressures from a calibrated pressure-scale tracing or a calibrated oscilloscope screen. If respiratory variation occurs in the PAP waveforms, the digital readout and printout will average pressures and frequently record a false low error.
3. Measure pressure complexes at the end of expiration, when the intrathoracic pressure is closest to a state of equilibrium with the intraventricular pressures.[1]
4. Obtain a strip recording of the PAP. In a spontaneously breathing patient, check for a fall in the baseline pressure caused by inspiration (respiratory variation) (Fig. 8-26).
5. Find the end of expiration two or three complexes before inspiration. Place a bar over the two or three pressure complexes that are most similar (Fig. 8-27). Measure the pressures at the peak of each complex, and average them. This is the *systolic* pressure.
6. Measure the pressures at the troughs of the waveforms, and average them. This is the *diastolic* pressure.
7. If a patient has a sustained dysrhythmia, average pressure from several waveforms.
8. If patient is on mechanical ventilation, note that end-expiration will appear on a different portion of the waveform as compared with a patient who is spontaneously breathing. When the ventilator delivers the machine breath, the monitored PAP waveform will increase (Fig. 8-28).
9. If patient is on PEEP on the mechanical ventilator, notice that PA systolic and diastolic pressures will go up during PEEP delivery. Correct by measuring two or three complexes before the rise. Do not discontinue mechanical ventilation or PEEP when obtaining readings.
10. To ensure more accurate measurements, remember that high values of PEEP above 10 cm H_2O can affect pressure readings, since a third of endobronchial pressure is distributed intrathoracically. Subtract a third of the PEEP value from the observed PA and wedge pressures. A patient on 15 cm H_2O PEEP with a PADP of 15 mm Hg has a real PADP of approximately 15 minus a third of 15, which is equal to a corrected PADP value of 10 mm Hg.
11. Correlate the digital values of the pressures with those obtained from the pressure-scale tracing. If there is a difference greater than 4 mm Hg, continue to obtain the pressures from the tracing.
12. Record PA pressures, and place pressure-scale tracing in patient's record.

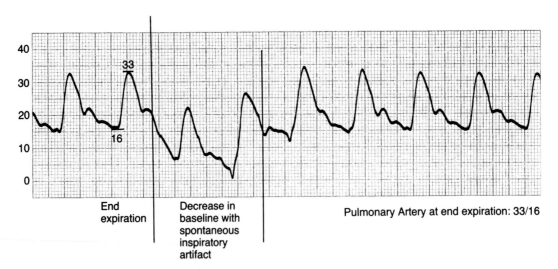

End
expiration

Decrease in
baseline with
spontaneous
inspiratory
artifact

Pulmonary Artery at end expiration: 33/16

Fig. 8-26   False decrease in pulmonary artery waveform during spontaneous inspiration. As spontaneous inspiration occurs, pleural pressures decrease, producing apparent fall in pulmonary pressures. (From Ahrens TS: Effects of mechanical ventilation on hemodynamic waveforms, *Crit Care Nurs Clin NA* 3:629, 1991.)

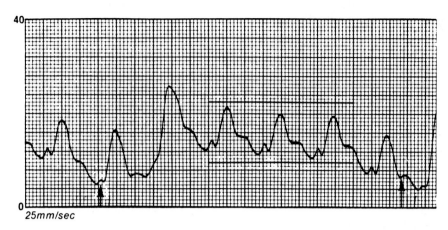

40

0

25mm/sec

Fig. 8-27 PAP tracing with respiratoy variation. Arrows indicate onset of inspiration. Complexes barred over are end-expiratory. PAP is 20/11 mm Hg. (From Ervin GW, Long S: *Memory bank for hemodynamic monitoring,* Baltimore, 1990, Williams and Wilkins.)

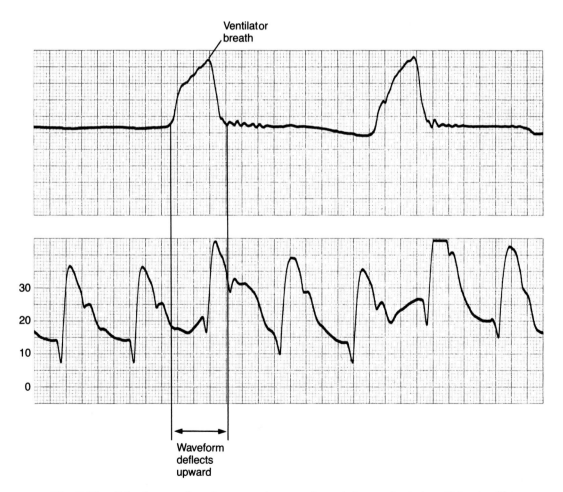

Ventilator
breath

30

20

10

0

Waveform
deflects
upward

Fig. 8-28 False increase in pulmonary artery waveform during mechanical ventilator (positive pressure) breath. As intrathoracic pressure increases, pulmonary pressures appear to increase. (From Ahrens TS: Effects of mechanical ventilation on hemodynamic waveforms, *Crit Care Nurs Clin NA* 3:629, 1991.)

Skill 8-12   Measurement of Pulmonary Artery Wedge Pressure

EQUIPMENT AND SUPPLIES

- 1-ml tuberculin syringe for a 0.75-ml balloon
- 3-ml syringe for a 1.5-ml balloon
- PA catheter
- Pressure monitor with strip chart recorder
- Transducer setup

NURSING INTERVENTIONS

1. Ensure that the transducer balancing port stopcock is level with the phlebostatic axis at the RA during pressure readings (see Fig. 8-7).
2. To avoid leaving the catheter wedged, always take readings in the sequence of PAWP first, PAP second, and RA third.
3. Place the monitor's digital readout knob on mean pressure.
4. Pull the pigtail on the continuous flush device to flush the line.
5. Plan to measure PAWP at end expiration (Figs. 8-29 and 8-30). If the patient has significant respiratory variation, plan to record pressures from a calibrated pressure-scale tracing.
6. Draw up correct amount of air into syringe. Check the side of the catheter for the maximum amount of air recommended by the manufacturer. Do not exceed 1.5 ml.
7. Open the balloon inflation valve and attach the syringe.
8. Slowly inflate the balloon with air, noting a slight resistance. If you do not feel resistance, suspect a ruptured balloon, and stop the procedure immediately.
9. Watch the oscilloscope screen closely, and stop injecting air as soon as the PAP waveform changes to a PAWP waveform (see Fig. 8-14). This indicates that the balloon is wedged in a narrow branch of the PA.
10. Observe the digital reading on end expiration.
11. Immediately remove the syringe, and let the air escape from the inflation valve by itself. Never aspirate the air with the syringe, since you may rupture the balloon.
12. Never inflate the balloon for more than 15 seconds because this may cause overwedging (falsely high pressure readings) and may damage the PA.
13. Close the inflation valve. Expel all air from the syringe, and reattach the syringe to the balloon inflation valve.
14. Record the digital PAWP reading or reading obtained from pressure-scale tracing. A true wedged position was obtained if the PAWP is lower than the mean PAP or PADP. The PAWP is never higher than the PADP.
15. Ensure that the PAWP waveform does not remain on the oscilloscope screen. If it does, the balloon may still be inflated, or the catheter tip may have become wedged in a small pulmonary capillary. Ask the patient to cough, place the patient on the right side, and move the arm to jolt the catheter tip free.
16. If the balloon remains wedged, notify the physician, and prepare the patient for a chest x ray. Prolonged wedging may cause a pulmonary infarction.
17. Observe for a damped PAP waveform on the oscilloscope screen. If this occurs, the balloon may still be partially inflated. Flush the line. If this does not help, notify the physician. A damped wedge tracing may also suggest that the catheter tip is in a zone 1 or 2 condition rather than zone 3 of the lung (see Fig. 8-16).
18. Observe for a RV waveform. If present, notify the physician immediately because of the risk of ventricular irritability if the catheter tip is in the ventricle.
19. If the balloon ruptures, close the port, tape it shut, and indicate on the tape that the balloon has broken, and notify the physician. The PADP may be used as a temporary substitute for the PAWP (normally the PADP is 1 to 3 mm Hg higher) as long as the patient has a normal pulmonary circulation and mitral valve.
20. Plan on limiting the number of balloon inflations to once every hour or less frequently, depending on the severity of the patient's condition. The average balloon can withstand approximately 72 inflations[4] (Table 8-3). The box on p. 192 provides guidelines for PAP monitoring.

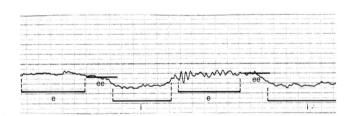

Fig. 8-29 Marked respiratory variation in the baseline of a PAWP tracing in a spontaneously breathing patient. Waveform decreases during inspiration; i = inspiration, e = expiration, ee = end expiration. (From Kinkade SL, Lohrman J: *Critical care nursing procedures: a team approach,* Philadelphia, 1990, BC Decker.)

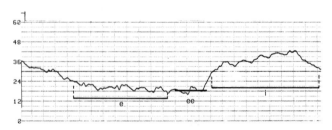

Fig. 8-30 Marked respiratory variation in the baseline of a PAWP tracing in a mechanically ventilated patient. Waveform increases during positive pressure inhalation. i = inspiration, e = expiration, ee = end expiration. (From Kinkade SL, Lohrman J: *Critical care nursing procedures: a team approach,* Philadelphia, 1990, BC Decker.)

Table 8-3 Troubleshooting Intravascular Catheters

Problem	Possible cause	Prevention	Remedy
Overdamped waveform	Clot at catheter tip	Use continuous flush device Use heparinized IV solution Use heparinized catheters Hand-flush occasionally	Aspirate, then flush catheter with heparin solution (not in PA wedge position) Remove catheter if unable to clear
	Air bubbles	Use care and attention to remove all air bubbles during equipment setup, particularly in the pressure transducer Use macrodrip versus microdrip	Flush system carefully (not to patient)
	Leak at some connecting point	Use Luer-Lok connectors and stopcocks Tighten securely	Check all connections, and tighten if necessary
	Kink in catheter	Loosely coil excess catheter Immobilize arm, if arm insertion Exercise caution during patient movement	Try to straighten kink Replace catheter if necessary
	Use of soft, compliant tubing	Use stiff connecting tubing	Replace soft tubing with stiff connecting tubing
"Noisy" underdamped waveform (with fling)	Use of lengthy tubing	Use no more than 2 or 3 ft of connecting tubing (preferably 18 inches or less) Use stiff connecting tubing	Decrease tubing length Use stiff connecting tubing
	Catheter tip near valve with turbulent blood flow	Position catheter distal to valve	Check catheter position by x-ray, and reposition if necessary Use commercial damping device
	Very rapid heart rate		Slow heart rate, if possible
Abnormally low or high pressures	Improper transducer level	Place air-fluid interface at phlebostatic level	Remeasure phlebostatic axis and reset transducer level accordingly
	Incorrect balancing of transducer and calibration of monitor to transducer	Balance and calibrate monitor to transducer correctly	Recheck zero and calibration of monitor
	Faulty transducer	Calibrate monitor to transducer, using known pressure; replace transducer if necessary	Recheck calibration with mercury or water manometer
"Over-wedged" or damped, elevated PAWP	Overinflation of the balloon	Slowly inflate balloon while closely observing waveform; inflate only enough to obtain PAWP; use a 3-ml plastic syringe with holes punctured at 1.5-ml to avoid injecting >1.5 ml air	Deflate balloon; reinflate slowly with only enough air to obtain a PA wedge waveform
	Eccentric inflation of the balloon	Check balloon inflation before insertion Do not inflate 7 F catheter with more than 1.0-1.5 ml air	Deflate balloon, reposition catheter, and slowly reinflate
	Location of catheter tip in zone 1 or 2 of the lung	Position catheter in zone 3 below the left atrium Maintain adequate LA pressure through volume administration Reduce airway pressure	Obtain lateral chest film to confirm catheter tip location; if in zone 1 or 2, reposition in zone 3, administer volume, or reduce airway pressure
PAWP with balloon deflated	Forward migration of catheter tip 2 degrees caused by excessive looping in RV or RA; inadequate suturing of catheter at insertion site; or excessive arm movement of catheter in antecubital vein	Advance catheter carefully, avoiding excessive catheter insertion Check catheter position on x-ray Suture catheter securely at insertion site Insert catheter in vein proximal to shoulder	Slowly withdraw catheter until PA waveform appears Obtain chest x-ray to determine excessive looping of catheter in RV or RA
PA balloon rupture	Overinflation of the balloon	Inflate slowly with only enough air to obtain PAWP	Remove syringe, and apply tape over stopcock to prevent further air injection
	Frequent balloon inflation	Monitor PADP as reflection of PAWP and LVEDP	Monitor PADP

Adapted from Tilkian AG, Daily EK: *Cardiovascular procedures: diagnostic techniques and therapeutic procedures,* St Louis, 1986, Mosby–Year Book.

Continued.

Table 8-3   Troubleshooting Intravascular Catheters—cont'd

Problem	Possible cause	Prevention	Remedy
	Active balloon deflation by withdrawing air into syringe	Allow balloon to deflate passively through stopcock Remove syringe after inflation	
Drastic change in pressure	Actual change in hemodynamic state		Carefully assess patient
	Air reference or transducer level changed	Maintain air fluid interface at phlebostatic level; rebalance before each reading	Reposition transducer at midchest level; rebalance
	Air or blood in transducer dome	Carefully remove all air bubbles during initial setup; maintain adequate pressure (300 mm Hg) in infusion bag	Carefully flush system to remove all air or blood (not into patient)
	Change in temperature of environment or IV solution	Use room temperature flush solution	Rebalance and calibrate
	Broken transducer cable	Carefully handle transducer and cable	Check transducer with known pressure of mercury or water; replace if faulty
No pressure	Power off	Check power	Turn power on
	Stopcock open to air	Always turn stopcock off to air after balancing (zeroing)	Turn stopcock off to air, open to catheter/transducer
	Transducer dome loose	Carefully tighten dome during setup, and check periodically	Tighten transducer dome
	Tubing connections loose	Carefully tighten all connections during setup, and check periodically	Tighten all connections
	Loose cable connections between transducer/monitor/oscilloscope	Carefully and firmly insert all connecting jacks during initial setup	Check all connecting jacks
	Transducer attached to wrong module or monitor	Carefully and accurately set up transducer and monitor	Attach transducer to appropriate module
	Gain setting too low	Correctly adjust gain setting of oscilloscope during initial monitor calibration	Reset gain on oscilloscope
	Incorrect scale selection	Select appropriate scale to correspond to monitored pressure	Select appropriate scale
	Faulty transducer	Calibrate monitor to transducer before patient use	Calibrate monitor to transducer; if faulty, replace

▼

Guidelines for Pulmonary Artery Pressure Monitoring

- Label lumens and lines.
- Balance transducer and calibrate monitor to transducer every 8 hours and PRN.
- Avoid drawing blood samples through the PA and RA ports, since fibrin accumulates and may eventually damp tracings.
- Use PA distal port for drawing mixed venous blood samples only.
- Avoid injecting medications through catheter unless absolutely necessary. If necessary, use venous infusion (cordis) or proximal ports only. Do not administer fluids or medications through the PA port. Pulmonary extravasation can occur.
- Ensure that pressure tubings and stopcocks are free of air and clots and that all connections are secure. Maintain sterility of all ports with sterile caps, and change caps regularly.
- Change central dressing site every 48 hours and the flush solution and tubing every 24 to 48 hours and transducer system every 2 to 4 days.

LEFT ATRIAL PRESSURE (LAP) MONITORING

Monitoring of the LAP is used in selected cases after major cardiac surgery, particularly in a failing heart, to assess the hemodynamic status of the left heart. LA catheters are also used in the postoperative management of the cardiac surgery patient who has significant pulmonary hypertension. After LVEDP, LAP is the most accurate index of volume status. The LAP will be increased in conditions such as pulmonary edema, left ventricular failure, mitral stenosis, and mitral insufficiency. During cardiac surgery, the left atrial catheter is placed in the superior pulmonary vein or the left atrium. It courses through the mediastinum and exits the body through a puncture incision in the upper abdominal wall. LA lines pose a number of serious hazards. Particulate embolism or air to the left side of the circulation (especially to the head or the coronary arteries) may occur while the catheter is in place. The LA catheter is removed percutaneously, and bleeding can occur from the atrial site, resulting in pericardial tamponade. Because of these risks, the LA catheter is rarely left in place for more than 48 hours (see Skill 8-13).

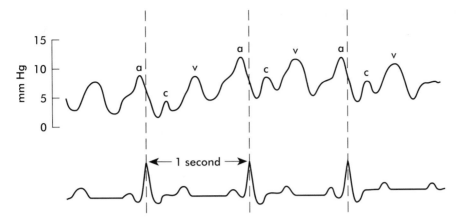

Fig. 8-31   Left atrial pressure waveform. At the point marked "*a* ", the patient's left atrium contracts and the mitral valve closes. At the point marked "*v* ", the left ventricle contracts, the mitral valve opens, and the left ventricle begins filling. *(Courtesy of Hewlett-Packard Company, Waltham, Mass.).*

Skill 8-13   Measurement of Left Atrial Pressure

EQUIPMENT AND SUPPLIES

- Single or multiple pressure transducer system
- Pressure monitor
- LA line
- Air filter

NURSING INTERVENTIONS

1. Ensure that the catheter is connected to an air filter close to the LA catheter insertion site to minimize the potential for air emboli.
2. Check that transducer balancing port stopcock is level with the phlebostatic axis during pressure readings each time the level of the head of the bed is changed (see Fig. 8-7). To ensure reliable readings, measure LAP at backrest elevations between 0 and 30 degrees.
3. Ensure that the transducer-monitor system has been balanced and calibrated at least once within the last 8 hours (see Skills 8-3 and 8-4).
4. Observe LAP waveform (Fig. 8-31). Check for heightened v waves, which may occur if the patient has mitral valve insufficiency, indicating regurgitative blood during ventricular contraction. Heightened v waves, accompanied by a rise of 2 mm Hg or more in LAP, may also indicate that the catheter has slipped through the mitral valve.
5. Place monitor pressure selector on MEAN setting.
6. Measure mean LAP at end expiration. The LAP will normally drop during inspiration in the spontaneously breathing patient and rise during inspiration of the mechanically ventilated patient. Do not discontinue mechanical ventilation or PEEP when obtaining the reading.
7. Evaluate the LAP reading. The normal LAP is 5 to 10 mm Hg, although readings vary from patient to patient. Establish a baseline reading for the patient, and determine the trend of values. Notify the physician if any subsequent readings rise or fall more than 2 mm Hg.
8. Maintain patency of LA line, controlling infusion rate of 3 to 4 ml/hr. Ensure that no other IV infusion is administered through the LA line to prevent risk of air emboli and infection.
9. Continuously assess catheter and pressure tubing for air bubbles. Aspirate all air bubbles.
10. If monitor shows dampened waveform, use standard troubleshooting measures (see Table 8-3). Then attempt to aspirate blood from the LA catheter. If there is no blood return, do not flush the catheter. Notify the physician, and prepare for line removal.
11. Change the dressing at the insertion site every 24 to 48 hours. Remove the dressing, and clean the site with povodine-iodine solution, observing strict aseptic technique. Check for redness, drainage, or broken sutures.
12. Change the flush solution and tubing every 24 to 48 hours.

MEASUREMENT OF CARDIAC OUTPUT

Cardiac output (CO) can be measured by the thermodilution method if a PA catheter has been inserted in the patient. This method uses the indicator dilution principle. A known quantity of a solution at a known temperature is injected into the right atrium and changes the temperature of the blood. When this blood reaches the pulmonary artery, a thermistor detects the temperature drop and sends a signal to the CO computer. The computer then calculates a time-temperature curve and displays CO in L/min. The volume of injectate used can vary (10, 5, 3, or 1 ml). The 10-ml boluses are generally used for adults.[8] The smaller volumes are used for pediatric patients or fluid-restricted adults who require frequent CO determinations.

The injectate can be at room temperature, or it can be iced. Iced injectate provides no particular advantage over room temperature injectate when the larger 10-ml volumes are used. Some patients, such as those classified as high volume, high mean arterial pressure, and high body temperature may continue to require iced injectate measures to ensure accuracy. Iced injectate decreases the variability in CO measurement by increasing the signal to physiological noise ratio. (Physiological noise is the respiration-induced change in the pulmonary artery temperature.) When the smaller volumes are used, iced injectates may result in greater reproducibility than those at room temperature. Some of the disadvantages of iced injectates include the following:

- Occurrence of cardiac dysrhythmias during injection.

- Increased time and cost in preparing iced temperature injectate.
- Increased time while waiting for temperature equilibration.
- Spurious values occurring because of warming of the injectate during handling.

Three types of injectate systems generally used in clinical practice for the delivery and maintenance of injectate include the prefilled syringes method, the open two-bag system, and the closed injectate delivery system (see Skills 8-14 through 8-16). Table 8-4 provides information on CO troubleshooting.

Skill 8-14   Measurement of Cardiac Output: Prefilled Syringes Iced Injectate Method

The major disadvantage of this type of system is the potential for catheter contamination. Bacterial growth can occur in an iced water bath after 3 hours. When syringes are chilled in ice baths, syringe hubs can become contaminated when the cap is removed, thereby contaminating the PA catheter or stopcock port. The chance of contamination increases with multiple interruptions of the catheter system to obtain CO measurements.

EQUIPMENT AND SUPPLIES

- Mask and sterile gloves
- PA thermodilution catheter
- Thermodilution CO computer with power source
- Cable for connecting PA catheter to computer
- 5 to 10 5-ml or 10-ml syringes
- Syringe needles and caps
- Alcohol sponges
- Injectate temperature probe
- Small sterile beaker, metal tubes, or sterile Ziploc bag to hold syringes
- Container for ice-slush solution
- Ice and water
- 100-ml IV bag of D_5W or NS
- Bottle of sterile NS

NURSING INTERVENTIONS

1. Place inner container that will hold syringes in container filled with ice and water. Fill inner container with NS.
2. Don mask. Open sterile packages of syringes (5 to 10) and IV solution. Don sterile gloves.
3. Withdraw from IV bag exact amount of solution into each syringe (5 or 10 ml), place cap on each syringe, and place in inner container. These syringes should remain sterile for at least 36 hours.
4. Remove plunger from one of the syringes, and insert temperature probe that leads to CO computer.
5. Allow the syringes 45 minutes to achieve the specified temperature range of 0 to 5° C (32 to 41° F).
6. Bring the CO computer to the bedside and turn it on. Attach the computer cable extension to the thermistor coupling of the catheter.
7. Determine the PA catheter model number, injectate temperature, volume to be injected, and type of injectate delivery system. Refer to the manufacturer's reference table to find the appropriate computation constant. Enter the appropriate constant on the CO computer.
8. Place the patient in the supine position, with the backrest angled from 0 to 20 degrees in elevation. CO measurements should be obtained in the same position in which

the other hemodynamic parameters were obtained. An upright posture may cause a change in CO because of possible venous pooling in the legs or an increased heart rate from the baroreceptor response.

9. Ensure that the PA catheter is in the correct position in the PA. Observe the oscilloscope for a characteristic PA waveform that changes to a wedge waveform during balloon inflation.
10. Record patient's heart rate, PA systolic, diastolic, mean, and wedge pressures, mean right atrial pressure, and MAP.
11. Ensure that continuous-drip medications are not being administered into the proximal port of the PA catheter. This prevents an inadvertent bolus administration of medication when performing the CO measurement.
12. Ensure that the computer is in the measurement mode and is ready.
13. Obtain a syringe from the ice bath. Avoid handling the barrel of the syringe to prevent heat gain. Inspect the syringe for proper volume and absence of air bubbles.
14. Attach the syringe to three-way stopcock at the proximal port of the PA catheter, and turn the stopcock open to the syringe.
15. Plan to inject the fluid during quiet respiration in the spontaneously breathing patient and at end expiration in the mechanically ventilated patient. This timing reduces the variability of CO results; although it does not accurately represent the average CO.
16. Push the *START* button on the CO computer. Rapidly inject the solution with a smooth and continuous action, without stopping or changing the injection rate. Complete the injection within 2 to 4 seconds, turn the stopcock back to a continuous infusion line, and remove the syringe.
17. Record the CO value (L/min) displayed on the computer. Evaluate the shape of the CO curve for accuracy (Fig. 8-32).
18. Repeat the procedure two more times, waiting at least 1 minute between injections. Average the three values if they are within 0.5 L/min of each other. If this criterion is not met, a fourth value may have to be obtained. The first measurement may be significantly higher than the subsequent measurements because of thermal loss in the catheter.
19. Record the type and amount of vasoactive drugs being administered at the time of the CO measurement. Graph the result on a CO curve, per unit protocol (Fig. 8-33).
20. Calculate the derived hemodynamic parameters as shown in Table 8-1. Such calculations can be performed on a hand-held computer.

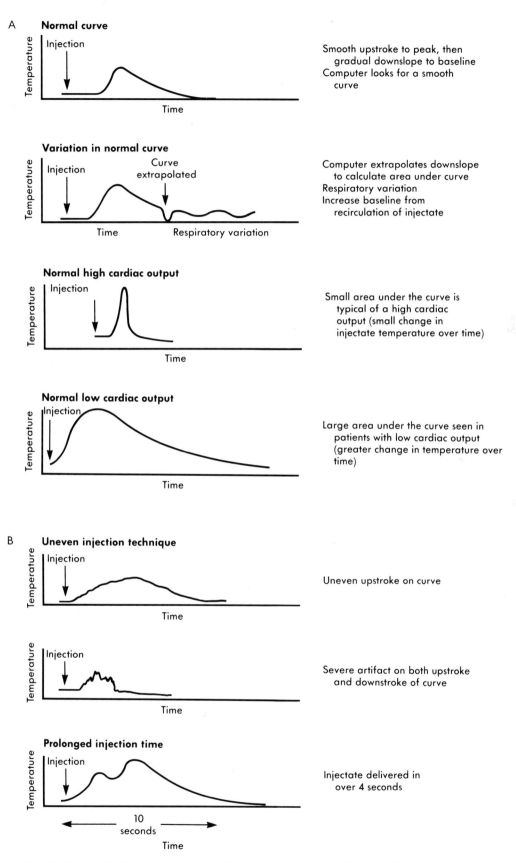

Fig. 8-32   A, Variations in the normal CO curve. **B,** Abnormal CO curves that will produce an erroneous CO value. (From Thelan LA, Davie JK, Urden LD: *Textbook of critical care nursing: diagnosis and management,* St Louis, 1990, Mosby–Year Book.)

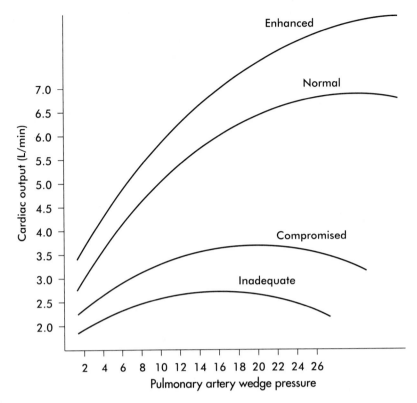

Fig. 8-33 Starling curves: Normal, enhanced, compromised, and inadequate responses to increases in preload. Starling curves can be plotted at the bedside by using the patient's cardiac output and PAWP to measure the response to specific interventions. (From Yee BH, Zorb SL: *Cardiac critical care nursing,* Boston, 1986, Little, Brown, and Company.)

Skill 8-15 **Measurement of Cardiac Output: Open Two-Bag System**

▼

This method can be performed with either iced or room temperature injectate immediately before measuring the CO. One bag of IV fluid will be used for aspiration of the injectate, and the other will be used for the temperature reference probe. When used for iced injectate preparation, the two bags would be placed in an ice-slush solution. The fluid would be withdrawn through an IV extension tubing or from the rubber port with a needle. Aspirating the cold solution into a room temperature syringe or IV tubing allows for some warming of the injectate, which may be a source of error. There is also more likelihood of contamination using this method because of the increase in breaks in the system.

EQUIPMENT AND SUPPLIES

- Mask and sterile gloves
- Two 100-ml IV bags of NS or D_5W
- Temperature probe
- Short IV administration set with attached stopcock
- Four 10-ml syringes with needles
- Large-gauge needle
- Alcohol pads
- Container of ice slush

NURSING INTERVENTIONS

1. If using iced injectate, put both IV bags in the ice slush without immersing the ports.
2. Open the main port of one IV bag, and pierce it with the large-gauge needle. Put the temperature probe into this port so that this bag can serve as the control temperature.
3. Spike the other IV bag with the IV tubing that has the attached stopcock. Hold the bag with the port upright, and squeeze air from the bag. Prime the IV tubing with fluid.
4. Follow steps 6 through 12 from Skill 8-14.
5. Don sterile gloves and mask. Attach the syringe to the stopcock, and aspirate injectate immediately before performing CO measurement.
6. Another option, without using IV tubing, is to aspirate injectate by inserting syringe needles into the rubber stopper at the end of the IV bag.
7. Follow steps 14 through 20 of Skill 8-14.

Skill 8-16   Measurement of Cardiac Output: Closed Injectate Delivery System for Cold Injectate

The closed injectate delivery system requires a special tubing setup, which can be used with either iced (Fig. 8-34) or room temperature injectate. The closed system maintains uninterrupted delivery of the injectate to the proximal port of the PA catheter, thereby reducing the necessity of multiple interruptions of the catheter system. Compared with the prefilled syringe method, the effort, time, and equipment required for nursing personnel to obtain CO measurements with the closed delivery system is also reduced. There is a very low rate of fluid contamination under in-use conditions. [22] An in-line thermistor located near the injection lumen port measures the injectate temperature as it is delivered into the catheter. Many of the temperature errors commonly associated with iced injectate are thereby minimized.

EQUIPMENT AND SUPPLIES

- CO-SET II
- PA thermodilution catheter
- Flow-through injectate temperature probe
- Cooling container
- Crushed ice and ice water
- 500-ml IV bag of D_5W or NS
- CO computer
- Connecting cable for CO computer
- Cooling container IV pole-mounting bracket
- Three-way stopcock and flush device

NURSING INTERVENTIONS

1. Suspend the injectate container no more than 3 feet above the catheter insertion site.
2. Remove CO-SET from its package, close the snap clamp, insert the nonvented spike into the vented injectate container, and pull apart the tubing coil (not the cooling coil) to get the desired tubing length between the IV container and the ice bucket.
3. Connect the 10-ml syringe assembly to the check valve (see Fig. 8-34). Open the snap clamp to allow solution to flow from the injectate container. To collect the discarded solution, hold the flow-through housing over an empty container.
4. Slowly pull and push the syringe plunger to prime the system; repeat five or six times until the system is completely free of air. The system may also be filled by squeezing the IV bag or plastic bottle. Remove the syringe from the check valve when using this method to fill the system.
5. Return the syringe plunger to the fully depressed position. Close the snap clamp.
6. Pack the container with crushed ice up to the inside ridge in the internal ribs, and seat the cooling coil on the first ridge. For maximum cooling, position the coil with the outlet at the bottom of the container.
7. Place the inlet and outlet tubing in the slots provided at the top of the container (see Fig. 8-34). Be sure that the white plastic tubing connector is inside the container.
8. Completely cover the cooling coil with crushed ice, and add iced water until the water is visible above the ice level.
9. Place any unused length of tubing coil inside the container to provide additional cold solution. Lock the lid on the container.
10. Verify that there is no air in the fluid path. Attach the flow-through housing to a three-way stopcock that has been attached to the proximal lumen hub of the catheter.
11. Insert the injectate temperature probe into the flow-through housing. Secure the system to minimize movement with respect to the patient.
12. Connect the injectate temperature probe cable to the Injectate Probe lead of the connecting cable.
13. To provide for accuracy, ensure that the injectate temperature falls within the following ranges: for 10-ml injectate, 6 to 12° C (43 to 54° F); for 5-ml injectate, 8 to 16° C (46 to 61° F). Plan to use an injectate volume of 10 ml unless clinically contraindicated.
14. Dial in the computation constant as in Skill 8-14, and prepare the computer for operation.
15. Open the snap clamp, and turn the stopcock at the catheter injectate hub to close the IV flush and to open the fluid path between the syringe and the catheter.
16. Perform a CO determination as in Skill 8-14. Space the injections at least 1 minute apart to allow the patient's blood temperature to return to normal.
17. At the end of the measurements, return the stopcock to its original (flush) position (assuring that the syringe is empty), and close the snap clamp.
18. Change the closed system every 48 hours to prevent contamination from bacterial growth.

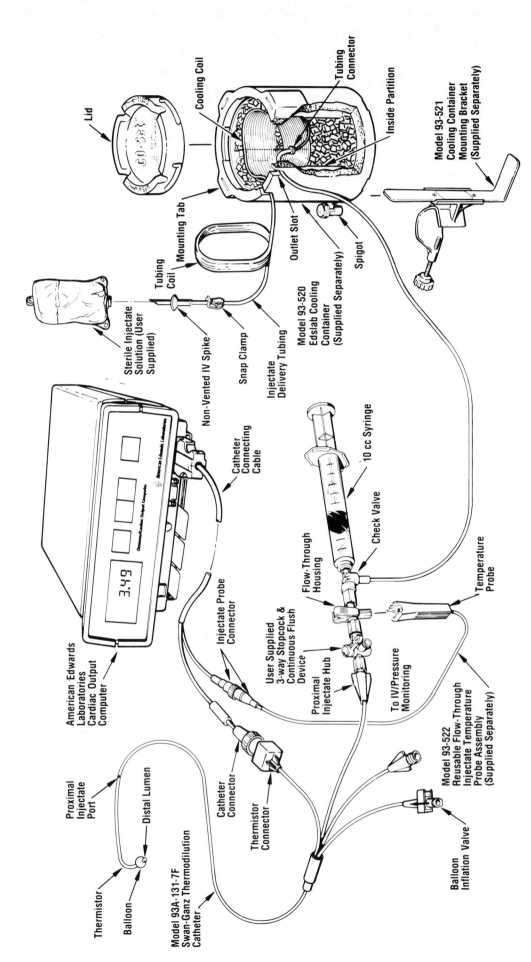

Fig. 8-34 CO-Set II, Closed Injectate Delivery System, Cold Injectate. *(Courtesy of Baxter Travenol Laboratories, Inc., Santa Ana, Calif.)*

Table 8-4   Cardiac Output Troubleshooting

Problem	Causes	Prevention	Remedy
CO reading higher than expected	Inaccurate injectate volume caused by air bubbles or loss of injectate	Carefully check for bubbles, and expel, if any	Check for exact volume of injectate before injection
	Wrong computation constant (CC)	Check appropriate CC on catheter insert, and set correctly on computer	For COs already done: correct CO = wrong CO × correct CC ÷ wrong CC
			Enter correct CC
	Warming of iced injectate in syringe before injection	If syringe method is used, handle syringe briefly, and hold only plunger and syringe flanges during injection	Perform outputs rapidly with minimal handling of syringe
			Use CO-SET with in-line temperature probe
	Migration of catheter tip toward PA wedge	Ascertain catheter tip position with x-ray	Withdraw catheter 1-3 cm
		Closely monitor PA pressure	
	Thermistor against wall of artery		Withdraw catheter 1-3 cm
	Uneven injection	Use two hands to deliver fast, even bolus	Use automatic injector
		Use automatic injector	Analyze curve on strip-chart recorder
	Right-to-left shunt	None	Use another method of CO determination (e.g., Fick)
	Low stroke volume with long lag time before onset of curve	None	Press *START* button after complete injection of indicator
CO reading lower than expected	Inaccurate injectate volume (more than indicated)	Use syringe of size that corresponds to injectate volume	Check for exact volume of injectate before injection
		Exercise care in filling syringe	
	Wrong CC	Check appropriate CC on catheter insert, and set correctly on computer	For cardiac outputs already done: Correct CO = wrong CO × correct CC ÷ wrong CC
			Enter correct CC
	Iced injections spaced < 1 minute apart	Wait approximately 1 minute between injections	Wait approximately 1 minute between injections
	Catheter kinked or partially obstructed by clot	Carefully protect catheter during patient movement	Try to straighten catheter
		Occasionally aspirate and flush manually	Aspirate and gently flush catheter
			Remove catheter if necessary
Scattered CO readings (poor reproducibility)	Cardiac dysrhythmias (e.g., ventricular ectopic beats, atrial fibrillation)	None	Try to inject during quiet period (i.e., without ventricular ectopic beats)
			Increase number of determinations (e.g., 5 or 6), and average readings
	Tricuspid regurgitation	None	Use another method of CO determination (e.g., Fick)
	Wide swings in intrapleural pressure (spontaneous respiration or mechanical ventilation)	Inject at same point in respiratory cycle	Inject at same point in respiratory cycle
		Increase number of determinations (e.g., 5 or 6), and average readings	Increase number of determinations (e.g., 5 or 6) and average readings
		Use iced injectate	Use iced injectate
	Electromagnetic interference	Isolate computer from other electromagnetic sources	Isolate computer from other electromagnetic sources
			Change power source (AC to battery or vice-versa)
			Wipe CO computer with damp cloth
	Migration of catheter tip toward pulmonary artery wall or thermistor against artery wall	Ascertain catheter tip location with x-ray	Withdraw catheter several cm to position in main PA
		Closely monitor PAP	
	Catheter looped in RV	Advance catheter carefully, avoiding excessive catheter insertion	Withdraw and reposition catheter
		Confirm catheter position with x-ray	

From Tilkian AG, Daily EK: *Cardiovascular procedures: diagnostic techniques and therapeutic procedures,* St Louis, 1986, Mosby–Year Book.

CLINICAL APPLICATION OF HEMODYNAMIC MONITORING

The ultimate goal in the monitoring and manipulation of hemodynamics is to provide the body with adequate amounts of oxygen while removing carbon dioxide and other waste products. Since this goal is achieved through adequate perfusion of the pulmonary and systemic circulations, it is important to review the determinants of arterial pressure. When working at the bedside with a patient who has a disturbance in tissue perfusion, the nurse will find that the patient's problem may be explained by an alteration in one or more of the components found in Fig. 8-35. When conceptualizing the cardiovascular system, nurses can simplify it by viewing it as a whole influenced by several basic hemodynamic components. The following factors that influence mean systemic arterial blood pressure are important to remember when monitoring and manipulating hemodynamic variables in the critical care patient:

- BP = cardiac output × systemic vascular resistance
- CO = heart rate × stroke volume
- Stroke volume = ventricular volume at end-diastole (EDV) minus the ventricular volume at end-systole (ESV)
- Preload and ventricular distensibility determine EDV
- Ventricular afterload and contractility determine ESV

Thus the five factors that determine CO, or the volume of blood that the heart ejects each minute, are the following (Fig. 8-36):

1. *Heart rate*—the number of times/min that the heart beats.
2. *Preload*—the filling pressure of the ventricles at the end of diastole, as generated by the volume of blood in the ventricles just before the next contraction. Preload is determined by the venous return, distribution of intravascular volume, and atrial contraction. The preload determines the initial stretch on the ventricles.
3. *Ventricular distensibility*—the degree to which the ventricle can stretch to accommodate volume. A scarred or chronically hypertrophied ventricle from chronic valvular disease, hypertension, or ischemic infarction will make the ventricle stiff. The stiff ventricle will not fill well at normal preload. Cardiac tamponade and pericardial constriction also restrict ventricular distensibility. The higher the preload and the more distensible the ventricle, the greater will be the EDV.
4. *Afterload*—The pressure the ventricles must pump against to eject blood. The lower the afterload, the more easily blood can be ejected from the heart. LV afterload depends on resistance of the systemic circulation and the condition of the aortic valve.
5. *Ventricular contractility*—the force with which the heart can contract. The contractility or inotropic state of the heart is the shortening ability of cardiac muscle fibers and determines the pumping ability of the heart.

An experienced nurse will not have to follow the steps of an algorithm in their proper order to determine the cause and necessary treatment of a patient's cardiovascular problems. For a new nurse, though, who is just learning about hemodynamic monitoring, it is important to be able to follow a systematic assessment. When assessing the cause of a patient's inadequate tissue perfusion, the nurse should first consider whether the patient has a low MAP. A determination should then be made as to whether or not the patient has either a decrease in systemic vascular resistance (such as caused by septic shock or rewarming after cardiac surgery) or a problem with cardiac output. If the hypotension is due to vasodilation, the problem can be remedied with extra fluids or a vasopressor, such as dopamine. If the patient's problem is not vasodilation, the next part of the equation, CO, should be examined. To evaluate the CO, the patient's heart rate should first be assessed for a possible pacemaker malfunction, bradycardia, or other dysrhythmia leading to hypotension. A bradycardia can be treated with atropine, a pacemaker, dopamine, or isoproterenol. If the heart rate is normal, the other part of the equation, stroke volume, should be assessed. If the patient has a PA catheter present, advanced hemodynamic monitoring can be performed. Assessment of the factors that determine an adequate stroke volume or cardiac output are as follows:[21]

1. Preload can be determined by the following:
   - Mean LAP—a direct measurement of LAP, a reflection of LVEDP
   - PAWP—a reflection of LVEDP
   - CVP—mean atrial pressure (MAP), a reflection of RVEDP
2. Ventricular distensibility can be determined by the following:
   - CVP
   - PAWP
   - Mean LAP
   - Mean systemic arterial pressure (MAP)
   - Heart rate
3. Afterload can be determined by the following:
   - Systemic vascular resistance (SVR)—resistance to LV systole. Also referred to as *peripheral vascular resistance* or *total peripheral resistance.*
   - Pulmonary vascular resistance (PVR)—resistance to RV systole.
4. Ventricular contractility can be determined by the following:
   - Left ventricular stroke work index (LVSWI)—indicator of the exertional work performance of the left ventricle adjusted for individual body size.
   - Right ventricular stroke work index (RVSWI)—indicator of the exertional work performance of the right ventricle adjusted for individual body size.
   - Stroke volume index (SVI)—stroke volume, adjusted for individual body size; indirect indicator of adequacy of stroke volume and contractility.

Three of these four factors—afterload, preload, and contractility—can be manipulated to optimize the CO (see Fig. 8-36). The fourth factor, ventricular distensibility, is

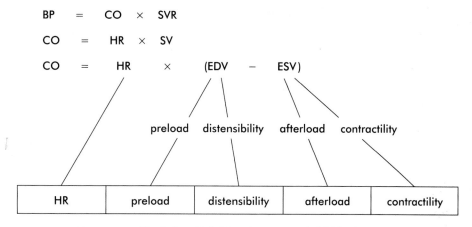

$$BP = CO \times SVR$$
$$CO = HR \times SV$$
$$CO = HR \times (EDV - ESV)$$

preload   distensibility   afterload   contractility

HR	preload	distensibility	afterload	contractility

Fig. 8-35   The factors that determine mean arterial blood pressure.

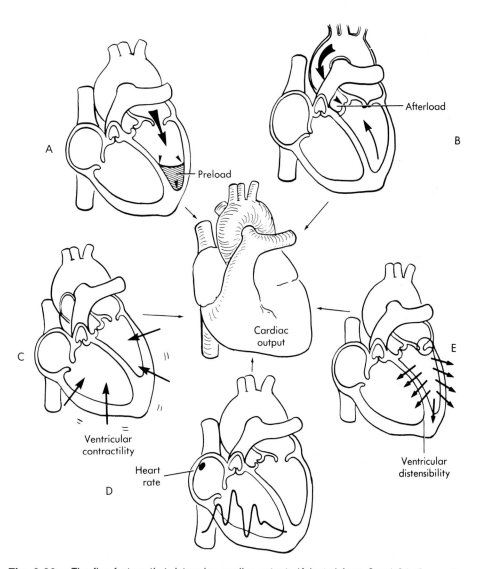

Fig. 8-36   The five factors that determine cardiac output. (Adapted from Quaal SJ: *Comprehensive intraaortic balloon pumping,* St Louis, 1993, Mosby–Year Book.)

largely determined by the long-term history of the ventricle and cannot be improved in the acute or postoperative setting unless a factor such as cardiac tamponade is causing the reduced distensibility.

Preload Manipulation

To know how to manipulate the preload, one needs to understand the Frank-Starling principle. This principle states that by increasing the length of ventricular fibers at the end of diastole, the stroke volume is increased, up to a finite point. The larger the diastolic volume of the heart, the more blood the ventricle will pump. If the ventricle is filled significantly beyond a certain plateau, though, overstretching muscle fibers, the CO may fall because of volume overload (Fig. 8-37). CO rises as preload is increased until the optimal preload on the Starling curve is exceeded. If a patient's CO is inadequate, the patient's fluid intake

can be increased to raise the preload or PAWP to as high as 18 to 20 mm Hg to optimize CO (see Fig. 8-33). A very sick heart may even need filling pressures higher than 18 to 20 mm Hg, but care must be taken not to force fluid out of the capillary lumen into the lungs. Overdistention of the postoperative heart is also very dangerous. According to Laplace's law, wall tension is proportional to pressure and diameter. The ventricle wall tension will increase as the ventricle is further filled. Wall tension has been positively correlated with myocardial oxygen consumption. As the ventricle is distended, myocardial oxygen demand increases, and the supply decreases because of impeded coronary blood flow.

The nurse's role in preload manipulation is to balance various factors, as ordered, and to increase or decrease the volume and pressure of the blood returning to the ventricle. Vasodilators, fluids, diuretics, and dysrhythmia control

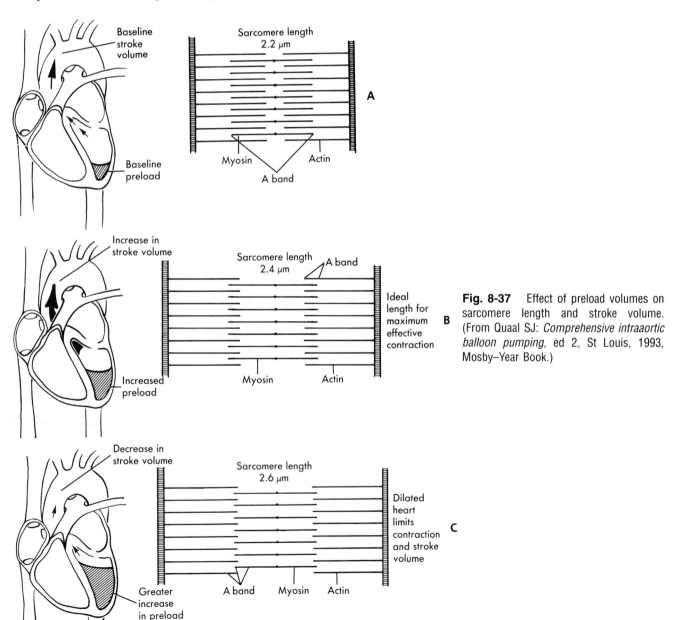

Fig. 8-37 Effect of preload volumes on sarcomere length and stroke volume. (From Quaal SJ: *Comprehensive intraaortic balloon pumping,* ed 2, St Louis, 1993, Mosby–Year Book.)

can all be used to manipulate preload (Fig. 8-38). The goal would be to determine the PAWP that produces the most optimal ventricular performance. One frequently used measure of ventricular performance is LVSWI. Fig. 8-39 shows the relative positions of patients in different types of shock on a ventricular function curve. By plotting the patient's PAWP and LVSWI on this type of curve, the nurse can assess the patient and determine what factors are needed to improve ventricular performance.

Afterload Manipulation

Afterload manipulation is usually directed at decreasing arterial pressure so that it becomes easier for the ventricle to eject blood, thereby increasing CO. Calcium channel blockers and peripheral arterial vasodilators can effectively decrease SVR, thereby reducing ventricular workload and myocardial oxygen demand (Fig. 8-40 and Table 8-5). If arterial pressure is dropped significantly, though, coronary, brain, and kidney perfusion may suffer. Afterload reduction should be performed cautiously if a patient is possibly fluid depleted. A patient should have an adequate fluid volume with a PAWP of at least 15 to 18 mm Hg before afterload reduction is attempted. The nurse should monitor the patient carefully, observing for reflex tachycardia. Afterload is usually adjusted to keep arterial BP at the 100 to 140 mm Hg systolic range. Mean BP may be adjusted as low as 70 mm Hg. Patients with severe heart failure can be placed on intraaortic balloon counterpulsation (IABC) to help decrease afterload. The IABC causes a decrease in peak systolic pressure because of deflation of the intraaortic balloon. Just before the beginning of systole, rapid balloon deflation occurs, creating a vacuum effect. This low-

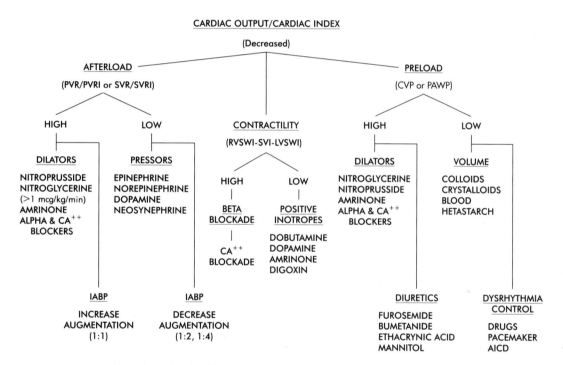

Fig. 8-38 Hemodynamic algorithm. (From Urban N: Hemodynamic clinical profiles, *AACN Clin Issues Crit Care Nurs* 1:119, 1990.)

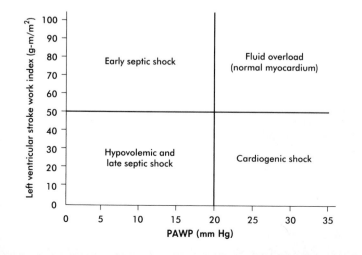

Fig. 8-39 Relative positions on the ventricular function curve of patients in different types of shock. (From Bustin D: *Hemodynamic monitoring for critical care,* Norwalk, Connecticut, 1986, Appleton & Lange.)

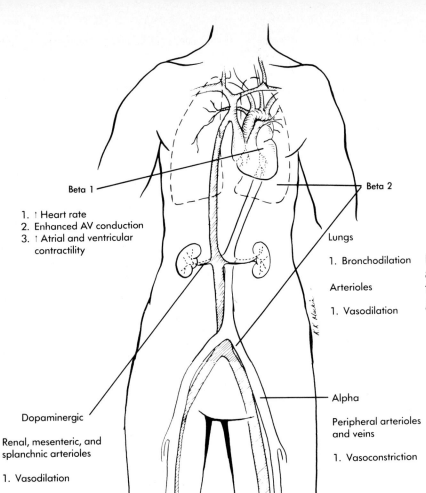

Beta 1

1. ↑ Heart rate
2. Enhanced AV conduction
3. ↑ Atrial and ventricular contractility

Beta 2

Lungs

1. Bronchodilation

Arterioles

1. Vasodilation

Alpha

Peripheral arterioles and veins

1. Vasoconstriction

Dopaminergic

Renal, mesenteric, and splanchnic arterioles

1. Vasodilation

Fig. 8-40 Cardiovascular effects of alpha and beta adrenergic and dopaminergic receptors. (Adapted from Quaal SJ: *Comprehensive intraaortic balloon pumping, ed 2*, St Louis, 1993, Mosby–Year Book.)

Table 8-5 Effect on Hemodynamic Parameters of Common Intravenous Medications for Monitored Patients

	HR	MAP	PAP	PAWP	CVP	SVR	SV	CO
Vasodilating agents								
Nitroglycerin	↑	↓	↓	↓	0/↓	↓	↑	↑
Nitroprusside	↑	↓	↓	0/↓	0/↓	↓	↑	↑
Hydralazine	↑	↓	↓	0/↓	0/↓	↓		↑
Phentolamine	↓	↓	↓	↓	↓	↓	↑	↑
Vasopressor agents								
Phenylephrine	0/↓	↑	↑	↑	↑	↑		↓
Metaraminol	0/↑	↑	↑	↑	↑	↑		↑/↓
Mixed activity agents								
Epinephrine	↑	↑	↑	↑	↑	↑/↓		↑
Norepinephrine	0/↑	↑	↑	↑	↑	↑		↑/↓
Ephedrine	↑	0/↑	0/↑	0/↑	0/↑	↑		↑
Dopamine	0/↑	0/↑	0/↑	0/↑	0/↑	↑		↑
Inotropic agents								
Dobutamine	0/↑	0/↑	0	0	0/↑	0/↑		↑
Isoproterenol	↑	0/↑	0/↑	0/↓	0/↓	0/↓	↑	↑
Amrinone	0	↓	↓	↓	0/↓	↓	↑	↑
Digoxin	↓						↑	↑
Antidysrhythmic agents								
Lidocaine	0	0/↓	0/↓	0	0	0/↓		0/↑
Quinidine	0/↓	↑	0/↓	0/↓	0/↑	0		↓
Procainamide	0	↓	0/↓	0/↓	0/↓	0		↓
Propranolol	↓	↓	0/↓	0/↓	0/↓	↓		↓
Labetalol	↓	↓	↓	↓	↓	↓		↓
Bretylium	↑/↓	0	0	0	0	0		0
Verapamil	↑/↓	0/↓	0/↓	0/↓	0/↓	↓		↑/↓

KEY: 0, Little or no change; ↑, increase; ↓, decrease. *CO*, cardiac output; *CVP*, central venous pressure; *HR*, heart rate; *MAP*, mean arterial pressure; *PAP*, pulmonary artery pressure; *PAWP*, pulmonary artery wedge pressure; *SV*, stroke volume; *SVR*, systemic vascular resistance.
Adapted from Darovic GO: *Hemodynamic monitoring: invasive and noninvasive clinical application*, Philadelphia, 1987, WB Saunders.

ers the systolic pressure in the aorta and makes it easier for the left ventricle to empty.

Contractility Manipulation

Contractility can be manipulated by adjusting the PAWP, which in turn determines the end-diastolic stretch of the myocardial muscle fibers. If the CO is still inadequate at normal filling pressures, the contractile strength of the heart is probably inadequate. Under these circumstances, it is appropriate to use a positive inotropic drug, such as Dobutamine (see Fig. 8-38 and Table 8-5). Increasing contractility, though, especially in a patient with impaired myocardial function, can be dangerous. When the force of contraction increases, myocardial oxygen requirements increase markedly.[10] If this increased demand for oxygen cannot be met, the patient may have angina, a myocardial infarction, dysrhythmias, or even a cardiac arrest (see box that summarizes factors influencing cardiac preload, afterload, and contractility).

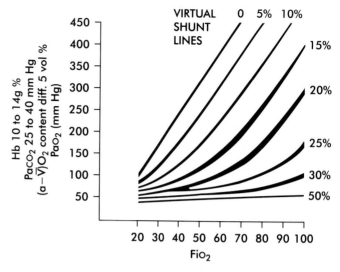

Fig. 8-41   Nomogram, Isoshunt lines: 1. Plot intersection of measured Pao_2 and present Fio_2. 2. Follow estimated shunt line to desired Pao_2 on the horizontal axis and read the Fio_2 required to deliver it on the vertical axis. (From Benetar SR: *British J Anesthesia* 45:711, 1973.)

Factors that Influence Preload, Afterload, and Contractility

Preload can be reduced by the following:
- Decreased intravascular fluid volume caused by vomiting, diarrhea, diuresis, diaphoresis, hemorrhage, or third spacing.
- Changed position reducing venous return caused by sudden change from lying to standing position or orthostatic hypotension.
- Dilated veins with pooling in extremities caused by sepsis, neurogenic shock, anaphylactic shock, hyperthermia, and drugs, such as nitroglycerin.
- Damaged right heart caused by myocardial infarction, cor pulmonale, or pulmonary embolus.
- Impaired atrial contraction caused by atrial fibrillation or myocardial infarction.
- Increased pericardial pressure, reducing cardiac filling caused by pericardial effusion or tamponade.
- Reduced negative intrathoracic pressure, reducing venous return caused by mechanical ventilation, high inspiratory pressures, high levels of PEEP, or tension pneumothorax.
- Reduced ventricular filling time caused by the tachycardia.

Preload can be increased by the following:
- Increased intravascular fluid volume caused by excess IV fluid, blood products, and renal failure.
- Reduced peripheral vascular resistance, augmenting venous return, caused by fever, anemia, or pregnancy.
- Constricted veins caused by anxiety, exercise, sympathomimetic drugs, hypothermia, or early hypovolemic and cardiogenic shock.
- Increased negative intrathoracic pressure, increasing venous return caused by deep inspiration.
- Improved gravity flow towards heart caused by changing to head down with legs elevated, Trendelenburg position.
- Increased ventricular filling time caused by bradycardia.

Afterload can be reduced by the following
- Reduced arterial resistance caused by arterial dilation from drugs, such as nitroprusside, and septic, anaphylactic, and neurogenic shock.
- Reduced impedance to blood flow through aortic valve caused by mitral regurgitation.
- Improved systolic unloading caused by vacuum effect of IABC, lowered blood viscosity.

Afterload can be increased by the following:
- Increased arterial resistance caused by arterial constriction with drugs, such as epinephrine, or early hypovolemic and cardiogenic shock, or atherosclerosis.
- Impeded blood flow through aortic valve caused by aortic stenosis.

Contractility can be reduced by the following factors:
- Acidosis.
- Ischemia.
- Heart failure.
- Anoxia.
- Local and general anesthetics.
- Barbiturates.
- Beta-blocker drugs.
- Calcium-antagonist drugs.
- Hyponatremia.
- Hyperkalemia.

Contractility can be increased by the following factors:
- Increased sympathetic nervous system stimulation.
- Increased circulation of epinephrine and norepinephrine.
- Cardiac glycosides.
- Beta-receptor stimulant drugs.
- Calcium.
- Glucagon.
- Caffeine.
- Increased preload.
- Increased afterload.

RESPIRATORY MONITORING

During the 1980s there were major advances in respiratory monitoring so that most ICUs now use a variety of technologies for evaluating a patient's respiratory status. Nurses are using computers and formulas at the bedside to estimate intrapulmonary shunting and to predict the results of ventilator changes. They are performing noninvasive monitoring of arterial oxygen saturation (Sao_2) with pulse oximetry (see Chapter 4), measuring end-tidal partial pressure of CO_2 ($Petco_2$) with capnography, evaluating trends in lung compliance, and performing transcutaneous Po_2 monitoring ($Ptco_2$) (see Chapter 4). Another promising respiratory-monitoring technique now available is continuous monitoring of mixed venous oxygen saturation (Svo_2).

RESPIRATORY FORMULAS

There are several condensed formulas that are useful at the bedside for respiratory monitoring. The equations that will be discussed include those that estimate intrapulmonary shunting so that adjustments in oxygenation can be made and formulas that predict the results of changes affecting ventilation.

Estimating Intrapulmonary Shunting

Intrapulmonary shunting ($\dot{Q}s/\dot{Q}t$) occurs when venous blood enters the lungs and is not exposed to functioning alveoli. As the blood leaves the lungs, it has not been well oxygenated so that the patient has a lower than normal Pao_2 level. The physiological shunt can be calculated using a sophisticated formula:

$$\frac{Cco_2 - Cao_2}{Cco_2 - Cvo_2}$$

▼ **Calculation of Alveolar Air Equation**

This equation is needed to determine the partial pressure of oxygen in the alveoli (PAo_2). Once you know the PAo_2 level, you can use it to find the Pao_2/PAo_2 ratio (a/A ratio).

SIMPLIFIED EQUATION

$PAo_2 = (P_B - P_{H_2O}) (Fio_2) - Paco_2$
Where:
- PAo_2 = partial pressure of alveolar oxygen (mm Hg)
- P_B = barometric pressure
- P_{H_2O} = pressure taken up by water vapor in the alveoli (47 mm Hg)
- Fio_2 = fraction of inspired oxygen, expressed in decimals
- $Paco_2$ = partial pressure of carbon dioxide in arterial blood, used as an estimation of partial pressure of alveolar carbon dioxide (mm Hg)
  Example: Mr. Smith has an Fio_2 level of 0.40 and a $Paco_2$ level of 50 mm Hg. He is at sea level where the barometric pressure is approximately 760 mm Hg (Adjust accordingly for high altitudes.)
  $PAo_2 = (760 - 47) \times (0.40) - 50$
  $= (713 \times 0.40) - 50$
  $= 285 - 50$
  $= 235$ mm Hg

This formula takes into account changes in CO, mixed venous oxygenation, and total blood-oxygen content but is not practical for performing at the bedside unless the nurse has access to a computer and all of the values necessary for the calculation. An easier estimate of intrapulmonary shunting to use is the Pao_2/PAo_2 ratio (a/A ratio), which is the ratio of arterial to alveolar partial pressure of oxygen.

The a/A ratio is useful in the critical care setting not only to estimate the intrapulmonary shunt but also to assess a patient's oxygenation status by predicting a patient's Pao_2 level at a given level of inspired oxygen (Fio_2). Use of the a/A ratio is helpful when a patient is on a mechanical ventilator and the nurse wants to change the patient's Fio_2 level to obtain a certain Pao_2 level. Calculation of the a/A ratio can help reduce the number of mechanical ventilator changes and drawing of arterial blood gases (ABGs)[5] (see boxes on calculation of a/A ratio and prediction of Pao_2 at a given Fio_2). A nomogram (Fig. 8-41) can also be

---

▼ **Calculation of Intrapulmonary Shunt (a/A Ratio)**

The a/A ratio can be used to estimate intrapulmonary shunting. This helps to assess a patient's oxygenation status.

$$a/A \text{ ratio} = \frac{Pao_2}{PAo_2}$$

Example: Mr. Smith has a Pao_2 level of 70 mm Hg and a PAo_2 level of 235 mm Hg. You already calculated his PAo_2 level by using the alveolar air equation (see box on the left)

$$a/A \text{ ratio} = \frac{70 \text{ mm Hg}}{235 \text{ mm Hg}}$$
$$= 0.3$$

This means that 30% of the oxygen available in the alveoli is reaching the arterial blood. The normal a/A ratio is approximately 0.80 to 0.85. The higher the a/A ratio, the better the lung function. In theory, if the a/A ratio is greater than 0.60, the patient would not need supplemental oxygen, since at this level the Pao_2 would be in excess of 60 mm Hg.

Example: Mr. Smith had been on an Fio_2 level of 0.40. After viewing his ABG measurements, the physician decided to increase the Fio_2 level to 0.50. Repeat ABG measurements showed a Pao_2 level of 80 mm Hg and a $Paco_2$ level of 50 mm Hg. These results suggest that the patient's oxygenation status has improved. To confirm this, check it with the ratio, as follows:

First, calculate PAo_2, using the alveolar air equation, based on the increased Fio_2.

$$PAo_2 = (713 \times 0.50) - 50$$
$$= 356 - 50$$
$$= 306 \text{ mm Hg}$$
$$a/A \text{ ratio} = \frac{80 \text{ mm Hg}}{306 \text{ mm Hg}}$$
$$= 0.26$$

This lower value shows that even less available oxygen is getting into the arterial blood. Even though the Pao_2 level has improved, the patient's oxygenation has deteriorated.

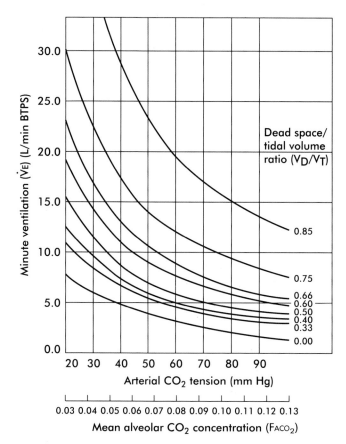

Fig. 8-42 Nomogram to estimate minute ventilation required to maintain a given Pa_{CO_2} when dead space/tidal volume ratio is known. To obtain the required minute ventilation needed to achieve a given Pa_{CO_2}, the minute ventilation is plotted against the Pa_{CO_2} (measured simultaneously) and the dead space/tidal volume ratio is read on the isopleth that corresponds to the intersection. The isopleth is then followed to the desired Pa_{CO_2} and the corresponding minute ventilation read off the vertical axis. (From Selecky PA et al: *Am Rev of Resp Dis* 117:181, 1978.)

used to estimate the Fio_2 level needed to achieve a desired Pao_2 level or the Pao_2 level that will be achieved at any given Fio_2 level.

Adjusting Ventilation to Change the pH and $Paco_2$ Level

When a patient on a mechanical ventilator has acute respiratory acidemia, the minute ventilation (V̇E) can be adjusted to obtain normal pH and $Paco_2$ levels. The V̇E is the sum of all of the air inhaled or exhaled in 1 minute and is equal to the respiratory rate times the tidal volume. The formula in the box on p. 208 or the nomogram in Fig. 8-42 can be used to calculate an adjusted V̇E. To change the V̇E, either the tidal volume or respiratory rate on the ventilator can be adjusted.

CAPNOGRAPHY

Capnography is a method of assessing ventilation by measuring the amount of CO_2 in exhaled gases. Its most frequent use is for intubated patients on mechanical ventilation. A sampling tube withdraws gas from the patient's airway, leading to a capnograph (Fig. 8-43). The capno-

---

Prediction of Pao_2 Level at a Given Fio_2 Level

The a/A ratio can be used to estimate Pao_2 at varying levels of Fio_2. This is especially useful in the ICU when making ventilator changes but is only accurate if the patient's oxygen consumption, Pao_2 level, cardiac output, ventilation-perfusion matching, and shunt remain constant. Suppose you have received a patient's ABG results and find that the Pao_2 level is too low. You have a *desired* level of Pao_2 that you would prefer. You realize that to obtain this Pao_2 level there is a *required* Fio_2 level that you will need to administer to the patient. You can begin with the following equation:

$$PA_{O_2} \text{ (required)} = \frac{Pa_{O_2} \text{ (desired)}}{\text{a/A ratio}}$$

Example: Mr. Brown has an a/A ratio of 0.4 and a Pao_2 level of 50 mm Hg. The nurse is concerned about his ABG results and would like for the patient to have a Pao_2 level of 80 mm Hg, thus plans to get an order to increase his Fio_2 level. Using the above equation,

$$PA_{O_2} \text{ (required)} = \frac{80}{0.4}$$
$$= 200$$

Solve for the new required Fio_2 level using the alveolar air equation:

$$PA_{O_2} = (P_B - P_{H_2O}) \times Fi_{O_2} - Pa_{O_2}$$
$$200 = (760 - 47) \times Fi_{O_2} - 50$$
$$250 = 713 \times Fi_{O_2}$$
$$250/713 = Fi_{O_2}$$
$$0.351 = Fi_{O_2}$$

Mr. Brown will need an Fio_2 level of approximately 35% to obtain a Pao_2 level of 80 mm Hg.

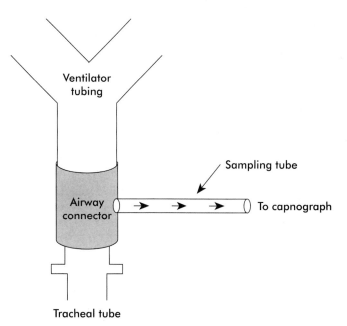

Fig. 8-43 Sidestream sampling technique where gas is withdrawn from patient's airway, leading to a capnograph.

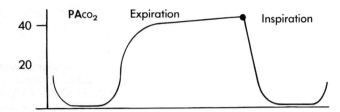

Fig. 8-44 Normal capnographic waveform. This capnogram graphically represents the amount of CO_2 in each of the patient's expirations.

▼ Estimating Ventilation Required to Maintain a Given pH and $PaCO_2$ Level

The following equation can be used to calculate new ventilator settings to manipulate a patient's pH and $Paco_2$ level. For every 10 mm Hg change in $Paco_2$ from 40 mm Hg, there is a corresponding change in pH of 0.08 from 7.40 in the opposite direction. As is shown in the equation that follows, the $\dot{V}E$ is inversely related to $Paco_2$. If PE decreases, $Paco_2$ increases and vice versa.

Example: Mr. Green is on a ventilator with a respiratory rate of 10 and tidal volume of 800 ml. His $Paco_2$ level is 60 mm Hg. The physician has requested that the $Paco_2$ level be decreased to 48 mm Hg.

$$\text{Present } Paco_2 \times \text{ present } \dot{V}E = \text{ desired } Paco_2 \times \text{ desired } \dot{V}E$$
$$60 \times (800 \times 10) = 48 \times \text{ desired } \dot{V}E$$
$$60 \times 8,000 = 48 \times \text{ desired } \dot{V}E$$
$$480,000 = 48 \times \text{ desired } \dot{V}E$$
$$10,000 \text{ ml} = \text{ desired } \dot{V}E$$

To obtain the 10,000 ml of $\dot{V}E$, you can leave the rate at 10 and increase the tidal volume to 1000 ml, or you can leave the tidal volume at 800 and increase the rate to 12. You can use the patient's weight to determine if the tidal volume is within the recommended range of 10 to 15 ml/kg. The above equation is effective only if the patient's condition remains stable without complicating pulmonary factors, such as intrapulmonary shunting.

---

graph then displays a breath-by-breath waveform (capnogram) of CO_2 concentration of gas in the airways (Fig. 8-44). This provides a measure of the end-tidal partial pressure of CO_2 ($Petco_2$). The methods of CO_2 gas analysis commonly used are mass spectrometry and infrared absorption spectrophotometry. Mass spectrometry is more expensive and is used for monitoring of multiple respiratory gases, including nitrogen, CO_2, and oxygen. The infrared absorption spectrophotometry is used more frequently in ICUs and is based on the principle that CO_2 absorbs infrared light. Clinical applications of capnography in critical care have grown in recent years, and The Society of Critical Care Medicine has recently recommended that all ICUs be capable of providing capnographic monitoring.

Having $Petco_2$ values available enables the nurse to assess changes in CO_2 production and reliably estimate the $Paco_2$. When ventilation and perfusion are evenly distributed, the $Petco_2$ closely approximates $Paco_2$. The $Petco_2$ also closely approximates the mean $PAco_2$. Therefore trends in $Paco_2$ values are reflected by $Petco_2$ values. The

difference between these two parameters, known as the *CO_2 gradient,* has been reported to be less than 6 mm Hg in healthy subjects.[17] When a patient is begun on capnography, it is important to correlate a $Paco_2$ measurement with the $Petco_2$ measurement to determine the CO_2 gradient. This correlation should then be repeated regularly, particularly when the patient's perfusion or respiratory status deteriorates. A low CO_2 gradient implies an optimal ventilation-perfusion relationship. This principle can be applied when determining adequate PEEP levels on the ventilator. If PEEP is raised too high, this can result in significant alveolar overdistention and widening of the CO_2 gradient.

$Petco_2$ measurements and capnograms provide the critical care nurse with information about changes in CO_2 production, ventilation-perfusion relationships, dead space ventilation, and other useful information about ventilation. A change in a patient's $Petco_2$ level can be caused by changes in CO_2 delivery to the lungs, a change in alveolar ventilation, or a new level of CO_2 production. Capnography is useful in many clinical conditions as a monitor to determine factors such as adequacy and safety of mechanical ventilation, increase in CO_2 production during rewarming after open-heart surgery, endotracheal tube (ET) positioning, optimal ventilation-perfusion relationship, and others (Table 8-6).

COMPLIANCE

Lung compliance is the change in volume per change in distending pressure and reflects the ease with which the lungs expand—their stiffness or, conversely, their distensibility. The higher the lung compliance, the greater the air volume that can be inhaled for a given change in distending pressure and the more distensible the lungs. Fig. 8-45 shows how compliance curves differ. In a patient with emphysema the lungs have lost some of their elastic recoil because of the destruction of alveolar-capillary membranes. They are therefore more easily expanded by a given amount of distending pressure. In pulmonary fibrosis the lung interstitium is infiltrated with scar tissue. Fibrotic lungs are stiffer and bring in less air for a given change in pressure.

It is important to monitor lung compliance in all patients on mechanical ventilation, since changes in compliance may indicate improvement or worsening of the lung disease. Some ventilators have in-line pneumotachographs available that constantly measure lung volume and pressures. These measurements are used to provide a pressure-volume curve that indicates lung compliance. Manual measurements of static compliance (Cst), taken at a point of no airflow, can also be performed (see Chapter 5). A Cst of 50 to 100 ml/cm H_2O is considered optimal.[14] The critical care nurse should monitor the trend of lung compliance changes. If compliance is decreasing, the patient could have problems such as ARDS, pneumothorax, atelectasis, pneumonia, pulmonary edema, pleural effusion, chest-wall restriction, or main-stem intubation.

Lung compliance should also be followed in the patient

Table 8-6   Clinical Interpretation of Capnography Measurements[12,17,20]

End-tidal CO_2 (Pet_{CO_2}) measurement	Physiological basis for change in Pet_{CO_2}	Clinical conditions
Increased Pet_{CO_2}	1. Hypermetabolic states causing increased CO_2 production 2. Hypoventilation	1. Multiple trauma, burns, hyperthyroidism, or malignant hyperthermia 2. Insufficient minute ventilation from mechanical ventilator; respiratory depression caused by increased intracranial pressure, pharmacological paralysis, and narcotics
Acute increase in Pet_{CO_2}	1. Sudden increase in CO_2 production caused by increased temperature, circulation, and metabolic rate 2. Improvement of circulation with improved CO_2 delivery to lungs 3. Increase in amount of CO_2 to be eliminated in lungs	1. Rewarming after major cardiovascular surgical procedures 2. Release of military antishock trousers 3. Administration of large doses of sodium bicarbonate
Waveform will fail to return to zero baseline on inspiration and will rise with each sequential inspiration	1. Rebreathing of CO_2	1. Incomplete seal of expiratory demand valve on ventilator; inadequate fresh gas flow through a T-tube; dislodged expiratory valve on self-inflating resuscitation bag
Increasing Pet_{CO_2} associated with increasing respiratory rate and a loss of plateau on capnogram	1. Inadequate spontaneous ventilation	1. Potential ventilator weaning failure
Decreased Pet_{CO_2}	1. Decreased metabolic rate with decreased CO_2 production 2. Decreased cardiac output resulting in reduction in pulmonary blood flow and inadequate elimination of CO_2 by lungs 3. Decreased systemic perfusion 4. Decreased pulmonary perfusion 5. Acute changes in respiratory gas exchange 6. Mechanical ventilator problem	1. Hypothermia, general anesthesia, or hypothyroidism 2. Acute heart failure or myocardial infarction 3. Hypovolemia with peripheral vasoconstriction 4. Pulmonary embolism 5. Atelectasis, endobronchial intubation, pneumothorax, or pulmonary edema or congestion 6. ET tube partially obstructed by mucous plug, cuff leak from ET tube, or kinked ET tube
Drop in Pet_{CO_2} to zero, and waveform disappears	1. Mechanical ventilator problem	1. Accidental intubation of esophagus, accidental extubation, or obstructed ET tube
Brisk drop in Pet_{CO_2}	1. Sudden cessation of cardiac output with lack of pulmonary blood flow or elimination of CO_2 by lung	1. Cardiac arrest

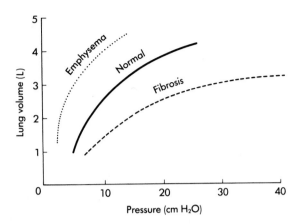

Fig. 8-45 Compliance curves. Compliance is high in emphysema and low in pulmonary fibrosis. (From Martin L: *Pulmonary physiology in clinical practice,* St Louis, 1987, Mosby–Year Book.)

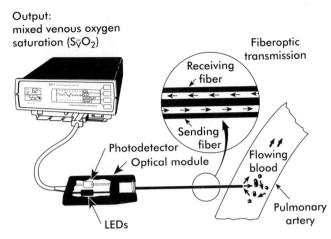

Fig. 8-46 Continuous monitoring of mixed venous oxygen saturation (Svo_2). The monitoring system consists of a fiberoptic catheter, an optical module, and an oximeter. Light of selected wavelengths is transmitted down one fiberoptic filament in the catheter body to the blood flowing past the catheter tip. The reflected light is then transmitted back through the second fiberoptic filament to a photodetector located in the optical module. Since hemoglobin and oxyhemoglobin absorb light differently at the selected wavelengths, the reflected light can be analyzed to determine the percent Svo_2. (*Courtesy of Baxter Travenol Laboratories, Inc., Santa Ana, Calif.*)

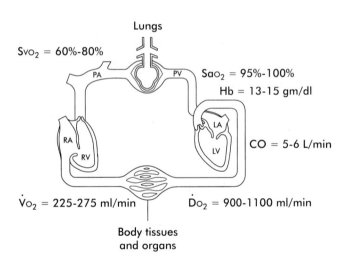

Fig. 8-47 Simplified diagram of the human circulatory system with normal values. Blood leaves the lungs with an arterial oxygen saturation (Sao_2) of 95% to 100%. Hemoglobin (Hb), at a concentration of 13 to 15 gm/dl, transports the oxygen in the blood. The left ventricle (LV) pumps the blood to body tissues at a cardiac output (CO) of 5 to 6 L/min. The oxygen delivery (Do_2) to the tissues is 900 to 1100 ml/min. At rest the body tissues use the oxygen at an oxygen consumption (Vo_2) rate of 225 to 275 ml/min. The venous blood carrying the remaining oxygen then returns to the heart and is pumped through the pulmonary artery (PA) towards the lungs. The mixed venous oxygen saturation (Svo_2) is measured in the pulmonary artery and reflects a mixture of all of the venous blood saturations from many body tissues. The normal Svo_2 is 60% to 80%. (*Courtesy of Baxter Travenol Laboratories, Inc., Santa Ana, Calif.*)

receiving PEEP. When PEEP gets too high the alveoli become overdistended, and Cst decreases. At this point, PEEP should be reduced to avoid pulmonary barotrauma. Following lung compliance values is also useful when weaning a patient from mechanical ventilation. Patients with Cst values less than 25 to 30 ml/cm H_2O may not be weaned successfully. This is because of the increased work required to expand poorly compliant lungs.

Continuous Monitoring of Mixed Venous Oxygen Saturation

Monitoring of mixed venous oxygen saturation (Svo_2) is becoming commonplace in ICUs across the United States. The technology for measuring Svo_2 is based on reflection spectrophotometry (Fig. 8-46). A modified PA catheter called a *fiberoptic flow-directed thermodilution PA catheter (Opticath)* is used for monitoring of Svo_2 (see Fig. 8-13). Svo_2 measurements reflect the body's ability to balance tissue oxygen demands with oxygen supply. When the Svo_2 value changes the nurse will need to determine which of the following four factors that maintain the oxygen supply-demand balance is affecting Svo_2:[6]

- Cardiac output (CO)
- Hemoglobin (Hb) concentration
- Tissue oxygen consumption (Vo_2)
- Arterial oxygen saturation (Sao_2)

Table 8-7 Interpretation of Sv_{O_2} Measurements[18]

Sv_{O_2} range	Physiological basis for change in Sv_{O_2}	Possible clinical causes
High (80%-90%)	1. Increased oxygen delivery	1. Increased Fi_{O_2} from mechanical ventilation, patient receiving more oxygen than required by clinical condition
	2. Decreased oxygen demand	2. Hypothermia, anesthesia, sepsis (decreased ability of tissues to use oxygen at cellular level), pharmacological paralysis, or left-to-right shunting
	3. Increased CO	3. Inotropic drug administration
	4. Artifact	4. Wedged catheter in PA
Normal (60%-80%)	1. Normal oxygen delivery and normal oxygen demand	1. Adequate tissue perfusion and oxygenation
Low (below 60%)	1. Increased oxygen demand	1. Shivering, seizures, severe pain, anxiety, hyperthermia, significant burns, multiple trauma, or nursing interventions, such as obtaining bed-scale weight and turning
	2. Decreased oxygen delivery caused by low hemoglobin	2. Anemia or bleeding
	3. Decreased oxygen delivery caused by low arterial oxygen saturation (Sa_{O_2})	3. Lung disease, hemorrhage, suctioning, disconnection from ventilator, inadequate Fi_{O_2} from ventilator, hypoxia
	4. Decreased oxygen delivery caused by low CO	4. Cardiogenic shock, hypovolemia, discontinuation of intraaortic balloon pump, or use of PEEP

It is helpful to observe the relationship of these variables in a simplified diagram of the human circulatory system (Fig. 8-47). Table 8-7 shows the interpretation of Sv_{O_2} measurements. An Sv_{O_2} level below 60% usually indicates cardiac decompensation; below 53%, lactic acidosis; below 32%, unconsciousness; and below 20%, permanent cellular damage. Guidelines important to know when caring for a patient on an Sv_{O_2} monitoring system are listed in the box at the right.

ASSESSMENT

The assessment of the patient on hemodynamic or respiratory monitoring is similar to that presented in Chapter 1 (see box on Guidelines for Conducting the Complete Assessment). During this assessment, the nurse would need to be alert for the complications of invasive respiratory and hemodynamic monitoring, such as infection, dysrhythmias, and pulmonary infarction (Table 8-8). Hemodynamic measurements are usually obtained every hour unless a patient is receiving a cardiac drug (e.g., dopamine or nitroprusside) through a continuous drip. In this case, measurements should be obtained every 15 minutes. Immediate postoperative patients and those in shock or who are deteriorating rapidly would also require every 15 minute hemodynamic and noninvasive respiratory monitoring. Normal hemodynamic pressures and calculated values are listed in Table 8-1. Table 8-2 lists the hemodynamic values that can be expected in various disease states. The nurse should be more concerned with establishing baseline values for the patient and following trends as opposed to focusing on normal and abnormal values.

▼ **Guidelines for the Sv_{O_2} Monitoring System**

- Calibrate the CO-oximeter on initial insertion, anytime the catheter is disconnected from the Optical Module, and routinely once a day.
- To calibrate, draw a mixed venous blood sample and send to laboratory for analysis (see Skill 8-17). Then compare the blood sample's value with the Sv_{O_2} value on the CO-oximeter at the time of sampling. Recalibrate if more than 4% difference between the two values occurs.
- Set alarm parameters at the keyboard at a range of 10% above and below the displayed Sv_{O_2} level. Update these parameters with any Sv_{O_2} change greater than 5% and whenever recalibration alters Sv_{O_2} readings.
- Document hourly Sv_{O_2} readings along with vital signs, and attach selected strips to the patient's chart. The strip recorder records the Sv_{O_2} level every 5 seconds. Intensity bars measure data transmission intensity every 2 minutes. Inadequate signal intensity causes the alarm to sound.
- Reassess patient if Sv_{O_2} falls below 60% or if it varies + or − 10% for 3 minutes or longer.
- Troubleshoot intensity alarm if it sounds. Check for catheter patency and placement, removing any air bubbles and kinks from the catheter. Attempt to withdraw blood from the catheter, and then try to flush the catheter. Reposition the patient.

Table 8-8   Complications of PA Catheters, Possible Causes, Prevention, and Interventions

Complication	Possible cause	Prevention	Interventions
Infection	Break in aseptic technique during catheter insertion, equipment setup, blood sampling, or tubing change Contamination through flow in transducer dome	Use careful aseptic technique Place sterile deadender caps on all stopcocks Use sterile sleeve over catheter Carefully check domes before use; never reuse disposable domes Sterilize transducer between patients Change disposable domes after defibrillation Do not use D_5W on transducer head or as IV flush solution	Remove all catheters if sepsis develops; administer antibiotics as indicated by culture and sensitivity Change transducer system every 2-4 days.
	Prolonged catheterization	Change flush solution and tubing every 24-48 hr Inspect and cleanse wound with bactericidal daily Minimize time catheter is in place	Apply iodophor ointment and sterile dressing to insertion site every 48 hr Remove catheter as soon as possible (replace after 4 days if necessary)
Cardiac tamponade	Perforation by catheter tip (usually during insertion)	Gently manipulate and advance catheter with balloon inflated Never advance catheter against resistance	Pericardiocentesis Reverse anticoagulation
Catheter coiling or knotting	Dilated RA or RV Softening of catheter secondary to prolonged insertion time with much manipulation Use of small (5 F) catheter	Advance catheter gently but swiftly before softening occurs; flush catheter with iced saline, or insert 0.025-inch guidewire to stiffen	Replace with new catheter
Balloon rupture	Excessive number of balloon inflations	Monitor PADP instead of PAWP (if close relationship); wedge catheter infrequently	Turn off stopcock of air lumen; place tape over stopcock to prevent further use Monitor PADP
	Overinflation of balloon	Inflate balloon only with amounts of air indicated on catheter (1.5 ml for 7 F)	
	Inflation of balloon with fluid Active deflation of balloon by withdrawing air back into syringe	Inflate balloon only with air or CO_2 Deflate balloon by removing syringe and allowing air to escape passively	
Dysrhythmias	Irritation of endocardium by unprotected catheter tip	Keep balloon inflated during advancement; advance gently	Administer lidocaine if necessary Defibrillate if ventricular fibrillation occurs Insert pacemaker for complete heart block
	Excess catheter loop in RV or RA Prolonged catheterization procedure with much manipulation	Obtain chest x-ray Insert catheter quickly, gently, and with minimal manipulation; use fluoroscopy, if possible	Withdraw catheter to remove loop
	Catheter tip withdrawn or fallen back into RV	Situate catheter well into main PA	Inflate balloon to encourage catheter passage out to PA
Thrombus/embolism	Clot from fibrin sheath around catheter	Use heparin-bonded catheters Use sheath with side arm infusion of heparin solution	
	Clot from within catheter	Maintain continuous flush with heparinized solution; manually flush every 4 to 6 hours	Anticoagulation and possible thrombolysis
	Occlusion of branch of PA by catheter	Systemic heparinization in high-risk patients Maintain catheter tip in main PA	
Pulmonary infarction/ PA rupture	Distal catheter tip migration (especially during first 24 hours)	Check x-ray immediately after catheter insertion and 12 hours later; remove catheter loop in RV or RA Continuously monitor PA waveform	Withdraw catheter tip to PA Supportive care Surgical repair if necessary
	Prolonged wedging of catheter	Wedge very briefly (<30 sec); leave balloon deflated with stopcock open and syringe removed; monitor PADP instead of PA (if close relationship)	
	Embolization of thrombus from catheters	Use heparin-bonded catheters; maintain adequate flush with heparinized solution	

Adapted from Tilkian AG, Daily EK: *Cardiovascular procedures: diagnostic techniques and therapeutic procedures*, St Louis, 1986, Mosby–Year Book.

Skill 8-17   Obtaining Samples for Mixed Venous Oxygen Determinations

▼

EQUIPMENT AND SUPPLIES

- Cup of ice
- Two 10-ml syringes
- 3-ml syringe
- Vial of heparin
- Syringe cap

NURSING INTERVENTIONS

1. Draw up 1 ml of heparin into the 3-ml syringe, and coat the inside of the syringe.
2. Expel excess heparin, leaving heparin to fill the dead space in the hub of the syringe.
3. Attach a 10-ml syringe to the sampling stopcock connected to the distal port of the pulmonary artery catheter.
4. Turn stopcock off to the flush solution.
5. Aspirate 5 ml into a 10-ml syringe to clear the line of flush solution. Close the stopcock to the halfway position, remove syringe, and discard.
6. Attach the heparinized syringe to the sampling stopcock.
7. Open the stopcock, and aspirate blood slowly. Aspirating too rapidly may result in withdrawing blood backward from the alveolar level where blood is reoxygenated.
8. Close the stopcock, and remove the syringe. Hold the syringe upright, and expel any air bubbles in the syringe. Cap the syringe, and roll it gently to mix the blood with the heparin. Submerge in cup of ice.
9. Attach the 10-ml syringe to the stopcock. Open the stopcock to the flush solution. Flush solution into the syringe to clear the stopcock. Turn the stopcock off to the sampling port, remove the syringe, and cap the port.
10. Flush the line until all traces of blood are removed.
11. Check the bedside monitor for reappearance of pulmonary artery waveform and patency of line.
12. Send sample to the laboratory as soon as possible.

NURSING DIAGNOSIS

Possible nursing diagnoses for patients requiring hemodynamic and respiratory monitoring might include the following:

- High risk for disturbance in pulmonary tissue perfusion related to potential problems of continuous wedge position of PA catheter balloon.
- High risk for infection related to presence of invasive lines.
- Impaired mobility related to attachment to monitoring equipment.
- High risk for injury related to air embolism secondary to presence of left atrial catheter.
- Potential disturbance in tissue perfusion of hand related to risk of impaired circulation secondary to presence of arterial catheter.
- Potential for impaired skin integrity related to presence of multiple invasive catheters.
- Sleep-pattern disturbance related to physical manipulation and noise associated with monitoring equipment.
- Anxiety related to fear of equipment and noises associated with hemodynamic monitoring.

PATIENT OUTCOMES

The following is a list of examples of patient outcomes that might be used in patients requiring hemodynamic and respiratory monitoring. Patient evidences:

- Lungs clear to bases, with evidence of PA catheter tip properly positioned in pulmonary artery.
- Low CO_2 gradient (correlation of $Paco_2$ and $Petco_2$).
- Improved Cst (normal is 50 to 100 ml/cm H_2O).
- Stable Svo_2 of 60% to 80% on continuous fiberoptic catheter monitoring system.
- Stable Sao_2 of $\geq$ 94% on pulse oximeter.
- Improvement in intrapulmonary shunt (a/A ratio) (normal is > 0.80 to 0.85).
- Stable heart rate of 60 to 100 beats/min.
- Stable BP of 100/60 to 140/90 mm Hg with MAP of 70 to 90 mm Hg.
- Stable CVP of 0 to 6 mm Hg (0 to 8 cm H_2O).
- Stable PAP of 20/6 to 30/12 mm Hg.
- Optimal PAWP to produce optimal CO for patient (normal PAWP range is 6 to 15 mm Hg).
- Improvement in CO (normal cardiac index is 2.5 to 4 $L/min/m^2$).
- SVR of 900 to 1200 dyne/sec/cm^5.
- PVR of 150 to 250 dyne/sec/cm^5.
- Improved LVSWI (normal is 50 to 62 g-m/m^2).
- Normal sinus rhythm on ECG monitor.
- Normal temperature of 36-38° C (97-100.5° F).
- White blood cell (WBC) count $\leq$ 11,000 ul and negative catheter and skin cultures.
- Clear, intact skin of normal color and temperature at catheter entry sites.
- Adequate perfusion to hands with brisk capillary refill (< 3 seconds) with normal color, warmth, sensation, and movement.

PEDIATRIC CONSIDERATIONS

Hemodynamic and respiratory monitoring equipment is being seen increasingly in pediatric ICUs because of the availability of miniaturized or scaled-down monitoring equipment. Conditions in which PA catheters are usually indicated in infants and children include:

- High peak pressures or high PEEP used with mechanical ventilation.
- Critical illness associated with severe pulmonary dysfunction (respiratory distress syndrome, pulmonary embolus, severe pneumonitis, or pulmonary artery hypertension).
- Conditions requiring afterload reduction therapy.
- Critical illness associated with definite myocardial dysfunction (myocarditis, structural abnormalities, cardiomyopathy, or myocardial infarction).

Children and infants have unique physiological characteristics. Their hemodynamic monitoring pressures will vary significantly from adult values (Tables 8-9 and 8-10).

Table 8-9   Comparison of Cardiovascular Characteristics of Children and Adults

Characteristic		Children		Adults	
ESTIMATED BLOOD VOLUME		80 ml/kg		65 ml/kg	
Heart rate (age related)	Infants	120 to 160 beats/min		60 to 100 beats/min	
	Toddlers	90 to 140 beats/min			
	Preschoolers	80 to 110 beats/min			
	School age children	75 to 100 beats/min			
	Adolescents	60 to 90 beats/min			
BP (age related)		*Systolic (mm Hg)*	*Diastolic (mm Hg)*	*Systolic (mm Hg)*	*Diastolic (mm Hg)*
	Neonates	60 to 90	20 to 60	100 to 140	60 to 90
	Infants	74 to 100	50 to 70		
	Toddlers	80 to 112	50 to 80		
	Preschoolers	82 to 110	50 to 78		
	School age children	84 to 120	54 to 80		
	Adolescents	94 to 140	62 to 80		
STROKE VOLUME	Neonates	5 ml/beat		60-130 ml/beat	
	Preschoolers	15 ml/beat			
	School age children	35 ml/beat			
Cardiac index		3.5 to 4 L/min/m^2 for neonates to school age children		2.5 to 4 L/min/m^2	
LV/RV weight ratio	Neonates	0.8:1		2.5:1	
	Infants	1.5 : 1			
	6 mo	2:1			

Adapted from Daily EK, Schroeder JS: *Techniques in bedside hemodynamic monitoring,* St Louis, 1985, Mosby–Year Book.

Table 8-10   Normal Hemodynamic Pressure Values in Neonates and Children

Hemodynamic parameter	Neonates (mm Hg)	Children (mm Hg)
LA pressure	1-4	5-10
a wave	—	3-7
v wave	—	5-15
LV pressure	60-100/5-10	80-130/10-20
RA pressure	0-3	1-5
a wave	—	3-7
v wave	—	2-5
RV pressure	30-60/2-5	15-30/2-5
PA pressure	30-60/2-10	15-30/5-10
Mean pressure	13-25	10-20

From Daily EK, Schroeder JS: *Techniques in bedside hemodynamic monitoring,* St Louis, 1985, Mosby–Year Book.

A small change in a parameter will also be more serious in a child than in an adult. For example, a drop in systolic blood pressure from 80 mm Hg to 74 mm Hg would be of much greater significance in a child than a similar drop in an adult.

Nurses need to be concerned about blood loss in children when there is frequent blood withdrawal from arterial lines. In infants weighing less than 10 kg (22 lbs) a record of the amount of blood withdrawn (including the initial discard) should be maintained.[21] Children can also become easily fluid and sodium overloaded if monitored lines are flushed frequently. When performing COs, injectates of 3 ml or less should be used.

One way to prevent some blood loss and the need for frequent tubing flushes is to use a T connector tube at the catheter insertion site (Fig. 8-48). When drawing blood a clamp is placed on the infusion line, distal to the T connector, and a small needle is inserted into the connector injection port. Three or four drops of fluid are allowed to drop out of the line; then a syringe is attached to withdraw the desired amount of blood. The pressure buildup within the infusion tubing during the clamping of the connector is sufficient to flush the line after the clamp is released. Therefore no fluids are administered.

High pressure bags with a continuous flush device are risky to use in pediatrics because the infusion rate can only be assumed, and the flush delivers an unknown quantity. For these reasons it is better to use a Holter pump system or syringe pump to maintain catheter patency and carefully control fluid delivery (Fig. 8-49). Most PA catheters can be maintained at infusion rates of 1 ml/hr.

Another problem with hemodynamic monitoring in children is that they have small vascular lumens and unpredictable anatomy so that cannulation is more difficult. CVP catheters may be inserted in the umbilical vein, external jugular vein, or less easily through the basilic or subclavian veins. In general the external jugular vein is the most accessible and is often distended and easily recognized in a crying infant. The right jugular vein is preferred because the course of the vein is less angled. Subclavian placements are difficult in a small child and can frequently lead to pneumothorax. PA catheters, which are larger, are in-

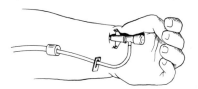

Fig. 8-48 Vascular infusion system with T connector. The T connector can be used to withdraw blood. (From Hazinski MF: *Nursing care of the critically ill child,* ed 2, St Louis, 1992, Mosby–Year Book.)

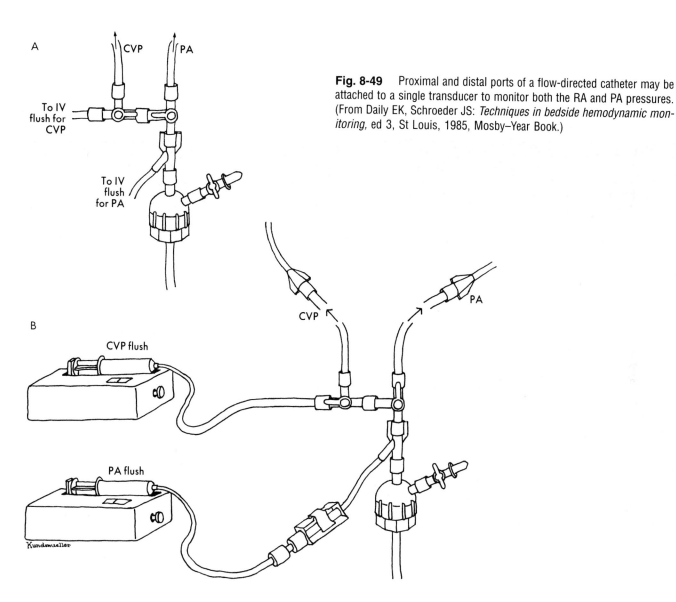

Fig. 8-49 Proximal and distal ports of a flow-directed catheter may be attached to a single transducer to monitor both the RA and PA pressures. (From Daily EK, Schroeder JS: *Techniques in bedside hemodynamic monitoring,* ed 3, St Louis, 1985, Mosby–Year Book.)

serted into the femoral or jugular veins in small infants and children. Use of the largest catheter possible improves the quality of hemodynamic pressures and decreases the risk of catheter lumen occlusion.

Because small children have smaller arteries, the incidence of thrombosis is greater in those less than 5 years of age. The frequency of arterial thrombosis increases when catheters are left in place for more than 3 days. When vigorous flushing of an arterial catheter occurs, this can cause retrograde embolization to the central circulation. This problem can be serious in infants, in whom the distance

from the peripheral site of cannulation to the aortic arch is small. Retrograde embolization can be reduced by limiting the amount of flush solution injected at any time to 0.5 ml in small children. Forceful injection of any amount of fluid should never be performed.

When preparing the heparin flush IV bag, the amount of heparin is reduced for the pediatric patient. Concentrations range between 0.25 to 1 unit heparin/1 ml IV solution. The lesser concentration is preferable, since inadvertent heparinization can occur in small infants if high concentrations are used.

PSYCHOSOCIAL CONSIDERATIONS

Patients in a highly technical ICU environment with the need for frequent monitoring are likely to suffer from psychosocial stress. In addition to emotional reactions such as fear, anxiety, depression, denial, and anger, ICU patients also experience sensory and perceptual problems. Being in an ICU environment causes a change in the variety and strength of sensory stimulation and can lead to sensory overload or deprivation. This can lead to problems, such as depersonalization, disorientation, psychotic behavior, hallucinations, labile moods, and panic. Patient response to the ICU environment can be identified by means of a thorough psychosocial assessment.

The ICU nurse has an important role in meeting the psychosocial needs of the critically ill patient. This role includes the following functions[2,3,15]:

- Communicating frequently with the patient, allowing the patient to verbalize fears.
- Thoroughly preparing the patient for procedures.
- Involving the patient in decisions about care.
- Respecting the patient's privacy.
- Helping the patient regain a sense of control by encouraging the performance of self-care activities.
- Providing cues for orientation, and eliminating sources of interference with the sleep/wake cycle.
- Touching, caring, listening, and attending to general comfort measures.

PATIENT AND FAMILY TEACHING

It is important to provide for teaching and psychosocial support for the family of the ICU patient, since the family plays a significant positive or negative role in the patient's response to illness. If the family's needs are ignored, the family could become a source of stress for the patient and the nurse. The positive presence of the family can aid in the recovery of the patient. Table 8-11 lists some of the strategies and nursing interventions available for providing teaching and support to the family.

HOME HEALTH CARE CONSIDERATIONS

Invasive hemodynamic and respiratory monitoring is not performed in the home health setting because of the risk of infection and critical condition of the patients. Noninvasive forms of monitoring, though, such as ECG and apnea monitoring are performed in the home. Home monitoring of an infant's respirations and heart rate has escalated to over 1% of all live births in some states.

Apnea Monitoring

Home apnea monitors provide important information about whether infants or adults are having continuing problems with episodes of apnea, in which ventilation ceases or drops below a preset level (usually 15 or 20 seconds). Some apnea machines can also simultaneously monitor the heart rate. A loud alarm on the monitor summons help for the individual each time the monitor senses pauses in chest wall motion, tachycardia (usually over 200 to 250 beats/min in infants), or bradycardia (usually 60 to 70

Table 8-11 Teaching and Support Strategies for the Family of the ICU Patient[11,13,16]

Method	Characteristics
Preoperative teaching	Can be performed as group teaching in classroom or individually at bedside; patient and families are present; presentation of preoperative and postoperative phase, including function of equipment, expected appearance, pain control, and role of patient and family; breathing exercises taught; tour of ICU included.
Perioperative liaison	A liaison nurse, who may be the patient's ICU admitting nurse, visits the surgical patient's family at preset intervals during the surgical procedure and after the transfer to the ICU; during the visits, emotional support and postoperative teaching are provided to the family.
Postoperative or post-ICU admission teaching	Includes family tour of unit, introduction to key personnel, explanation of equipment and patient's condition, provision of brochure with unit policies and phone numbers, and discussion of family role.
Family conference	Multidisciplinary meeting conducted with family of an ICU patient; increases relatives' coping mechanisms and improves patient care; helps with patient care decisions and planning for future.
Mutual-peer family support group	Provides interactive social support group for family members in the critical care setting; helps to alleviate social isolation; provides for sharing of feelings, interpersonal learning, problem solving, and learning of coping strategies.
Educational family support group	Formal presentation followed by question-and-answer period of topics such as disease process, coping skills, available resources, and illness management; not a forum for emotional sharing and individual problem solving.

beats/min in infants). The indications for in-patient and home health apnea monitoring are listed in the box on p. 217. There are two types of apnea monitors. The impedance pneumographer records changes in resistance of an electrical field (impedance) that occur with variations in thoracic volume. Impedance is measured by placing two electrodes on each side of the patient's chest in basic ECG patterns (Skill 8-18). The other apnea monitor, the pressure transducer, is placed between the patient's mattress and box springs. It detects the slight shift in the center of gravity that occurs during normal respiration. Once an infant returns home on apnea monitoring, decisions for stopping home monitoring will be based on clinical criteria. Most likely the monitor will be discontinued when the infant has had 2 or 3 months free of events requiring vigorous stimulation, mouth-to-mouth resuscitation, or CPR.

▼
Indications for Apnea Monitoring

INFANTS AND CHILDREN

- Infants with one or more severe apparent life-threatening events (ALTE) requiring vigorous stimulation, mouth-to-mouth resuscitation, or cardiopulmonary resuscitation (CPR).
- Preterm infants with apnea of prematurity who are otherwise ready for discharge.
- Siblings of two or more victims of sudden infant death syndrome (SIDS).
- Central hypoventilation, tracheostomy, or neurological disorders.

ADULTS

- Neuromuscular disease (e.g., Guillain-Barré syndrome)
- Traumatic injury, not requiring mechanical ventilation
- Acute exacerbation of COPD
- Inhalation of certain toxic chemicals
- Narcotic or central nervous system (CNS) depressant overdose

Skill 8-18   Infant Apnea Monitoring
▼

EQUIPMENT AND SUPPLIES

- Apnea monitor
- Lead wire receptor and cable
- Two lead wires
- Two electrodes
- Sterile gauze pad
- Alcohol swabs

NURSING INTERVENTIONS

1. Ensure that the monitor is plugged into the wall outlet.
2. Depress the POWER button on the face of the monitor to turn it on.
3. Prepare infant for procedure by talking to infant and cuddling.
4. Peel off the paper backing on an electrode. Check the sponge pad in the center to see if it is still moist with conductive jelly.
5. Apply an electrode to each side of the infant's abdomen, just below the rib cage.
6. Connect the lead wires to the electrodes, using the manufacturer's color code.
7. Attach the two lead wires to the lead wire receptor, matching the lead wires with their color-coded mates.
8. Plug the lead wire cable into the outlet labeled PATIENT CABLE, on the back of the monitor.
9. Push the ALARM SOUND button. To test the alarm, disconnect the lead wire cable from the monitor. If the alarm does not sound, get another monitor. If the alarm does sound, reconnect the lead wire cable, and reset the alarm.
10. Set the ALARM DELAY selector at 10, 15, or 20 seconds. The alarm will sound if the patient does not breathe within the time you have set.

REFERENCES

1. Ahrens TS: Effects of mechanical ventilation on hemodynamic waveforms, *Crit Care Nurs Clin North Am* 3(4):629, 1991.
2. Caine RM: Families in crisis: making the critical difference, *Focus Crit Care* 16(3):184, 1989.
3. Clochesy JM: *Essentials of critical care nursing,* Rockville, Maryland, 1988, Aspen.
4. Darovic GO: *Hemodynamic monitoring: invasive and noninvasive clinical applications,* Philadelphia, 1987, WB Saunders.
5. Dettenmeier PA, Johnson TM: The art and science of mechanical ventilator adjustments, *Crit Care Nurs Clin North Am* 3(4):575, 1991.
6. Enger, EL: II. Perspectives on the interpretation of continuous mixed venous oxygen saturation, *Heart Lung* 19(5):578, 1990.
7. Enger EL: Pulmonary artery wedge pressure: when it's valid, when it's not, *Crit Care Nurs Clin North Am* 1(3):603, 1989.
8. Gardner PE: Cardiac output: theory, technique, and troubleshooting, *Crit Care Nurs Clin North Am* 1(3):577, 1989.
9. Gibbs NC, Gardner RM: Dynamics of invasive pressure monitoring systems: clinical and laboratory evaluation, *Heart Lung* 17(1):43, 1988.
10. Halfman-Franey M, Bergstrom D: Clinical management using direct and derived parameters, *Crit Care Nurs Clin North Am* 1(3):547, 1989.
11. Halm MA: Strategies for developing a family support group, *Focus Crit Care* 18(6):444, 1991.
12. Hess D: Noninvasive respiratory monitoring during ventilatory support, *Crit Care Nurs Clin North Am* 3(4):565, 1991.
13. Hill M: Teaching after CABG surgery: a family affair, *Crit Care Nurse* 9(8):58, 1989.
14. McCauley MD, Von Rueden KT: Moninvasive monitoring of the mechanically ventilated patient, *Crit Care Q* 11(3):36, 1988.
15. Meijs CA: Care of the family of the ICU patient, *Crit Care Nurse* 9(8):42, 1989.
16. Stanik JA: Caring for the family of the critically ill surgical patient, *Crit Care Nurse* 10(1):43, 1990.
17. Szaflarski NL, Cohen NH: Use of capnography in critically ill adults, *Heart Lung* 20(4):363, 1991.
18. Thelan LA, Davie JK, Urden LD: *Textbook of critical care nursing. Diagnosis and management,* St Louis, 1990, Mosby–Year Book.
19. Urban N: Hemodynamic clinical profiles, *AACN Clin Issues Crit Care Nurs* 1(1):119, 1990.
20. Von Rueden KT: Noninvasive assessment of gas exchange in the critically ill patient, *AACN Clin Issues Crit Care Nurs* 1(2):239, 1990.
21. Webster H: *Hemodynamic monitoring in children.* In Daily EK, Schroeder JS, editors: *Techniques in bedside hemodynamic monitoring,* St Louis, 1985, Mosby–Year Book.
22. Yonkman CA, Hamory BH: Sterility and efficiency of two methods of cardiac output determination: closed loop and capped syringe methods, *Heart Lung* 17(2):121, 1988.

CHAPTER 9

Defibrillation and Implantable Cardioverter Defibrillators

Objectives

After completing this chapter, the reader will be able to:

- Identify dysrhythmias treated by cardioversion and defibrillation.
- Discuss the physiological conditions contributing to tachydysrhythmias.
- Describe the safety precautions that must be considered with the use of cardioversion and defibrillation.
- Discuss the indications and complications associated with cardioversion and defibrillation.
- Describe the procedure of defibrillation, internal defibrillation, and cardioversion.
- Describe the operation and complications of an implantable cardioverter defibrillator (ICD).
- Devise a plan of care for the patient with an ICD.
- Discuss the teaching, pediatric, psychosocial, and home health considerations of caring for a patient with an ICD.

Electrical defibrillation is the delivery of an electrical current through the heart to depolarize a critical mass of the left ventricular myocardium. When the cardiac fibers repolarize, they will hopefully return to a normal synchronized pattern permitting coordinated electrical conduction and myocardial contraction. Defibrillation is presently the most effective method of terminating ventricular fibrillation (VF) and pulseless ventricular tachycardia (VT). Defibrillation is also used for asystole if the rhythm is unclear and the tracing may possibly represent fine VF. *Synchronized cardioversion* is the delivery of an electrical current lower than used in defibrillation and timed to occur during the QRS complex of the cardiac cycle rather than the vulnerable period of the T wave. This therapy is used to treat unstable VT with a pulse or supraventricular tachydysrhythmias. Certain tachydysrhythmias are responsive to lower levels of electrical energy that cause less damage to the myocardium (see Chapter 6 for discussion of automaticity, altered conduction, and reentry).

INDICATIONS FOR DEFIBRILLATION

Defibrillation is indicated for the following conditions:
- VF.
- Ventricular flutter.
- Pulseless VT.
- Asystole where the rhythm is unclear and possibly VF.
- Reentry circuits.
- Reentry dysrhythmias.

INDICATIONS FOR CARDIOVERSION

Cardioversion is indicated for the treatment of sustained VT with a pulse or supraventricular tachydysrhythmias. There are two types of cardioversion: urgent synchronized cardioversion and elective synchronized cardioversion. The indications for using each procedure will be based on the assessment of the patient (Table 9-1).

COMPLICATIONS OF DEFIBRILLATION AND CARDIOVERSION

The complications associated with the procedures of defibrillation and cardioversion can be kept to a minimum by using extreme caution. Because of higher current requirements, complications are likely to be more severe with defibrillation, and in some cases, life threatening. Complications for both include the following:
- Dysrhythmias—asystole, bradycardia, AV block, VF following SVT.
- Embolic episodes.
- Skin burns.
- Electrical accidents.
- Inappropriate defibrillations—no malignant dysrhythmia present.
- Ineffective treatment of the dysrhythmia.
- Myocardial damage.
- Hypotension.
- Muscle pain.
- Pulmonary edema.

Table 9-1 Assessment of Tachydysrhythmias for Appropriate Treatment

Assessment	Intervention
Sustained VT with a pulse	
Hemodynamically stable and asymptomatic: systolic BP > 90 mm Hg, no complaints of chest pain, awake, alert, oriented, lungs clear, and respiratory rate 12-20 breaths/min.	Trial of pharmacological therapy (Lidocaine is drug of choice).
Hemodynamically unstable: dyspnea, chest pain, history of myocardial ischemia or MI, or CHF.	Urgent synchronized cardioversion with an amnestic sedative.
Severely unstable and has deteriorated: systolic BP < 90 mm Hg, crackles in lungs (indicative of pulmonary edema), or unconsciousness.	Unsynchronized cardioversion (defibrillation) without an amnestic sedative.*
Supraventricular tachydysrhythmias (SVT)†	
Possible VT due to wide-complex tachycardia; ensure that it is not ventricular in origin or due to preexcitation.	If in doubt, treat as in VT.
Unstable, does not respond to vagal maneuvers or drug therapy (Verapamil), and dysrhythmia is not caused by digitalis toxicity; SVT causes or exacerbates cardiovascular instability with: hypotension, dyspnea, chest pain, signs of ischemia, or CHF; patient has condition (acute MI or acute ischemic heart disease) that is aggravated by the tachycardia.	Patient requires urgent synchronized cardioversion.
Stable but unresponsive to medical therapy.	Elective synchronized cardioversion only after initial mechanism of dysrhythmia is controlled.

*Unsynchronized cardioversion (defibrillation) avoids the delays of waiting for the unit to synchronize. When VT is rapid, the T wave may not be easily distinguished from the QRS complex, so a nonsynchronized shock may be safer, being less likely to fall on the T wave.
†Supraventricular tachydysrhythmias originate primarily above the bifurcation of the bundle of His. They include atrial fibrillation, atrial flutter, paroxysmal atrial tachycardia, junctional tachycardia, paroxysmal supraventricular tachycardia, nonparoxysmal atrial-ventricular (AV) junctional tachycardia, and AV nodal reentry tachycardia.

ELECTRICAL SAFETY DURING DEFIBRILLATION AND CARDIOVERSION

Electrical safety is a foremost consideration when treating dysrhythmias with defibrillation equipment.

Process of Defibrillation

- Avoid placing excess amounts of conductive paste on the chest or paddles. The gel forms a conductive bridge on the skin causing skin burns when the defibrillator discharges.
- Avoid using alcohol or alcohol pads on the skin for defibrillation. Electrical current passing through the alcohol pads can burst into flames.
- Avoid charging the defibrillator until ready to discharge the current.
- Avoid placing the paddles near the monitoring electrodes to prevent sparks that can cause skin burns.
- Do not tilt the paddles during use to avoid arcing.
- Maintain good contact with the skin to prevent dissipation of the current.
- Maintain the appropriate amount of pressure on the paddles for discharge of the device, a range of 12 to 25 pounds of pressure.
- Stand clear from the patient and bed when discharging the device.
- Do not make contact with any grounded metal object during operation of the defibrillator.
- Be aware of idiosyncracies of the defibrillator in use.

Care of Equipment

- Frequently examine the paddles for pitting and buildup of an oxide film.
- Do not discharge the paddles when pressed together or into the air.
- The defibrillator is not deactivated by disconnection of the power cord if it is also battery operated.
- Maintain battery status of the device by keeping it plugged in during periods of inactivity.

Environment

- Eliminate the presence of oxygen in concentrations greater than 60%. Electrical arcing under these conditions will encourage combustion.
- Operate the equipment only in a dry area.
- Disconnect electrical equipment from the patient. Be sure that the patient is not in contact with any grounded metal object.
- Do not use a defibrillator in the presence of flammable substances or anesthetic agents.

Skill 9-1   Application of External Defibrillation

EQUIPMENT AND SUPPLIES

- Defibrillator
- Defibrillation paddles
- Recording paper
- Conductive gel or disposable pads
- Code cart
- Airway support equipment
- Cardiac monitor
- Emergency pacing equipment
- Documentation record

NURSING INTERVENTIONS

1. Assess for the presence of VF, VT, or asystole on the patient's cardiac monitor, the indications for defibrillation, and call for help.
2. Check the carotid pulse. If no pulse is present in a witnessed arrest and a defibrillator *is not available,* perform a precordial thump. Deliver the thump to the center of the sternum with the hypothenar aspect of the fist and from a height of no more than 12 inches. After the precordial thump, reassess the status of the pulse and call for a defibrillator if no pulse has returned.
3. If no pulse is present and a defibrillator *is readily available* at the bedside, defibrillate patient before administering CPR.
4. If the patient is not on a cardiac monitor and has the symptoms of a cardiac arrest, check for an absent pulse, begin CPR, and call for a defibrillator. Apply the feature of the "quick look" paddles to determine the patient's rhythm.

5. Prepare for defibrillation immediately by plugging in the machine and ensuring that the unit is in the nonsynchronized mode.
6. Apply a thin coat of conductive paste to the entire surface of the paddles. The paste decreases transthoracic resistance, preventing skin burns. Ensure that the paste does not drip down the chest wall to prevent arcing of current across the surface of the chest.
7. For the initial defibrillation attempt, set the energy level to 200 J.
8. Charge the capacitors. In some units, there is a charge button right on a paddle, the machine, or both. Charging may take several seconds. When the full charge is reached, this will be indicated on a digital display or an indicator light on the paddles.
9. Place paddles in appropriate location on the patient's chest. For standard or anterolateral placement, place one electrode paddle to the right of the upper sternum just below the right clavicle. Place the other just to the left of nipple in the anterior axillary line (Fig. 9-1). Ensure that the paddles are not placed too close together (Fig. 9-2).
10. If using an anteroposterior paddle position, place one paddle anteriorly over the precordium, just to the left of the lower sternal border and place the other on the back behind the heart below the left scapula (Fig. 9-3).

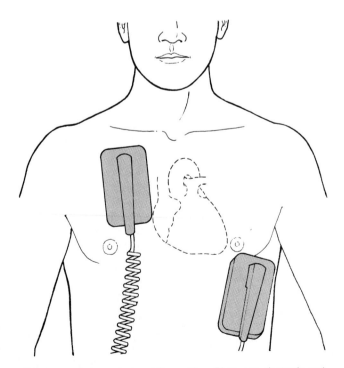

Fig. 9-1   Anteroapical paddle position. Place one electrode paddle to the right of the upper sternum just below the right clavicle. Place the other just to the left of the nipple in the anterior axillary line.

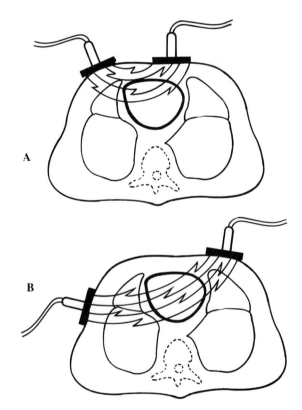

Fig. 9-2   A, When the electrode paddles are placed too close together, a substantial amount of current shunts between them and an insufficient amount reaches the heart. **B,** Wider spacing of the paddles allows a sufficient amount of current to reach the left ventricle. (From Tilkian AG, Daily EK: *Cardiovascular procedures,* St Louis, 1986, Mosby–Year Book.)

11. Rotate slightly for firm position and even distribution of the gel. Apply a firm even pressure (approximately 11.4 kg [25 lb]) for good contact with the skin.
12. Warn personnel to "stand clear" of the bed and any equipment that is in contact with the patient. Observe the area to ensure that everyone is clear.
13. Deliver the electrical current by depressing both discharge buttons on the paddles simultaneously.
14. Assess cardiac rhythm and pulse. Observe for spontaneous breathing with return of pulse and take blood pressure.
15. If unsuccessful, repeat steps for a second defibrillation. Increase the charge level to 200 to 300 J. Should a third shock be required, charge the machine to the maximum current level of 360 J.
16. Reapply conductive gel if necessary to prevent skin burns and to decrease the skin resistance.
17. Administer cardioactive drugs, such as epinephrine or antidysrhythmics, to supplement unsuccessful defibrillation.
18. If there is no response to the defibrillation attempt, assess the patient's airway and ventilation, patency of IV lines, pulse generated with CPR, ABG values, electrolyte levels, and presence of hypothermia, or toxic drug or alcohol levels. Variables affecting the outcome of defibrillation can be found in the box on this page.
19. Monitor for asystole. Confirm asystole in at least two lead configurations, evaluating the straight line for fine VF. Shock the patient again for fine fibrillation.
20. Plan to administer emergency pacing that may be required until patient's rhythm stabilizes.
21. Once patient attains a life-sustaining rhythm, initiate preventive measures to minimize the possibility of recurrence of the dysrhythmia.
22. Document the event.

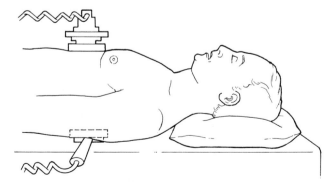

Fig. 9-3 Anteroposterior paddle position. Place one paddle anteriorly over the precordium, just to the left of the lower sternal border and place the other on the back behind the heart below the left scapula.

▼ **Factors Affecting the Outcome of Defibrillation**

TRANSTHORACIC IMPEDANCE

High over bone
Increased during inspiration
Influenced by energy level used
Affected by total number of shocks

PADDLES

Size
Placement
Pressure
Interface

PROCEDURE

Dose
Total number of shocks
Delay between shocks

OTHER

Digitalis
Duration of VF
Myocardial environment

Skill 9-2 **Defibrillation During Open-Chest Resuscitation**
▼

EQUIPMENT AND SUPPLIES

- Cardiac arrest cart
- Cardiac arrest tray
- Defibrillator
- Sterile internal paddles
- Bottle of sterile normal saline
- Tray of 4 × 4 gauze sponges

NURSING INTERVENTIONS

1. Using sterile technique, unwrap sterile cover of internal defibrillator paddles and place where physician (in sterile gloves, gown, cap, and mask) can reach them.
2. Attach the cable from the internal paddles to the defibrillator.
3. Open tray of 4 × 4 gauze sponges, pour sterile normal saline into tray, and hand tray so that physician can obtain sponges.
4. The physician will place the sponges between the paddles and epicardium of the heart and will place one paddle at the apex and the other paddle over the right atrium or ventricle.
5. Set the defibrillator energy level to 5 to 10 J.[6]
6. When the physician is ready, press the charge button to charge the capacitors.
7. Ask all bystanders to "stand clear" of the bed and equipment in contact with the patient. Observe the area.
8. When asked by the physician, press the discharge button on the defibrillator to deliver the countershock.
9. Assess the pulse and monitor patient's rhythm.
10. If fibrillation continues, charge the capacitors 5 J higher up to a maximum of 40 J and repeat the procedure.
11. If procedure is successful, cover chest with sterile towels and prepare to transport to operating room for closure of incision.

Skill 9-3   Assistance with Elective Cardioversion

EQUIPMENT AND SUPPLIES

- Cardioverter-defibrillator
- Conductive gel or disposable pads
- Cardiac monitor and electrodes
- Emergency pacing equipment
- 12-lead ECG machine
- Medications for sedation
- IV infusion equipment
- Code cart with resuscitation board
- Bag-valve-mask unit and suction equipment
- Intubation tray with airways
- Documentation record

NURSING INTERVENTIONS

1. In elective cardioversion, withhold diuretics and short-acting digitalis preparations for 24 to 36 hours before cardioversion, as ordered. The risk of lethal dysrhythmias must be considered in the presence of digitalis toxicity.
2. Have patient fast for 6 to 8 hours before the procedure. This is helpful in the prevention of vomiting and aspiration.
3. Notify the anesthesiologist of the procedure, if appropriate. The anesthesiologist will be administering light sedation for transient amnesia and will be present to intubate the patient in the event of a cardiac arrest.
4. Plug cardioverter-defibrillator into an electrical outlet and test it (see the specific product manual) to avoid failure of the unit during the procedure.
5. Explain the procedure to the patient. Avoid using the word "shock", since this may increase the patient's anxiety level.
6. For elective cardioversion, witness the patient's consent or check the chart for a signed, witnessed consent.
7. Insert IV line.
8. Assess and record the patient's cardiovascular status, heart rhythm, mentation, respiratory status, and peripheral pulses.
9. Obtain the results of any significant laboratory tests ordered (i.e., digitalis and potassium levels).
10. Connect the patient to the cardiac monitor. If a separate monitor is used, the patient must also be connected to the defibrillator to provide the signal for synchronization of the shock. Avoid placement of the monitoring electrodes in the same position required for the defibrillator paddles.
11. Select a monitor lead producing a tall upright R wave (usually lead I). Ensure that a clear, readable tracing is being monitored without artifact or interference.
12. Obtain a 12-lead ECG to confirm persistence of the dysrhythmia.
13. Remove artificial devices (e.g., dentures, eyeglasses, or contact lenses)
14. Administer oxygen for 15 minutes before cardioversion unless contraindicated. This prevents hypoxia that may occur during the procedure if a 1 to 2 minute period of apnea occurs.
15. Remove the patient's oxygen mask to a safe distance before discharging the defibrillator because oxygen is potentially combustible with electrical arching.
16. Prepare the patient. Be sure the chest area is clean and dry. Remove any time-release medication patches from the chest, such as nitrate pastes. Defibrillation over a nitroglycerin patch has been known to cause a small explosion.[11]

17. Inspect the skin for broken areas. Open skin wounds and moisture lower electrical resistance and may cause arching with decreased energy delivery to the myocardium.
18. Inspect the environment for potential electrical hazards. Disconnect unnecessary electrical equipment. Other grounded equipment attached to the patient may redirect the current through its ground and damage the equipment.
19. Administer sedation, as ordered. IV diazepam or Versed may be given. The anesthesiologist may want to give a short-acting anesthetic.
20. Place disposable electrode pads on the patient's chest. If gel is used, cover entire paddle surface. Avoid excessive gel, as it may result in an electrical accident to the patient or operator.
21. Set up the defibrillator. Turn it on and set the control to synchronized mode.
22. Set the energy level requested by the physician (Recommended current requirements for tachydysrhythmias are listed in Table 9-2).
23. Charge the capacitor (can also be done by the physician at the paddles). Cardioversion is a procedure performed in most hospitals only by a physician.
24. Notify physician when full charge has been reached or physician may check the indicator light on the paddles.
25. The physician will apply the paddles to the patient's chest in the same location as that used for defibrillation.
26. Warn personnel to "stand clear" before the paddles are discharged.
27. The physician will depress the discharge buttons on the paddles simultaneously. The device will discharge an electrical current 10 ms after the inscription of the R wave once appropriate synchronization with the patient's QRS complex is achieved (Fig. 9-4).
28. Observe the cardiac rhythm immediately postcardioversion. The ensuing rhythm may indicate asystole, severe bradycardia, or idioventricular rhythm until the SA node resumes its pacemaker function.
29. If the initial shock is ineffective, more shocks will need to be administered no closer than every 3 minutes, increasing the energy level in increments up to 360 J.
30. Should the rhythm deteriorate to VF, turn off the synchronized mode, charge the unit to 200 J, and defibrillate the patient immediately.
31. Maintain airway support and nothing by mouth (NPO) status until the patient is fully awake and it is certain that the procedure will not be repeated.
32. Discuss the results of the procedure with the patient and assess for postconversion complications. Check the skin for signs of irritation or burns. Apply burn cream as ordered.
33. Administer oxygen postcardioversion if not contraindicated.
34. Administer medications, as ordered, to enhance the maintenance of sinus rhythm. Delay in administration of the medication may result in return of the dysrhythmia.
35. Obtain a 12-lead ECG to record conversion rhythm.
36. Maintain full CPR readiness and monitor for dysrhythmias for 4 hours postcardioversion.

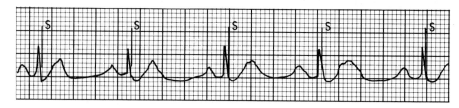

Fig. 9-4   Synchronizer spikes superimposed on the R wave of the ECG.

Table 9-2   Recommended Energy Levels for Cardioversion and Defibrillation

Dysrhythmia	Energy level
Cardioversion	
Paroxysmal SVT	75-100 J
Atrial flutter	25-50 J
Atrial fibrillation	First shock: 100 J
	Second shock: 200 J
	Third shock: 360 J
Unstable VT (with a pulse)	First shock: 50 J
	Second shock: 100 J
	Third shock: 200 J
	Fourth shock: 360 J
Defibrillation	
Pulseless VT and VF	First shock: 200 J
	Second shock: 200-300 J
	Third shock: 360 J
	Subsequent shocks: 360 J

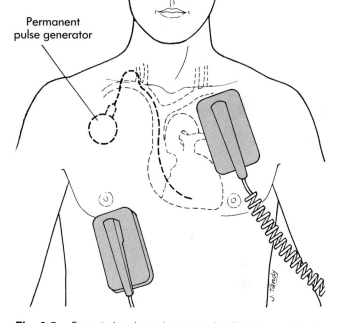

Fig. 9-5   For anterior chest placement of defibrillator paddles in a patient with a pacemaker, position the paddles along a line perpendicular to a line formed between the generator and the lead.

DEFIBRILLATION OF THE PACEMAKER PATIENT

Delivery of an electrical shock can damage an implanted pacemaker temporarily or permanently. Pacemaker complications postshock therapy include the following: the need to reprogram, failure to pace, failure to sense, exit block, noncapture, reversion to end of pacemaker life characteristics, and complete failure of the device. Precautions to be taken include the following:[3,8]

- Be aware of the type of pacemaker in use.
- Determine the location of the hardware in the chest.
- Remember that a unipolar system may be more susceptible to the electromagnetic interference (EMI) from the defibrillator.
- Position the paddles at least 12.5 cm (5 inches) away from the pulse generator of the pacemaker. Anteroposterior paddles are preferable.
- If an anterior chest placement is used, position the paddles along a line perpendicular to a line formed between the generator and the lead (Fig. 9-5). This directs the current perpendicular to the sensing vector of the system. Paddle considerations decrease the amount of potential endocardial burn that can occur with the current passing down the implanted lead.
- Use as low a current setting as possible, less than 300 J for the pacemaker patient.
- Have a transcutaneous or transvenous pacing system on standby.
- Have the appropriate pacemaker programmer on standby in case of noncapture.
- Analyze pacemaker function postprocedure.
- Consider that pacemaker pulses or spikes may be counted by the defibrillator and give a false rate during arrest situations.

THE IMPLANTABLE CARDIOVERTER DEFIBRILLATOR

The purpose of the implantable cardioverter defibrillator (ICD) is to provide for immediate termination of VF and VT in patients whom these dysrhythmias cannot be controlled by pharmacological or surgical therapies (Fig. 9-6 shows treatment options). Because of technological advancements and improved survival rates, even nurses working in general practitioners' offices need the skills to care for patients with an ICD.[5] Two basic principles should be considered in the care of the patient with an ICD: know the patient and know the device.

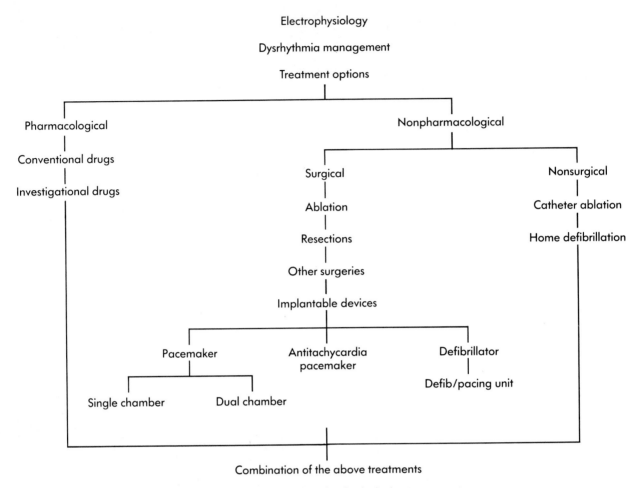

Fig. 9-6   Treatment options for dysrhythmia management.

INDICATIONS FOR THE ICD

The ICD device is recommended for the following categories of patients[1]:
- Patients whose VT or VF is inducible during programmed electrical stimulation despite antidysrhythmic medication trials.
- Survivors of cardiac arrest, not associated with acute MI, whose dysrhythmia cannot be induced by programmed electrical stimulation.

In this last situation, the usefulness of medications cannot be evaluated if the VT or VF cannot be reproduced during electrophysiological testing. Some of the patients for whom drug therapy has failed are candidates for subendocardial resection of the arrhythmogenic focus rather than the ICD. A composite of the typical ICD patient is a male, 55 years of age who has experienced one or more episodes of aborted sudden cardiac death (SCD), failed serial electrophysiological testing, tried three to five antidysrhythmic drugs, has an ejection fraction of less than 32%, and has associated coronary artery disease, cardiomyopathy, or CHF.

CONTRAINDICATIONS TO THE ICD

Contraindications to the ICD include the following patient conditions:

- Frequent episodes of VT or VF (more than two events per month). They may not be candidates because of frequent triggering of the device.
- Uncontrolled CHF, because the ICD probably will not prolong their lives.
- Less than 6 to 12 months of productive life expectancy.
- A history of noncompliance to medical treatment.
- Extreme psychological barriers to the device.

THE ICD SYSTEM

The ICD system consists of the generator, a multi-lead system, and the patient (Fig. 9-7). The generator consists of a power source (2 lithium-silver vanadium pentoxide cells connected in a series) capable of shocking the patient approximately 200 times, depending on joule setting and frequency of shocks. The generator has a capacitor to store the energy and deliver the charge and the logic circuits to tell the device what to do. Two criteria used to determine defibrillator function include heart rate and probability density function (PDF). The PDF, also called morphology sensing, diagnoses VT or VF based on the amount of time the QRS complex spends away from the isoelectric base-

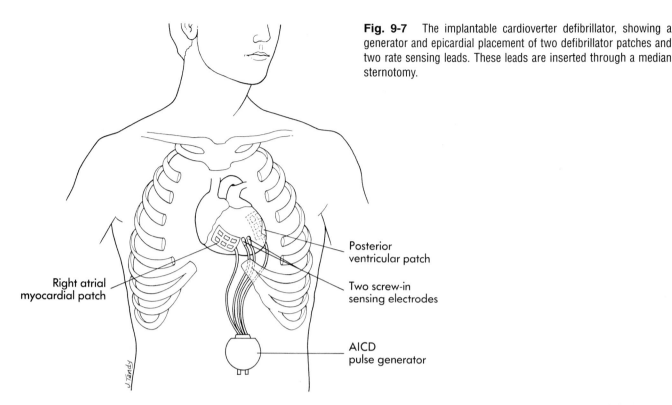

Fig. 9-7 The implantable cardioverter defibrillator, showing a generator and epicardial placement of two defibrillator patches and two rate sensing leads. These leads are inserted through a median sternotomy.

Right atrial myocardial patch

Posterior ventricular patch

Two screw-in sensing electrodes

AICD pulse generator

line. Wide complex VT or coarse VF are away from the baseline a high percentage of the sense time as compared to the ECG in sinus rhythm. If it cannot detect adequate durations of isoelectric segments the rhythm meets the defibrillation criteria. Although this technology is sophisticated, it cannot always differentiate between the wide QRS complex tachydysrhythmias, such as SVTs with aberration and VT or VF.

There are several lead systems in current use (Fig. 9-8). The final lead combination is determined by the size and condition of the heart, the approach for the procedure, and the preference of the surgeon.

1. *SVC Spring lead.* This lead is entered into the subclavian vein and threaded to rest in the superior vena cava (SVC) and right atrium. The spring lead provides the defibrillation shocks and has a tendency to retract into the superior vena cava causing inappropriate shocking of the heart.
2. *Patch lead.* One or two patches are sewn to the pericardium or myocardial surface of the left ventricle through a surgical incision into the chest. The patches function like the paddles of a defibrillator. One patch is used for morphology sensing with the PDF function.
3. *Bipolar lead.* This lead is threaded through the subclavian vein and wedged into the right ventricular apex. The bipolar lead is used for rate sensing (similar to a pacing lead). Preferred method of rate sensing is myocardial screw-in lead.
4. *Myocardial screw-in lead.* Two screw-in leads are used for rate sensing. They are attached to the epi-

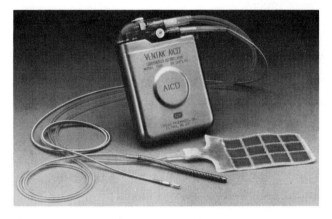

Fig. 9-8 The triple lead system of an implantable cardioverter defibrillator, showing the spring lead, bipolar lead, and patch lead. *(Courtesy of Cardiac Pacemakers, Inc., St. Paul, Minn.)*

cardial surface of the left ventricle.

5. *Endotak-C catheter.* Evolution of the defibrillation lead systems is progressing quickly to percutaneous insertion of defibrillation catheters. This approach will all but eliminate the need for the open chest insertion techniques.

Implantation of the ICD

The operative technique for implantation of an ICD is an open chest procedure performed under general anesthesia. The patient may also undergo associated forms of open heart surgery, such as a bypass, valvular, or antidysrhythmic surgery with the ICD, if deemed necessary.

Operation of the ICD

The basic device cardioverts VT and defibrillates VF. The ICDs currently in use take approximately 2 minutes to deliver a complete treatment sequence. Fig. 9-9 diagrams the timing and event sequence for the CPI Ventak 1550. If there are problems with the operation of the device one should call the physician who implanted the unit or call the technical service of the manufacturer or the local representative. These companies will usually have a 24-hour, toll-free hotline for emergency service. The following considerations are included in the daily patient assessment and evaluation of the device:

- The device is turned on (active) and off (inactive) with a doughnut-shaped magnet (Fig. 9-10). Audible tones are heard from the ICD when it is active and affected by a magnetic field. The tones are synchronized with the patient's heart rate. It identifies events being sensed. (This is sometimes called a *beep-o-gram*).
- Rate or rate and morphology criteria must be met to trigger the device.
- The ICD must be active to treat dysrhythmias. To determine whether the device is active, a magnet is applied over the ICD and the tones emitted are evaluated. A steady tone indicates deactivation; R wave synchronous beeping tones indicate the device is active.
- Administration of cardioactive drugs that alter electrophysiological properties of the heart modify the information presented to the device. Detection criteria may not be met. Defibrillation thresholds can also be changed beyond the capacity of the defibrillator.
- The ICD cannot differentiate supraventricular from ventricular dysrhythmias.
- Once the ICD is fully charged, it is committed to fire. A magnet can cause a shock to be redirected into itself rather than into the patient, but one must act quickly to redirect the shock.
- If there are ICD patients on the unit, a magnet should be available for use.
- The ICD must be charged periodically to maintain a normal charge time. Clinic visits for follow-up are to be scheduled every 2 months for the first year and thereafter every month. During the visit the capacitors are reformed using the programmer. Long periods of inactivity increase the charge time. Newer devices will contain timers to automatically reform the capacitors.

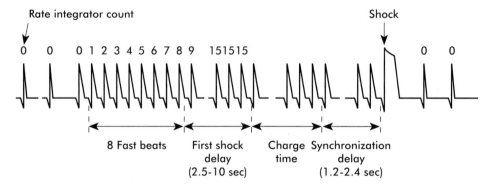

Fig. 9-9   After detection, the Ventak 1550 pulse generator waits 2.5 seconds to be sure the dysrhythmia is sustained before charging and delivering a shock.

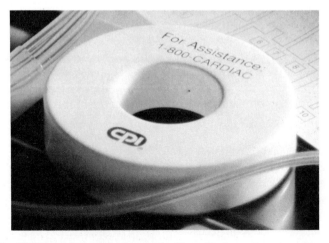

Fig. 9-10   The ICD device is turned on and off with a doughnut-shaped magnet. *(Courtesy Cardiac Pacemakers, Inc., St. Paul, Minn.)*

- The energy discharged from the ICD can be felt to varying degrees by someone in contact with the patient. The sensation has been described as a "buzzing" feeling. Wearing rubber gloves may assist in insulating bystanders.
- The ICD treats the dysrhythmia; it does not prevent it. Consequently, the cause or precipitating event must be investigated.
- In the CPI Ventak 1550 and higher numbered series, the device will emit tones when charging if it is near end of life.
- Normal operation of a pacemaker under certain circumstances can interfere with operation of an ICD. Most often, it will double count and fire inappropriately or detect the pacemaker spikes and not treat the VT or VF.
- The device should be inactive if the patient has an AV sequential temporary pacemaker in use, if the patient is going for a surgical procedure, and on removal of the device.

Complications of the ICD

Complications of ICDs are divided into three categories: the system, patient/system interface, and the patient (see the box on the right). The nurse plays a major role in management of complications by the following:
- Assessing the patient and the environment accurately.
- Reporting and recording events that affect the operation of the device.
- Initiating preventive measures for safe care of the patient on the unit, including posting the following:
  1. *No Magnet* signs on the patient's door.
  2. An ICD status sign over the patient's bed or on the door.
  3. A diagram in the room of the patch locations to facilitate CPR.
- Completing the patient education program.
- Incorporating device precautions into the patient's treatment program.
- Recognizing complications.
- Monitoring effectiveness of programming changes made in device operation, such as the following:
  1. Change in rate recognition criteria.
  2. PDF on or off.
  3. Joule setting for first shock.
  4. Shock delay time.
  5. Alterations in existing dysrhythmia.
  6. New dysrhythmias.

Preoperative Preparation for ICD Implantation

Preoperative preparation consists of the following:
- Provide patient and family education.
- Obtain results of any laboratory or diagnostic tests performed.
- Do not administer new cardioactive medications. Current antidysrhythmic medications must be in a steady state to avoid a negative impact on defibrillation thresholds.

Complications of the Implantable Cardioverter Defibrillator

SYSTEM

Lead fracture
Electromechanical interference
Component failure
Radiation effects
Insufficient energy for shocks

SYSTEM/PATIENT INTERFACE

Lead migration
False positive shocks
    Malsensing
    New dysrhythmias
Concomitant drug therapy
    Alters defibrillation threshold
    Alters rate
    Alters QRS complex morphology
    Depletes potassium
Ventricular tachycardia with magnet test (Misdirect)
Pacemaker interactions
    Detection inhibition
    Double counting
Skin potentials
Cardiac perforations

PATIENT

Operative death
Infections
Ventricular tachycardia death
Psychological effects
Pain
Bleeding
Thrombosis
Hematoma
Acceleration of ventricular tachycardia
Pack migration
Fluid accumulation in pocket
Postoperative dysrhythmias
Twidler's syndrome

- Check the patient for any remote sites of infection.
- Instruct the patient on coughing, deep breathing, and the use of incentive spirometry to prevent respiratory complications.
- Orient the patient to the surgical ICU and its routine.
- Complete an extensive skin prep by washing with an antibacterial soap 2 to 3 times a day for several days to decrease the chance of infection.
- Do not apply ECG monitoring leads near potential incision sites.
- Witness the operative permit.
- Administer preoperative medications as ordered.
- Complete the preoperative checklist for surgical procedures.
- Monitor the ECG.
- Insert a Foley catheter, arterial line, and pulmonary artery catheter.
- Ensure that cardiopulmonary bypass equipment is on standby.

- Check the ICD for function and status (i.e., active or inactive).

The remaining preparation is the usual for a surgery of this nature and takes into account procedures to be performed that relate to the ICD.

Postoperative Care of the ICD Patient

The immediate postoperative period for the ICD patient is spent in the ICU. Patients are then transferred to a step-down unit for the remainder of the hospital stay. Care of the patient is much the same as it is for any patient having open heart surgery. Nursing care specific to the postoperative patient with an ICD is as follows:

- Alert all staff members as to the status of the device, for example, active or inactive. The ICD is usually activated when the patient is transferred to the step-down unit, 24 to 48 hours postimplant. Time should be allowed for the postprocedural ectopy to diminish.
- Anticipate treatment of potential dysrhythmias.
- Monitor closely for postoperative complications from the procedure and ICD.
- Do not initiate AV sequential pacemaker therapy with an active device.
- Document all the following with shock events:
  1. ICD may not be clearly recorded. Some hospital telemetry or computerized monitoring systems cannot record a deflection with the ICD discharge.
  2. Rescue shocks (from an external defibrillator).
  3. Drug administration.
  4. Patient symptoms.
- Secure a doughnut-shaped magnet to keep on the emergency care cart.

ASSESSMENT

After surgical implantation of the ICD, the nurse should perform a complete ICU admission assessment. The patient's condition and environment will need the following to be assessed for events that could precipitate dysrhythmias:

- Monitor blood pressure, central venous pressure, and pulmonary capillary wedge pressure for low values, indicating decreased blood volume.
- Listen to breath sounds and monitor oxygen levels for hypoxemia, possibly due to atelectasis from lack of deep breathing and coughing.
- Observe for a decreased cardiac output, less than 4 L/min.
- Assess for WBC count greater than 12,000, indicating sepsis.
- Check for appropriate drug levels (i.e., digoxin, quinidine, and procainamide).
- Evaluate ABG results for metabolic and acid-base imbalances.
- Check laboratory reports for electrolyte imbalances, especially of K^+, Ca^{++}, and Mg^{++}.
- Observe 12-lead ECG for signs of ischemia; attachment of the patches generates some ST segment changes.

- Assess patient's surgical site for signs of infection. The ICD implantation results in a moderate degree of swelling. The appearance of swelling is accentuated by the size of the device.
- Observe for the ability to perform activities of daily living.
- Note fatigue, chest pain, and increase in heart and respiratory rates with exertion.
- Check for potential hazards in the environment.
- Assess the psychosocial, rehabilitative, and educational needs of the ICD candidate preoperatively and periodically postoperatively.
- Assess patient's coping mechanisms, observing for abnormal anxiety levels as demonstrated by negative stress responses.
- Evaluate patient's perceptions of quality of life.
- Assess patient's emotional state for pain and anxiety.
- Observe for inappropriate levels of pain shown by frequent, vague complaints, pain of longer duration than expected, or minimal responses to medications.
- Assess patient responses to ICD shocks and whether they are appropriate for the device.
- Determine patient's awareness of negative outcomes related to the implant procedure.
- Observe family interactions and note the presence of social support.

NURSING DIAGNOSIS

The following are examples of nursing diagnoses for patients with ICDs:

- Decreased cardiac output related to dysrhythmias.
- Ineffective breathing pattern related to splinting secondary to pain from cardiothoracic surgical procedure.
- High risk for infection related to surgical incisions, sternal wound, and abdominal pocket for the ICD.
- High risk for injury related to ICD malfunction.
- Self-care deficit related to a compromised cardiovascular response.
- Pain related to surgical incision.
- Activity intolerance related to fear of exertion with an implanted cardioverter defibrillator (ICD).
- Knowledge deficit related to comprehension difficulties of regimen for an ICD.
- Ineffective individual coping related to depression secondary to fear of death.
- Ineffective rest-activity pattern related to poor adjustment to the ICD.
- Disturbance in body image related to ICD implant.
- Social isolation related to a perceived hazard by others of shocks from the ICD.
- Powerlessness related to dependency on the ICD.

PATIENT OUTCOMES

The following are possible patient outcomes for patients with ICDs. Before discharge, the ICD patient evidences:

- Clear and equal bilateral breath sounds.
- Spontaneous, unlabored respirations, of normal pattern, 12 to 20 breaths/min.

- Chest x-ray within normal limits for patient with fully expanded lungs.
- Chest x-ray showing heart of normal size for patient with patches for internal defibrillator in the correct position on the heart.
- Normal heart sounds without friction rub after adaptation of the heart to the epicardial patches.
- Stable heart rate between 60 to 100 beats/min.
- Stable BP within range of 100/60 to 140/90 with mean arterial pressure of 70 to 90 mm Hg.
- Temperature between 36.1° to 38° C (97° to 100.5° F) for 24 hours before discharge.
- Surgical site with moderate swelling and of normal skin color and temperature with a clean and dry incision line.
- Performs activities of daily living within the limits of cardiovascular status, response to the procedure, and duration of illness.
- Records own daily weight and reports weight gains of greater than 0.5 kg (1 lb) in a 24-hour period.
- Reports adequate pain relief with prescribed analgesics.
- Articulates feelings related to acceptance and adaptation to the ICD.
- Reports signs and symptoms of complications.
- Identifies potentially hazardous situations in the environment that might affect the ICD.
- Describes the effect of a magnet on the ICD.
- States actions for management of an ICD shock.
- States the date for first clinic visit.

PEDIATRIC CONSIDERATIONS

Children can tolerate faster heart rates with dysrhythmias better than many adults even at rates close to 200 beats/min. In the pediatric age group, cardiac arrest is most often secondary to respiratory arrest. When no pulse is present, one should first provide an infant or child with adequate ventilation and oxygenation while administering external chest compressions. In the treatment of supraventricular dysrhythmias with cardioversion, avoid shocking children unless they are showing signs of decompensation. If VF is present, the recommended energy level for defibrillation is 2 J/kg (1 J/lb) and double the level with unsuccessful defibrillation. For cardioversion in children the recommended energy level is 0.2 to 1 J/kg (0.1 to .05 J/lb). Other considerations are the size of the paddles. Using too small a paddle has the effect of concentrating the energy with the potential to damage the conduction system. Pediatric paddles are available with 8 cm (3⅛ in) diameter electrodes for children and 4.5 cm (1¾ in) diameter electrodes for infants.

Implantation of an ICD in a small child would be difficult because of the size of the device, rate cutoff, and narrow range of energy levels. Children do not have the muscle mass on their bodies to support the weight and extensive hardware. The muscle mass of a child's heart is smaller, a consideration for current levels delivered directly to the heart muscle. The ICD has been implanted in children who tolerated the procedure well. Until the devices are smaller and there is a broader selection of rates and energy levels, the ICD in children will be limited.

PSYCHOSOCIAL CONSIDERATIONS

Studies have examined the psychosocial aspects of ICD implantation. It has been found that patients with chronic VT and their families feel overwhelmed by the following:[4]
- The length of hospital stay.
- The intensive testing, electrophysiological studies, cardiac catheterization, and scans.
- The need for many medications.
- The limited number of options available, and the risk/benefit ratio of each.
- The impact of VT on the individual's lifestyle and personal goals.

Patients in a support group identified the following issues of significance to them and their families:
- Fear of cardioversion.
- Fear of experimental medication and surgery.
- Competence of local physicians.
- Lengthy hospital stays.
- Emotional stability.
- Concern for the family's well-being.
- A need to express their own experiences.
- An affirmation of mutual needs and feelings.
- Conflicting treatment plans among physician groups.
- Boredom.
- Physical symptoms related to diagnostic and treatment procedures.
- The possibility of surgery.
- Adaptation to lifestyle.

Negative changes in lifestyle include less physical activity, less sexual activity, memory loss, depression, dependency, and thoughts of death.

When meeting the emotional needs of patients surviving sudden cardiac death (SCD), the caring nurse would need to address the issues of fear related to the possibility of cardiac arrest out of the hospital, fear and confusion secondary to recollections of resuscitation or of the "near death phenomenon", and fear of hospital discharge with the potential for a recurrent cardiac arrest. Patients with ICDs also have a fear of being shocked and are concerned that the shocks will embarrass them in public. Never knowing when the ICD may fire, patients have been known to feel imprisoned by fear.[7] Patients describe an ICD shock as a sudden blow to the chest or back. It is helpful if the nurse explains that the discharge is more of a startling sensation than a painful one. Nursing interventions might include encouraging the patient to (1) think positively, (2) gradually increase social outings and activity level, (3) listen to calming music, (4) make plans for the future and lists of things to do, and (5) share fears and concerns with others. Spouses tend to be concerned about the patient's pain and are concerned about panic and death. They need to know that touching an ICD patient during a discharge will not harm them, as the shock is transferred as a skin potential of approximately 2 J.[5]

A team approach to long term follow-up with easy access to the support structure should be developed. Emphasis should be placed on communication, support groups, education, stress management, and definitive support for the spouses.[2] Even with all of the ensuing problems, the vast majority of the patients would have the device implanted again if given the choice.

PATIENT AND FAMILY TEACHING

Patient education is one of the most critical needs of ICD patients and often requires several hours of intense, individualized instruction. The educational program begins long before the ICD implant. Treatment has taken the patient through months, and in some cases, years of problems, diagnostic tests, hospitals, and physicians of different specialties. A patient educational record may be helpful to facilitate communication among the educators (Fig. 9-11).

Preoperative Instructions

- Review dysrhythmia information.
- Present benefits of an ICD.
- Discuss realistic expectations from the ICD. The ICD does not prevent the dysrhythmia, it treats the dysrhythmia.
- Provide model to demonstrate operation and implantation of an ICD.
- Show the video *A Gift of Time* available from Cardiac Pacemakers, Inc.
- Set up an album that takes the patient and family on a picture tour of the experience. The album should contain copies of all the materials they will receive.
- Ensure that patient receives the ICD patient manual.
- Interview patient to identify potential hazards in lifestyle at home, work, leisure activities, and hobbies.
- Prevent respiratory complications by teaching patient to cough, deep breathe, and use incentive spirometer.
- Instruct in the need to ambulate early.

Postoperative Instructions

- Review preoperative instructions for self-care.
- Provide emotional support.
- Follow-up on electrophysiological studies or dysrhythmia induction studies will be done utilizing the device to trigger and treat the dysrhythmia.
- Teach patient to inspect the incision and implant sites for signs of infection, drainage, swelling, redness, and skin warm to touch (temperature above 38° C [100.5° F]).
- Inform patient to protect the implant site from irritation by clothing or belts, to avoid scrubbing the site vigorously, to avoid tub baths for the first week, and to shower with a safety chair.
- Remain on prescribed medications and diet.

Safety precautions

- Carry an identification card that includes the patient's, physician's, and manufacturer's phone number, the ICD lead and model information, rate cut-off of the device, use of an external defibrillator, deactivation instructions, and shock sequence.
- Obtain a Medic Alert bracelet.
- Carry an instruction letter at all times.
- Retain a copy of the warranty.
- Avoid magnets and large magnetic fields since they turn the device on and off.
- Avoid equipment such as electrocautery, diathermy, arc welding, large transformers, running electric motors, transcutaneous electrical nerve stimulation (TENS) units, biomagnetic products, lithotripsy, and magnetic resonance imaging (MRI). These devices can affect operation of the ICD.

Healthcare system notification and follow-up

- Call physician if audible tones are heard from the ICD. The tones mean the ICD has been exposed to a magnetic field.
- Keep scheduled clinic visits every 2 months the first year and monthly thereafter as the end of life of the ICD occurs. Anticipate approximately 3 years of ICD battery life. Replacement of the ICD will not be a major surgical procedure unless the lead system requires changing. The generator pocket will be reopened and a new generator will be inserted into the same pocket.
- Use transtelephonic monitoring for dysrhythmia evaluation and psychological support.
- Notify members of the health care team about the ICD (i.e., surgeons, dentist, emergency personnel, etc). The patient's physician should be contacted before any procedures are done. Deactivation of the device is recommended before any surgical procedure.
- Report recurrence or new symptoms to physician.
- If any symptoms are experienced during activity, stop and notify physician. Symptoms include the following: shortness of breath, chest pain, fatigue, weakness, rapid heart rate, shocks, nausea, or syncope.
- Keep a diary of the shocks (pulses) received (Fig. 9-12). Notify physician of each shock to evaluate appropriate versus inappropriate shocks.

HOME HEALTH CARE CONSIDERATIONS

Home health care should be an integral part of the support system for the patient with an ICD. Development of the hospital-based program includes members of the frequently used home health agencies. Home health nurses will need to develop an in-depth understanding of the patient and the device.

Home health nurse's role

The nurse should assess the home for environmental safety (i.e., use of magnets, small electrical tools, etc.).

ICD INSTRUCTION STATUS   Patient ID:

Purpose: To provide communication and documentation of patient education.

	Date	Init.	Understand		Recommendation	
			Yes	No	Review	Other
Preadmission:						
Patient manual						

Preimplant:						
Preop instructions						
Physical therapy						

Postimplant:						
Temporary ID card						
Generator warranty						
Medic alert						

Instruction Sheets – Going Home With Your ICD:

#1a General reminders/ follow-up						
#1b AICD activity diary						
#2 Activity						
#3 Surgical site						
#4 Emergency plan						

Discharge:						
Prescriptions						
Clinic appointments						
Emergency letter						

Other:

Education level upon completion: Level 1 __ 2 __ 3 __ 4 __ 5 __

Summary:

Fig. 9-11   ICD education record.

AT HOME WITH YOUR ICD

ICD Instruction Sheet #1a

ICD Activity Diary

Name: _____ Dr. Telephone #: _____

Explanation: shock# = number of shocks received, date, time, indicate any symptoms observed or felt during the shock event, activity in progress at the time, and note information or instructions given to you by the doctor.

Shock#: _____ Date: _____ Time: _____

Symptoms: _____

Activity: _____

Information from doctor (If needed): _____

Shock#: _____ Date: _____ Time: _____

Symptoms: _____

Activity: _____

Information from doctor (If needed): _____

Shock#: _____ Date: _____ Time: _____

Symptoms: _____

Activity: _____

Information from doctor (If needed): _____

Shock#: _____ Date: _____ Time: _____

Symptoms: _____

Activity: _____

Information from doctor (If needed): _____

Fig. 9-12 Diary of ICD shocks received.

The home health nurse should do the following:

- Reinforce the education begun in the hospital and complete the teaching program.
- Be the liaison to the physician until the patient returns for the first clinic visit and is more independent.
- Monitor wound care.
- Monitor the effects of cardioactive medications.
- Assess adaptation to the device.
- Identify potential or actual device complications.
- Initiate an interim activity program until the patient attends cardiac rehabilitation.
- Transmit ECG recordings to the physician if dysrhythmias develop during home health care visits.
- Set up an emergency plan for the members of the family.

Family emergency plan

- Post an emergency plan at home in the event of cardiac arrest. Ensure that family knows not to wait for ICD to discharge but to initiate CPR, phone 911, continue CPR, unlock doors, and return to CPR.
- Inform significant others and family members of the potential to detect skin potentials when the device discharges.

Activity levels

- Participate in cardiac rehabilitation, phase I and II. This includes developing an exercise prescription (i.e., type of exercise, frequency, and duration), pulse monitoring (i.e., demonstration and return demonstration), target heart rates (consider the rate cut off of the ICD), risk factor analysis, and lifestyle adjustments. A monitored program provides the incentive and support needed by the patient to resume an active lifestyle.
- Take pulse with any new activity or if an abnormal rhythm is suspected. (Give pulse demonstration and return demonstration.) Compare the rate to your rate cutoff.
- Restrict lifting to 3.6 to 4.5 kg (8 to 10 lbs) for 4 to 6 weeks if sternal incision was performed, as it takes the sternum this length of time to heal.
- Avoid strenuous activities. Once the surgical site is healed the patient can continue with previous lifestyle.
- Sit down and rest when feeling of onset of dysrhythmia occurs.
- Do not drive for the first 6 months. A person who experiences syncope should not be driving. The delay in driving is to evaluate the patient's response to the shocks and to control the syncope with medications if possible.
- Do not be concerned with travel restrictions, there are none. Just notify airport security of the ICD. The handcheck device does contain a magnet. Keep it 25 cm (10 in) away from the ICD.
- Return to work when approved by physician.
- Enjoy and get on with life.

Skill 9-4   Initiation of a Rescue Shock for an ICD Patient in Cardiac Arrest

▼ ....

EQUIPMENT AND SUPPLIES

- Defibrillator
- Defibrillation paddles
- Recording paper
- Conductive gel or disposable pads
- Code cart
- Lidocaine bolus
- Doughnut-shaped magnet
- ICD programmer

NURSING INTERVENTIONS

1. Anticipate a possible cardiac arrest. Be prepared with the equipment and information on whom to call (i.e., surgeon, electrophysiologist, or both).
2. Observe the cardiac monitor. For the active ICD, allow it 60 seconds to convert the lethal dysrhythmia. Time the ICD shocks accurately. A complete treatment sequence is 5 shocks in approximately 2 minutes. Time for the second through the fifth shocks is shorter than for the initial shock since repeated charging requires less time. The device will not recycle to deliver additional shocks until there has been a 35 sec period of a nondysrhythmic state. (Table 9-3).
3. If the ICD does not convert the lethal dysrhythmia, initiate CPR without delay. Consider the use of rubber gloves for CPR. The rescuer may be startled by a shock generated from the ICD. The shock will not be dangerous to the rescuer.
4. Administer lidocaine as the dysrhythmic drug of choice, or as ordered by unit protocol.
5. After waiting the initial 60 seconds, perform an external defibrillation protocol suggested in Skill 9-1. The output of the ICD was probably insufficient to defibrillate the heart. Position external paddles 12.5 to 15 cm (5 to 6 in) away from the generator.
6. If the initial shock is unsuccessful, consider rotating the paddles to direct the current between the defibrillation patches attached to the heart. The patches shunt the current from the heart. Higher energy levels may be required.
7. Following return of normal rhythm, monitor the patient's rhythm closely. Cardioversion or defibrillation can be performed externally without damage to the device but may cause tissue damage around the rate sensing leads and affect rate recognition.
8. If shocks are inappropriate or occuring frequently because of uncontrolled irritability, deactivate the device (performed by the physician or ICD nurse). The following dysrhythmias may cause the device to inappropriately discharge:
   - VT not meeting morphology criteria.
   - VT slower than the rate cutoff.
   - SVT with aberrancy.
   - SVT meeting the rate cutoff—atrial fibrillation.
   - Spikes from a dual chamber pacemaker.
   - Unipolar pacemaker (contraindicated with an ICD).
   - Nonsustained VT.
9. Change status sign if the device remains inactive.
10. Obtain a chest x-ray to verify lead integrity and cardiac status.
11. Document the initiating dysrhythmia, the number of shocks delivered, dysrhythmia tracings, data intergated from the ICD through the programmer, status of the device, rescue shocks delivered (i.e., energy level and number), medications, and the patient's response.

Table 9-3   Operation of An ICD

Device capabilities	1550	1600
Energy Level 1 (J)	26/30	.1, .5, 1, 2, 3, 4, 6, 8, 10, 12, 14, 17, 20, 23, 26, 30
2 (J)	30	30
Programmable	Yes	Yes
Rate Range	125-200	110-200
Programmable	Yes	Yes
PDF	On/off	On/off
Shock Delay (sec)	2.5	2.5, 5, 7.5, 10
Programmable	No	Yes
EOL	Status display tone with charging CT > 35.8 Redirects charge internally = No patient shock (BOL charge time × 1.33 = ERI)	Same
Number of shocks Rx sequence	1-5, Stat shock	Same
Detection time (sec)	2-5 (8 cycles)	Same
Magnet test	On/off	On/off
Redirect (sec)	2-3	2-3
Recycle to next sequence	35	Same
Charge time (sec)	6-7	Same

*1555, same capabilities as the 1550, except only high energy (30 J) shocks. On/off with magnet, place over device 30 sec. (Listen for continuous tone for off).

REFERENCES

1. Arteaga WJ, Drew BJ: Device therapy for ventricular tachycardia or fibrillation: the implantable cardioverter defibrillator and antitachycardia pacing, *Crit Care Q* 14(2):60, 1991.
2. Badger JM, Morris PL: Observations of a support group for automatic implantable cardioverter-defibrillator recipients and their spouses, *Heart Lung* 18(3):238, 1989.
3. Cardiac Pacemakers, St Paul, Minn: *Physician's manual. Ventak Model 1550,* St Paul, Minn, 1988.
4. DeBasio N, Rodenhausen N: The group experience: meeting the psychosocial needs of patients with ventricular tachycardia, *Heart Lung* 13(6):597, 1984.
5. DeBorde R, Aarons D, Biggs M: The automated implantable cardioverter, *AACN Clin Issues Crit Care Nurs* 2(1):170, 1991.
6. Kinkade SL: *Open-chest resuscitation.* In Kinkade SL, Lohrman J, editors: *Critical care procedures: a team approach,* Philadelphia, 1990, BC Decker.
7. Meek J: The dreaded defibrillator, *Am J Nurs* 91(5):32, 1991.
8. Sager DP: Current facts on pacemaker electromagnetic interference and their application to clinical care, *Heart Lung* 16(2):211, 1987.
9. Wrenn K: The hazards of defibrillation through nitroglycerin patches, *Ann Emerg Med* 19(11):1327, 1990.

CHAPTER 10

Advanced Cardiac Life Support

Objectives

After completing this chapter, the reader will be able to:

- List the common causes of sudden cardiac death.
- Describe the stages of a resuscitative attempt.
- Describe situations requiring the use of the precordial thump.
- Discuss the algorithms for treating lethal dysrhthmias.
- Describe the stabilization process of the arrested patient.
- Outline the nurse's role in situations requiring advanced cardiac life support (ACLS).
- List the methods for starting and maintaining ACLS intravenous (IV) drips.
- Describe the nurse's role during "no-code" situations.
- Identify the required documentation during and after an arrest.
- Compare and contrast the adult code with the pediatric code.

Each year approximately one million Americans die of diseases of the heart and blood vessels.[7] Roughly one half of these deaths are associated with heart attack and one third of these deaths occur outside of the hospital, usually within 2 hours of symptom onset.[28]

Sudden death or death within 1 hour of the onset of symptoms is usually caused by a cardiac dysrhythmia.

Even in the best emergency situations, a delay can occur in actually beginning advanced cardiac life support (ACLS). This delay can prove fatal if defibrillation is delayed beyond 8 minutes. Cardiopulmonary resuscitation (CPR) should only be administered when defibrillation is not available or after the initial shocks have failed to restore circulation.

In-hospital cardiac arrest occurs in 1% to 2% of all patients admitted to the hospital.[23] Survival of an in-hospital arrest is lower than that of the arrest out of the hospital, since hospitalized patients are generally sicker and carry a poorer prearrest prognosis. Half of the patients in the hospital who arrest are resuscitated; one third of those survive for 24 hours. Approximately 15% survive to leave the hospital.[4,32]

One important factor in predicting the outcome of an in-hospital cardiac arrest is the length of the resuscitation attempt. The longer the attempt, the higher the death rate.[4,32] The highest survival rate has been seen in codes that last fewer than 15 minutes. Few patients survive resuscitation attempts that last longer than 30 minutes. This should be considered when deciding to terminate resuscitation attempts in adults when the code continues longer than 30 minutes. This is especially true if the patient has shown no signs of responding, unless he or she is hypothermic.[20] The probability that a patient will survive more than one code during a hospital stay is extremely small.[10]

▼ Troubleshooting During a Code

The ACLS or critical care nursing team leader should anticipate and plan for the following during most codes:
- Speak clearly and succinctly because communicating above the noise and confusion will be difficult.
- Ensure that the medication nurse articulates the type, amount, and name of the drug prepared.
- Obtain necessary equipment, anticipating that some of the equipment (e.g., suction, oxygen, monitors, and defibrillators) may not function properly.
- Always label IV infusions with at least the name of the drug and the amount.
- Use preprinted drip charts for medication regulation.
- Keep all used vials and other medication containers that were used in a clean trash can so that they can be checked against the recorded data of the code.
- Secure the IV site carefully and monitor frequently for infiltration.
- Anticipate possible problems and have a backup plan for all aspects of the code.
- Ensure that the recording nurse is able to see and hear the code activities.

THE RESUSCITATION PROCESS

The management of a cardiac arrest victim is difficult and stressful. Many problems arise during the resuscitation process. See the box on p. 235 for troubleshooting tips during the code situation.

The code situation can be divided into the following stages independent of the cause of the arrest:

- The ABCs (basic cardiac life support).
- Precordial thump.
- Quick-look defibrillation.
- Stabilization.
- Specific therapy.
- Cardiac arrest outcome management.
- Postresuscitation management.

The ABCs—Basic Cardiac Life Support

The goal of basic cardiac life support (BCLS or CPR) is to maintain sufficient perfusion of the brain and other vital organs until an adequate, spontaneous cardiac output can be established. There is a window of approximately 4 minutes after loss of the victim's pulse and respirations before anoxic brain injury begins. CPR, however, supplies only 20% of the normal cardiac output, even when expertly administered. This blood flow is not evenly distributed. The majority of the blood flow from CPR goes to the head and the upper extremities because of the distribution of the venous valves at the inlet to the thorax. The heart muscle normally receives its blood flow during diastole as the muscle relaxes. This blood flow is driven by the pressure gradient between the coronary ostia at the root of the aorta and the coronary sinus in the right atrium. During normal CPR the gradient between the aorta and the atria essentially disappears so that there is almost no coronary perfusion. The heart continues to develop progressive cellular hypoxia and acidosis despite the presence of an effective pulse with CPR. This effect is demonstrated by the increased mortality seen in patients despite prompt CPR if ACLS measures are delayed beyond 12 minutes[2] and by the increased resistance of ventricular dysrhythmias to defibrillation with prolonged CPR. The effects of prolonged cardiac hypoperfusion can be avoided by prompt defibrillation and/or administration of epinephrine.

The patient is rapidly assessed to determine unresponsiveness, lack of respirations, and pulse. BCLS measures are started and the cardiac arrest team is notified. The basic algorithms for BCLS can be found on Fig. 10-1.

Precordial Thump

The precordial thump is a forceful blow delivered to the sternum (Fig. 10-2). The precordial thump is used for a patient in asystole or who demonstrates an abnormal rhythm, e.g., VF, VT, or complete AV block.[2] Such a thump delivers a low-level electric depolarization (approximately 25 joules [J]) that is able to interrupt and reentrant pathway if delivered at an opportune moment in the cardiac cycle.[6,25]

Since the myocardium becomes anoxic soon after a car-

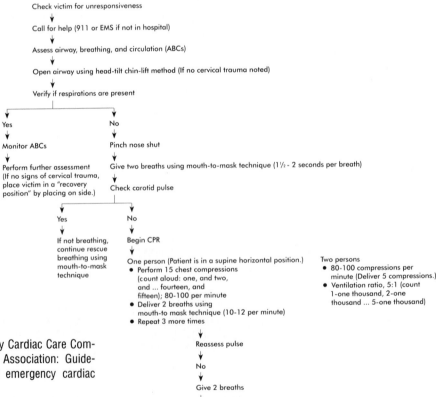

Fig. 10-1   BLS algorithm. (From Emergency Cardiac Care Committee and Subcommittees, American Heart Association: Guidelines for cardiopulmonary resuscitation and emergency cardiac care, *JAMA* 268:2172, 1992.)

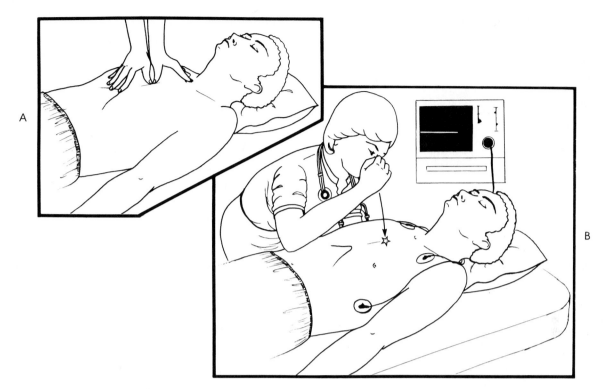

Fig. 10-2 **A,** Measurement of the midsternum for the precordial thump. **B,** Administration of precordial thump to a monitored patient in ventricular fibrillation. (From Guzzetta CE and Dossey BM: Cardiovascular nursing: bodymind tapestry, St Louis, 1984, Mosby–Year Book.)

diac arrest, a precordial thump should be delivered within 1 minute of the arrest. A solitary precordial thump is recommended in patients with (1) monitored VF [6], (2) witnessed cardiac arrests when a defibrillator is not present, (3) ventricular tachycardia, if pulse is present, (4) asystole, or (5) marked bradycardia. The precordial thump is not considered a part of BCLS. It is indicated only when the patient is monitored or can be monitored quickly.

Defibrillation

The treatment of choice for VT is prompt delivery of an electrical shock (200 to 300 J) to simultaneously depolarize cardiac tissue, allowing the normal cardiac pacemakers to resume.[29]

Rapid early defibrillation is endorsed by the AHA.[7] First responders are trained to use the automated external defibrillator (AED). See Appendix A for the algorithm.

The voltage required to return the heart to a normal rhythm rises rapidly during a cardiac arrest. As the dysrhythmia persists, the heart becomes increasingly hypoxic and acidotic, leading to increasing voltage requirements to defibrillate the heart. Eventually the heart becomes unresponsive to defibrillation attempts without other adjunctive measures.

Internal, or direct, defibrillation is used operatively or in an emergency situation when the chest has been opened. Direct defibrillation requires much less energy (3 to 5 J) than the external shock.[1,35] No more than 50 J should be used.[1]

If the initial dysrhythmia is not VF or VT, or the patient has not responded to three defibrillation attempts for VF or VT, the rescue team should resume CPR and attempt to improve the victim's physiological status before initiating further therapy. Refer to Chapter 9 for additional information and skill.

Stabilization

If defibrillation is unsuccessful or a rhythm other than VF or VT is seen using the quick-look paddles, one should attempt to improve the metabolic environment of the cardiac cells by securing the airway and administering 100% oxygen, continuing effective cardiac compressions, administering the appropriate drugs, and correcting any metabolic or life-threatening, acid-base disorders that are discovered. During this phase the patient should be placed on a continuous cardiac monitor and blood can be sent for measures of arterial blood gases, electrolytes, calcium, and magnesium.

Airway Management with 100% Oxygen

It is critically important to secure the patient's airway and provide adequate ventilation with 100% oxygen early in every cardiac arrest. Early intubation is preferable if it can be accomplished simultaneously with other techniques. It is more important, however, to ensure that the patient has been defibrillated and has received epinephrine.

It is helpful to have two people provide bag-valve-mask

Skill 10-1   Bag-Valve-Mask Resuscitation

EQUIPMENT AND SUPPLIES

- Mask (clear if possible)
- Self-inflating bag-valve-mask device
- System for delivery of supplemental oxygen

NURSING INTERVENTIONS

1. When the victim is first discovered, provide mouth-to-mouth or mouth-to-mask resuscitation until a bag-valve-mask system with supplemental oxygen becomes available.
2. Insert oral airway if necessary to prevent the tongue from falling back against the pharynx and obstructing the airway.
3. Gently extend the neck and lift the mandible.
4. Seal the mask securely over the face to prevent leakage of the air with resulting underventilation of the patient.
5. Place thumb and index finger of same hand on either side of the mask and exert pressure to create a tight seal around the patient's mouth.
6. Using an even squeezing motion, compress the bag with the free hand.
7. Ventilate the victim at a rate of at least 12 breaths/min with at least 200 ml of oxygen (800 ml of air).
8. Assess ventilation initially by observing movement of the patient's chest and auscultating over both lung fields to confirm air movement. Check abdomen for gastric distention.
9. Obtain blood gases early in the arrest, if possible, to assess the adequacy of oxygenation and ventilation as well as the patient's acid-base status.

ventilation so that one person can maintain the sealed open airway while the other person ventilates the patient. Improper bag-valve-mask technique can lead to (1) gradual inflation of the stomach with impairment of ventilations and increasing risk of aspiration of gastric contents or (2) posterior esophageal rupture resulting from increased intragastric pressures during chest compressions. For these reasons, early intubation is recommended in most arrest situations to secure the airway against aspiration, improve the efficiency of ventilations, and provide an alternate route for the delivery of ACLS medications.

The patient should be hyperventilated before intubation and no attempt at intubation should last longer than 30 seconds without resuming CPR and ventilation. After intubation, proper placement of the ET tube should be determined by auscultating over lung fields and the stomach along with observation of the chest-wall movement during ventilations. The ET tube should be taped securely in place to prevent undesired movement during the resuscitation attempt. One hand should also be kept on the ET tube to prevent slippage. When personnel step away from the bed during defibrillation, tugging on the ET tube must be avoided. Persistent hypoxia or hypercarbia should prompt the team to reassess the airway including the connections from the wall oxygen source to the bag-valve-mask device, the adequacy of delivered ventilations, the ET tube placement, or the possibility of embolism.

Intravenous Access

Access to the circulation is necessary to deliver drugs. Although some drugs (i.e., epinephrine, atropine, and lidocaine) can be delivered via the ET tube. Medications administered via ET tube, require doses 2 to 2.5 times greater than the recommended IV doses and should be diluted in 10 ml of normal saline or distilled water.[7] Intramuscular drugs should be avoided in a cardiac arrest, since muscle tissue is relatively underperfused until a stable cardiac rhythm can be established.

The administration of intracardiac medications used to be advocated to assure rapid delivery of the drug to the heart. This technique is now felt to be too hazardous for most arrest situations. The use of IV medications has been shown to have acceptable efficacy in both animal models and clinical trials without the risks of intracardiac injections.

If no vein has been accessed prior to the arrest, a peripheral vein should be used since CPR would have to be stopped to begin a central IV. Drugs administered peripherally require 1 to 2 minutes to reach the central circulation. Therefore if peripheral venous access is used during a code, IV medications should be administered via bolus followed by a 20 ml bolus of IV fluid and elevation of the extremity.[7]

If initial drug administration through a peripheral line does not rapidly restore the circulation, a central line should be placed with minimum interruption of CPR. Distal saphenous veins in the legs, and distal wrist and hand veins should be avoided, since the delivery of drugs administered by these routes is markedly delayed. To have a large-bore access for rapid drug delivery, a 16- or 18-gauge angiocath should be inserted. It is critical to carefully secure the IV catheter to the patient to prevent accidental removal.

In life-threatening emergencies, IV access should not be unduly delayed while the site is being prepared and draped. The need for IV access is critical. If the resuscitation attempt is successful, the IV sites can be rotated to new, sterile sites in the intensive care unit under more controlled conditions.

Acid-Base Management

A major cause of refractory dysrhythmias in cardiac arrest is untreated acidosis and hypoxia, especially for patients with delayed CPR. Untreated acidosis or hypoxia should always be suspected in the victim with asystole, fine VF, high-grade heart block, or severe unresponsive bradycardia.

The cardiac arrest victim will develop acidosis on both a respiratory and a metabolic basis until adequate CPR is initiated. After CPR is initiated and adequate ventilations are begun, the victim can remain in a stable acid-base status for a considerable period of time. Cardiac arrest victims can be maintained with prompt CPR alone for up to 45 minutes before any sodium bicarbonate is required to treat developing acidosis.[5]

It is currently recommended that no sodium bicarbonate be given in most arrest situations, especially in the witnessed arrest. Complications associated with sodium bicarbonate therapy include the following:

- Paradoxical intracellular acidosis (because of more rapid diffusion of CO_2 into cells than bicarbonate).
- Hyperosmolarity.
- Alkalosis.
- Hypernatremia.
- Shift in the oxyghemoglobin saturation curve.

If acidosis is strongly suspected, therapy should be guided by blood-gas results. If severe acidosis is seen (pH < 7.20), treatment can be initiated as follows:

- Increase rate/volume of ventilations.
- Check for placement of the endotracheal tube.
- Check adequacy of CPR.
- Check x-ray for pneumothorax.

If severe acidosis persists despite these maneuvers, the team leader may consider sodium bicarbonate at an initial IV dose of 1 mEq/kg followed by no more than half the initial dose at intervals of no less than every 10 minutes. The importance of adequate ventilation and circulation cannot be overemphasized.

Specific Therapy

If the patient remains pulseless and apneic, specific therapy for the dysrhythmia encountered can be given. Dysrhythmias commonly encountered in ACLS situations are VF, VT, asystole, electromechanical dissociation (EMD), bradycardia, paroxysmal supraventricular tachycardia (PSVT), and ventricular ectopy. Code drugs are used at this point to treat these dysrhythmias in the adult victim.

Drugs Used in Cardiac Arrest

The following are several objectives of drug therapy of ACLS:

- To optimize cardiac function.
- To reestablish spontaneous circulation.
- To correct hypoxemia.
- To correct acidosis.
- To suppress sustained ventricular dysrhythmia.
- To relieve pain.
- To treat congestive heart failure.

When giving ACLS drugs after the first defibrillation, CPR must be continued in the unresponsive patient to ensure circulation of the drugs before attempting subsequent defibrillations. The sequence in which drugs are administered depends on the cause of the cardiac arrest, length of time that the patient has been without effective cardiac output and ventilation, and response to other therapies[19] (Tables 10-1 and 10-2).

During the code, drugs are initially given IV by bolus injection. They are then added to IV solutions and administered via a continuous IV infusion when the patient has an established heart rate.

Table 10-1 Advanced Cardiac Life Support Drugs*

Drug	Dose† and route	Indications	Action

Lidocaine (do not administer in same line with sodium bicarbonate)	IV
	Bolus (loading dose)
	  1-1.5 mg/kg (usually 50-75 mg) initially
	  0.5-1.5 mg/kg every 5-10 min to 3.0 mg/kg maximum dose
	Continuous infusion (no continuous infusion during cardiac arrest) with return of perfusion, continuous infusion 2-4 mg/min
		Frequent PVCs
		VT
		VF
		Complex ectopy in acute myocardial ischemia
		Not recommended in uncomplicated acute MI or ischemia without PVCs
			Depresses automatically and conduction of ectopic impulses in ventricles, particularly in ischemic tissue.
			Serves as a local anesthetic of the amide type that suppresses dysrhythmias of ventricular origin

Epinephrine (should not be administered in same IV lines with alkaline solutions)	IV
	1.0 mg (10 ml of a 1:10,000 solution)
	Bolus
	  repeated every 3-5 min during resuscitation
	ET tube
	  Optimal dose unknown but 2-2.5 times IV bolus dose recommended.
	Intracardiac administration (only during open cardiac massage)
	  1.0 mg only when other routes of administration are impossible
		Cardiac arrest
		VF
		VT
		Asystole
		PEA (EMD)
			Increases myocardial and central nervous system blood flow
			Increases heart rate
			Strengthens myocardial contractility

*Refs 1, 2, 3, 7, 13-15, 21, 34.
†Doses given by peripheral veins should be followed by a 20 ml normal saline flush.

Continued.

Table 10-1   Advanced Cardiac Life Support Drugs—cont'd

Drug	Dose and route	Indications	Action

Atropine (use with caution with myocardial ischemia or infarction)	IV
	Bolus
	  Asystole
	    1 mg repeated in 3-5 min
	      (to a total dose of 2.0 mg)
	  Bradycardia
	    0.5-1 mg every 3-5 min
	      (to total of 2.0 mg)
	Not recommended for continuous IV infusion
	ET tube
	  1.0 mg in 10 ml sterile water or saline
		Sinus bradycardia
		Asystole
		AV node block
			Enhances rate of discharge of SA node
			Increases heart rate
			Facilitates AV conduction
			Decreases AV block

Dopamine (is inactivated by alkaline solutions)	IV Never give bolus Continuous infusion (only) 2.5-5 µg/kg/min initially then titrated to the desired effect	Hypotension Shock	Increases cardiac output, renal blood flow, and blood pressure May cause tachydysrhythmias
Bretylium	IV Bolus 5 mg/kg followed by defibrillation; can be increased if VF continues to 10 mg/kg and repeated at 5 min intervals to a maximum dose of 30-35 mg/kg Continuous infusion for persistant recurring VT 5-10 mg/kg, diluted to 50 ml D$_5$W given over 8-10 min. Once this loading dose has been administered, a maintenance dose of 1-2 mg/min can be infused.	VT or VF unresponsive to lidocaine Ventricular ectopy when lidocaine is contraindicated or ineffective.	Causes initial release of norepinephrine, followed by adrenergic blocking Raises VF threshold Increases action potential duration and effective refractory periods in normal tissue
Calcium chloride (precipates in alkaline solutions such as sodium bicarbonate)	IV Bolus 2-4 mg/kg of 10% solution (2.72 mEq) over 1-2 min. May repeat dose every 10 min	Only recommended for hyperkalemia, hypocalcemia, calcium channel blocker toxicity, and pretreatment for verapamil in treatment of SVT Hyperkalemia, hypocalcemia, and calcium channel blocker toxicity	May increase myocardial contractile force May enhance ventricular automaticity minimizes risk of hypotension when given with Verapamil Increases the force of myocardial contraction
Calcium gluconate (precipates in alkaline solutions such as sodium bicarbonate)	IV Bolus 5-8 ml of 10% solution over 1-2 min. May repeat dose every 10 min		
Dobutamine HCL (inactivated by alkaline solutions)	IV Continuous infusion 2-20 µg/kg/min	Heart failure or cardiogenic shock	Improves myocardial contractility

Amrinone	IV
	Bolus
	  0.75 mg/kg over 2-3 min
	Infusion
	  5-15 µg/kg/min
		Increases cardiac function
		Induces vasodilation
			Improves myocardial contractility.

Sodium Bicarbonate (contraversial)	IV Bolus (when used) 1 mEq/kg initially over 3-5 min Repeat ½ the initial dose every 10 min thereafter or as directed by the ABGs only use when pH < 7.1	Preexisting metabolic acidosis Cardiac arrest, only after more definitive treatment has been established	May counteract metabolic acidosis (controversial)
Verapamil	IV Bolus 2.5-5 mg over 2 min initially and 5-10 mg dose every 15-30 min (to a maximum of 20 mg) if PSVT persists and there is no adverse response to initial dose	PSVT with a narrow QRS complex Atrial flutter Atrial fibrillation	Slows conduction through AV node Produces vasodilation Calcium channel blocker

Table 10-1   Advanced Cardiac Life Support Drugs—cont'd

Drug	Dose and route	Indications	Action
Adenosine	IV Bolus 6 mg over 1-3 sec followed by 20 ml NS. If no response within 1-2 min, repeat dose of 12 mg over 1-3 sec followed by 20 ml NS.	Dysrhythmia due to reentry involving the AV node or sinus node. PSVT	Depresses AV node and sinus node activity.
Isoproterenol (Isuprel) (Do not mix with sodium bicarbonate, barbituates, epinephrine, calcium, or amirophylline)	IV Continuous infusion 2-10 μg/min titrate to produce heart rate of 60 or systolic BP of ≥ 90 Do not give IV push Do not mix with another drug	Indicated only for temporary control of severe bradycardia unresponsive to atropine Refractory torsades de pointes	Increases heart rate Increases cardiac output Enhances automaticity and accelerates conduction Raises blood pressure Promotes bronchodilation

Procainamide	IV
	Bolus
	  20 mg/min until:
	    Dysrhythmia is suppressed, hypotension occurs, QRS complex is widened by 50% of its original width, or total of 17 mg/kg of drug is given
	Continuous infusion
	  1-4 mg/min (maintenance dose)
		Ventricular ectopy when lidocaine is contraindicated or ineffective
		Recommended when lidocaine is contraindicated or has failed
			Depresses automaticity and conduction
			Prolongs refraction in the atrial and the ventricles

Table 10-2   Drugs Used in Cardiac Arrest by Route

Drug	IV bolus*	Continuous infusions†	Endotracheal	Intracardiac‡	Intraosseous
Lidocaine	+	+	+	−	+
Epinephrine	+	+	+	−	+
Atropine	+	−	+	+	+
Dopamine	−	+	−	+	*
Bretylium	+	+	−	−	−
Calcium	+	−	−	+	−
Dobutamine	−	+	−	−	−
Isoproterenol	−	+	−	−	−
Procainamide	+	+	−	−	+
Sodium Bicarbonate	+	−	−	−	+
Verapamil	+	−	−	−	−

*+Yes, −No
†After establishing a pulse.
‡Controversial

Table 10-3   Unit Composition of Drug Mixtures for Continuous Infusions and Usual Doses

Drug	Unit dose/250 ml D₅W	Concentration (per ml)	Usual dose per min*	Ml/hr†
Lidocaine hydrochloride (Xylocaine)	1000 mg (1 gm)	4 mg	2-4 mg	30-60
Epinephrine	1-8 mg	4-32 μg	1-4 μg	Depends on unit dose
Dopamine	400 mg	1600 μg	400 μg	15
Bretylium	1000 mg (1 gm)	4 mg	1-2 mg	15-30
Dobutamine	500 mg	2 mg	200-1000 μg	6-30
Isoproterenol	1 mg	4 μg	2-10 μg	60-300
Procainamide	1000 mg (1 gm)	4 mg	1-4 mg	15-60
Sodium bicarbonate	1 mEq/ml	1 mEq/ml	18 mEq	IV push

*Usually stated as low dose and increased or titrated as needed.
†Microdrops, check manufacturers for number of drops/min (60 microdrops/min were used here).

Mixing IV Infusions During a Cardiac Arrest

The method most commonly used when mixing ACLS drugs is known as the *Rule of 250*. This means that one unit of a drug is added to 250 ml of D_5W. Table 10-3 shows unit concentrations. Infusion rates are set at 15 to 30 ml/hr initially on an infusion pump.

During a code, it will be primarily the nurse's responsibility to locate, calculate, mix, label, hang, and time IV drips, such as lidocaine and dopamine. Codes run much more smoothly when IV drips are properly set up and maintained.

IV drip rate charts should be readily available during any code. Usually they are prominently displayed in the critical care settings and on crash carts. Appendices B to F show common drugs and drip rates. Unless directed otherwise by the medical staff, mix the IV drips in D_5W in the smallest containers available, preferably 250 ml. This may prevent administration of excess fluid. In addition, volume control chambers should be used to prevent an accidental bolus administration of a drug. Further, it is recommended that an IV pump be used, as well as one with a line separator.

Initial Adult IV Drip Rates

Once the infusion has started, monitor the patient carefully (ECG, arterial and pulmonary artery pressures, respiratory and central nervous system status, urine output, and neuromuscular responses) for the response to the drip rate. The nurse should adjust the infusion rate in small increments (3 to 5 drops/min or ml/hr). Do not adjust the drip rates in large increments. Most IV push/drip medications are designed to act quickly. Major shifts in dosages are enormously difficult to correct.

CARDIAC ARREST OUTCOME MANAGEMENT

After the patient's physiological status has been optimized, the individual should be reevaluated and the electrical rhythm confirmed (Fig. 10-3). In the ACLS situation, there are the following typical situations:

- Ventricular fibrillation (VF) and pulseless ventricular tachycardia (VT)
- Asystole
- Pulseless electrical activity (PEA)* [electromechanical dissociation (EMD)]
- Sustained ventricular tachycardia (VT) with a pulse
- Bradycardia
- Ventricular ectopy

Each of these conditions requires different, specific drug therapy for management of the arrest victim.

VF and Pulseless VT

If VF or pulseless VT is confirmed, defibrillation should be attempted (Fig. 10-4). If unsuccessful, the patient can be treated with either lidocaine or bretylium, if

lidocaine is ineffective, to attempt to raise the fibrillation threshold. Lidocaine is currently the preferred agent since more health care providers are aware of the dosages and complications associated with lidocaine than with bretylium. The initial dose of lidocaine is 1-1.5 mg/kg, which can be given either IV or via the ET tube. CPR should be administered for 1 to 2 minutes to circulate the drug followed by defibrillation. If unsuccessful, the lidocaine can be repeated in doses of 0.5-1.5 mg/kg boluses every 5-10 minutes up to a total dose of 3 mg/kg. An alternative is to give bretylium at a dose of 5 mg/kg followed by another defibrillation attempt of 360 J. If still unsuccessful, bretylium can be increased to 10 mg/kg IV push up to a maximum dose of 30-35 mg/kg. The patient should be repeatedly reassessed for return of pulse and rhythm, adequacy of ventilation and chest compressions, acid-base status, adequacy of IV access, and lead placement. In a prolonged arrest a central venous access should be considered to improve delivery of drugs to the central circulation. No cardiac resuscitation should be terminated until cardiac unresponsiveness has been determined by the physician in charge of the resuscitation effort.

Asystole

Persistent asystole after attempts to normalize the patient's physiological state carries a grave prognosis. This rhythm is associated with end-stage heart disease, severe metabolic disarray, or a prolonged cardiac arrest. Defibrillation should be considered if there is any doubt whether the rhythm is asystole or fine VF. If asystole is confirmed in two leads (to rule out fine VF), the patient can be treated with epinephrine 1:10,000, 1.0 mg IV push, repeated every 3-5 minutes (Fig. 10-5). Recent research suggests that doses of epinephrine up to 10 times larger than those recommended by ACLS guidelines produce improved hemodynamics and defibrillation rates and increase the likelihood of a successful resuscitation.[14] If ineffective, atropine 1.0 mg IV push (repeated every 3-5 minutes) may be successful, since asystole can result from increased parasympathetic tone. A central venous access can be placed and the patient should be repeatedly reassessed. Correcting metabolic problems with sodium bicarbonate should be addressed in the hope of obtaining any electrical activity. As a final measure, a pacemaker should be considered.

Pulseless Electrical Activity

Pulseless electrical activity (PEA) occurs when there is electrical activity of the heart that should produce a pulse but no palpable carotid pulse is present. PEA comprises a group of rhythms that are associated with clinical states, but these should be rapidly assessed and corrected if possible. Treatable causes include severe hypovolemia (usually resulting from hemorrhage), tension pneumothorax, pericardial tamponade, and severe hypoxia or acidosis.

Less correctable causes of PEA include cardiac rupture, pulmonary embolism, and massive MI. These patients rarely survive.

---

*The 1992 guidelines have incorporated EMD and a heterogeneous group of rhythms (e.g., ventricular escape rhythm) under a new summary term PEA.

Lead II

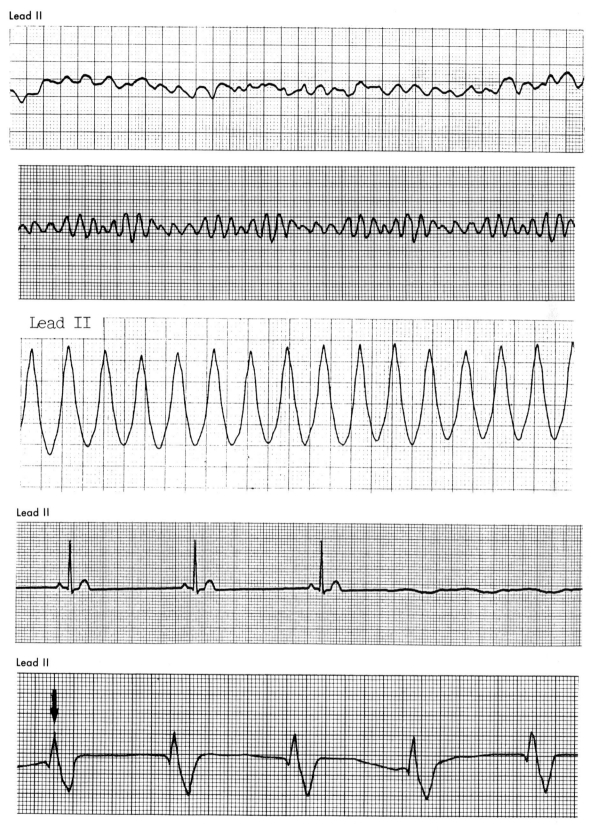

Fig. 10-3 Lethal dysrhythmias. **A,** Fine VF. **B,** Coarse VF. **C,** VT converted to VF by precordial thump. **D,** Bradycardia leading to asystole. **E,** PEA (EMD). (From Grauer K, Cavallaro DL: *ACLS: certification preparation and a comprehensive review,* ed 2, St Louis, 1987, Mosby–Year Book.)

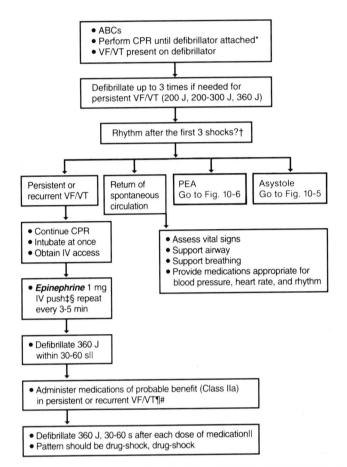

- ABCs
- Perform CPR until defibrillator attached*
- VF/VT present on defibrillator

Defibrillate up to 3 times if needed for persistent VF/VT (200 J, 200-300 J, 360 J)

Rhythm after the first 3 shocks?†

| Persistent or recurrent VF/VT | Return of spontaneous circulation | PEA Go to Fig. 10-6 | Asystole Go to Fig. 10-5 |

- Continue CPR
- Intubate at once
- Obtain IV access

- Assess vital signs
- Support airway
- Support breathing
- Provide medications appropriate for blood pressure, heart rate, and rhythm

- **Epinephrine** 1 mg IV push‡§ repeat every 3-5 min

- Defibrillate 360 J within 30-60 s‖

- Administer medications of probable benefit (Class IIa) in persistent or recurrent VF/VT¶#

- Defibrillate 360 J, 30-60 s after each dose of medication‖
- Pattern should be drug-shock, drug-shock

Class I: definitely helpful
Class IIa: acceptable, probably helpful
Class IIb: acceptable, possibly helpful
Class III: not indicated, may be harmful
*Precordial thump is a Class IIb action in witnessed arrest, no pulse, and no defibrillator immediately available.
†Hypothermic cardiac arrest is treated differently after this point. See section on hypothermia.
‡The recommended dose of **epinephrine** is 1 mg IV push every 3-5 min. If this approach fails, several Class IIb dosing regimens can be considered:
- Intermediate: **epinephrine** 2-5 mg IV push, every 3-5 min
- Escalating: **epinephrine** 1 mg-3 mg-5 mg IV push (3 min apart)
- High: **epinephrine** 0.1 mg/kg IV push, every 3-5 min
§ **Sodium bicarbonate** (1 mEq/kg) is Class I if patient has known preexisting hyperkalemia
‖Multiple sequenced shocks (200J, 200-300J, 360 J) are acceptable here (Class I), especially when medications are delayed

¶ • **Lidocaine** 1.5 mg/kg IV push. Repeat in 3-5 min to total loading dose of 3 mg/kg; then use
- **Bretylium** 5 mg/kg IV push. Repeat in 5 min at 10 mg/kg
- **Magnesium sulfate** 1-2 g IV in torsades de pointes or suspected hypomagnesemic state or severe refractory VF
- **Procainamide** 30 mg/min in refractory VF (maximum total 17 mg/kg)
• **Sodium bicarbonate** (1 mEq/kg IV):
Class IIa
- if known preexisting bicarbonate-responsive acidosis
- if overdose with tricyclic antidepressants
- to alkalinize the urine in drug overdoses
Class IIb
- if intubated and continued long arrest interval
- upon return of spontaneous circulation after long arrest interval
Class III
- hypoxic lactic acidosis

Fig. 10-4   Algorithm for VF and pulseless VT.

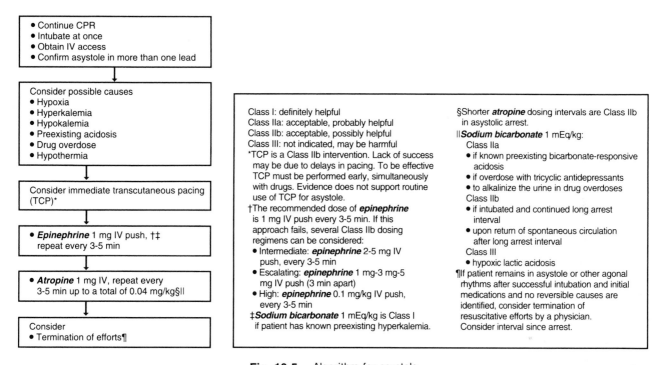

- Continue CPR
- Intubate at once
- Obtain IV access
- Confirm asystole in more than one lead

Consider possible causes
- Hypoxia
- Hyperkalemia
- Hypokalemia
- Preexisting acidosis
- Drug overdose
- Hypothermia

Consider immediate transcutaneous pacing (TCP)*

- *Epinephrine* 1 mg IV push, †‡ repeat every 3-5 min

- *Atropine* 1 mg IV, repeat every 3-5 min up to a total of 0.04 mg/kg§‖

Consider
- Termination of efforts¶

Class I: definitely helpful
Class IIa: acceptable, probably helpful
Class IIb: acceptable, possibly helpful
Class III: not indicated, may be harmful
*TCP is a Class IIb intervention. Lack of success may be due to delays in pacing. To be effective TCP must be performed early, simultaneously with drugs. Evidence does not support routine use of TCP for asystole.
†The recommended dose of *epinephrine* is 1 mg IV push every 3-5 min. If this approach fails, several Class IIb dosing regimens can be considered:
- Intermediate: *epinephrine* 2-5 mg IV push, every 3-5 min
- Escalating: *epinephrine* 1 mg-3 mg-5 mg IV push (3 min apart)
- High: *epinephrine* 0.1 mg/kg IV push, every 3-5 min
‡*Sodium bicarbonate* 1 mEq/kg is Class I if patient has known preexisting hyperkalemia.

§Shorter *atropine* dosing intervals are Class IIb in asystolic arrest.
‖*Sodium bicarbonate* 1 mEq/kg:
Class IIa
- if known preexisting bicarbonate-responsive acidosis
- if overdose with tricyclic antidepressants
- to alkalinize the urine in drug overdoses
Class IIb
- if intubated and continued long arrest interval
- upon return of spontaneous circulation after long arrest interval
Class III
- hypoxic lactic acidosis
¶If patient remains in asystole or other agonal rhythms after successful intubation and initial medications and no reversible causes are identified, consider termination of resuscitative efforts by a physician. Consider interval since arrest.

Fig. 10-5   Algorithm for asystole.

The major issue in patients with PEA is to aggressively seek a correctable cause. A patient can start out with a dysrhythmic arrest and develop traumatic PEA even with properly administered CPR. Hypovolemia, tension pneumothorax, and cardiac tamponade must be addressed before declaring a patient cardiac unresponsive in this circumstance (Fig. 10-6).

Hypovolemia is addressed with a rapid volume challenge with a volume expander such as normal saline via two large-bore IV access sites (central access preferred).[19] The patient should receive volume and not vasopressors in this situation.

Tension pneumothorax is assessed by listening over the lung fields, observing the movement of the chest during ventilation, and looking for tracheal shift or neck vein distention. If a tension pneumothorax is suspected, it can be treated with chest tube insertion and/or needle aspiration. The goal is to prevent the buildup of pressure in the chest with resulting mediastinal shift.

If a patient has had obvious external chest trauma, has prominent neck veins, and a brisk backflow from a central IV line, pericardial tamponade should be suspected. Cardiac tamponade is usually a diagnosis of exclusion during a cardiac arrest. If no other cause of PEA is found, a needle pericardiocentesis should be attempted followed by a thoracotomy if evidence of tamponade is found. The most common cause of failure of a needle pericardiocentesis is the use of a needle that is too short. The needle should be at least 16 gauge and 9 cm long (the needle on a spinal tap tray is available in most areas of the hospital). No patient should be in PEA without ruling out cardiac tamponade as a possible cause.

Severe acidosis or hypoxia is detected with a blood gas measurement during the stabilization phase and is addressed with intubation, 100% O_2, CPR, and hyperventilation of the patient. The patient should be repeatedly reassessed for adequate ventilation and chest compressions. Blood gases should be obtained as needed. Drug treatment of PEA includes epinephrine IV push repeated at least every 3-5 minutes. Current research is exploring the notion of increasing this dose (see algorithm).

If marked bradycardia is present with PEA, atropine

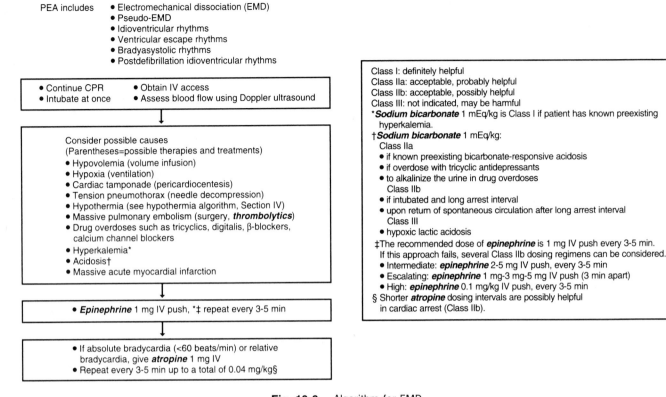

PEA includes
- Electromechanical dissociation (EMD)
- Pseudo-EMD
- Idioventricular rhythms
- Ventricular escape rhythms
- Bradyasystolic rhythms
- Postdefibrillation idioventricular rhythms

| • Continue CPR | • Obtain IV access |
| • Intubate at once | • Assess blood flow using Doppler ultrasound |

Consider possible causes
(Parentheses=possible therapies and treatments)
- Hypovolemia (volume infusion)
- Hypoxia (ventilation)
- Cardiac tamponade (pericardiocentesis)
- Tension pneumothorax (needle decompression)
- Hypothermia (see hypothermia algorithm, Section IV)
- Massive pulmonary embolism (surgery, *thrombolytics*)
- Drug overdoses such as tricyclics, digitalis, β-blockers, calcium channel blockers
- Hyperkalemia*
- Acidosis†
- Massive acute myocardial infarction

- *Epinephrine* 1 mg IV push, *‡ repeat every 3-5 min

- If absolute bradycardia (<60 beats/min) or relative bradycardia, give *atropine* 1 mg IV
- Repeat every 3-5 min up to a total of 0.04 mg/kg§

Class I: definitely helpful
Class IIa: acceptable, probably helpful
Class IIb: acceptable, possibly helpful
Class III: not indicated, may be harmful
* *Sodium bicarbonate* 1 mEq/kg is Class I if patient has known preexisting hyperkalemia.
† *Sodium bicarbonate* 1 mEq/kg:
  Class IIa
  - if known preexisting bicarbonate-responsive acidosis
  - if overdose with tricyclic antidepressants
  - to alkalinize the urine in drug overdoses
  Class IIb
  - if intubated and long arrest interval
  - upon return of spontaneous circulation after long arrest interval
  Class III
  - hypoxic lactic acidosis
‡The recommended dose of *epinephrine* is 1 mg IV push every 3-5 min. If this approach fails, several Class IIb dosing regimens can be considered.
  - Intermediate: *epinephrine* 2-5 mg IV push, every 3-5 min
  - Escalating: *epinephrine* 1 mg-3 mg-5 mg IV push (3 min apart)
  - High: *epinephrine* 0.1 mg/kg IV push, every 3-5 min
§ Shorter *atropine* dosing intervals are possibly helpful in cardiac arrest (Class IIb).

Fig. 10-6 Algorithm for EMD.

may be given to induce cardioacceleration and possibly increase the effectiveness of cardiac contractions.

MANAGEMENT OF LIFE-THREATENING DYSRHYTHMIAS WITHOUT CARDIAC ARREST
Sustained VT with a Pulse

The management of sustained VT is based on whether or not the patient is stable or unstable. Fig. 10-7 shows this algorithm. Patients are considered unstable if they have hypotension, symptoms of chest pain, dyspnea, congestive heart failure, infarction, or ischemia.

Bradycardia

Bradydysrhythmias are rhythm disorders ranging from simple sinus bradycardia to PEA and asystole (Fig. 10-8). No specific treatments other than oxygen and IV access are needed for simple sinus bradycardia. If signs and symptoms occur, such as hypotension, premature ventricular contractions (PVCs), chest pain, dyspnea, or altered mental status, atropine 0.5 mg every 5 minutes up to 2 mg can be administered intravenously. As a temporizing measure, an external pacemaker can be applied or the patient can be started on an isoproterenol drip of 2 to 10 μg/min. Transvenous pacemaker therapy may be required if the bradydysrhythmia continues.

Ventricular Ectopy

When a viable cardiac rhythm is detected during CPR, the victim should be evaluated for the presence of a pulse, adequate blood pressure and respirations. Oxygen (100%) should be maintained and bag ventilation continued if needed.

If the victim's underlying rhythm was either VF or VT during the arrest, lidocaine, procainamide, or bretylium should be provided IV with additional boluses as needed. The usual dose of lidocaine is an initial 1 mg/kg bolus, and a continuous infusion of 2 to 4 mg/min. Additional boluses of 0.5 mg/kg, as needed, may be administered every 2 to 5 minutes up to 3 mg/kg or until the ectopy is suppressed. If adequate suppression of ectopic beats cannot be obtained with lidocaine or if the drug is not well tolerated, procainamide may be tried. Procainamide must be administered slowly, however, to avoid hypotension. A loading dose sufficient to suppress the ectopic beats up to a maximum dose of 1000 mg may be given, followed by a continuous infusion of 1 to 4 mg/min[2] (Fig. 10-9). If these drugs are ineffective, Bretylium can be given. Current American Heart Association (AHA) ACLS guidelines suggest that routine use of antidysrhythmic drugs in AMI patients is disputed since such therapy has not been shown to improve mortality following MI.[7]

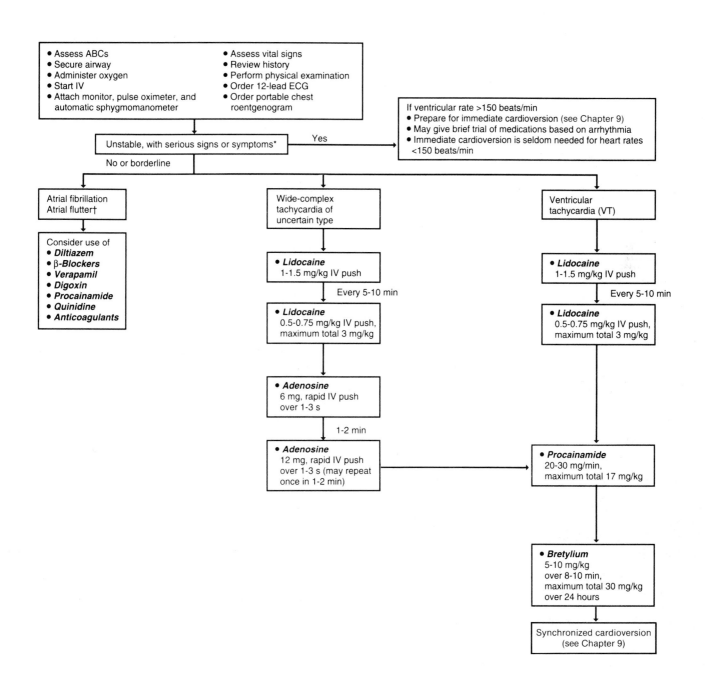

Fig. 10-7   Algorithm for sustained VT.

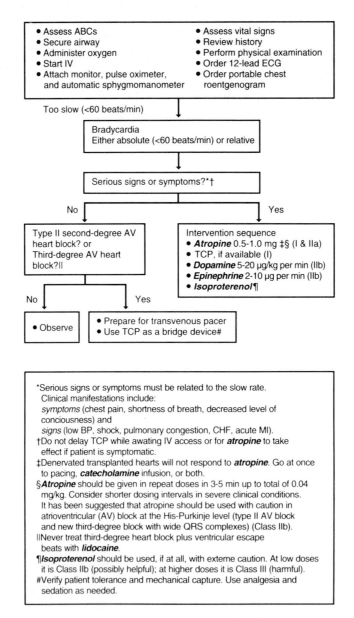

Fig. 10-8 Algorithm for bradycardia.

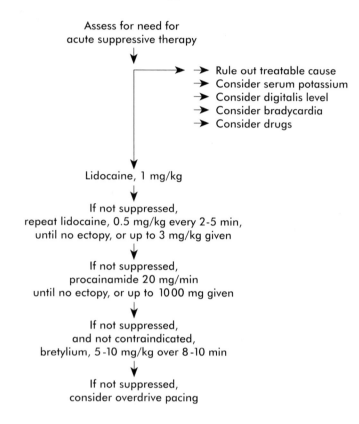

Once ectopy is resolved, maintain as follows:
After lidocaine, 1 mg/kg .... Lidocaine drip, 2 mg/min
After lidocaine, 1-2 mg/kg .... Lidocaine drip, 3 mg/min
After lidocaine, 2-3 mg/kg .... Lidocaine drip, 4 mg/min
After procainamide .... Procainamide drip, 1-4 mg/min
(Check blood level.)
After bretylium .... Bretylium drip, 2 mg/min

Ventricular ectopy: acute suppressive therapy. This sequence was developed to assist in teaching how to treat a broad range of patients with ventricular ectopy. Some patients may require care not specified herein. This algorithm should not be construed as prohibiting such flexibility. Such therapy has not been shown to improve mortality after MI.[7]

Fig. 10-9 Algorithm for ventricular ectopy.

Paroxysmal Supraventricular Tachycardia (PSVT)

There are many supraventricular tachydysrthymias that are encountered in the emergency room or critical care unit. Cardioconversion of the patient who displays serious signs and symptoms should be done immediately. Patients are usually hemodynamically stable and the dysrhythmia can be managed with drugs. Fig. 10-10 shows the algorithm for paroxysmal supraventricular tachycardia.

Postresuscitation Management

The first goal of postresuscitation management is to maintain adequate ventilation and circulation. The patient should be maintained on 100% oxygen and assessed for spontaneous respirations. If the patient cannot breathe adequately, bag-valve-mask ventilation should be maintained and intubation considered if not performed during the resuscitation effort. The position of the ET tube should be verified to ensure that it has not slipped into the right main bronchus. One should listen over both lung fields and then the tube should be secured in place. Blood gases should be obtained to ensure adequate ventilatory management and assess the patient's acid-base status.

The patient's circulatory status should be assessed by checking the pulse and blood pressure. Patients frequently

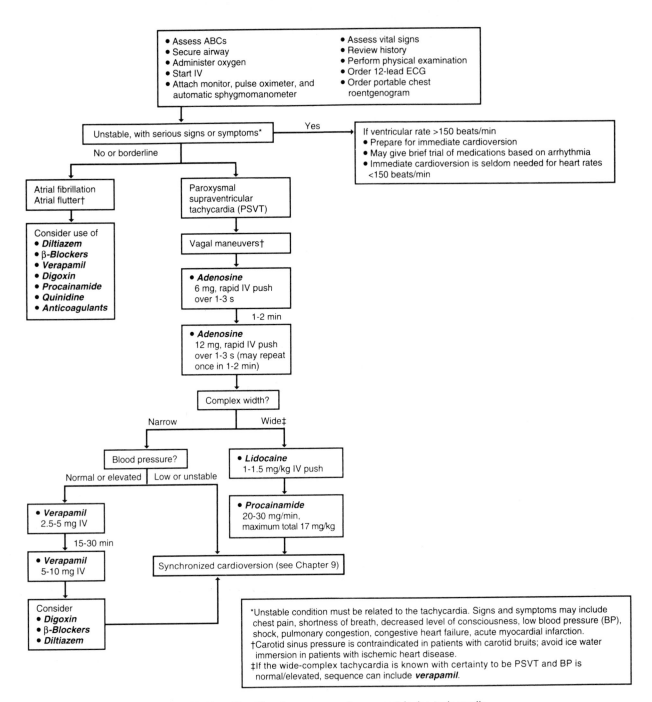

Fig. 10-10 Algorithm for paroxysmal supraventricular tachycardia.

ly present with hypotension after an arrest. If the blood pressure does not start to rise after several minutes, a dopamine drip can be initiated to raise the systolic pressure above 90 mm Hg. If there is a persistent bradycardia with hypotension, the patient should be evaluated for acidosis and hypoxia. Atropine should be considered. Serum electrolytes including calcium and magnesium should be assessed.

Every patient should have lead placement verified in the postresuscitation period and be maintained on a continuous cardiac monitor. A 12-lead ECG should be obtained and read when possible. The patient's history should be reviewed with emphasis on current medications. A flow sheet should be maintained to monitor the patient's vital signs and urinary output.

If the patient is not in a critical care unit, arrangements should be made for transfer to an intensive care setting for continued monitoring, close observation, and interventions, if necessary. This is a critical period during the resuscitation effort that is often neglected. After arrangements for transfer are made, the patient should be accompanied to the intensive care unit by a team of at least four health care providers. One provider watches the cardiac monitor and uses the defibrillator if necessary. A second provider observes the IV drips and administers any needed medications. The third manages the airway, oxygen, and ventilates, if needed. The fourth provider performs CPR, if necessary.

After the patient has been safely transferred to an intensive care setting the circumstances surrounding the arrest and management by the cardiac arrest and unit teams should be reviewed.

The patient should be closely monitored and assessed in the intensive care unit for at least 72 hours. A careful head-to-toe postarrest physical assessment is necessary to determine the patient's physiological status.

Patients who are awake and alert should be monitored and have an IV line and supplemental oxygen. Those who are unconscious generally have an ET tube in place and may be on a ventilator. The ET tube needs to be suctioned at least every 1 to 2 hours and as needed. Hemodynamically unstable patients with cardiac failure or hypoperfusion should have a pulmonary artery catheter inserted to monitor pulmonary artery wedge pressures (PAWP) and cardiac outputs. After an MI, the PAWP is optimally raised to 15 to 18 mm Hg. If the PAWP is above this range and the patient demonstrates signs of pulmonary edema, diuretics, morphine, and vasodilators are usually ordered by the physician. Patients are generally catheterized after an arrest and urinary output is monitored hourly. The patient and family will also need psychological support after a code. This experience is an extremely frightening event for the patient and for the patient's family.

ASSESSMENT

The initial assessment of the cardiac arrest victim takes only a few seconds. All other assessments are delayed or carried out simultaneously until the patient is resuscitated (see Skill 10-2).

NURSING DIAGNOSIS

Following are sample nursing diagnoses for the patient who requires advanced cardiac life support:
* Acid-base imbalance related to inadequate perfusion during cardiac arrest.
* Decrease in arterial blood pressure related to low blood volume.
* Decrease in cardiac output related to cardiogenic shock.
* Decrease in cardiac output related to VT.
* Disturbance in cardiac rhythm related to cardiac arrest.
* Disturbance in gas exchange related to cardiac arrest.
* Fluid volume deficit related to hemorrhage.
* Ineffective airway clearance related to pulmonary secretions.
* Decrease in tissue perfusion related to VF.
* Anxiety related to cardiac arrest event.

PATIENT OUTCOMES

The following is a list of desired outcomes for patients receiving advanced cardiac life support.
Patient evidences:
* Normal sinus rhythm.
* Pulse rate and blood pressure within normal limits for the patient.
* Patent airway.
* Normal respiratory pattern bilateral; even, clear chest movement; clear and equal breath sounds.
* Clear chest x-ray.
* Urinary output ≥30 ml/hr.
* Normothermia.
* Glasgow coma scale score of 15.
* Palpable peripheral pulses.

Skill 10-2 Conducting the Postarrest Assessment

NURSING INTERVENTIONS

1. Auscultate the lungs to determine that breath sounds are bilateral and equal. Assess breath sounds for adventitious sounds. Observe chest movements. Auscultate heart sounds. Assess rate and rhythm.
2. Evaluate arterial blood gases, serum electrolytes, protein, albumin, hematocrit, and hemoglobin.
3. Evaluate chest x-ray to determine position of ET tube, cardiac silhouette, presence of broken ribs, pulmonary edema, or pneumothorax.
4. Obtain sputum culture and sensitivity in case aspiration occurred during arrest.
5. Monitor pulse and blood pressure every 5 to 15 minutes until the patient is stabilized. Inspect neck veins. Assess peripheral pulses for perfusion.
6. Auscultate heart sounds. Assess rate and rhythm.
7. Obtain 12-lead ECG. Compare with previous ECG if available. Continue to monitor for ventricular ectopic activity and changes in ECG intervals (i.e., PR, QRS, and QT).
8. Assess cardiac output and pulmonary artery wedge pressure, if pulmonary artery catheter is in place.
9. Review other laboratory results, if appropriate (e.g., echocardiogram).
10. Assess level of consciousness.
11. Assess memory.
12. Check pupils (note what drugs were given during code).
13. Note seizure activity.
14. Test muscle strength and reflexes.
15. Assess psychological status.
16. Conduct skin assessment for burns from defibrillation.
17. Perform gastrointestinal assessment noting nasogastric tube placement.
18. Measure urine output hourly.
19. Monitor intake.
20. Monitor additional laboratory data (e.g., serum electrolytes, serum urea nitrogen, creatinine, protein, albumin, osmolality; urine electrolytes, urea nitrogen, creatinine, and osmolality). Evaluation of urine electrolytes should not be made immediately after the administration of diuretics. A minimum of 12 hours (24 hours preferably) should elapse before urinalysis.

MEMBERS AND ROLES OF THE CODE TEAM

The person who first discovers or witnesses the cardiac arrest and the second person on the scene become the initial members of the resuscitation team and carry out CPR until relieved. When the code team arrives, these roles are assumed by team members.

Variations on the size of the code team depend on the time of day and the hospital's staffing patterns, acuity of patient care, availability of ACLS certification programs, and the number of codes occurring during the month. Usually a code team consists of 7 to 8 individuals. If more than 7 or 8 members of the arrest team are at the patient's bedside, communications and coordination can break down quickly. Most patient care rooms simply are not large enough to contain a full code team, airway equipment, crash cart, ECG monitors, and visitors or onlookers. The physician and nursing team leaders must ensure there is adequate space for the code team to function smoothly and rapidly.

TERMINATION OF RESUSCITATION

CPR, once initiated, must continue until determined to be no longer necessary by the physician, until the patient recovers, or until the CPR providers are exhausted. The following criteria can be used to assist in making the decision to terminate CPR[7,33]:

- A preexisting contraindication to initiating CPR (e.g., a Do-Not-Resuscitate (DNR) order).
- Cardiac death: electric asystole (documented by a properly functioning ECG monitor) of 15 minutes or more in a normothermic patient (may be longer in a hypothermic patient), in spite of ACLS measures.

Brain death cannot be determined during CPR. Checking pupils for light reflex during CPR lends unclear findings, since drugs administered during the code situation, such as atropine, dopamine, and epinephrine, result in pupillary dilation during the postresuscitation period. Additionally, hypoperfusion may prolong the routine half-lives of such drugs.[21,34]

The issue of when to terminate a cardiac resuscitation effort is a difficult area for which no hard and fast guidelines have been established. The decision rests primarily with the physician who is running the cardiac arrest team and should be based on cardiovascular unresponsiveness. The idea behind this concept is that with prompt CPR, correction of acid-base disorders, pharmacological therapy, and defibrillation (where appropriate), a patient who can respond develops an effective pulse. With prolonged treatment, without evidence of return of effective cardiac electrical activity or pulse, the patient is determined to have no evidence of cardiac or cerebral viability, and the determination is made that death has occurred. At this time resuscitation efforts can be discontinued because the patient is considered clinically dead.

The outcome of CPR is determined by a combination of the following factors:

- The patient's age.
- Condition at the time of the arrest.
- The underlying cause of the arrest.
- Cardiac rhythm at the time of the arrest.
- Preexisting cardiac disease.
- Speed and ease of ACLS institution.

Empirical data indicate that there are the following predictors for a poor outcome of resuscitation[7]:

- An unwitnessed arrest or a delay in the resuscitation attempt.
- Severe underlying disease.
- Prolonged resuscitation.
- An asystolic arrest.

Since termination of resuscitation is a clinical decision based on cardiovascular unresponsiveness in the face of appropriate resuscitation efforts, good documentation is critical to allow adequate evaluation of the arrest team.

DECISION-MAKING IN ACLS: DNR DILEMMA

Critical care nurses are confronted with a complex and agonizing ethical dilemma: whether or not to begin or withhold resuscitation efforts from critically ill patients.

Situations involving withholding resuscitation can place nurses in a precarious position. The nurse is often the one who must understand the decisions, carry out the physician's orders or hospital's policy, and interact with the family and visitors. At best, the guidelines for DNR or "no-code" situations are ambiguous and vary among institutions and even between practitioners. At worst, there is considerable confusion regarding when, where, or how DNR orders are to be carried out.

Whatever the patient care setting, the nurse should know policies and protocols regarding resuscitation. Policies serve a protective function for the patient, the nurse, the physician, and the health care agency.

Successful resuscitation requires both the reestablishment of effective cardiovascular function and the restoration of complete neurological function. These successful outcomes necessitate the making of difficult ethical decisions by the physician, including whether or not to institute CPR and whether or not to discontinue CPR. A patient classification system was created to aid health care providers to make decisions in this difficult area (see the box on p. 253.

DNR or "no-code" orders are required for those patients who are not to be resuscitated. A DNR order essentially means that cardiopulmonary resuscitative measures will be withheld in the event of an acute cardiac or respiratory arrest.[24] The determining factors for resuscitative status should be clear and individually prepared for each patient. The following questions should be answered when determining code status:

- Is there any reason not to resuscitate the patient?
- Is the patient now competent?
- Does the patient want to be resuscitated?
- Was the patient competent in the past?
- Does the family or legal guardian want to have the patient resuscitated?

▼ **Patient Classification System**

Whenever appropriate, critically ill patients should be classified according to the following system:

CLASS A

Maximal therapeutic effort without reservation.

CLASS B

Maximal therapeutic effort without reservation but with daily evaluation because probability of survival is questionable.

CLASS C

Selective limitation of therapeutic measures. The criterion that determines every aspect of the therapeutic regimen continues to be the overall welfare of the patient. Certain procedures may cease to be justifiable and become contraindicated. The therapeutic plan must be clearly detailed to the other members of the care team so that all understand and are united about their caring efforts and responsibilities. As an integral part of caring for the patient, appropriate notes specifically describing the therapeutic plan should be made in the patient's record. The patient's resuscitation status should be similarly recorded following the policy governing orders limiting full cardio-pulmonary resuscitation.

A Class C patient is not an appropriate candidate for admission to an intensive care unit. A decision to transfer the patient out of the intensive care unit is based on the needs of the patient, and transfer is appropriate only after required comfort measures become manageable in a nonintensive care setting. Whatever the patient's location, however, and irrespective of the specific therapeutic measures that have been selectively limited, a Class C patient and his family require and must be given full general support.

CLASS D

All therapy can be discontinued. Any measures which are indicated to insure maximum comfort of the patient may be continued or instituted.

From Critical Care Committee, Massachusetts General Hospital: Optimum care for hopelessly ill patients, *New Engl J Med*, 295:362-364, 1976.

• Was there an advance directive (e.g., a living will)? If the answer to these questions is "no", then the patient is not the best candidate for CPR. Once the decision to make the patient a "no code" has been made by the physician, in collaboration with the patient and/or family, the DNR or no-code order must be written on the patient's chart. Unless nurses have these written orders, they must perform CPR for all patients who suffer cardiac arrest. In many institutions, these orders are passed by word-of-mouth or implied by euphemisms, such as "routine care only" or "comfort measures only," for patients who should not receive CPR (e.g., those with terminal cancer). Also confusing the issue are the "slow-code" orders. This means code the patient but go about the procedure slowly. Essentially, allow the patient to die while setting up the code.

Verbal, indirect DNR, or slow-code orders create for the nurse legal, professional, moral, and ethical dilemmas. The nurse is encouraged to review hospital policy regarding DNR orders to facilitate clarification of unclear verbal or written orders regarding code status.

ACLS/CARDIAC ARREST DOCUMENTATION AND EVALUATION

During most cardiopulmonary arrests, the registered nurse is responsible for documenting the ACLS activities. Documentation forms vary widely among hospitals, clinics and paramedic units. In its purest form the arrest record describes the flow, conduct, and outcome of the arrest. Any notations made by the nurse must reflect that flow (Fig. 10-11).

PEDIATRIC CONSIDERATIONS

The majority of cardiac arrests in children are caused by respiratory arrest. The precipitating events are frequently respiratory obstruction and anoxia. There is a 25% mortality rate for those children who experience a respiratory arrest without cardiac involvement.[22,25] When respiratory arrests progress to full cardiac arrests, greater than 80% mortality has been reported.[22,30] Since mortality rate is high and asystole is difficult to treat in children, keeping a respiratory arrest from progressing to a cardiac arrest is of prime importance.[11]

Children at risk for an arrest include those who:
• Have an unstable cardiovascular status.
• Have a rapidly progressing pulmonary disease.
• Are heavily sedated.
• Have an artificial airway.
• Have a deteriorating neurological status.
• Tend to put items in their mouths.
• Have an overwhelming severe infection.

Resuscitation

Cardiopulmonary resuscitation of the pediatric patient places increased demands on the individuals involved in running the code. Children are not little adults, and although the basic elements of the code situation apply to children, there are modifications in procedures, medication dosages, and equipment.[17]

The ABCs

Resuscitation in children focuses on airway management and breathing, since most arrests are respiratory. A foreign body lodged in the airway should be suspected in children under 4 years of age who are basically healthy. If a foreign body is present, standards approved by the American Heart Association should be used. If this occurs in a hospital setting, one should suction the patient.

When positioning the child for CPR, one should not hyperextend the neck because a small child's vertebrae are so supple that they may actually block the airway posteriorally. The child's airway can be opened by using the head-tilt, chin-lift method or by using the jaw thrust, placing the child in the sniffing position. If a neck injury is suspected, the head-tilt should be avoided.

CARDIOPULMONARY RESCUSCITATION DATA RECORD

Date: _____

Name	Age	Sex	ED Number	Time arrived in ED:	Mode of arrival	Approximate time of arrest:	Code called:

Etiology of arrest:
  ☐ Respiratory   ☐ Cardiac   ☐ Other: _____   CPR started: _____   Notification of: By: _____   ☐ Yes
Initial   ☐ V. Fibrillation   ☐ Asystole   ☐ Other   Family @ _____   _____   Time:
Rhythm: ☐ V. Tachycardia ☐ EMD   ☐ Time: _____   By: _____   Physician @ _____   _____
☐ Witnessed   ☐ Unwitnessed   By: _____   Monitor to Pt. @ _____   Chaplain @ _____   _____   ☐ No
Local physician: _____

Respiratory Management

Method	Time	By
Airway		
Oxygen		
M to M		
Ambu/Mask		
Ambu/ET		

Intubation

Tube size: _____   Time: _____
By: _____

Placement checked*			
Time			

*Breath sounds

Circulatory Assistance

Time			
Method			
By			
Pulse Ck			

Prehospital Care

☐ None ☐ BCLS @ _____
☐ ACLS @ _____ ; Meds, IV's, etc.: _____
_____
_____

Precordial Thump: ☐ No ☐ Yes Time: _____ Response: _____

Defibrillation or Cardioversion

Arrhythmia				
Time				
Watts/Sec				
Response				

Lab	Time

X-ray	Time

Blood Gases

Time			
Site			
By			
O2 Con.			
pH			
P_{CO_2}			
P_{O_2}			
Base Ex			

History/Prior Condition:
_____
_____
_____
_____
_____
_____

Intravenous Therapy

Solutions & Amount	Site	Needle	Time	Rate	Medications added	Amt. rec.	By

Medications

Epinephrine	Dose/Rt							
	Time							
Na Bicarb	Dose/Rt							
	Time							
Ca. Chloride	Dose/Rt							
	Time							
Atropine	Dose/Rt							
	Time							
Isoproterenol	Dose/Rt							
	Time							
Lidocaine Bolus	Dose/Rt							
	Time							
Lidocaine Drip	Dose/Rt							
	Time							
Bretylium Bolus	Dose/Rt							
	Time							
Pronestyl	Dose/Rt							
	Time							
Dopamine Drip	Dose/Rt							
	Time							
Dobutamine	Dose/Rt							
	Time							
Levophed	Dose/Rt							
	Time							
Verapamil	Dose/Rt							
	Time							
	Dose/Rt							
	Time							
	Dose/Rt							
	Time							
	Dose/Rt							
	Time							
	Dose/Rt							
	Time							
	Dose/Rt							
	Time							

Comments: _____
_____
_____
_____
_____
_____
_____
_____
_____
_____
_____
_____
_____
_____
_____
_____
_____
_____
_____
_____
_____
_____
_____
_____
_____

Vital Signs

Time			
B/P			
Pulse			
Resp.			
Temp.			
Pupils			

Procedures Time Size By

NG			
Foley			
Pacemaker			

Neuro Status By GCS

Time		
Eyes Open		
Best Verbal Response		
Best Motor Response		
Total Score		

Outcome: Time CPR Stopped: _____
  ☐ Survived
Disposition: _____
Time of Transfer: _____
Condition @ Transfer: _____
_____
Disposition of Valuables: _____
_____

☐ Expired @ _____
Autopsy Requested: ☐ Yes ☐ No
Medical Examiner Notified:
  ☐ No ☐ Yes Time: _____
  By: _____
Organs Donated: ☐ Yes ☐ No
Consent Signed: ☐ Yes ☐ No
Physician Summary/Impression: _____

CPR Team:
M.D. in Charge: _____
Others: _____
_____
_____
_____

Total Time of Resuscitation: _____
**Attach Representative ECG Strips to Back.
Signatures:

_____   _____   _____
Recorder   Nurse   Physician

Fig. 10-11 Cardiopulmonary resuscitation data record. (From Judith Y. Bradford: A new CPR form you can use, *Nursing '86* 16(9):40, 1986.)

Table 10-4 Differences in CPR for Infants, Children, and Adults*

	Infants	**Children**	**Adults**
Age	Under 1 year	1-8 years	Above 8 years
Compression delivery	2 fingers	Heel of 1 hand	Heels of both hands
Compression depth	1.25-2.5 cm (½-1 inch)	1-1½ inches	1½-2 inches
Compression rate	100-120/min	80-100/min	80-100/min
Ventilations/min	20	15	12
Compression-ventilation ratio	5:1	5:1	15:2

*These are general guidelines and may need to be adjusted for children who are very small or unusually large.

The rescuer's mouth covers and seals the infant's mouth and nose. If the victim is a child, the nose is pinched and only the mouth is covered. The volume of air in an infant's or child's lungs is smaller than that of an adult and the air passages smaller, making resistance to flow potentially high. Therefore the appropriate volume to breathe into the child is the amount that will make the chest rise and fall (Table 10-5). If the airway is free of a foreign body and the child does not breathe spontaneously, it may be necessary to intubate the child. If no pulse is felt, chest compressions are begun (see Fig. 10-12 and Table 10-4). Assessing the apical pulse by placing one's ear against the chest is faster and more accurate than feeling for the pulse.

Defibrillation

Most cardiac dysrhythmias after a respiratory arrest in children are bradycardia, asystole, or agonal rhythm. VF is rarely seen. As a result, defibrillation is rarely needed. If defibrillation is needed, the recommended energy for the initial countershock is 2 J/kg. A paddle of 4.5 cm in diameter is appropriate for infants while an 8 cm diameter is adequate for children weighing over 10 kg (22 lbs).[7] If unsuccessful, a second and, if necessary, a third countershock of 4 J/kg is recommended[1,7]. If this dose does not work, treatment should be directed toward correction of acidosis, hypoxemia, and hypothermia, if present. Defibrillation of children should be performed only if the child is monitored because VT is rare in children.

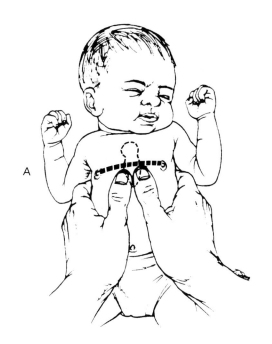
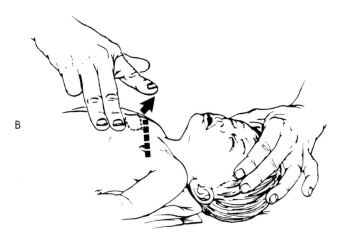
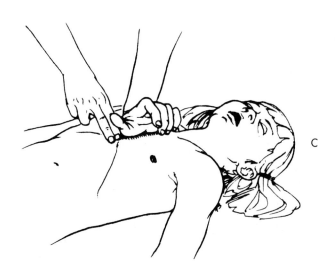

Fig. 10-12 Compression sites. Locating finger position for: **A,** Small neonates; **B,** Infants; **C,** Children. (From Standards and guidelines for cardiopulmonary resuscitation (CPR) and emergency cardiac care (ECC), *JAMA* 255:2905, 1986.)

Stabilization

Improved delivery of oxygen is achieved by using either a bag-valve-mask or bag-valve-tube device. The resuscitation bag should permit oxygenation with 100% oxygen.

Specific therapy

Most cardiac dysrhythmias in children occur as a result of hypoxia, acidosis, or electrolyte disturbance. These precipitating factors must be corrected as soon as possible to prevent further deterioration. Cardiac dysrhythmias and common treatments used during cardiac arrest can be found in Table 10-5.

Many times IV access is difficult to achieve. Whenever possible, central venous access is preferred to peripheral access. The three sites commonly used for central venous access during a code are the subclavian vein, the internal jugular vein, and the femoral vein. Neck veins are difficult to cannulate in children, however, because of the short length of their necks, and the femoral vein is no longer

Table 10-5 Pediatric Dysrhythmias and Treatment

Dysrhythmia	Treatment/comments
Primary treatment: Airway, breathing, and circulation	
Correct: hypoxemia, acidosis, hypoglycemia, potassium and calcium imbalance, hypothermia, and vagal stimulation	
Asystole	Atropine
Idioventricular rhythm	Bicarbonate
	Epinephrine
	Isoproterenol
	(Defibrillation is worthless)
Bradycardia	Atropine/Isoproterenol
	Bicarbonate
	Epinephrine
Second-degree heart block	Atropine (type I)
	Isoproterenol/pacemaker (type II)
Third-degree heart block	Pacemaker
	If unavailable:
	Atropine, isoproterenol
	Bicarbonate, and epinephrine
PVCs	Lidocaine
	Procainamide
	Bretylium
	Propranolol
	Phenytoin
	Amiodarone
Ventricular tachycardia	Cardioversion at 0.2 to 1.0 J/kg
Ventricular fibrillation	Defibrillation at 2 J/kg
	Repeat doubling J
	Consider: bicarbonate, epinephrine, lidocaine, and bretylium
Low cardiac output	Dopamine (? tamponade)
Regular rhythm	Dobutamine
Normovolemic	
Low cardiac output	5% albumin
Regular rhythm	Plasma
Hypovolemic	Blood
	Normal saline or lactated Ringers
	Hetastarch

Adapted from Curley MAQ. In Kelly S, editor: *Pediatric emergency nursing*, Norwalk, Connecticut, 1988, Appleton & Lange.

recommended as a cannulation site because of decreased subdiaphragmatic venous return during cardiac resuscitation.[13] In light of this, peripheral venous access is most often chosen as the initial route of IV and drug administration.[13] Peripheral sites most commonly used include external jugular veins, antecubital veins, and long saphenous veins. The umbilical vein can be used in newborns. Intraosseous vascular access can be used during a code if IV access cannot be obtained. Intraosseous access is obtained by placing a rigid needle (bone marrow needle or spinal needle with stylet) into the anterior tibial bone marrow. In the absence of all of these routes the ET route may be used for administration of epinephrine, atropine, or lidocaine.[1,2]

Drugs used in a pediatric cardiac arrest

Dextrose is administered IV to combat hypoglycemia because hypoglycemia contributes to acidosis. In addition, dextrose is a direct stimulant of contractile force and is an osmotic diuretic. A 25% dextrose solution is used as treatment. The standard 50% dextrose solution can be diluted 1:1 with sterile water to obtain a 25% solution. The initial dose is 2 ml/kg.[12,31] This dose is given as a bolus.[3] To maintain adequate glucose levels, an infusion of 10% dextrose in 0.25% normal saline can be run at a rate not to exceed 4 ml/kg/hr.[3] Blood-glucose levels should be monitored by Dextrostix or another blood-glucose monitor. Colloid volume expanders such as albumin, blood and plasma, or crystalloid solutions such as Ringer's lactate or normal saline, can be administered to the hypovolemic child. If hypovolemia is suspected, Ringer's lactate at 10 to 15 ml/kg can be administered over 10 to 15 minutes.[3]

The drugs used to treat children receiving pediatric resuscitation are basically the same as those used for adults. The medications most commonly used in pediatric ACLS are atropine, epinephrine, and dopamine. Lidocaine, procainamide, and bretylium are infrequently used since children rarely go into VT or VF. Sodium bicarbonate, calcium, and isoproterenol are deemphasized in pediatric resuscitation. Drug administration is complicated by the need to adjust doses to the child's body weight. Pediatric dosages are based on body weight expressed in kilograms.

Since drug calculations for the pediatric patient can be a tedious procedure, it is useful to post a chart of commonly used drugs and dosages for pediatric ACLS on the code chart or other location where drugs will be prepared. Table 10-6 contains information useful for preparing pediatric code drugs. Additionally, individual emergency drug sheets can be prepared for each child.[16] Since children are smaller than adults, they experience fluid overload with much less fluid. Therefore it is helpful to mix drugs in 100 ml of fluid.

Postresuscitation management requires careful monitoring of all body functions. This includes monitoring vital signs, auscultation of heart and lungs, intake and output, and all tubes and lines. Assessment will determine the patient's response to the hypoxic event and determine any tissue or system damage. Any abnormal or sluggish re-

Table 10-6   Pediatric Drug Dosages
....

EPINEPHRINE

Dose = 0.01 mg/kg (comes in 10-ml syringes [0.1 mg/l ml] of 1:10,000 solution)

	Weight of patient	Dose for IV bolus (or ET)
	10 kg	0.1 mg (1 ml)
	20 kg	0.2 mg (2 ml)
	30 kg	0.3 mg (3 ml)
	Adult	0.5-1.0 mg (5-10 ml)

IV Infusion Dose of Epinephrine = 0.1-1.0 μg/kg/min
  Mix 0.6 × body weight (kg) in mg in 100 ml of D_5W.
    Then 1 drop/min = 0.1 μg/kg/min; Titrate to effect

Weight of patient	How to mix	Initial rate*	Maximum rate
10 kg	6 mg in 100 D_5W	1 drop/min (= 0.1 μg/kg/min)	10 drops/min
20 kg	12 mg in 100 D_5W	1 drop/min (= 0.1 μg/kg/min)	10 drops/min
30 kg	18 mg in 100 D_5W	1 drop/min (= 0.1 μg/kg/min)	10 drops/min
Adult	1 mg in 250 D_5W	15-30 drops/min (1-2 μg/min)	Titrate up

ATROPINE

Dose = 0.02 mg/kg (minimum dose = 0.1 mg; maximum single dose = 1.0 mg)
May repeat 0.02 mg/kg every 5 min up to 1.0 mg (for child) and 2.0 mg (for adolescent)

	Weight of patient	Single dose (IV or ET)
	10 kg	0.2 mg
	20 kg	0.4 mg
	30 kg	0.6 mg
	Adult	0.5-1.0 mg

LIDOCAINE

Dose = 1.0 mg/kg IV bolus

	Weight of patient	Dose for IV bolus
	10 kg	10 mg
	20 kg	20 mg
	30 kg	30 mg
	Adult	50-100 mg

IV Infusion Dose of Lidocaine = 20-50 μg/kg/min
  Mix 120 mg in 100 ml of D_5W = 1200 μg/ml
    Then 1 drop/kg/min = 20 μg/kg/min (initial rate) 2.5 drops/kg/min = 50 μg/kg/min (maximum rate)

Weight of patient	How to mix	Initial rate*	Maximum rate
10 kg	120 mg in 100 D_5W	10 drops/min	25 drops/min
20 kg	120 mg in 100 D_5W	20 drops/min	50 drops/min
30 kg	120 mg in 100 D_5W	30 drops/min	75 drops/min
Adult	1000 mg in 250 D_5W	30 drops/min = 2 mg/min	4 mg/min

DOPAMINE

IV Infusion Dose = 2-20 μg/kg/min
  Mix 6 mg × body weight (kg) in 100 ml of D_5W
    Then 1 drop/min = 1.0 μg/kg/min
        5 drops/min = 5 μg/kg/min (= usual initial rate)
        20 drops/min = 20 μg/kg/min (= maximum rate)

Weight of patient	How to mix	Initial rate*	Maximum rate
10 kg	60 mg in 100 D_5W	5 drops/min (50 μg/min)	20 drops/min
20 kg	120 mg in 100 D_5W	5 drops/min (100 μg/min)	20 drops/min
30 kg	180 mg in 100 D_5W	5 drops/min (150 μg/min)	20 drops/min
Adult	(80 kg) 200 mg in 250 D_5W	30 drops/min (400 μg/min)	Titrate up

NOTE—when infusing the small quantities of drug required for pediatric IV infusions, it is essential to use an infusion pump to ensure accuracy.
From Grauer K, Cavallaro DL: ACLS: Certification preparation and comprehensive review, ed 2, St Louis, 1987, Mosby–Year Book.

Continued.

Table 10-6   Pediatric Drug Dosages—cont'd

ISOPROTERENOL

IV Infusion Dose = 0.1-1.0 μg/kg/min
   Mix 0.6 mg × body weight (kg) in 100 ml of D_5W.
      Then 1 drop/min = 0.1 μg/kg/min; Titrate to effect

Weight of patient	How to mix	Initial rate*	Maximum rate
10 kg	6 mg in 100 D_5W	1 drop/min (= 0.1 μg/kg/min)	10 drops/min
20 kg	12 mg in 100 D_5W	1 drop/min (= 0.1 μg/kg/min)	10 drops/min
30 kg	18 mg in 100 D_5W	1 drop/min (= 0.l μg/kg/min)	10 drops/min
Adult	1 mg in 250 D_5W	30 drop/min (2 μg/min)	20 μg/min

SODIUM BICARBONATE

Respiratory failure is the most common cause of cardiac arrest in children. The most important treatment priority is to improve ventilation, *not* to administer sodium bicarbonate. Epinephrine is the drug of choice for the arrested heart. Sodium bicarbonate should be considered only if the arrest is prolonged or if the patient was known to have an underlying metabolic acidosis.
   Dose = 1 mEq/kg (50 ml of 8.4% solution = 50 mEq)

Weight of patient	Dose (IV or intraosseous)
10 kg	10 mEq (⅕ ampule, 10 ml)
20 kg	20 mEq (⅖ ampule, 20 ml)
30 kg	30 mEq (⅗ ampule, 30 ml)
Adult	50-100 mEq (1-2 ampules)

DEFIBRILLATION

Dose = 2 J/kg for initial countershock
   If this is unsuccessful, double the dose (to 4 J/kg) and repeat × 2

Weight of patient	Initial shock (2nd shock-3rd shock)
10 kg	20 J (then 40 J- 40 J)
20 kg	20 J (then 80 J-80 J)
30 kg	60 J (then 120 J-120 J)
Adult	200 J (then 300 J-360 J)

OXYGEN

Inadequate oxygenation is the most common cause of cardiac arrest in children! Oxygen should be administered to all children exhibiting cardiac arrest even if measured arterial oxygen tension is high.

---

sponses should be carefully assessed particularly neurological status, cardiac and respiratory functioning, and renal output. Assess the child for complications of CPR, such as fluid and electrolyte imbalance, acid-base imbalances, cardiac dysrhythmias, cardiac tamponade, pneumothorax or hemothorax, abdominal distention, or liver laceration.

Termination of Resuscitation[11]

The difficult decision to end resuscitation is made by the physician in charge of the team and/or the attending physician in collaboration with the parents. Consideration is given to the child's cerebral and cardiovascular status, along with the precipitating event and/or underlying diagnosis. For example, vigorous efforts may continue if the arrest was precipitated by cold water submersion and/or hypothermia.

If there is a low probability of recovery or high probability of survival with significant disability, efforts may be stopped. Ominous signs include coma, absence of spontaneous respirations and brainstem reflexes, and fixed, dilated pupils for 20 to 30 minutes.

If resuscitation fails, the parents will require much staff support. Accurate and timely information during the code should be provided. If possible, let the parents see the child during the code. This reassures them that everything is being done. When all activity ceases, the family will need time to spend with the child. The nurse should stay with them. There may not be a need for dialogue, but the presence of the nurse is supportive.

Before parents leave the hospital, it is important to discuss feelings and physical events that will ensue in subsequent days and weeks. Refer them to available support groups.

Staff responses are also intense. No one is ever prepared for a child's death. Feelings of helplessness and guilt usually prevail. Members of the staff and the pediatric code team also need to be supported after the crisis.

PSYCHOSOCIAL CONSIDERATIONS

A cardiac arrest is one of the most stressful events that can occur. It is stressful for all involved: the patient, the family, and the staff. Emotional support will be needed by all persons involved.

Surviving the event has many psychological effects on the patient. These patients experience fear, anxiety, anger, depression, tenseness, sleeplessness, irritability, memory lapses, violent dreams, and an uneasy feeling of uniqueness.[8,9,15]

Patients who recover from a cardiac arrest describe several common experiences.[9,15,26,27] Patients relate having a feeling of separation of mind and body, where the mind was able to observe the resuscitation efforts. This is known as *otoscopic observation.* Many patients describe the mind as traveling through a long dark tunnel with a bright light at the end. Occasionally patients report meeting a dead friend, relative, or deity while journeying toward the light.

As the resuscitative event restores the patient's cardiovascular function, patients relate a feeling of traveling back toward their bodies, oftentimes associated with pain and distress. Many later express wanting to tell the physician to stop the code. Many wish to return to the peace of the bright light and long for the loved one or friend who served as their guide. Other patients relate the near-death episode as a frightening experience. They report sights of hell, strange creatures, feelings of doom, helplessness, and loneliness.

All patients experience the reality of their own mortality. Patients and families have fears of arrest recurrence.

Nursing intervention should address the needs of the cardiac arrest patient. During the code, the patient can be addressed and the activities explained. When the patient regains consciousness, emotional support should be provided. Once the patient has been stabilized, the resuscitation should be discussed with the patient. Many patients do not wish to discuss their near-death episode for fear of being thought as crazy.

Families need information about loved ones during the cardiac arrest. They feel lost and helpless. Information helps the family gain perspective. If family members witnessed the cardiac arrest, they may feel guilty that they did not or could not do more. They need emotional support as well.

Regardless if the patient is revived or not, the staff participating in the code also needs emotional support.

PATIENT AND FAMILY TEACHING

Teaching CPR and the use of the emergency medical system should be directed to all individuals but especially to those who are at risk. Family members should be taught to recognize apnea, impending MI, and other events that can lead to cardiac arrest. Family members should be taught CPR procedures and should be encouraged to take the American Heart Association or American Red Cross course.

HOME HEALTH CARE CONSIDERATIONS

Many emergencies occur in the home. When the cardiac patient, critical care patient, or other at-risk patients are cared for in the home, the family should be able to perform CPR, should know what the patient's drugs are used for, and should write down all emergency phone numbers and keep them posted by the phone.

The decision to initiate or not to initiate CPR must be made before going home. If the decision is made to make the patient a no code, a DNR order, written by the physician, is necessary. Unless there is a written order to the contrary, CPR must be initiated in cardiac arrest situations.

REFERENCES

1. American Heart Association: Standards and guidelines for cardiopulmonary resuscitation and emergency cardiac care, *JAMA* 255:1843, 1986.
2. *American Heart Association: Textbook of advanced cardiac life support,* Dallas, 1987, The Association.
3. Baker FJ, Strauss R, Walter JJ: Cardiac arrest. In Rosen P, Baker FJ, Braen GR et al: *Emergency medicine,* Vol 1, St Louis, 1983, Mosby–Year Book.
4. Bedell SE, Pelle D, Maher PL et al: Do-not-resuscitate orders for critically ill patients in the hospital: how are they used and what is their impact? *JAMA* 256:233, 1986.
5. Bishop RL, Weisfeldt ML: Sodium bicarbonate administration during cardiac arrest: effect on arterial pH, Pco_2, and osmolality, *JAMA* 235:506, 1976.
6. Caldwell G et al: Simple mechanical methods of cardioversion: a defense of the precordial thump and cough version, *Br Med J* 291:627, 1985.
7. Emergency Cardiac Care Committee and Subcommittees, American Heart Association: Guidelines for cardiopulmonary resuscitation and emergency cardiac care, *JAMA* 268:2171, 1992.
8. Featherston RG: Care of the sudden cardiac death survivors: the aberrant cardiac patient, *Heart Lung* 17(3):242, 1988.
9. Finkelmeier BA, Kenwood NJ, Summers C: Psychologic ramifications of survival from sudden cardiac death, *Crit Care Nurs Q* 7(2):71, 1984.
10. Frost E: Tracing the tracheostomy, *Ann Otol Rhinol Laryngol* 85:618, 1976.
11. Gildea J: A crisis plan for a pediatric code, *Am J Nurs* 86(5):557, 1986.
12. Goodwin BA: Pediatric resuscitation, *Crit Care Nurs Q* 10(4):69, 1988.
13. Grauer K, Cavallaro D: *ACLS, Certification preparation and a comprehensive review,* ed 3, St Louis, 1992, Mosby–Year Book.
14. Gulanick M: Upgrading resuscitation procedures, *Focus Crit Care* 10(3):24, 1983.
15. Guzzetta CE, Dossey BM: Cardiovascular nursing: holistic practice, St Louis, 1992, Mosby–Year Book.
16. Hazinski MF: Reducing calculation errors in drug dosages: the pediatric critical information sheet, *Pediatr Nurs* 12(2):132, 1986.
17. Hazinski MF: *Nursing care of the critically ill child,* ed 2, St Louis, 1992, Mosby–Year Book.
18. Holloway NM: The updated ACLS standards. I. The lethal dysrhythmias, *Crit Care Nurse* 7(3):18, 1987.
19. Jones S, Bugg AM: LEAD drugs for cardiac arrest, *Nursing '88* 18(1):34, 1988.
20. Kouwenhoven WB, Jude JR, Knickerbocker GG: Closed-chest cardiac massage, *JAMA* 173:1064, 1960.
21. Lewis FR, Trunkey DD: Pupillary reactivity in circulatory arrest, *Surg* 95:380, 1984.
22. Lewis JK, Menter MG, Eshelman SJ et al: Outcome of pediatric resuscitation, *Ann Emerg Med* 12:297, 1983.
23. Lowenstein SR, Sabyan EM, Lassen CF et al: Benefits of training physicians in advanced cardiac life support, *Chest* 89:512, 1986.

24. Miles SH, Cranford R, Schultz AL: The do-not-resuscitate order in a teaching hospital, *Ann Intern Med* 96:660, 1982.

25. Miller J, Trech D, Horwitz L et al: The precordial thump, *Ann Emerg Med* 13:791, 1984.

26. Moody R: *Life after life,* Atlanta, 1975, Mockingbird Books.

27. Oakes AR: Near death events and critical care nursing, *Topics Clin Nurs* 3:61, 1981.

28. Persons CB: *Critical care procedures and protocols,* Philadelphia, 1987, JB Lippincott.

29. Rosen P, Baker FJ, Braen GR et al: *Emergency Medicine,* Vol I, St Louis, 1983, Mosby–Year Book.

30. Rosenberg NM: Pediatric cardiopulmonary arrest in the emergency department, *Am J Emerg Med* 2:497, 1984.

31. Rudnitsky GS, Cahill LJ: Pediatric and neonatal resuscitation, *Topics Emerg Med* 11(1):68, 1989.

32. Scaff B, Munson R, Hastings DF: Cardiopulmonary resuscitation at a community hospital with a family practice residency, *J Family Practice* 18:561, 1984.

33. Tilkian AG, Conover MB: Cardiopulmonary resuscitation. In Tilkian AG, Daily EK: *Cardiovascular procedures,* St Louis, 1986, Mosby–Year Book.

34. Vallerand AH, Deglin JH: *Drug guide for critical care and emergency nursing,* Philadelphia, 1991, WB Saunders.

35. Vertiglia WJ, Hamilton GC: Electrical interventions in cardiopulmonary resuscitation, defibrillation, *Emerg Med Clin N Am* 1:515, 1983.

CHAPTER 11

Intraaortic Balloon Counterpulsation

Objectives

After completing this chapter, the reader will be able to:

- Differentiate between inflation and deflation of the intraaortic balloon (IAB) in relationship to the mechanical cardiac cycle.
- Discuss the primary and secondary effects of intraaortic balloon counterpulsation (IABC).
- Identify the types of patients who may require IABC, the contraindications of IABC, and the complications of IABC.
- Describe the nursing assessment of potential complications associated with IABC.
- Formulate the nursing diagnoses, patient outcomes, and nursing interventions specific to patients undergoing IABC.
- List the steps in the insertion and care of the central lumen of the IAB and the initial setup of the intraaortic balloon pump (IABP).
- Describe the appropriate steps in triggering, timing, and troubleshooting of the IABP.
- Discuss the weaning process and the steps in the removal of the percutaneous IAB.
- Describe the possible psychosocial responses and teaching needs of patients undergoing the stress of IABC.
- Differentiate between pediatric and adult IABC patient care requirements and precautions.

THE CONCEPT OF IABC

Currently, intraaortic balloon counterpulsation (IABC) is the most widely used temporary circulatory assist device. The *intraaortic balloon* is an inflatable plastic device mounted on a vascular catheter that is usually inserted percutaneously through the common femoral artery. The balloon is positioned in the descending thoracic aorta with its tip just distal to the left subclavian. The bottom of the balloon is positioned above the renal arteries (Fig. 11-1). Once inserted, the balloon is attached to the intraaortic balloon pump (IABP) console, which monitors both the ECG and arterial pressure. The console shuttles a gas, usually helium, in and out of the IAB, resulting in balloon counterpulsation. *Counterpulsation* refers to the alternating inflation and deflation of the intraaortic balloon during diastole and systole, respectively. The console relies on a trigger event, most commonly the R wave, to identify the beginning of the next cardiac cycle and deflate the balloon. Since there is a normal physiological electrical mechanical delay, the intraarterial waveform is used for timing of inflation and deflation.

The balloon is inflated in diastole and deflated in systole (Fig. 11-2). The inflation and deflation of the balloon provides for diastolic augmentation and systolic unloading (Fig. 11-3). *Diastolic augmentation* is the resultant elevation of peak diastolic pressure because of inflation of the intraaortic balloon. The balloon is rapidly inflated at the beginning of diastole, when the aortic valve closes. When this occurs, the balloon displaces a volume of blood equal to the balloon volume of 40 cc. This raises the diastolic pressure in the aorta, and some of the displaced blood volume passes down the coronary arteries. Since the majority of coronary artery blood flow occurs during diastole, the heart greatly benefits from inflation of the balloon. Increased coronary blood flow improves myocardial oxygen supply, thereby improving ventricular contractility in the ischemic regions.

Systolic unloading is the resultant decrease in peak systolic pressure because of deflation of the intraaortic balloon. Just before the beginning of systole, rapid balloon deflation occurs, creating a "vacuum" effect. This lowers the systolic pressure in the aorta and makes it easier for the left ventricle to empty. This workload reduction of the left ventricle is called *decreasing the afterload* and reduces the myocardial oxygen requirements.

The primary beneficial effects of IABC are: (1) improved coronary artery flow and myocardial oxygen supply because of diastolic augmentation and (2) decreased

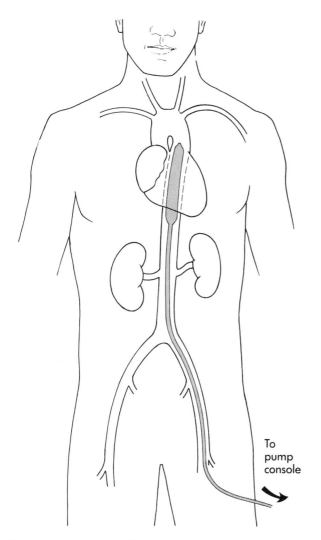

Fig. 11-1   Intraaortic balloon positioned in the descending aorta distal to the left subclavian artery and above the renal arteries.

afterload and myocardial oxygen demand because of systolic unloading. Secondary effects include an increased cardiac output and cardiac index, decreased heart rate, decreased pulmonary artery diastolic and pulmonary artery wedge pressures, improved peripheral perfusion, and increased urine output.

INDICATIONS FOR IABC

Specific indications for use of the IABC include support of the patient:

- With a failing heart in post-MI (cardiogenic) shock.[1,4]
- With an acute anterior infarction, to contain the area of injury.
- With mechanical complications of an acute MI, such as papillary muscle rupture, ventricular septal rupture, or acute mitral regurgitation.
- Who is preoperative, in the coronary care unit, who continues to have unstable angina pectoris resistant to β-blockers, nitrates, and calcium antagonists.

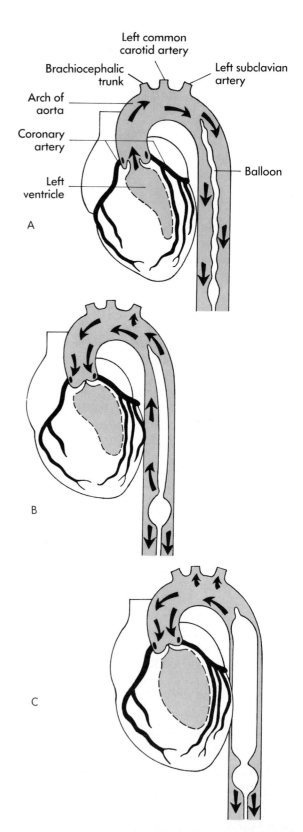

Fig. 11-2   **A,** During systole the balloon is deflated, which facilitates ejection of the blood into the periphery where systemic arterial resistant vessels are perfused. **B,** In early diastole, the balloon begins to inflate. **C,** In late diastole, the balloon is totally inflated, which augments pressure in the proximal aorta and increases the coronary perfusion pressure with the end results of increased coronary and cerebral blood flow.

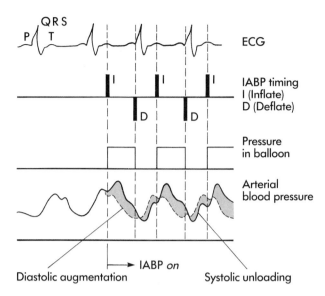

Fig. 11-3 Timing of the IABP. Top tracing shows ECG. Second tracing marks balloon inflation and deflation. Third tracing shows pressure in the balloon itself. Final tracing represents intraarterial blood pressure, showing the diastolic augmentation and systolic unloading. (From Elefteriades JA, Geha AS: *House officer guide to ICU care,* Rockville, Md, 1985, Aspen.)

- After open heart surgery, to assist a weak heart after coming off cardiopulmonary bypass.
- With hemodynamic decompensation before heart transplantation.
- At high risk during coronary arteriography or other surgical procedures.
- Receiving a percutaneous transluminal coronary angioplasty or thrombolytic therapy.[3]
- In noncardiac shock.
- Requiring circulatory assistance, in combination with extracorporeal membrane oxygenation (ECMO) or venoarterial bypass (VAB) pumping.[5]

CONTRAINDICATIONS OF IABC

Contraindications for IABC include the following:
- Irreversible brain damage, because of the poor prognosis of the patient.
- Chronic end-stage heart disease.
- Advanced or terminal neoplastic disease.
- Aortic regurgitation, since inflation of the balloon in diastole may increase the regurgitation from the aorta to the left ventricle, possibly overwhelming the ventricle.
- Dissecting aortic or thoracic aneurysm because of danger of passing the balloon.
- Peripheral vascular disease that limits insertion of the balloon.

COMPLICATIONS OF IABC

During percutaneous insertion of the IAB, some of the following problems may occur: dislodgement of athero-

sclerotic plaques or thrombi, inability to insert the IAB because of tortuous vessels, and difficulty in finding the femoral artery because of lack of a strong femoral pulse. Some of the complications that can occur during IABC are as follows:
- Asymptomatic vascular complication.
- Limb ischemia.
- Thromboembolism.
- Obstruction of major arteries.
- Compartment syndrome.

ASSESSMENT

When performing an ongoing assessment of the patient receiving IABC, in addition to the routine assessment, the nurse will need to:
- Measure the respiratory rate for signs of tachypnea that could be caused by sepsis.
- Auscultate for decreased breath sounds resulting from atelectasis that is caused by restriction in ability to elevate head of bed >30 degrees in presence of balloon catheter.
- Assess for temperature differences in legs. Be alert for cool legs or toes with pain, decreased sensation, loss of motor function, pallor, cyanosis, mottling, or poor capillary refill, indicating limb ischemia. Grade capillary refill as immediate (<3 sec) or delayed.
- Palpate or use a doppler to assess posterior tibial, dorsalis pedalis, and popliteal pulses. Mark location with felt tip marker. Weak or absent pulses will occur because of peripheral embolism, transient arterial spasm, or impedance of blood flow in femoral artery by balloon or thrombus.
- Assess left radial pulse (Allen's test) (Fig. 11-4). Weak or absent pulse may be caused by inappropriate positioning of IAB with possible obstruction of left subclavian artery.
- Assess ulnar arterial pulse. Weak or absent pulse with inadequate perfusion to hand may be caused by occlusion from radial artery catheter.
- Apply blood pressure cuff around ankle and use a doppler to measure the systolic ankle blood pressure. Use either posterior tibial or dorsalis pedis pressures. Record the ratio of the ankle BP to the brachial BP (ankle-arm index). Arterial occlusion may exist if the ratio is less than 1.0.
- Ask patient if back or chest pain exists. This could be caused by aortic dissection, thoracic or abdominal aneurysm, or MI.
- Monitor for increase in heart rate or decrease in cardiac output caused by sepsis or cardiovascular deterioration (Table 11-1 shows the expected effects of IABC on failing heart).
- Observe for acute change in mean arterial pressure caused by possible problems with timing or fluid volume depletion.
- Note increase in pulmonary artery wedge pressure

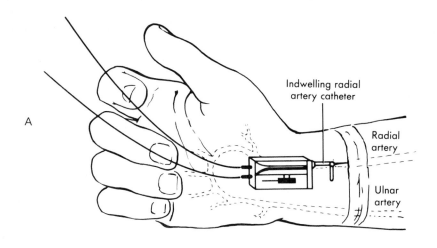

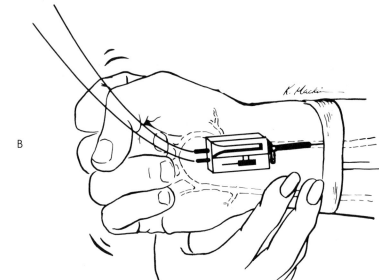

Fig. 11-4 Allen's test for radial artery patency when indwelling monitoring catheter is in place in radial artery. **A,** Catheter is in place in radial artery. **B,** Patient makes fist while examiner manually compresses ulnar artery or positions hand in fist if patient is unable to cooperate. **C,** Examiner maintains compression on ulnar artery while patient opens fist. Hand should flush and resume pink color if blood perfusion through radial artery is adequate with catheter in place. (From Quaal SJ: *Comprehensive intraaortic balloon pumping,* St Louis, 1992, Mosby–Year Book.)

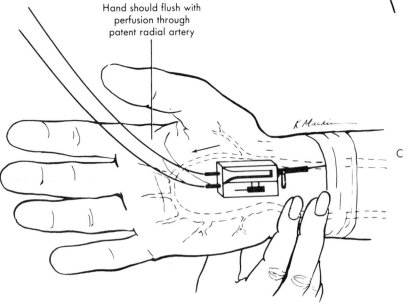

Table 11-1 Effects of Intraaortic Balloon Counterpulsation on the Failing Heart

IABC decreases	IABC increases
Heart rate	Diastolic aortic pressure
Preload (left ventricular end-diastolic pressure)	Stroke volume
Afterload (aortic end-diastolic pressure)	Ejection fraction
Myocardial oxygen consumption	Cardiac output and index
Left atrial pressure	Coronary perfusion pressure
Pulmonary artery wedge pressure	Peripheral tissue perfusion
Pulmonary artery diastolic pressure	Urine output
Systolic pressure	
Systemic vascular resistance	

caused by possible fluid volume overload or cardiovascular deterioration.

- Observe ECG monitor for cardiac dysrhythmias. Dysrhythmias will necessitate more frequent assessment of timing of IABC.
- Check for decreased mentation.
- Ask if patient has a tingling sensation, pain, or numbness of catheterized extremity; such sensations could be caused by neuropathy.
- Measure hourly urine outputs. A decrease below 20 to 30 ml/hr may indicate inadequate cardiac output or volume depletion.
- Test urine for hematuria. This may be caused by excessive coagulation therapy.
- Observe for flank pain, elevated BUN and creatinine levels, and acute drop in urine output. This may be indicative of catheter migration down aorta with obstruction of renal arteries or of presence of renal artery emboli.
- Measure temperature, observing for fever from catheter-related sepsis.
- Observe patient for chills from sepsis.
- Evaluate serum laboratory results for hemolysis, anemia, and thrombocytopenia caused by destruction of formed blood elements by balloon movements.
- Check for elevated levels of creatinine kinase (CK) from 1000 to 5000 IU. This may be a sign of compartment syndrome and muscle damage.
- Check lab reports for leukocytosis. This may indicate catheter-related sepsis.
- Check catheter insertion site dressing for excessive bleeding caused by coagulation therapy.
- Test stools and NG drainage for guaiac positive results caused by coagulation therapy or stress ulcers.

- Ask if patient has any abdominal pain possibly caused by mesenteric artery occlusion.
- Measure patient's girth for abdominal distension.
- Palpate abdomen for rigidity.
- Auscultate for decreased bowel sounds, indicative of bowel ischemia secondary to emboli.
- Take thigh and calf measurements, observe for edema, and palpate extremity for tenseness to rule out compartment syndrome.
- Ask patient about complaints of continuous limb pressure and deep throbbing pain, indicative of compartment syndrome.
- Determine if limb pain is induced with passive stretching of affected muscle.
- Observe skin for petechiae caused by coagulation therapy.
- Observe for pale skin color, indicative of decreased perfusion and inadequate cardiac output.
- Observe leg and foot for pale, shiny skin and loss of hair, and signs of decreased perfusion.
- Observe IAB catheter insertion site for purulent drainage.
- Observe for skin breakdown especially in affected extremity, caused by immobility of extremity with balloon catheter.
- Assess patient for feelings of hopelessness possibly caused by inability to be weaned from IABC.
- Assess patient's stress, anxiety level, and fear of death.
- Observe for irritability, confusion, and other signs of sleep deprivation that can be caused by frequent manipulation of patient and presence of many environmental noises preventing sleep.
- Check for disorientation and other signs of sensory overload caused by excessive manipulation, pain, noise, and discomfort.

NURSING DIAGNOSIS

Possible nursing diagnoses for patients with IABC include the following:

- Decreased peripheral tissue perfusion distal to catheter insertion site related to obstruction from balloon catheter.
- High risk for decreased tissue perfusion related to clot formation or arterial damage secondary to presence of balloon, catheter, sheath, or graft.
- Decreased tissue perfusion related to gas embolism secondary to balloon leak.
- Disruption of platelet integrity related to mechanical trauma of balloon inflation.
- High risk for blood volume deficit related to bleeding secondary to anticoagulation therapy and coagulopathies.

PATIENT OUTCOMES

The following are examples of possible outcomes for the patient with IABC:

Patient evidences:

- Lungs clear and equal to bases on auscultation.
- Normal ABGs for patient's inspired oxygen level.
- Clear mentation with orientation to time, person, place.
- Decreased preload or left ventricular end-diastolic volume as shown by decreased pulmonary artery wedge pressures and pulmonary artery diastolic pressures.
- Decreased assisted aortic end-diastolic pressure (afterload reduction).
- Adequate urinary output of > 30 ml/hr.
- Normal mean arterial pressure of 70 to 90 mm Hg.
- Decreasing reliance on inotropic and vasopressor agents.
- Normal 12-lead ECG and normal sinus rhythm of heart rate 60 to 100 beats/min.
- Minimal bleeding at balloon catheter insertion site.
- Adequate pulses in all extremities through palpation or doppler.
- Normal color, appearance, turgor, capillary refill, temperature, and sensation in all extremities and skin pressure points.
- Positive Allen's test.
- Assisted arterial pressure wave shows balloon inflation at the dicrotic notch and balloon deflation before next systolic event.

TRIGGERING AND TIMING OF THE IABP

The *trigger* is the signal used by the IABP to identify the beginning of the next cardiac cycle and deflate the IAB. Most IABPs now have five choices of trigger. These are the following:

1. *ECG:* The R wave of the ECG is the trigger event.
2. *Pacer AV:* The ventricular spike of an AV sequential pacemaker is the trigger event. This should be used only when the ECG trigger is unobtainable in the presence of an AV pacer and 100% paced rhythm.
3. *Pacer V:* The ventricular spike of the ventricular pacemaker is the trigger event. This should be used only when the ECG trigger is unobtainable in the presence of a ventricular pacer and a 100% paced rhythm.
4. *Pressure:* The upslope of the arterial pressure waveform is the trigger event.
5. *Internal:* The IAB is inflated and deflated asynchronously at a preset rate determined by the IAB frequency switch. This is used only when the patient does not have a cardiac cycle, such as during cardiopulmonary bypass.

Timing is the inflation and deflation of the IABP in concert with the mechanical cardiac cycle. When the balloon inflates and deflates, the configuration of the arterial wave-

Text continued on p. 270.

Skill 11-1   Insertion of the IAB

Insertion of the IAB may be performed at the bedside, in the cardiac catherization laboratory, or in the operating room. The most common method of insertion is percutaneously through the right or left femoral artery using the Seldinger technique. There are alternate means of inserting the IAB surgically, such as through a graft sewn to the side of the femoral artery. Depending on its availability, fluoroscopy may or may not be used to determine the position of the balloon.

EQUIPMENT AND SUPPLIES

- Intraaortic balloon catheters
- IABP console
- Transducer and pressure tubing setup (for dual lumen IAB)
- IV poles, blood, and IV fluids
- Antibiotics, anticoagulants, analgesics, and sedatives
- Sterile gloves, gowns, drapes, masks, and caps
- Percutaneous insertion set
- Surgical instrument tray and suture material
- Povidone-iodide solution and ointment
- Xylocaine and syringes
- Occlusive tape and sterile dressings
- Protective underpads
- Sterile basin and sterile saline
- ECG monitor, defibrillator, and pacemaker
- Emergency intubation equipment and emergency drug cart
- Fluoroscopy equipment

NURSING INTERVENTIONS

1. Apply face mask and wash hands.
2. Prepare transducer and pressure monitoring setup for monitoring of arterial pressure.
3. Turn IABP console on (Skill 11-2).
4. Examine the patient's 12-lead ECG to determine which lead maximizes the R wave and minimizes the other wave forms. Establish direct ECG to IABP console.
5. Put on gown, mask, and cap.
6. Assist physician in shaving, cleansing, and draping the insertion site.
7. Check distal pulses of extremities (pedal, popliteal, and posterior tibial).
8. Mark pedal and posterior tibial pulse sites with a marker. This simplifies assessment of pulses postinsertion.
9. Open sterile trays and supplies.
10. After IAB is inserted, connect pressure tubing to central lumen (Skill 11-3).
11. Set appropriate inflation at beginning of diastole (Skill 11-4).
12. Set appropriate deflation before the next systole.
13. Initiate IABC.
14. Assist with suturing the catheter to the skin.
15. Apply povidone-iodide solution to site, according to agency policy.
16. Don sterile gloves and apply occlusive dressing over insertion site.
17. Assess distal pulses frequently and notify physician if significant changes occur.
18. Check that chest x-ray has been done to verify position of the IAB. Tip of the IAB should be at the level of second or third intercostal space.

Note: Management of the IABP console may or may not be a nursing function. Consult hospital standards and policies.

Skill 11-2   Initial Setup of IABP

EQUIPMENT AND SUPPLIES

- Intraaortic balloon pump (Datascope System 90 will be used as example)
- Power source
- ECG cable
- Arterial line cable
- IAB catheter with 6-foot extender

NURSING INTERVENTIONS

1. Establish power by plugging power cord into AC outlet (omit for startup in portable operation). Turn rear panel *main* switch to *on.*
2. Pull and turn *trigger select* switch to *ECG.* Datascope System 90 will automatically perform system check. Alarm lights will illuminate and then each illuminate for 2 seconds in the following order:
   - *Trigger*
   - *Gas loss*
   - *IAB catheter*
   - *Pneumatic drive*
   - *Low helium tank*

   When check is complete, *System test OK* will appear on monitor screen.
3. Establish gas pressure by opening helium tank in rear of IABP.
4. Set initial control settings on front panel. Begin by setting *IAB frequency* at *1:1.*
5. Set *IAB augmentation* to *Min.*
6. Set *IAB inflation* at midpoint.
7. Set *IAB deflation* at midpoint.
8. Set *Delay marker* at *Preset.*
9. Check that rear panel controls are set the following ways:
   - *Timing Auto*
   - *IAB fill Auto*
   - *Slow gas loss alarm—On.*

10. Establish ECG by plugging *ECG cable* into *ECG* on rear of Datascope System 90.
11. Establish pressure. Attach arterial line to Datascope compatible transducer and plug into *pressure transducer* of System 90. *XXX* will flash on monitor screen next to *sys.*
12. Zero transducer. Open transducer to air. Push *zero* button for 3 seconds. Note: —two audible clicks and spike on pressure trace.
    —mean pressure only now displayed on monitor screen.
13. Adjust initial timing. Adjust *IAB inflation* and *IAB deflation* controls to position intensified portion of arterial waveform to correspond to diastole as shown below.

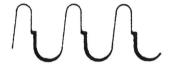

14. Attach IAB catheter with 6-foot extender to safety chamber.
15. Depress *IAB fill* for 1 second. *Auto filling* message will appear on monitor screen. Wait until message clears before proceeding.
16. Initiate IABP. Depress *assist/standby.*
17. Rotate *IAB augmentation* clockwise until IAB augmentation is optimal. Observe that augmentation occurs during diastole.
18. Fine tune inflation and deflation point for optimal augmentation and unloading as necessary (see Skill 11-4 on timing the IABP).
19. Depress *delay marker.* Observe intensified mark occurs at dicrotic notch. All arterial pressure values now appear on the monitor screen.
20. Depress *aug alarm set.* Adjust if desired.

Skill 11-3   Care of the Central Lumen of the Intraaortic Balloon

IAB catheters may be single or dual lumen. The single lumen catheter is a smaller French size and may be beneficial in reducing limb ischemia in patients with a smaller vasculature. The dual lumen catheter is most commonly used. It allows for insertion over a J-tipped guide wire and continuous pressure monitoring from the tip of the IAB.

EQUIPMENT AND SUPPLIES

- IV heparin flush solution according to hospital policy for maintaining arterial line patency
- Arterial pressure monitoring apparatus with 3 ml/hr continuous flush device
- Transducer for arterial pressure monitoring

NURSING INTERVENTIONS

1. Aspirate 3 ml initially from central lumen before making a fluid to fluid connection between the pressure tubing and the central lumen. Use careful and cautious technique to prevent thrombus or air from embolizing off the tip of the catheter. Such an embolus could potentially enter the carotid or coronary arteries from the aortic arch.
2. Do not pulsate the IAB when manipulating the central aortic pressure line or central lumen of the IAB.

3. Do not manually flush the central aortic pressure line or central lumen with a syringe.
4. Fast forward flush once every hour using the 3 ml/hr flush device to maintain patency of the central aortic line.
5. Always aspirate 3 ml initially if the central aortic pressure line or central lumen becomes dampened. Should resistance be met on aspiration, consider the lumen to be occluded. Discontinue use of the central aortic pressure line and central lumen by placing a sterile Luer Lok syringe on the port.
6. Perform ABG sampling cautiously with careful technique according to hospital policy.
7. Troubleshoot the central aortic pressure line with the same considerations as that of a standard arterial line.

Skill 11-4   Timing the IABP

EQUIPMENT AND SUPPLIES

- Intraaortic balloon pump
- Arterial line connection to IABP monitor
- Clear ECG signal on monitor

NURSING INTERVENTIONS

1. Plan to check timing at least every 2 to 4 hours or if the following occur:
   - Dysrhythmias.
   - Triggering mode changes.
   - Cardiac index decreases.
   - Heart rate changes by 20%.
2. Review where systole and diastole begin on an arterial waveform (Fig. 11-5). Systole begins where the sharp upstroke begins. Diastole begins at the dicrotic notch, which represents aortic valve closure.
3. Determine when balloon inflation should occur by observing Fig. 11-5. The balloon is inflated at the onset of diastole (at the dicrotic notch) and deflated before the next systole.
4. Obtain a paper strip recording or have the machine console freeze the arterial waveform. The strip recording should appear similar to the one in Fig. 11-6.
5. Identify the following points on the ideal arterial pressure waveform of Fig. 11-7:
   - End-diastolic pressure.
   - Systolic pressure.
   - Dicrotic notch (balloon inflation begins).
   - Diastolic augmentation (peak diastolic pressure caused by balloon inflation).
   - Balloon-assisted end-diastolic pressure.
   - Balloon-assisted systolic pressure.

6. Assess the strip recording for the ideal balloon timing features. Compare to Fig. 11-6. Ensure that balloon inflation occurs at the dicrotic notch (C), the beginning of diastole. This should result in a sharp V configuration between the patient's systolic pressure (B) and diastolic augmentation (D).
7. Using the appropriate knob or slide, adjust inflation, creating a V appearance rather than a U shape (Fig. 11-8)
8. Ensure that the diastolic augmentation (D) is equal to or greater than the patient's systolic pressure (B).
9. Ensure that the balloon-assisted end-diastolic pressure (E) is less than the patient's end-diastolic pressure (A).
10. Ensure that the balloon-assisted systolic pressure (F) is lower than the patient's systolic pressure (B).

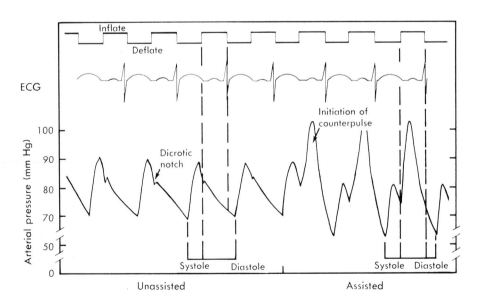

Fig. 11-5 Systole begins where the sharp upstroke begins. Diastole begins at the dicrotic notch, which represents aortic valve closure. The balloon is inflated at the onset of diastole (at the dicrotic notch) and deflated prior to the next systole, at the beginning of the QRS complex. (From Daily EK, Schroeder JS: *Techniques in bedside hemodynamic monitoring,* ed 4, St Louis, 1989, Mosby–Year Book.)

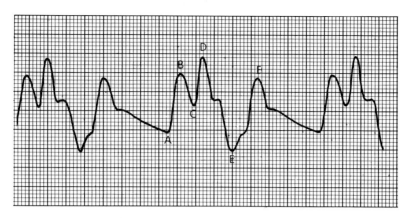

Fig. 11-6 Paper strip recording of arterial pressure waveform in 1:2 assist frequency. Note V wave appearance to dicrotic notch. (From Quaal S: *Comprehensive intraaortic balloon pumping,* St Louis, 1993, Mosby–Year Book.)

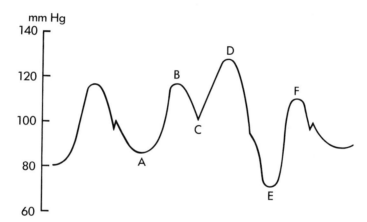

Fig. 11-7 Ideal alterations in arterial pressure waveform during initiation of intraaortic balloon counterpulsation. **A,** Patient's end-diastolic pressure. **B,** Patient's systolic pressure. **C,** Dicrotic notch (balloon inflation begins here). **D,** Diastolic augmentation (peak diastolic pressure caused by balloon inflation). **E,** Balloon assisted end-diastolic pressure. **F,** Balloon assisted systolic pressure.

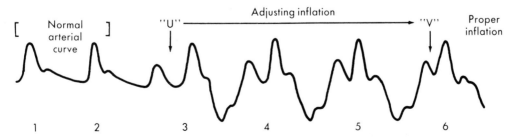

Fig. 11-8 Beats 1 and 2 represent normal arterial pressure curve. Beats 3, 4, 5, and 6 represent adjustment of inflation (adjusted to gradually occur earlier with each beat) so that U shape of dicrotic notch forms V, signifying proper inflation by beat 6. (From Quaal S: *Comprehensive intraaortic balloon pumping,* St Louis, 1993, Mosby–Year Book.)

form changes. The nurse can tell whether the IABP is properly timed by evaluating the waveform. The IABP should be set to inflate at the dicrotic notch and deflate before the next systole. Because inflation and deflation affect both systolic and diastolic pressures, the mean arterial pressure is a more accurate reflection of pressure changes. The mechanics of timing the IABP depends on the manufacturer. Regardless of how the IABP is timed, the anticipated alterations in the assisted arterial pressure waveform are the same. The timing of the inflation-deflation sequence must be precisely correlated with certain points on the arterial waveform. This ensures maximal hemodynamic benefit from counterpulsation.

Improper Timing

Improper timing of the IAB may result in a negative or less than therapeutic impact on patient hemodynamics. For example, if the balloon inflates during late systole, there will be an increase in afterload. Early inflation and late deflation are the timing errors that cause the most harm. Fig. 11-9 shows tracings of improper balloon-assisted arterial pressure waves juxtaposed on the patient's arterial tracing. Figs. 11-10 through 11-13 show how improper balloon-assisted arterial pressure waves appear on the IABP pressure monitor. The physiological effects of improper timing are included in each figure.

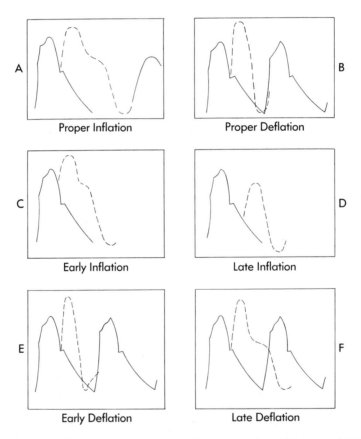

Fig. 11-9   The dotted line represents balloon assisted pressure waveform superimposed on the patient's normal arterial pressure waveform (solid line). **A,** Proper inflation—balloon inflates at dicrotic notch, appearing as sharp V configuration. **B,** Proper deflation—occurs prior to next systole. **C,** Early inflation—balloon inflates before (instead of at) dicrotic notch. **D,** Late inflation—the sharp V that should occur at the dicrotic notch takes on a U shape. **E,** A sharp drop in the waveform occurs after diastolic augmentation. **F,** Late deflation—diastolic augmentation appears as a widened arterial waveform. (Adapted from Yee BH, Zorb SL: *Cardiac critical care nursing,* Boston, 1986, Little, Brown, & Co.)

Inflation of the IAB prior to aortic
valve closure

Waveform Characteristics:
- Inflation of IAB prior to dicrotic notch
- Diastolic augmentation encroaches onto systole (may be unable to distinguish)

Physiological Effects:
- Potential premature closure of aortic valve
- Potential increased LVEDV and LVEDP or PAWP
- Increased left ventricular wall stress or afterload
- Aortic Regurgitation
- Increased MVO$_2$ demand

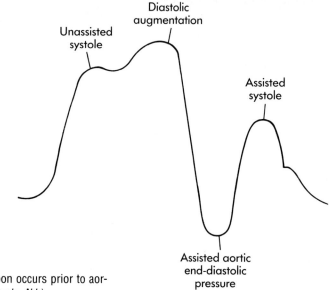

Fig. 11-10   Early inflation. Inflation of the intraaortic balloon occurs prior to aortic valve closure. *(Courtesy of Datascope Corporation, Montvale, NJ.)*

Inflation of the IAB markedly after
closure of the aortic valve

Waveform Characteristics:
- Inflation of the IAB after the dicrotic notch
- Absence of sharp V
- Suboptimal diastolic augmentation

Physiological Effects:
- Suboptimal coronary artery perfusion

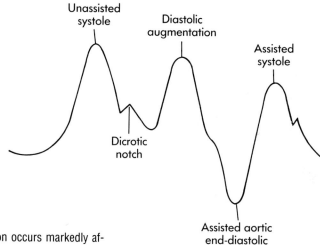

Fig. 11-11   Late inflation. Inflation of the intraaortic balloon occurs markedly after closure of the aortic valve. *(Courtesy of Datascope Corporation, Montvale, NJ.)*

Premature deflation of the IAB
during the diastolic phase

Waveform Characteristics:
- Deflation of IAB is seen as a sharp drop following diastolic augmentation
- Suboptimal diastolic augmentation
- Assisted aortic end-diastolic pressure may be equal to or greater than the unassisted aortic end-diastolic pressure
- Assisted systolic pressure may rise

Physiological Effects:
- Suboptimal coronary perfusion
- Potential for retrograde coronary and carotid blood flow
- Angina may occur as a result of retrograde coronary blood flow
- Suboptimal afterload reduction
- Increased MVO$_2$ demand

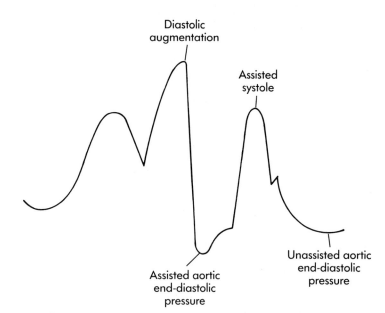

Fig. 11-12   Early deflation. Premature deflation of the intraaortic balloon occurs during the diastolic phase. *(Courtesy of Datascope Corporation, Montvale, NJ.)*

Deflation of the IAB late in diastolic phase as aortic valve is beginning to open

Waveform Characteristics:
- Assisted aortic end-diastolic pressure may be equal to the unassisted aortic end-diastolic pressure
- Rate of rise of assisted systole is prolonged
- Diastolic augmentation may appear widened

Physiological Effects:
- Afterload reduction is essentially absent
- Increased MVO_2 consumption due to the left ventricle ejecting against a greater resistance and a prolonged isovolumetric contraction phase
- IAB may impede left ventricular ejection and increase the afterload

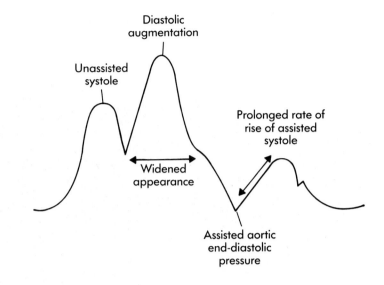

Fig. 11-13   Late deflation. Deflation of the intraaortic balloon occurs late in diastolic phase as aortic valve is beginning to open. *(Courtesy of Datascope Corporation, Montvale, NJ.)*

TROUBLESHOOTING IABC
Patient Conditions

1. *Decreased diastolic augmentation*
   - Refill IAB. Some balloons need to be refilled every 2 hours and when necessary, since helium can diffuse across the balloon membrane over time or leak out of tubing connections.
   - Check for IAB leak. Most leaks are caused by atherosclerotic plaques abrading the balloon.
   - Verify IAB position. A change in the position can alter the appearance of the augmented pressure waveform.
   - Assess for an improvement in patient's hemodynamic status causing the systolic and diastolic augmented pressures to move toward each other. The augmentation pressure wave may not exceed the patient's systolic peaks.
   - Assess for deterioration in patient's hemodynamic parameters (i.e., increased heart rate and decreased cardiac output) that can make it more difficult to achieve the appropriate augmented pressure.
   - Assess arterial pressure waveform for damping.
2. *Ventricular standstill or prolonged cardiac arrest*
   - Establish adequate trigger to ensure IAB movement during the arrest. The IAB should not remain immobile for more than 30 minutes in the same position to prevent thrombus formation.
   - Use ECG or arterial pressure trigger during CPR. Trigger will synchronize to chest compressions. If chest compressions do not provide an adequate trigger to allow balloon movement, the following settings may be used to move IAB:
     - *Trigger select*—internal.
     - *IAB frequency*—1:2.
   - *IAB augmentation*—to a level that movement of safety chamber balloon is still observed.
   - Readjust timing once ECG is reestablished.
3. *Ventricular fibrillation*
   - When the patient is defibrillated, no action dealing with the IABP is required. The IABP is electrically isolated and no danger of harm to unit or patient exists during defibrillation.
   - Assure safety by standing clear of IABP during defibrillation.
4. *Atrial fibrillation*
   - Irregularity of the R-R interval may pose a timing problem.
     - Use *auto* timing.
     - Adjust *IAB inflation* and *IAB deflation* controls to position the intensified portion of waveform to correspond to diastole.
     - The *IAB deflation* slide control may be moved to the extreme right allowing deflation of the balloon on the R wave. This prevents inflation during any systolic event, regardless of timing.
     - Investigate the need for verapamil or digoxin.
5. *Tachycardia greater than 120 beats/min*
   - Verify that helium is the fill gas being used rather than carbon dioxide because helium, a lighter gas, has a quicker response time.
   - Set assist frequency at 1:2. This increases the machine's ability to follow the rapid rate with increased effectiveness.
6. *Ventricular tachycardia*
   - Decrease assist frequency to 1:3. Ventricular tachycardia can usually trigger the IABP.
   - Initiate antidysrhythmic therapy or cardioversion.

7. *Ectopy*
   - No action required; treat the ectopy.
8. *Heart rate below 40 beats/min*
   - Check for poor electrode pickup. Adjust electrodes.
   - Increase rate of IABP.
9. *Patient's AV pacemaker is pacing over 110 beats/min or AV interval is <50 msec or >250 msec:*
   - Check for selection of wrong pacer trigger.
   - Adjust pacemaker settings.

Mechanical IABP Problems*

1. Arterial waveform artifact
   - Optimize arterial pressure tubing setup.
   - Use a damping device if necessary.
2. *Dampened arterial waveform*
   - Check for air bubble in transducer.
   - Fast flush arterial line.
   - Check to see if an excessive length of pressure tubing might be dampening the waveform.
3. *No trigger*
   - Check for wrong trigger mode. Change trigger select.
   - If ECG is trigger event, reattach or reposition electrodes. Pumping restarts automatically.
   - If amplitude of R wave is too low, change lead placement.
4. *Large leak in IAB*
   - Check for blood in tubing; if present, contact physician and prepare for removal of IAB. Balloon will have to be removed to prevent possibility of gas embolus or balloon entrapment.
5. *Small gas loss or slow leak in IAB*
   - Check for blood in tubing; check that fittings in pneumatic circuit are not loose.
   - If no blood in balloon, restart pumping by pushing *IAB fill.* Once IAB is filled, restart pumping.
   - Check for excess moisture in balloon catheter and extender. Dispel moisture and refill.
6. *IAB or extension tube is disconnected*
   - Reattach IAB or extension tube. Refill balloon by pushing *IAB fill.* Once IAB is filled, restart pumping.
7. *IAB kinked*
   - Check catheter and tubing. Straighten kink. Restart pumping.
8. *Component failures in pneumatic system*
   - Attempt to restart. If alarm repeats, contact service department.
9. *Low helium tank*
   - Make sure helium tank is turned on. If not, open helium tank.
   - Check to see if less than 24 fills are left in helium tank. If so, replace helium tank.

10. *Microprocessor or other electronic failure*
    - Turn IABP off and restart it. If *system test OK* message appears, initiate IABP. If *system test fails* displayed, contact service department.
11. *Hospital power failure or need to unplug for patient transport*
    - IABP will automatically switch to portable operation.

INTRAAORTIC BALLOON COUNTERPULSATION MONITORING CHECKLIST

In addition to routine ICU procedures and assessments, the patient with IABC will need the following special care. Before balloon catheter insertion:
- Record quality of peripheral pulses.
- Make note of temperature, color, and mobility of extremities.
- Record baseline vital signs and hemodynamic monitoring parameters.
- Obtain results of blood studies to rule out serious bleeding problems.

Immediately after balloon catheter insertion:
- Obtain portable chest x-ray.
- Ensure that head of bed is elevated less than 30 degrees.
- Ensure that affected extremity does not bend at knee or hip, which can move the balloon tip up in the aorta or kink the IAB catheter.
- Assess need for analgesics or sedation.
- Assess vascular sufficiency of extremities every 15 minutes for 1 hour, every 30 minutes the next 2 hours, and then every hour for the next 8 hours.
- Assess catheter dressing for excessive bleeding.

Every hour:
- Have patient flex feet to avoid venous stasis.
- Obtain vital signs and hemodynamic monitoring measurements including arterial pressures, left atrial pressure, pulmonary capillary wedge pressure, pulmonary artery pressures, and cardiac output or index.
- Compare hemodynamic measurement changes with expected hemodynamic effects listed in Table 11-1.
- With patient on 1:1 mode, record pressures in the following order: patient's systolic pressure/balloon-assisted end-diastolic pressure and diastolic augmentation/mean arterial pressure (e.g., 80/50 and 120/74).
- Measure and record urine output.

Every 2 hours:
- Perform range of motion to uninvolved limbs.
- Encourage coughing and deep breathing.
- Change patient's position, using a partial turn and avoiding movement of catheter site.
- Assess extremities for temperature, color, capillary refill, tingling, numbness, movement, and pain.
- Assess dorsalis pedalis, posterior tibial, popliteal, femoral, radial, and ulnar pulses bilaterally by palpation or doppler.
- If loss of any pulses, rule out IAB catheter migration.

---

*These brief troubleshooting instructions are based on the Datascope System 90 Intraaortic Balloon Pump.

- Assess respiratory rate, pattern, rhythm, and breath sounds.
- Verify correct IAB trigger event and timing every 2 to 4 hours and adjust inflation and deflation accordingly.
- Observe for diastolic augmentation (dependent on diastolic time) and afterload reduction every 2 to 4 hours.
- Observe, monitor, and document unassisted and assisted arterial waveforms every 2 to 4 hours (see section on documentation below).

Every 4 hours:
- Perform Allen's test.
- Assess neurological status.
- Assess for flank, back, or chest pain.

Every 8 hours:
- Guaiac or hematest nasogastric drainage, stool, and urine.
- Assess skin for petechiae or ecchymoses.

Every 24 hours:
- Obtain, record, and evaluate laboratory studies.
- Change balloon catheter dressing every 24 to 48 hours according to hospital policy (similar to changing a central line dressing).

Continuously:
- Identify irregular heart rhythms and administer prescribed antidysrhythmic agents.
- Evaluate timing with decrease in cardiac output, change in triggering mode, or with variation of heart rate by 20%.
- Initiate fill cycle for tachycardias, elevated temperatures, and irregular heart rate if diastolic augmentation is reduced.
- Provide for temporary pacing to override bradycardia, tachycardia, or ectopy.
- In the event of asystole, chose a trigger that will assure balloon movement.
- Ensure that IAB is not immobile for > 30 min in the same position.
- Wean patient from inotropic and vasopressor agents as ordered.
- Administer fluid, as ordered, to maintain adequate filling pressures as diastolic filling pressures fall.
- Administer peripheral vasodilators, as ordered, to further decrease afterload and increase peripheral perfusion.
- Administer heparin, as ordered, to prevent thrombus formation on balloon catheter.
- Administer antibiotics, as ordered, to prevent infection.
- Apply antiembolism stocking or elastic bandages to uninvolved leg, as ordered.

DOCUMENTATION

When the nurse is documenting arterial pressures, the values are more consistent if they are taken from the IABP monitor. The bedside monitor identifies peak pressure as systole. During counterpulsation the peak pressure in the aorta may be the diastolic augmentation pressure. Most IABP monitors can clearly differentiate the difference between the two pressures.

In addition to the standard charting required of the ICU patient, the following measurements should be included when charting on the patient with IABC:
- *Inflation point*—the point on the arterial waveform where balloon inflation occurs.
- *Deflation point* — the point on the arterial waveform where balloon deflation occurs.
- *Assist frequency* — ratio of balloon inflations to heart beats.
- *Unassisted systole (UAS)* — systolic pressure that does not follow deflation of the IAB.
- *Unassisted aortic end-diastolic pressure* — aortic end-diastolic pressure without IABP intervention.
- *Unassisted mean arterial pressure* — the time-averaged pressure throughout each cycle of the heartbeat without IABP intervention.
- *Assisted systole (AS)* — systolic pressure that follows an assisted aortic end-diastolic pressure. Characteristically it is lower than the unassisted systolic pressure.
- *Diastolic augmentation* — resultant elevation of peak diastolic blood pressure caused by inflation of the IAB.
- *Assisted aortic end-diastolic pressure (AOEDP)* — the lowest diastolic pressure in the aorta that is affected by deflation of the IAB.
- *Assisted mean arterial pressure* — the time-averaged pressure throughout each balloon-assisted cycle of the heartbeat.
- When the balloon is refilled.
- Absence of blood in the IAB catheter and extender.

Peripheral Circulation Checks

- Skin color (i.e., normal, erythema, mottling, pallor, cyanosis, or jaundice).
- Temperature (i.e., normal, warm, or cool).
- Sensation (i.e., normal, decreased, pain, deep throbbing, pressure, numbness, or tingling).
- Movement (i.e., strong, weak, or none).
- Capillary refill (i.e., immediate or delayed).
- Pulses (i.e., by doppler or palpable, 3+, 2+, 1+, 0).
- Thigh and calf measurements.
- Ankle and brachial BP (ankle/arm index [AAI]).

WEANING FROM IABC

The duration of IAB therapy varies, depending on the patient condition. Patients who received IABP therapy for postoperative low cardiac output support usually recover completely within 72 hours. The physician will decide to wean from the IABP based on the following general guidelines:
- Cardiac index greater than 2.0 L/min.
- Pulmonary capillary wedge pressure less than 20 mm Hg.
- Systolic blood pressure greater than 100 mm Hg.
- Decrease in heart rate and absence of dysrhythmias.

- Absence of signs of myocardial ischemia.
- Pharmacological intervention at normal or below normal dosages.

The weaning method depends on physician preference and the type of pump being used. The most common method is to change assist frequency from 1:1 pumping to less frequent assistance (1:2, 1:3, 1:4). Decreasing balloon volume can also be used as a means of weaning (from 40 to 30 to 20 ml). Another weaning approach is to decrease the IAB augmentation. This results in decreased diastolic augmentation pressure, which should be tolerated by the patient who is ready for weaning. Regardless of the weaning method used, it is important to monitor the patient closely at each stage for signs of deterioration in hemodynamic status, angina, and ECG changes. If the patient does not tolerate weaning, the physician should be notified immediately and the weaning process should cease. The IAB is removed if function is satisfactory on 1:3 frequency.

PATIENT AND FAMILY TEACHING

The possibility of needing IABC postoperatively after open-heart surgery should be discussed with the preoperative patient. Pictures and flip charts can be used to help the patient visualize what to expect. A common misconception shared by patients and their families is that IABC replaces the action of the heart. They may become anxious when the IABP stops for any reason and should be informed ahead of time of the function of IABC. It is important to reassure the patient and family that the pump is assisting, not pumping for, the heart. The patient should be taught to keep the affected leg straight, without flexing at the groin. The patient will need to report pain, numbness, or tingling in the affected limb immediately. The patient should be told the importance of informing the nurse of chest, back, abdominal, or incisional pain. It will be the patient's responsibility to cooperate with position changes, coughing and deep breathing, and range of motion exercises, which should be taught preoperatively. Embolism may occur even after the IAB catheter is removed and the patient has returned home. Therefore the patient and family members should be taught to continue with assessments of limb circulation.

PEDIATRIC CONSIDERATIONS

The physiological goals of IABC are the same in the pediatric population as in adults. Children demonstrate greater aortic compliance than adults, which may diminish the degree of augmentation achieved. Diastolic augmentation may not be the essential effect of IABC in children. Afterload reduction may be the principal effect. The IABP is used mainly in major medical centers where pediatric open-heart surgery is frequently performed. The major indication of use in children is in treating low cardiac output and left ventricular dysfunction in the postoperative period.[2] IABC may also be indicated in selected myocardiopathies, congenital heart lesions, myocarditis, and sepsis that cause intractable failure. Contraindications include brain

Skill 11-5 Removal of the Percutaneous IAB Catheter

The IAB catheter is removed by a physician at the bedside or in the operating room if it was surgically inserted. Removal can be closed using pressure to control the arterial site or open with direct repair of the arterial site. The main problem associated with removal of the balloon catheter is the potential release of thrombi as the catheter is withdrawn. These thrombi may form around the catheter site where the blood flow is reduced.

EQUIPMENT AND SUPPLIES

- Protective underpads
- Sterile gloves
- Sterile gauze dressings
- Elastic pressure tape

NURSING INTERVENTIONS

1. Explain procedure to the patient, noting that manual pressure will be applied for 30 minutes after removal and bedrest will continue for 24 hours after removal.
2. Use protective underpads. The IAB catheter and introducer sheath are removed as a unit. Bleeding both proximal and distal to the insertion site is encouraged to expel any potential clots.
3. Once the IAB catheter is removed, apply manual pressure to both the proximal and distal portions of the femoral artery for at least 30 minutes.
4. After achieving hemostasis, apply a gauze pressure dressing and stabilize with elastic tape.
5. Instruct patient to alert the nurse for any complaints of pain or wetness around insertion site.
6. Check insertion site every 15 minutes until patient is stable and then every hour for swelling, bleeding, or hematoma formation.
7. Check pedal and posterior tibial pulses bilaterally every hour. Diminished or absent pulses may indicate a need for an embolectomy.
8. Apply a new sterile occlusive dressing every 24 hours until the wound is healed.

death, patent ductus arteriosus, aortic valve insufficiency, and aortic aneurysms.

Balloons ranging from 2.5 to 20 cc in volume are used. Insertion of the IAB is performed through a side-arm graft anastomosed to either the common femoral or internal iliac artery. Because the catheter length is shorter, the logistics of transporting a pediatric IABP patient can be difficult, posing a risk of movement of the catheter. If the balloon catheter is too long, it may occlude the renal or mesenteric vessels that arise from the descending aorta. The complication of renal failure should be monitored postinsertion by observing for urine outputs of less than 0.5 to 1.0 ml/kg/hr and by observing the urine for hematuria. To detect bowel ischemia from mesenteric occlusion caused by emboli or the balloon catheter, one should observe for abdominal distension and gastric bleeding. The child's girth should be measured every 2 to 4 hours.

The ECG is the most common trigger used. Increased heart rates necessitate a console with a sensitive mechanism, allowing a trigger to be achieved from a rapid QRS signal. The pump console should be set in the manual mode. The rapid heart rates also require a quick response gas flow to maximally inflate and deflate the balloon. Helium, rather than carbon dioxide, may inflate the balloon more effectively, since it is a lighter gas. The nurse will need to preload the pediatric balloon more frequently than in the adult. During the manual-fill process a loss of helium may occur.

The predominant determinant of stroke volume in a child is heart rate; the heart rate may vary, requiring the operator to make frequent adjustments in timing. When irregular rhythms or tachyarrhythmias occur, the nurse may need to decrease the frequency of balloon inflation. The balloon timing should be readjusted with changes in the heart rate plus or minus 10 beats/min.[2] The best evidence for optimal timing are measurable hemodynamic changes as seen on the arterial waveform and in the clinical setting.

PSYCHOSOCIAL CONSIDERATIONS

Patients on IABC are exposed to a great deal of external stimuli, including noise and painful manipulation, which may cause sensory overload and sleep deprivation. They may also become accustomed to the noise of IABC and become anxious when it stops. Providing music through earphones that is selected by the patient may help to induce relaxation. Patients may become restless and attempt to get out of bed. This behavior can be caused by several factors including denial of the illness, cerebral hypoxia secondary to low cardiac output, or confusion caused by sensory overload or sleep deprivation. Emotional support and appropriate sedation are important to ensure the patients' own safety. One should plan nursing care activities to allow for uninterrupted periods of rest whenever possible.

Study results have shown that the most significant stressors of patients on IABC are admission to the ICU, the limited mobility their treatment necessitates, and the lack of knowledge and understanding of their illness and treatment.[6] Patients should be given ample opportunity to voice their concerns and ask for comfort measures, such as position changes and back rubs. Every attempt should be made to give the patient as much control as possible. Some patients may see the need for the IABP as a sign of a worsening condition. The fear of death may be very real to them. The nurse should continually provide caring support and information that diminishes the threat of being on IABC. Patients should be informed clearly of the temporary need for the machine and the eventuality of the weaning process. Nurses should not hold conversations about the patient's condition in the room. Denial may be their best stress management strategy that permits them to cope with a situation that might otherwise be intolerable.

REFERENCES

1. Allen JN, Wewers MD: Acute myocardial infarction with cardiogenic shock during pregnancy: treatment with intraaortic balloon counterpulsation, *Crit Care Med* 18(8):888, 1990.
2. Anella J, McClosdey A, Vieweg C: Nursing dynamics of pediatric intraaortic balloon pumping, *Crit Care Nurse* 10(4):24, 1990.
3. Kahn JK et al: Supported "high risk" coronary angioplasty using intraaortic balloon pump counterpulsation, *J Am Coll Cardiol* 15(14):1151, 1990.
4. Maccioli GA, Lucas WJ, Norfleet WA: The intraaortic balloon pump: a review, *J Card Anesthesia* 2:365, 1988.
5. Nawa S, Yamada M, Teramoto S: Evaluation of conventional circulatory assist devices, *Chest* 95(2):261, 1989.
6. Patacky MG, Garvin BJ, Schwirian PM: Intraaortic balloon pumping and stress in the coronary care unit, *Heart Lung* 14(2):142, 1985.

CHAPTER 12

Intracranial Pressure Monitoring, Seizure Control, and Cervical Spine Traction

Objectives:

After completing this chapter, the reader will be able to:

- Describe a neurological assessment.
- Discuss nursing management of a patient during and after a seizure.
- State the acceptable range for intracranial pressure (ICP).
- Calculate cerebral perfusion pressure (CPP).
- State normal ICP and CPP values.
- Describe CPP and autoregulation.
- Discuss the importance of maintaining sterility when caring for all intracranial monitoring devices.
- Identify potential problems that can occur with varied ICP monitoring devices.
- Formulate appropriate nursing diagnoses for the patient with intracranial hypertension.
- Discuss the importance of immobilization for cervical spine fractures.
- Describe safety measures employed when caring for patients in cervical traction.
- Describe safety measures when turning a patient on a Sukoff board.

Approximately 2 million people a year suffer from head injury. Of these, 500,000 receive severe head injuries, approximately 70,000 of these victims endure lifelong disabilities of loss of function, and 50,000 die of their injuries.[2] The highest incidence of victims is among males ages 15 to 24.

The nurse's ability to assess and immediately intervene with head-injured patients is a key element in the prevention of further damage and complications. Some fundamental points in the care and management in this chapter will focus on the patient who sustains a head injury resulting in increased intracranial pressure (ICP), the patient who exhibits seizure activity, and the patient who requires cervical traction, since spinal cord injuries are relatively common among the head-injured population.

ASSESSMENT

To carry out a comprehensive health assessment, a careful medical history should be taken. Because of past or present neurological impairments and treatments, the patient may be unable to communicate an accurate medical history. A family member or close friend then becomes a vital source of patient information (Skill 12-1).

The respiratory patterns will assist in the assessment of the level of brain stem function. One should note the quality, rate, rhythm, and respiratory effort displayed. The following are abnormal breathing patterns associated with altered levels of consciousness:

- *Posthyperventilation apnea*—A brief period of apnea following several deep breaths, which lowers Pco_2 below resting level. Rhythmic breathing returns after Pco_2 level returns to normal.[12]
- *Cheyne-Stokes respiration*—Hyperpnea alternating with apnea in a smooth crescendo-decrescendo pattern. Hyperpnea usually lasts longer than the apnea.
- *Central neurogenic hyperventilation*—Sustained, regular, and rapid breathing.
- *Apneustic breathing*—Prolonged inspiratory cramp or end-inspiratory pause of 2 to 3 seconds.
- *Cluster*—Various patterns of gasping respirations, deep "all-or-none" breaths, usually at a slow rate.
- *Ataxic*—Irregular, random pattern with deep and shallow breaths.

NURSING DIAGNOSIS

The following are possible nursing diagnoses for the patient with neurological impairment:

- Decrease in cerebral tissue perfusion related to in-

Skill 12-1   Neurological Assessment

EQUIPMENT AND SUPPLIES

- Newspaper, telephone book, menu, or other reading material
- Paper, pencil, and pen
- Wristwatch
- Safety pin and wisp of cotton (e.g., cotton swab)
- Tongue blade
- Reflex hammer
- Penlight or flashlight
- Aromatic substances (e.g., lemon, coffee, oil of wintergreen or peppermint, salt, and vinegar)
- Common objects (e.g., a key or coin)
- Test tubes of hot and cold water
- Stethoscope
- Tuning fork

NURSING INTERVENTIONS

1. Obtain the patient history[33]
   a. The chief complaint—major symptoms. (Note complaints of headache, vomiting, or visual problems.)
   b. The present problem including the following:
      - Onset.
      - Progression.
      - Time, frequency, and location of symptoms.
      - Combination of symptoms, such as headache and fever (when and how often).
      - Dizziness, vertigo, or syncope.
      - Factors that improve or worsen problem.
      - Convulsions, twitching, and difficulty remembering.
      - Change in vision.
      - Change in ability to control bowel or bladder.
      - Any body numbness.
      - Any paresis.
   c. Past history including the following:
      - Intellectual development.
      - Education.
      - History of central nervous system (CNS) infections (e.g., meningitis, sinusitis, acne, abscessed teeth, chronic middle ear infections, seizures, or head injury).
   d. Headache.
   e. Vomiting.
   f. Medications, particularly those that may effect pupillary size.
   g. Source of information.
   h. Related hereditary diseases, such as seizures or neurological diseases.
2. Systematically examine patient head-to-toe.
3. Prepare patient. Assist with gown. Position and drape.
4. Evaluate in sitting, standing, and lying positions.
5. Assess level of consciousness (LOC) (e.g., awake and alert, somnolence, or coma). Ambiguous terms, like semicomatose, are sometimes used to describe the LOC. It is not as important to find a label for the patient's LOC, as to describe the patient's best response to the stimulus used (i.e., voice, shout, or pain). Specific descriptions of the behaviors exhibited allow for a more consistent monitoring of the LOC. If a change in stimulus is needed to elicit the same response from the patient, a change in the LOC has occurred.
6. Assess mentation and thought processes. To test cortical function, observe the patient for orientation to person, place, time, and situation. Time and situation are the first components of orientation the patient will loose. Assess the ability to respond to the immediate environment through verbal, visual, and tactile stimulation. Note insight

and perceptual skills. Measure judgmental abilities by posing a situation to the patient requiring the patient to provide a solution. For example, tell the patient "It is raining outdoors. What will you gather before leaving your house?" Short- and long-term memory evaluation indicates not only cerebral cortical but also reticular activating system functioning. Short-term memory may be assessed by listing a sequence of 3 to 4 items (e.g., apple, orange, banana, and pear) and asking the patient to repeat them in the same order. Long-term memory includes information known for greater than 24 hours. Common questions used to test long-term memory are siblings' names and ages, place of birth, and schools attended.[33]

7. Assess the mental status during the interview process and note speech patterns, thought processes, and memory capabilities. Note slurred speech, incomprehensible words, confusion or repetitive speech patterns. Also note reading, writing, spelling, and comprehension abilities. Ask the patient to repeat words and complete sentences, testing the ability to recall information.
8. Observe behavior for emotional status, affect, and mood. How does the patient react to the environment? Is the patient answering questions appropriately? Observe for inappropriate laughing or crying and also note bizarre or uncontrollable behaviors.
9. Test the function of the 12 cranial nerves.[3] This assessment gives the most information about the function of the brain stem. Refer to Table 12-1 for a complete guide to cranial nerve assessment.
10. Assess the patient's coordination and balance (i.e., cerebellar function). Observe the patient walking heel-to-toe on a straight line. Watch the patient dress or undress. Ataxia, tremors, and the inability to perform rapid alternating movements or coordinated movements are symptoms of cerebellar dysfunction. Perform a Romberg test. The patient stands with feet slightly apart and closes the eyes, thus removing visual aid for balance. If there is a cerebellar problem, the patient will sway and possibly fall toward the side of the lesion.
11. Determine system function response by checking motor strength in all extremities.
    a. Test motor response to verbal stimuli (Table 12-2).
    b. Describe the quality of motor movement in detail, following commands uniformly with all four extremities. decorticate or decerebrate posturing (Fig. 12-1), flexion or extension, limited or asymmetrical movement, or flaccid paralysis of any extremities.
    c. Monitor patient for any spontaneous jerking, twitching, or involuntary movement indicative of seizure activity.
    d. Observe for patient's ability to demonstrate strength, for example, gripping the examiner's fingers. Assess whether motor strength is symmetrical. The patient may have a grasp reflex, but this is a false indicator of strength. A grasp reflex commonly occurs in patients with frontal lobe damage. The patient will be able to squeeze the examiner's hands but will not be able to release the grasp (like the grasp of an infant). A better method to assess the upper extremity strength is the palmar drift test. In this test, ask the patient to raise the arms in front with palms turned up and to close eyes. If there is any weakness in the extremity, the palm will turn down and the arm will slowly drop on the affected side. Watch the patient ambulate to evaluate leg strength. If the patient is not ambulatory, have the patient flex each leg. Muscle strength should be

Skill 12-1   Neurological Assessment—cont'd

tested against the examiner's resistance, against gravity, or with the effects of gravity removed. Weakness of the legs will be determined by the inability to bend the leg against gravity or pressure.[33] Observe the performance of activities of daily living (ADLs). This will provide a great deal of information regarding thought processes, coordination of movement, and strength.

12. Assess sensory function. Ask patient to close eyes. Check the response by pinprick, touch, or cotton. Check all areas of the patient's body for intact sensation. Test position sense (i.e., toe-up or toe-down) and point discrimination. Sensation should be tested on arms, legs, and trunk using the following stimuli: pain, temperature, light, touch, and vibration.

13. Percuss the deep and superficial reflexes. Reflexes give information about the functioning of the spinal cord. Elicit the deep reflexes of the biceps, triceps, brachioradialis, patellar, and achilles tendons using a reflex hammer (Fig. 12-2). Tapping the tendons lightly causes the reflex stretching of muscles and the reflexes are graded according to response. Babinski's sign can also be tested (Fig. 12-3).

The symmetry of the reflex response from one side of the body to the other is assessed and recorded. Any differences noted may aid in location of lesions. A convenient method for recording is the use of a stick figure (Fig. 12-4). Reflex responses are indicated at all reflex sites.

The superficial reflexes include the corneal, abdominal (upper and lower), cremasteric, and gluteal. These re-flexes are generally tested by use of cotton wisps or finger pressure.

14. Assess skin integrity. Note lacerations, contusions of the head or neck, leaking of fluid from ears (otorrhea), nose (rhinorrhea), or frequent swallowing that could be signs of cerebrospinal fluid (CSF) leakage. Ecchymosis around the eyes ("raccoon eyes") or bruising behind the ears ("battle sign") can be indicative of basilar skull fractures or head trauma.[33]

15. Inspect for signs of trauma. Look at the major muscle groups for atrophy or wasting. Observe the spine for deformities and mobility. Watch the patient walk and talk.

16. Palpate the spinal vertebra. Beginning with C3, gently tap down the midline of each vertebra. Note any pain over a particular area of the spine.

17. Auscultate to detect vascular abnormalities, such as arteriovenous malformations, a carotid-cavernous fistula, or poor carotid flow. Place a stethoscope over all aspects of the skull, the eyes, and along the carotid arteries. Normally, no sound is detected when the stethoscope is placed over the skull. If a vascular malformation exists, a bruit can be heard.

18. Monitor vital signs. Hypothermia (i.e., decreased body temperature less than 35° C [95° F]) decreases the overall metabolic rate and decreases cerebral blood flow and oxygen consumption. Hyperthermia (i.e., increased body temperature greater than 38.4° C [101° F]) increases metabolic rate, oxygen, and glucose demand on the body. A patient with hypothalamic dysfunction will have altered temperature-regulating capabilities.

---

creased ICP secondary to intercerebral bleeding.[22]

- Decrease in adaptive capacity: intracranial, related to increased brain mass.
- Impaired physical mobility related to hemiparesis.
- Potential fluid volume deficit related to hyperthermia.
- Self-care deficit: feeding, bathing and hygiene, dressing and grooming, and toileting secondary to reduced level of consciousness (LOC).
- Disturbance in self-esteem related to altered ability to perform activities of daily living (ADL).
- Speech pattern disturbance related to hemiparesis.
- Potential for infection related to ICP monitoring.
- Potential for injury related to poor balance secondary to cerebrovascular accident (CVA).
- Pain related to surgical incision.
- Disturbance in bowel elimination related to immobility.
- Impaired home maintenance management related to decreased mobility.
- Ineffective family coping related to severe disability of patient.
- Dysreflexia related to excessive autonomic response to noxious stimuli secondary to spinal cord injury (SCI).
- Hypothermia related to SCI.

PATIENT OUTCOMES

The following are sample expected outcomes for patients with neurological impairment:

The patient evidences:

- Increased LOC and motor and sensory responsiveness.
- ICP at rest within normal limits (i.e., 0 to 15 mm Hg).
- Cerebral perfusion pressure (CPP) > 60 mm Hg.
- Arterial blood gases (ABGs) of Po_2 80 to 100 mm Hg; Pco_2 of 35 to 45 mm Hg; HCO_3^- of 22 to 26 mEq.
- Bilateral equal and clear breath sounds on auscultation.
- Systolic arterial pressure between 100 and 160 mm Hg.
- Clear chest x-ray and no further injury to spinal cord after immobilization of fracture site.
- Minimal complications from spinal cord damage.

SEIZURES

Seizures are uncontrolled electrical discharges from the neurons in the cerebral cortex that cause brief, jerky contractions of a muscle group or the whole body. However, electrical discharge can occur with or without clinical manifestation, depending on the part of the brain involved and

Text continued on p. 284.

Table 12-1   Assessment of Cranial Nerve Function[2]

Nerve	Function	Technique of assessment	Maladaptive findings
Olfactory (I) (Sensory)	Sense of smell	Lemon packets, coffee, and peppermint water have specific odors that can be identified through the sense of smell. Test only one nostril at a time with the patient's eyes closed. Ammonia or ether should not be used since they irritate the nasal mucosa and are not really smelled.	A frontal lobe lesion is suspected in patients with unilateral loss of smell in the absence of nasal disease.
Optic (II) (Sensory)	Sight	The optic nerve is tested for visual acuity and visual fields. Finger testing can be used as a rough test for both acuity and field of vision. Another test for visual acuity is asking the patient to read something, such as a newspaper or informational booklet.	Visual field defects can be produced by lesions along the visual pathway. Partial or complete blindness with sluggish or absent pupillary response, Marcus-Gunn pupils.
Oculomotor* (III) (Motor)	Raise eyelid, control inward, upward, and downward movement of the eyeball. Parasympathetic components constrict pupil control ciliary muscles.	Have the patient raise eyebrows; follow the examiner's finger with eyes. Check the pupillary response to light. The pupil should react briskly when the light is shown in the eye, this is called a direct response. The size, shape, and symmetry are also assessed. To demonstrate the connection between the two oculomotor nerves, a consensual light response should also be assessed. A consensual response occurs in the eye opposite to the one the light is shined into — a slight constriction should be seen.	Inability to look up, down, or inward (medially) with the affected eye. Eye turns down and out. Ptosis (dropping) of the lid. Dilation or sluggish pupillary response.
Trochlear (IV)* (Motor)	Controls downward and outward movement of the eyeball.	Have the patient follow the examiner's finger in a down and outward direction. Often associated with head tilt to compensate.	Failure of the affected eye to move down and out or down and in.
Trigeminal (V) (Mixed-both motor and sensory)	The motor portion controls opening and closing of the jaw. The sensory portion has three divisions concerned with pain, temperature, and light touch sensation from the scalp and face. (Division 1 - above the eye and cornea. Division 2 - upper lid. Division 3 - lower lip and chin.)	*Motor* - Observe the muscles of mastication for symmetry. Place the examining hand at the temporal-mandibular joint and have the patient open and close mouth (a good method of testing these muscles). *Sensory* - A pin can be used to test the integrity of the sensory portion of the C5. Avoid using pins and use wisps of cotton to do the testing. During all sensory testing the patient must be tested with the eyes closed. Testing of the corneal reflex can also be done at this time. A wisp of cotton lightly touching the cornea will elicit this reflex. The corneal reflex is a test of two cranial nerves, V and VII. V perceives that there is something on the cornea and VII blinks the eyelid.	Paraesthesias.
Abducens (VI)* (Motor)	Outward movement of the eyeball	Ask the patient to follow the examiner's finger with the eyes.	Loss of lateral movement. Diplopia on lateral gaze.
Facial (VII) (Mixed)	*Sensory* - Taste to the anterior two-thirds of the tongue. *Motor* - Facial muscle movement.	*Sensory* - A small amount of salt or sugar can be used to test this function. With the patient's eyes closed, place the substance in the patient's hand, and ask the patient to taste it. *Motor* - Ask the patient to "make faces" for you. Smiling, showing the teeth, winking, whistling, and wrinkling the forehead. Observe for symmetry or weakness of the facial muscles.	*Sensory* - Inability to taste on the anterior two-thirds of the tongue. *Motor* - Facial weakness or paralysis.

*Cranial nerves III, IV, and VI: The oculomotor, trochler, and abducens are tested together. These nerves supply the muscles of eye movement.
†Cranial nerves IX and X are usually tested together.

Table 12-1   Assessment of Cranial Nerve Function[2]—cont'd

Nerve	Function	Technique of assessment	Maladaptive findings
Acoustic (VIII) (Vestibulocochlear) (Sensory)	Hearing and regulates balance.	To test the patient's hearing, hold a wrist watch to the ear and ask if it can be heard. A command whispered at the foot of the bed is another effective way to test the hearing. If this test is chosen, multiple modlities can be tested such as the ability to hear; the ability to interpret what is said; and the ability to follow a simple command. The vestibular portion of this cranial nerve is usually not tested as part of a routine admission assessment. The critical care nurse should be aware of at least one way of evaluating this part of the C8. The most commonly performed test is the ice water caloric or (oculovestibular) test in which 30-60 ml of water is placed in to the ear canal. The ice water works to speed up the motion of the semicircular canal in the ear being tested and this simulates spinning. The eyes begin a rhythmic searching pattern to try to orient the cerebellum in space so balance can be maintained. This searching movement of the eyes is called nystagmus and is normal when ice water is placed in to the ear. Electronystagmography can also be used to test this function. The rationale behind any test of vestibular function is that the balancing mechanism used is a very complex system involving the inner ear (C8); the eyes (C2); the extraocular movements (C3, C4, and C5); and the cerebellum. For the patient to be balanced, the entire system must be intact.	Tinnitus. Decreased hearing or deafness lesion. Loss of balance. Vertigo.
Glossopharyngeal IX† (Mixed)	Gag reflex, taste, (posterior one-thirds of the tongue) and salivating (parotid gland).	Testing the gag reflex can be accomplished with a tongue blade or a small (#10) suction catheter. Asking the patient to forcefully cough is another way to check the gag reflex.	Loss of taste in the posterior one-third of the tongue. Lesions in the parotid gland thereby decreasing salivation. Loss of sensation on the affected side of the soft palate.
Vagus (X)† (Mixed)	Taste, swallowing, lifts palate, talking, and maintains cardiac muscle tone and rate of contraction. Constricts bronchial muscles and stimulates muscles and glands.	The vagus nerve is impossible to test fully. Innervation from the vagus nerve extends from the oral cavity to the rectum. It stimulates salivation; is involved in swallowing and talking; innervates the muscles of respirations as well as maintaining cardiac muscle tone and rate of contraction; and finally vagal stimulation increases the production of hydrocholoric acid in the stomach, and increases peristalsis. This cranial nerve is critical to survival. The nurse is restricted to checking the patients ability to swallow, and speak without any hoarseness or weakness of voice and inspection of the soft palate.	*Dysphonia* - Impairment of the voice. Hoarseness due to paralysis of the vocal cords. *Dysphasia* - Impairment in swallowing. Weakness or sagging of the soft palate. Deviation of the uvula from midline.
Spinal Accessory (XI) (Motor)	Lifts the shoulder by innervating the trapezius and sternocleidomastoid muscles. Turns the head.	Nurse places a hand on either side of the patients chin and asks the patient to push against the examiner's hand. Ask the patient to shrug their shoulders. The nurse should be alerted to the symmetry of the trapezius and sternoclediomastoid muscles.	Atropy of the innervated muscles.
Hypoglossal (XII) (Motor)	Tongue movement.	Ask the patient to stick out tongue; the tongue deviates towards the abnormal side. Note strength of the tongue and any signs of atrophy or tremors.	Deviation, atrophy, or tremoring of the tongue are signs of dysfunction of the nerve.

Table 12-2   The Glasgow Coma Scale Response Chart

Examiner's test	Stimulus	Patient's response	Assigned score
Eye opening (Assesses arousal ability.)	Spontaneous	Eyes open spontaneously without stimulation.	4
	Speech	Eyes open when asked.	3
	Pain	Eyes open with noxious stimuli.	2
	Pain	Eyes do not open, regardless of stimuli.	1
Best motor response (Measures appropriateness of speech or LOC.)	Commands	Follows simple commands; able to repeat performance.	6
	Pain	Pulls examiner's hand away when patient is pinched.	5
	Pain	Pulls a part of body away when pinched.	4
	Pain	Flexes body inappropriately to pain.	3
	Pain	Body becomes rigid in an extended position when examiner pinches.	2
	Pain	Has no motor response to pinch.	1
Verbal response (Measures overall awareness and ability to respond to external stimuli.)	Speech	Carries on a conversation correctly and can tell examiner about time, place, and self.	5
	Speech	Seems confused or disoriented.	4
	Speech	Examiner understands patient's talk but it makes no sense.	3
	Speech	Makes sounds that examiner cannot understand.	2
	Speech	Makes no noise.	1

From Flynn J-BMcC, Hackel R: *Technological foundations of nursing,* Norwalk, Conn, 1990, Appleton & Lange.

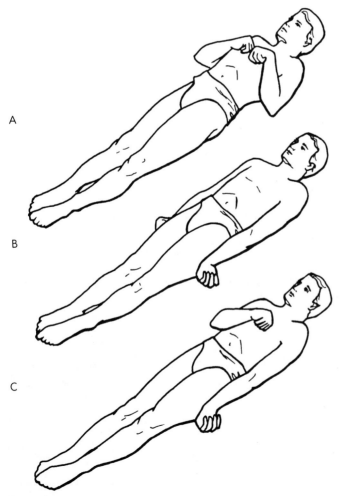

Fig. 12-1   Decorticate and decerebrate responses. **A,** Decorticate response. Flexion of arms, wrists, and fingers with adduction in upper extremities. Extension, internal rotation, and plantar flexion in lower extremities. **B,** Decerebrate response. All four extremities in rigid extension with hyperpronation of forearms and plantar extension of feet. **C,** Decorticate response on right side of body and decerebrate response on left side of body. (From Zschoche D: *Mosby's comprehensive review of critical care,* ed 3, St Louis, 1986, Mosby–Year Book.)

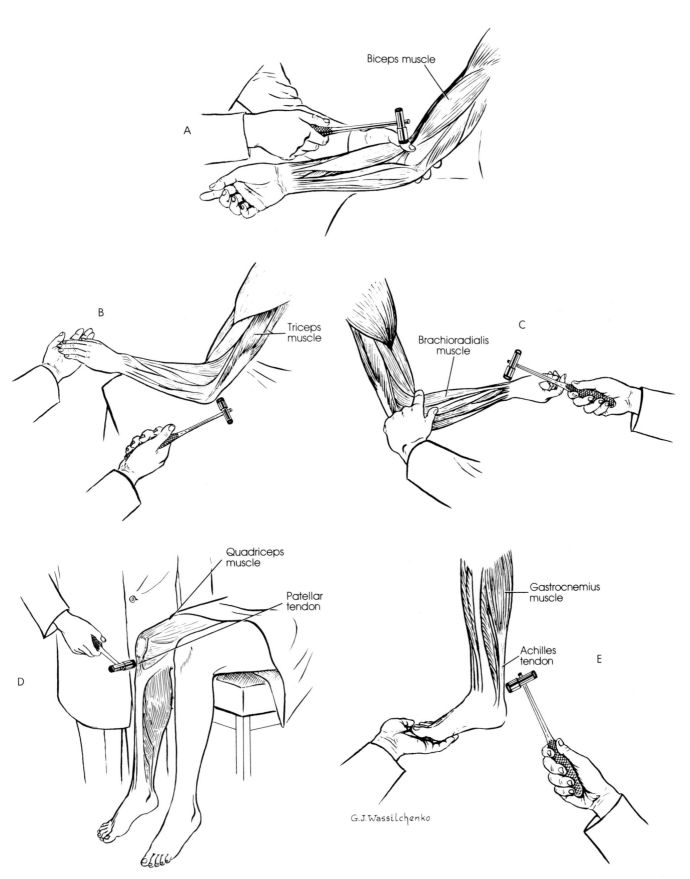

Fig. 12-2   Deep tendon reflexes. **A,** Biceps reflex. **B,** Triceps reflex. **C,** Brachioradialis reflex. **D,** Patellar reflex. **E,** Achilles reflex. (From Rudy EB: *Advanced neurological and neurosurgical nursing,* St Louis, 1984, Mosby–Year Book.)

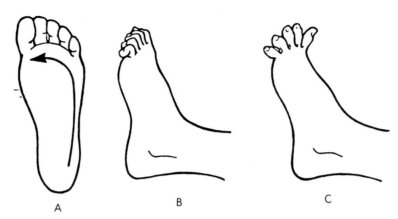

Fig. 12-3 Babinski's sign. **A,** Test maneuver. **B,** Normal response (negative Babinski's sign). **C,** Abnormal response (positive Babinski's sign). (From Zschoche D: *Mosby's comprehensive review of critical care,* ed 3, St Louis, 1986, Mosby–Year Book.)

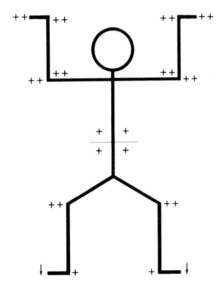

Fig. 12-4 Record reflex responses using a stick figure.

Grade 0	0	Absent
Grade 1	+	Diminished
Grade 2	+ +	Normal
Grade 3	+ + +	Brisker than normal
Grade 4	+ + + +	Hyperactive

(From Malasanos L, Barkauskas V, Stoltenberg-Allen K: *Health assessment,* ed 4, St Louis, 1990, Mosby–Year Book.)

the path of the electrical discharge. The discharge is associated with an immediate disturbance of sensation, LOC, and convulsive movement.

An International Classification of Epileptic Seizures has been developed to assist in the categorization of seizures. The terminology in this system is widely used for the diagnosis and classification of seizures.

Partial or Focal Seizures

Partial or focal seizures occur when electrical activity involves only one part of the brain. They may present with a wide variety of symptoms depending on which area of the cortex is involved. Partial seizures are classified as simple partial seizures, complex (i.e., temporal lobe or psychomotor) partial seizures, and partial seizures that are secondarily generalized.[9]

Simple partial seizures are caused by localized cortical electrical stimulation resulting in a variety of symptoms, depending on the site of the focus. Simple seizures may be manifested by motor, sensory, or autonomic symptoms. Motor symptoms include focal jerks of any muscle but particularly the face and hands. The person loses control of the affected areas during the 5 to 15 seconds of the seizure. Sensory symptoms may include hallucinations, sensory illusions, burning, numbness, tingling, or crawling sensations.[23] Autonomic symptoms present with flushing, increased heart rate, sweating, increased or decreased blood pressure, and pupillary changes.

Complex partial seizures are focal seizures arising from the anterior temporal lobe. These seizures usually present with an aura. Cognitive effects of the aura include déjà-vu, fear, and paranoia. Psychomotor symptoms include smacking the lips, chewing, swallowing, grimacing and picking at the clothing.

Partial seizures that are secondarily generalized and complex partial seizures may generalize into tonic-clonic seizures if both hemispheres are involved.

Generalized Seizures

Generalized seizures involve both sides of the brain. They are classified as tonic-clonic, (grand mal) absence attacks (petit mal), tonic, clonic, myoclonic, atonic, akinetic, and status epilepticus.

Patients who have *tonic-clonic seizures* often experience auras that are either physical (i.e., spasm of an extremity) or sensory (i.e., a smell or hearing a sound signal from the body). There is an alteration in the LOC with tonic-clonic seizures that includes loss of all awareness to surroundings. Tonic-clonic seizures have four phases. The seizure begins with a preictal (aura) phase followed by a stiffening of all four extremities, lasting about 1 minute. Patients then experience severe generalized clonus or jerking movement and frothing at the mouth, followed by a postictal phase. Not all patients undergo the tonic-clonic phases of the seizure; some may only have either tonic or clonic movements. Many times the patient is incontinent of the bowels or bladder.[1,28]

Patients who are prone to tonic-clonic seizures are at the greatest risk for accidental harm, either by biting their tongues or suffering from multiple bruises, lacerations, or contusions. Those who experience the clonic state will often display the following symptoms after the seizure: flaccid, comalike appearance; pupils that are fixed and dilated; no corneal or deep tendon reflexes; and a positive Babinski's reflex. Symptoms of the postictal phase include confusion, disorientation, fatigue, falling into a deep sleep, and amnesia for the seizure, except for the aura.[9]

Absence seizures are characterized by a loss of awareness (but not an aura), LOC, or loss of muscle tone. The individual appears to be staring. This type of seizure lasts for 10 to 30 seconds and may occur infrequently or up to hundreds of times a day.

Tonic seizures are rare; no clonic movements are seen. This type of generalized seizure is characterized by a sudden rigidity of the muscles, LOC, flushing, increased heart rate and blood pressure, sweating, and pupillary changes.

Clonic seizures do not have the phases of tonic-clonic seizures. They are characterized by generalized brief spasms followed by asymmetrical, bilateral jerks lasting up to several minutes. They generally occur in children between the ages of 4 and 8 years old.

Myoclonic seizures are characterized by brief sudden muscle contractions in the arms, legs, or trunk. There is little or no LOC. Myoclonic seizures are associated with biochemical alterations, fevers, or spinal cord lesions.

Atonic or akinetic seizures present with a loss of body tone and are associated with a feeling of falling. Generally, persons with this type of seizure disorder do not lose consciousness and are able to catch themselves before falling.

Status epilepticus is recurrent, continual seizure activity. The patient does not fully regain consciousness between seizures. This is an emergency situation that requires immediate medical attention. If status epilepticus is left untreated, the patient is at risk for possible respiratory affect or aspiration along with cerebral impairment from ischemic hypoxia. Patients with the following history are more susceptible to status epilepticus: patients with a known seizure disorder who are noncompliant with medication regime or on subtherapeutic doses of anticonvulsant therapy and patients suffering any of the following: encephalitis, subarachnoid and intracerebral hemorrhage, hypoglycemia, acute alcohol withdrawal, or cerebral edema.[1]

INCREASED INTRACRANIAL PRESSURE (ICP)

Normal ICP is the reflection of the total intracranial volume against the rigid adult skull. Intracranial volume is

Skill 12-2 Seizure and Postictal Care[2,9,20,28]

EQUIPMENT AND SUPPLIES

- Oral airway
- Crash cart and suction device
- IV setup (i.e., IV catheter, fluid, tubing, and IV pole)
- Blood tube
- Gloves

NURSING INTERVENTIONS

1. Stay with patient (see the box on Seizure Environmental Precautions). If patient is standing, lower patient to the floor and logroll patient to one side.
2. Call for assistance.
3. Note time, onset, duration, and type of seizure.
4. Note area of initial muscle contraction.
5. Note patient's LOC.
6. Do not place anything in the patient's mouth when teeth are clenched. This can cause harm to patient's teeth or nurse's fingers.
7. Insert airway only if possible. Use the head tilt–chin lift maneuver to maintain a patent airway.
8. Loosen all clothes. Do not restrain patient.
9. Prepare for potential emergency situation.
10. Call physician stat for seizure activity lasting 3 minutes in duration or cessation of pulse or respirations.
11. Note time the postictal phase begins.
12. Place patient on side, if not able to do so earlier, to decrease chances of aspiration.
13. Assess airway and breathing.
14. Insert airway prn and assist with breathing (if necessary).
15. Begin oxygen therapy as needed.
16. Start peripheral IV prn.
17. Examine the patient for vomiting, mouth or tongue lacerations, and bowel or bladder incontinence.
18. Monitor vital signs (no oral temperatures) and neurological status.
19. Monitor for additional seizures that may be indicative of status epilepticus.
20. Observe and document return of responsiveness.
21. Provide quiet and restful environment.
22. Provide patient with reassurance and orientation to events to decrease psychological impact of seizure disorder.
23. Draw blood work to obtain anticonvulsant levels, if patient is on medication therapy. Report results to physician.
24. Record the following data: type, progression, duration, and precipitating event; location of onset and frequency; medication type, amount, and effect; presence or absence of continence; eye movement during seizure; pupillary responses; and state of consciousness.

comprised of three constituents: brain tissue (88.5%), cerebral spinal fluid (CSF) (8% to 9%), and blood in arteries and veins (2.5%). Intracranial volume (ICV) is equal to the sum of the brain volume (BV), cerebrospinal fluid volume (CSFV), and cerebral blood volume (CBV). This can be expressed by the following formula:

$$ICV = BV + CSFV + CBV$$

The volume within the intracranial compartment is limited because the structure of the skull. The easiest pressure to measure is that of the CSF. This pressure is referred to as the ICP.[12]

▼
Seizure Environmental Precautions[20]

- Have airway at the bedside at all times.
- Pad siderails and maintain in the up position whenever the patient is in bed.
- Remove loose sharp objects from the patient's immediate area.
- Avoid use of restraints.

The CSF, produced in the four ventricles of the brain, fills the ventricles and serves to cushion the external surface of the brain and spinal cord. It is secreted at a rate of about 0.5 ml/min with a total volume in the system of 135 to 140 ml.[30] CSF is constantly replenished, causing an entire volume turnover about every 5 hours. This process nourishes the nervous tissue and assists in the removal of the by-products of metabolism. The CSF is absorbed through the arachnoid granulations and is deposited in the venous sinuses to be returned to the vascular circulation (Fig. 12–5). In the lateral recumbent position, the normal ICP is 0 to 15 mm Hg.[30] Healthy individuals experience transient elevations of ICP during the day when doing Valsalva's maneuvers. Elevations are usually brief and self-limited. Generally, the higher and more sustained the elevation of the ICP, the more severe the significance. A sus-

tained ICP greater than 15 mm Hg is regarded as abnormal.[11] Intracranial hypertension is defined as an ICP of greater than 20 mm Hg.

Increased ICP occurs when there is an increase in volume of any of the three major constituents without a compensatory reduction in one of the other constituents. The chief compensatory mechanism is the reduction in the CSF by increased reabsorption or a decreased production. Vasoconstriction of the blood vessels to reduce blood volume and shifting of brain tissue are also compensatory mechanisms but are temporary and of limited value.

The concept of compliance also contributes to the understanding of intracranial hypertension. Compliance is an index of the volume-pressure relationship within the skull. When compensatory mechanisms are operational, compliance is normal. As compensatory mechanisms fail, compliance is minimal and a small increase in volume will cause a large increase in pressure.[27]

The brain itself is able to regulate blood flow by autoregulation and by initiating elevations in systemic blood pressure. Autoregulation is accomplished by three main physiological mechanisms: pressure changes, cerebral vasoconstriction, and metabolic factors.[30]

Various autoregulatory mechanisms maintain primary control over ICP. Head injury interferes with some of these

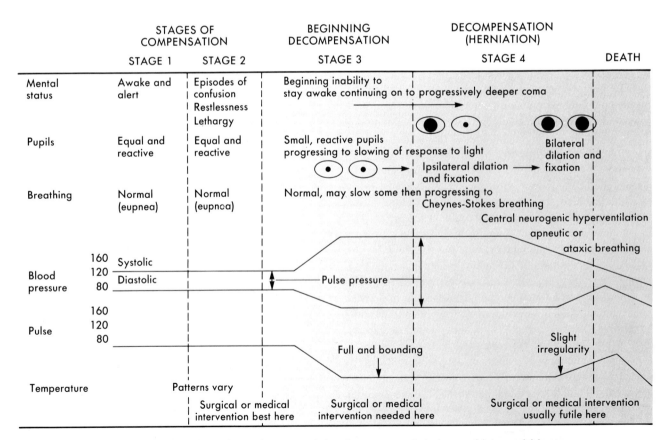

Fig. 12-5 Clinical correlates of compensated and uncompensated phases of intracranial hypertension. Mosby–Year Book.) (From Beare PG, Myers JL: *Principles and practice of adult health nursing,* St Louis, 1990, Mosby–Year Book.)

mechanisms not allowing for maximum functioning. Most medical and nursing interventions for controlling increased ICP are aimed at supporting the compensatory mechanisms of the brain.

Increased ICP is a major complication of many neurological dysfunctions, including head trauma, brain tumors, intracranial hemorrhage, and brain abscess. The nurse caring for the neurological patient must be constantly on the alert for the development of increased ICP.[32]

Causes of Increased ICP

There are many causes and pathological conditions that increase ICP. Changes in CSF absorption or production, alterations in the cerebrovasculature, or conditions that involve the brain parenchyma can often result in cerebral edema. Cerebral edema is the abnormal accumulation of fluid from one of the three intracranial compartments (i.e., brain parenchyma, cerebrovascular volume, or CSF). Cerebral edema can cause compression of brain tissues and blood vessels or block CSF pathways, all of which contribute to the increase in ICP. Cerebral edema is usually greatest within the first 72 hours of the injury.

A concussion is a closed head injury with some degree of neurological dysfunction, although LOC may not occur. This condition occurs immediately following the trauma, not days later, and complete recovery of neurological function routinely occurs within 6 to 12 hours or sooner.

A contusion is a closed head injury caused by a bruise usually found on the crest of the gyrus. The occurrence is usually in the temporal poles and the inferior aspect of the frontal lobes. A contusion normally extends only to the white matter. The brain becomes hyperemic and swollen following a contusion.[2]

Hematomas may result in ICP. There are four major types of hematomas: acute subdural, chronic subdural, epidural, and intracerebral (Fig. 12-6). Acute subdural hematoma results from a violent injury to the brain. The epidural hematoma is often a result of a skull fracture over the meningeal vascular channels, causing an arterial bleed. This is often the most dangerous, since the patient presents as only confused or extremely agitated and deteriorates rapidly because of the arterial nature of the bleed. An intracerebral hematoma is a type of clot occurring within the substance of the brain. It is usually found to occur in the frontal or temporal lobes beneath a contusion.[30]

An open head injury is classified as a fracture, with a tear in the dura (Fig. 12-7). This may lead to CSF leakage often detected in the ears (otorrhea) or in the nares (rhinorrhea) (Fig. 12-8).

Another important condition resulting in ICP is herniation of the brain through an opening in the wall of the cranial cavity. Progressing in a head-to-toe direction, the expanding brain will herniate through the falx, tentorium, or the foramen magnum. There are three types of herniation: central downward, uncal, and downward cerebellar (Fig. 12-9).

Management of Intracranial Hypertension

Intracranial hypertension must be treated aggressively to prevent severe morbidity and mortality in the head-injured population. A threshold of 20 mm Hg is the most widely adopted level at which ICP therapy is initiated in head-injured patients.[35] The goals of medical and nursing management of intracranial hypertension are to identify and treat the pathophysiological signs of increased ICP.

Assuring adequate oxygenation is the first step in the management of intracranial hypertension.[12,29] To maintain adequate ventilation, an ET tube or tracheostomy may be

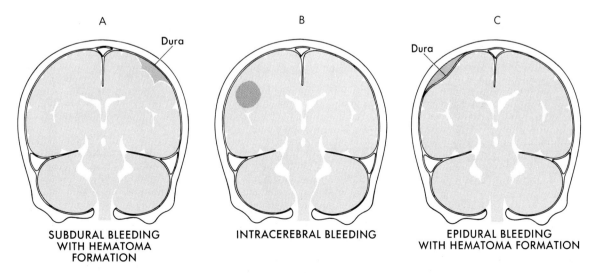

Fig. 12-6 Types of hematoma. **A,** Subdural bleeding with hematoma formation. **B,** Intracerebral bleeding. **C,** Epidural bleeding with hematoma formation. (From Beare PG, Myers JL: *Principles and practice of adult health nursing,* St Louis, 1990, Mosby–Year Book.)

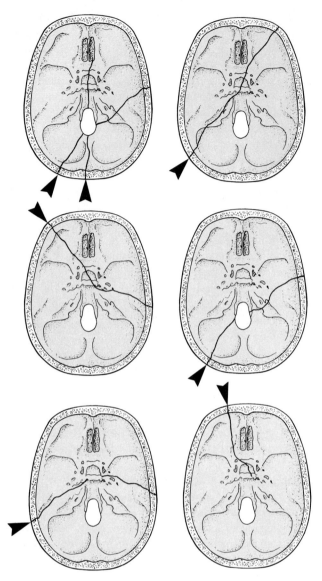

Fig. 12-7   Basilar skull fractures. Contracoup forces go in the opposite direction along similar paths.

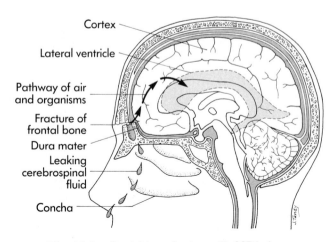

Fig. 12-8   Frontal bone fracture with CSF leakage.

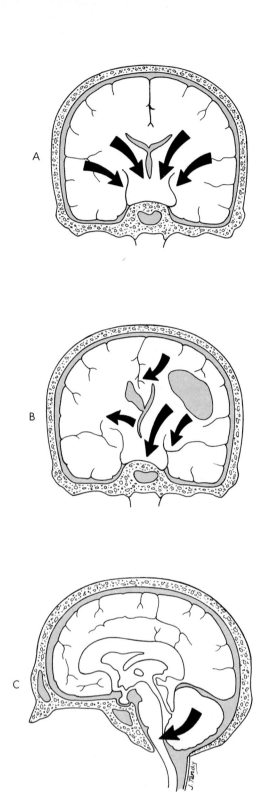

Fig. 12-9   Herniation of the brain: **A,** Central downward. **B,** Uncal herniation. **C,** Downward cerebellar. The central herniation is characterized by stupor, irregular respirations, pupil constriction (initially) leading to moderate fixed dilation, decerebrate and decordicate postures, and coma. The uncal type is characterized by third cranial nerve palsy on the side of the lesion, decreased LOC, Cheyne-Stokes respirations, bilateral Babinski, and decerebrate posture. Cerebellar herniation is characterized by respiratory disturbance, coma, cardiac irregularity, and arching of neck and back.

necessary. ABG analysis will guide the oxygen therapy. The goal is to maintain the Pao_2 greater than 70 mm Hg. A mild hyperventilation, to maintain an arterial CO_2 tension ($Paco_2$) of 25 to 30 mm Hg, can have an effect on cerebral blood flow.[12,13] The lowering of the $Paco_2$ will lead to a constriction of the cerebral blood vessels, reducing cerebral blood flow, thereby decreasing the ICP. This positive effect assumes a brain healthy enough to respond to hypocapnia by vasoconstriction.

Determining cerebral perfusion pressure (CPP) is the most rapid means to determine the pressure at which the cells of the brain are being perfused with oxygen and other essential nutrients. The formula to determine CPP is: CPP = mean arterial blood pressure − ICP.[24]

$$CPP = \frac{(\text{diastolic blood pressure} \times 2) + \text{systolic pressure}}{3} - ICP$$

Normal values range from 60 to 90 mm Hg.[1] Ideally, CPP in the brain injured should be 70 to 90 mm Hg.[1] A CPP of less than 50 mm Hg results in a significant decrease in cerebral blood flow.

Many factors can influence CPP. In the healthy adult, the autoregulation mechanism maintains the cerebral blood flow at a consistent rate in the presence of varying systolic blood pressure changes. Autoregulation is able to do this by dilation and constriction of the cerebral arteries. A loss of this regulatory mechanism may follow local or diffuse vascular damage resulting in complications such as hypoxia, vascular collapse, progressive cerebral edema, petechial hemorrhages, and cell death.

Despite the widespread controversy over the value of steroid therapy in treating certain forms of cerebral edema, glucocorticosteroids have been used extensively in the prevention and treatment of cerebral edema. Untreated cerebral edema can lead to increased ICP or complicate potential ICP problems. Dexamethasone (Decadron), a semisynthetic steroid, is the most commonly used steroid, and studies demonstrate that it reduces the quantity of vasogenic edema.[15]

The mode of action of steroids is not universally agreed on, but it is felt that their effect on edema is mainly through the stabilizing effect on the cell membrane. Steroids are also thought to improve neuronal function by improving cerebral blood flow and restoring autoregulation. The benefit from steroids is considered most useful in patients with tumors.[5]

Osmotically active agents have been used for over 50 years to treat cerebral tissue swelling. The principle governing the use of hypertonic solutions is the removal of fluid from the cerebral tissues in response to a vascular osmotic gradient. To be effective, the agent must remain in the intravascular compartment, meaning that in brain injury and damage to the blood-brain barrier the effect of osmotic withdrawal is from normal rather than edematous tissue. The beneficial effects must be attributed to a decrease in the bulk of normal tissue. If there is a major disruption of the blood-brain barrier, this form of therapy may be more harmful than beneficial, since the hypertonic solution could pass into the edematous tissue and lead to a rebound phenomenon.[15]

Recent studies have demonstrated the positive effect of loop diuretics (nonosmotic), such as furosemide (Lasix) and ethacrynic acid (Edecrin) on ICP. These diuretics cause a reduction in CSF production by 40% to 70%, thus reducing the ICP. This lowering of pressure enhances the clearance of tissue fluid.[15]

The pharmacological control of cerebral metabolic rate has been shown to be effective in controlling ICP.[16] High dose barbiturates (i.e., pentobarbital and thiopental) were the first agents introduced and they have been shown to cause a decrease in ICP. A secondary effect of this regimen is a reduction in cerebral edema and a more uniform blood supply to the brain.

Barbiturate therapy is appropriate for severe intracranial hypertension (ICP greater than 40 mm Hg) for at least 15 minutes or a reduction in mean CPP to less than 50 mm Hg. The EEG and serum barbiturate levels should be monitored daily.

Current investigation is underway on other agents that may be useful in controlling metabolic rate. These agents include phenytoin, lidocaine, and dimethyl sulfoxide. The mechanisms of these therapeutics are not well understood, but their effect on preventing the formation of cerebral edema and controlling ICP is promising.[7]

Proper positioning is mandatory as a management method. All patients with head trauma should be positioned to prevent flexion of the neck or hips. Head, neck, and extreme head flexion increase ICP. Head rotation of 90 degrees to either side may also result in increased ICP.[8,12,30] In the presence of increased ICP, the head of the bed should be elevated 30 to 45 degrees to improve venous drainage from the head.[8,12,30]

Concentrating nursing care activities into scheduled blocks of time to avoid overstimulation of the patient is a useful technique. Long periods of patient activity without rest may increase ICP and is not recommended. Talk about the patient's condition in the presence of the patient should be avoided.

Valsalva maneuvers, such as straining at stool, turning in bed, or sitting up, increase ICP. A Valsalva maneuver alone may not be sufficient to cause a sustained increase in ICP but may accelerate a deteriorating condition with other pressure-producing conditions.[30] Avoiding the cough reflex will also help to prevent rises in ICP. The nurse can administer lidocaine endotracheally when suctioning to prevent coughing.

ICP and CPP should be monitored during all activities. All ICP monitoring devices should be carefully maintained to obtain accurate readings.

The nurse caring for a severe closed-head injury patient is faced with the need to simultaneously minimize rises in ICP and to prevent the complications of immobility. To provide adequate nursing care for the patient with increased ICP, the nurse should be able to identify and prioritize the patient's problems (i.e., potential and actual) to assist in the development of nursing diagnoses.

CONTINUOUS ICP MONITORING

Continuous ICP monitoring began in the 1960s and is now considered commonplace in most critical care units. ICP monitoring is a continuous, direct measurement technique that uses an intracranial sensor, transducer, and recording device.[21] ICP monitoring has allowed for the early detection of intracranial hypertension as a complication of head trauma and for aggressive treatment of these patients. ICP monitoring devices also allow for the evaluation of the treatments and nursing care activities being used to prevent or control intracranial hypertension.[15] Pressures above 20 mm Hg for 30 minutes or more, or levels above 40 mm Hg for 15 minutes that do not respond to conventional therapy are considered evidence of uncontrolled ICP levels.[30]

ICP monitoring devices measure the volume of the following three compartments encased in the dura matter and

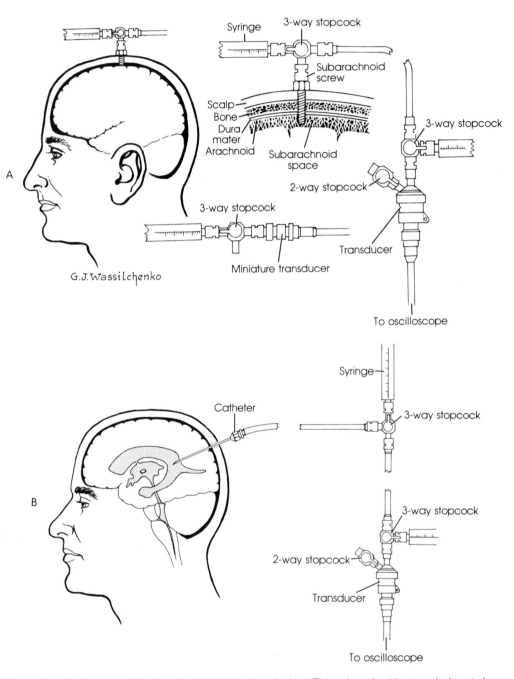

Fig. 12-10 **A,** Subarachnoid screw pressure monitoring. The subarachnoid screw is inserted through a burr hole in the skull and attached to a transducer and oscilloscope for continuous monitoring. **B,** Ventricular pressure monitoring. Catheter is inserted through burr hole in skull into lateral ventricle and attached to a transducer and oscilloscope to monitor ICP. (From Rudy EB: *Advanced neurological and neurosurgical nursing,* St Louis, 1984, Mosby–Year Book.)

skull: the brain parenchyma, the cerebrovascular system, and the CSF system.

There are several risks and complications related to the use of ICP monitoring, such as the inability to tap the ventricle, hemorrhage, continued leak of CSF, and infection. The techniques for measuring ICP vary, but the most frequently used include the following:
- Subarachnoid screw monitoring.
- Intraventricular monitoring.
- Epidural monitoring.

Subarachnoid Bolt/Screw Pressure Monitoring

A subarachnoid bolt/screw is inserted by a physician under sterile conditions (Fig. 12-10, *A*). A twist drill opening is made through the dura into the subarachnoid space, behind the hairline anterior or posterior to the coronal suture, usually in the nondominate hemisphere. A stopcock is attached to the bolt with pressurized tubing and a transducer, both filled with normal saline solution.[28] The transducer is balanced every 12 hours or whenever the system is disconnected or tampered with (e.g., irrigated by neurosurgeon with normal saline to dislodge blood, air, or brain tissue that may be disrupting the system). The subarachnoid bolt/screw method provides direct pressure measurement and does not penetrate the cerebrum.

Intraventricular Pressure Monitoring

An intraventricular catheter (IVC) or cannula is inserted in the anterior horn of the lateral ventricle, usually in the nondominant hemisphere by a neurosurgeon under sterile conditions (see Fig. 12-10, *B*). It is used in both adults and children, with special care being taken with children because of the small size of the ventricles.[4,24] The IVC transducer is balanced and recalibrated every 12 hours and as needed if the following conditions exist: dampened waveform, blood at transducer, unusually high or low readings according to patient status, or possible equipment malfunction.

Epidural, Fiber-Optic Transducer-Tipped Catheter Monitoring

The epidural, fiber-optic catheter tip transducer or radio transmitter is a device implanted through a burr hole in the

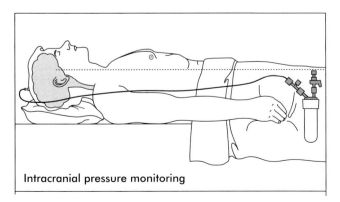

Intracranial pressure monitoring

Fig. 12-11 Position of patient for ICP monitoring.

Skill 12-3 Balancing a Transducer for Monitoring a Subarachnoid Bolt/Screw[17]

EQUIPMENT AND SUPPLIES
- Bolt device, monitor, and stopcock
- Spinal needles
- 2 sterile barriers (fenestrated if available)
- 2 4 × 4 gauze pads with alcohol, and antiseptic solution
- 2 dry 4 × 4 gauze pads
- 2 pairs of sterile gloves
- Masks
- Xylocaine
- Twist drill

NURSING INTERVENTIONS
1. Position patient (Fig. 12-11). Wear sterile gloves. Prepare sterile field with mask in place.
2. Open sterile barrier and place a small hole the size of the bolt in the middle of the barrier (if fenestrated unavailable).
3. Untape previous dressing.
4. Remove gloves.
5. Place monitor alarm in *standby* and *balance* mode.
6. Don second pair of sterile gloves.
7. Wipe stopcock and bolt* with one alcohol 4 × 4 gauze pad. Inspect stopcock, bolt, and transducer for blood or foreign material. Notify neurosurgeons of any abnormalities.
8. Maintain the balancing port at the proper level throughout monitoring. If the patient moves, reposition and rebalance the transducer. Position the top of the balancing port level with the foramen of Monro, which is at a point between the end of the patient's eyebrow and the tragus of the ear.
9. Turn stopcock *off* to the patient and remove the cap from the balancing port stopcock to open the transducer to atmospheric pressure.
10. *Balance (zero)* the transducer to atmospheric pressure by depressing the zero button on the monitor.
11. Return the stopcock to original position with deadhead in place, open to the patient and transducer closed to air. Observe oscilloscope for acceptable tracing with monitor in the *mean* mode, and turn alarms on to monitor ICP and ensure curve is present for patency. When the transducer is balanced, there will be a flat wave at zero.
12. Wipe stopcock and bolt as in step 7 and replace dressing.
13. Redress bolt with 1 to 2 sterile 4 × 4 gauze pads and apply occlusive sterile dressing to create a closed system.
14. Remove sterile barrier. Time, date, and initial dressing.
15. Record the following data: Glasgow Coma Scale ratings, reflexes, otorrhea, rhinorrhea, ecchymoses, nuchal rigidity, ICP readings and waveforms, dressing site, drainage, pain, sedation, respiratory and ventilatory pattern, thought processes, mood, and affect.

*Do not change bolt insertion site dressing.

epidural space (Fig. 12-12), rarely is it placed subdurally. The adjacent dura must be free from the inner table of the skull to avoid a wedge effect. Note that this system has a lower risk of infection than an IVC or subarachnoid bolt. Balancing and recalibration are not necessary with this system. All calibrations are done in the surgery by the physician at the time of insertion. Table 12-3 reviews the different types of monitoring devices and the advantages and disadvantages of each[14,31].

Skill 12-4   Balancing a Transducer During IPC Monitoring with an Intraventricular Catheter[16]

EQUIPMENT AND SUPPLIES

- Sterile 25-gauge prepackaged needle
- Sterile barrier
- 10-pack sterile 4 × 4 gauze pads
- Sterile gloves
- Mask
- Alcohol
- Drainage control bag (if appropriate)

NURSING INTERVENTIONS*

1. Prepare sterile field with mask in place.
2. Check system for air bubbles, blood, or tissue. Notify neurosurgeon of any abnormalities. It is normal to have air in the tubing below the drip chamber.
3. Check all exposed connections to ensure they are tight each time the system is manipulated to avoid leakage of CSF and contamination of the system or inaccurate readings.
4. Clamp tubing between the three-way stopcock and drip chamber. Turn three-way stopcock *off* to the patient.
5. Wear one sterile glove, separate 10-pack of 4 × 4 gauze pads. With unsterile hand, pour a small amount of alcohol over half of the 4 × 4 gauze pads.
6. Place two 4 × 4 gauze pads under self-sealing cap of the IVC.
7. Don other sterile glove.
8. With sterile gloves in place, remove needle's protective cap by disengaging needle by the hub. Return needle to sterile field.

9. Wipe self-seal cap with one 4 × 4 gauze pad with alcohol.
10. With sterile gloved hand, insert 25-gauge needle into self-sealing cap. (Inserting needle into cap at this time prevents direct route from air to patient's ventricles, as system is shut off to the patient by three-way stopcock.)
11. Place monitor alarm in *standby* and *balance* mode.
12. With unsterile hand, *zero* transducer by pressing the zero button on the monitor.
13. Turn monitor knob back to *mean* mode, range of the monitor should be on 25 to 50, depending on waveform.
14. Remove needle with sterile hand and rewipe self-sealing cap with alcohol 4 × 4 gauze pad. Remove needle gently so as not to dislodge IVC. It is important to remove the needle before turning the stopcock to prevent any inadvertent drainage of CSF and contamination by air having a direct route to the patient's ventricles.
15. Turn stopcock to position reading *open* to patient, transducer, and drainage system. Return monitor alarms to the *on* position. Check level of system to ensure that it coincides with the level ordered by the physician for drainage purposes.
16. Observe monitor for waveform and ICP reading. If ICP and waveform are unsatisfactory, recheck system and notify neurosurgeon. The waveform will be more accurate and clear when the three-way stopcock is *off* to drainage.

*Procedure may vary with agency. Check agency policy.

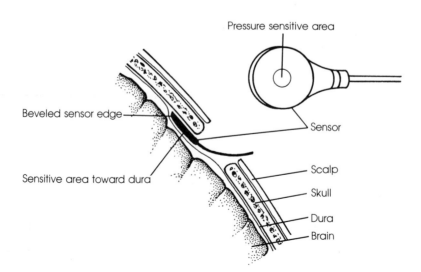

Fig. 12-12   Fiberoptic epidural pressure monitoring system. (From Ivan LP, Choo SH, Ventureyra ECG: *Child's Brain* 7:306, 1980.)

Skill 12-5 Care of the Patient with a Ventriculostomy[8,18]

EQUIPMENT AND SUPPLIES

- IVC
- Drip chamber
- Collection bag
- Sterile tube for daily cultures of CSF

NURSING INTERVENTIONS

1. Maintain and balance system as stated in Skill 12-4. Do not change IVC dressing.
2. Check position of drip chamber every hour or whenever patient or bed position is changed to ensure proper functioning of the system and avoid rapid loss of CSF.
3. Check and record volume drained every hour. Avoid tugging or pulling on the catheter. If the constant flow of CSF is impeded to the bag and an increase of pressure buildup occurs, a potential backflow to the patient can occur that increases the chance of infection, chamber collapse, or subdural hematoma.
4. Maintain drip chamber at ordered level, usually between the 10 to 15 cm mark, according to the physician's order. This mark should be level with the ventricle (Fig. 12-13). Start *0* point at the highest level of the drip chamber. Level of the ventricle is located at the halfway point of the tragus of the ear to the outer corner of the eye. If the reservoir is allowed to slip below ventricular level, excessive CSF will drain out. If the reservoir is placed too high, the ventricular pressure will not be relieved.
5. For safety purposes, place the chamber on the side of the pole attached to the bed to avoid additional pressure.
6. The physician will order a specific height (in cm) to maintain the IVC. Continuous or intermittent drainage should occur when the patient's ICP exceeds the level ordered (e.g., ordered IVC at 15 then CSF should drain when ICP is greater than 15).
7. Exception to above instance would include a conversion factor because of different units (e.g., drainage bag at 15 cm and monitor reads 15 mm Hg). If ICP reads 18 to 19 mm Hg, call neurosurgeon to check the system. If monitor reads negative numbers, the system is not functioning properly.
8. CSF sampling is performed by neurosurgeon under sterile procedure. The sample (approximately 4 ml) is taken from self-sealing port, placed in sterile tube, and sent for culture and sensitivity. Take samples daily to monitor results closely for infection.
9. Maintain strict aseptic technique when changing dressings and when caring for the ventricular catheter.
10. Prevent tension on the tubing when moving and turning the patient.
11. Check patency of tubing.
12. Monitor patient for the following: irritability, decreased LOC, increased white blood cell count, positive CSF culture results, nuchal rigidity, positive Kernig's sign, photophobia, and bleeding or infection at the insertion site.
13. Drainage bag changes include the following:
    - Turn IVC *off* to drainage.
    - Wear mask and gloves.
    - Disconnect at Luer-Loc syringe connection.
    - Discard bag and replace with new bag.
    - Label new bag with date, time and initials.
14. Record data (see Skill 12-3).

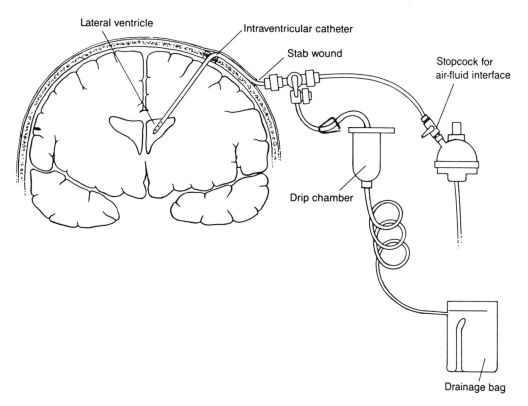

Fig. 12-13   Drip chamber is level with ventricle. (From Kinkade SL, Lohrman J: *Critical care nursing procedures: a team approach*, Toronto, 1990, BC Decker.)

Table 12-3   Methods of Monitoring*

Type	Placement	Advantages	Disadvantages
Subarachnoid bolt/screw	Hollow metal screw/bolt inserted through 1.27 cm twist drill hole (½ inch) beneath dura into the subarachnoid space (usually placed in the nondominant hemisphere).	Useful with small ventricles, no penetration of brain parenchyma, access volume/pressure response, access CSF sample, easy to insert, reliable, and easily balanced and calibrated with external pressure transducer.	Unreliable at high ICP levels (brain herniates into bolt), requires intact skull, 1%-2% infection risk, unable to withdraw significant amount of CSF, need for recalibration, risk of bleeding at insertion site, dura must be open, high profile of screw exteriorly (74 mm), and single lumen may become occluded.
Intraventric catheter (IVC) or cannula	A small rubber or polyethylene catheter is introduced through a burr hole into the anterior horn of the lateral ventricle (usually in the nondominant hemisphere).	Easy CSF sample/removal, reliable measurement, access of volume/pressure response, easy instillation of medication or contrast media, and most reliable and accurate way to determine ICP.	Placement problems with small ventricles/midline shift, possible damage to brain parenchyma (intracerebral bleeding or edema along the tract), 1%-6% infection rate, catheter occlusion with blood and brain tissue, need to realign transducer with head after any change in position, and ventricular collapse with rapid CSF drainage.
Epidural sensor	Balloon radio transmitter or a fiber-optic transducer placed through a burr hole between skull and dura. (The adjacent dura must be free from the inner table to avoid wedge effect.) Can also be placed subdurally.	Easy insertion, low risk of infection, no penetration of the dura, no external connection sites, no need for recalibration, and sensor/ICP readings not altered by blood or air.	Questionable accuracy of measurement, inability to calibrate after insertion, inability to determine volume/pressure response or sample CSF, wave form may become dampened, and wedge effect from the dura.
Fiber-optic transducer-tipped catheter (FTC) (Ex-Camino catheter)	Placed through subarachnoid bolt with the catheter extending just beyond the tip of the bolt. Placed in CSF or brain parenchyma. (A miniature transducer is located at the end of the tip of the catheter and light fibers sense movement in response to pressure.)	No need to recalibrate, can be used because of its size and versatility-intraventricular, subarachnoid, and subdural, smaller burr hole needed for insertion, no artifactual interference, able to monitor ICP during patient transfer, and lack of static fluid column.	Caution in handling—risk damage to light fibers and need to replace entire catheter if damaged, risk of infection, and zero drift.
LADD pneumatic sensor (Continuous monitoring used with monitor and printer system)	Epidural space	Dura remains intact, rapid response to pressure changes, no wire or fluid connection to patient, disposable and durable, and radiopaque disc permits x-ray verification.	Similar to epidural sensor.

*Refs 3, 8-10, 12, 25, 26.

Table 12-3   Methods of Monitoring —cont'd

Type	Placement	Advantages	Disadvantages
LADD intracranial pressure monitor (Used with newborns and infants)	No accepted method for the application of the sensor of this instrument to the anterior fontanel (which is critical for accurate measurement). The head is shaved over the area of the anterior fontanel and the sensor is gently applied to the skin. First half of the foam adhesive is applied, then the sensor and is checked for the ICP reading. Apply the remaining foam and see if the numbers correlate. Both of these readings should correlate with the reading obtained when the sensor was held gently against the skin before starting the application. For continuous use, reapplication may need to occur every 1-2 hours.	No penetration of the dura required, quick and easy, infection rate low, routine care easy to administer, monitoring cable can be detached from monitor, and easy to adjust.	ICP values can be influenced markedly by the amount of external pressure applied to the sensor.
Telemetric pressure sensor (Used in children 2 years of age and older)	Connect in-line with any closed ventricular shunt system.	No more risk or discomfort than the shunt itself, detects cardiac or respiratory related variations of the IVP that offers an indication that the ventricular catheter is unobstructed, can save costs and risks of CT scans, shunt taps, or unnecessary shunt revisions, no wires or tubes through the skin, barometric pressure compensation, in vivo zero point calibration, minimal drift problems, ICP readings can detect shunt malfunctioning, uses telemetric pressure balanced method analagous to the sphygmomanometer and fast response to detect cardiac related pulsations of ICP.	Adverse effects are similar to that of the shunt itself, foreign body rejection, shunt obstruction, mechanical failure, and excessive lowering of ICP.

Intracranial Pressure Waveforms

Three types of intracranial waveforms can be seen when monitoring: A, B, and C waves (Fig. 12-14). The A wave, or plateau wave, varies in intensity and amplitude. These waves usually range from 50 to 100 mm Hg and last from 5 to 20 minutes. The A waves usually occur when the mean ICP is in excess of 20 mm Hg and indicate advanced ICP. Once A waves have occurred, they tend to recur often and with greater amplitude. They persist for long periods of time and are associated with headache, decreased LOC, agitation, nuchal rigidity, restlessness, and general neurological decline. B waves are thought to be related to respirations. They fluctuate every 30 seconds to 2 minutes. They may rise as high as 50 mm Hg, but these elevations are never sustained. The C wave correlates with changes in blood pressure. C waves elevate, but the elevations are not sustained.

The ICP waveform occurs as the result of the transmission of systolic and diastolic arterial pressures in the brain tissue. The wave formations may signify specific changes occurring in the brain but may also indicate failure in the monitoring system, resulting in a dampened waveform (see Fig. 12-14,C). One should be familiar with the normal waveforms and, after troubleshooting the dampened waveform, should also be able to identify abnormal wave patterns. Table 12-4 discusses troubleshooting a dampened waveform.

SPINAL CORD INJURY

Approximately 10,000 persons a year sustain permanent injuries to the spinal cord. Almost one third of these die before reaching the hospital. Of those who survive, one half become paraplegics and one half become quadriplegics.[10]

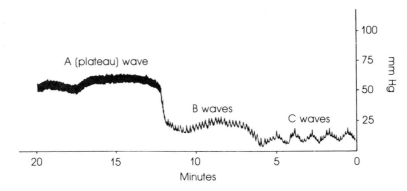

Fig. 12-14   Composite drawing of ICP waveforms. A (plateau) wave, B waves (normal ICP waveforms), C waves (dampened waveform).

Table 12-4   Troubleshooting a Dampened Waveform[9,28]

Problem	Remedy
Loss of waveform	Reposition catheter tip (withdraw slightly).
Air in line	Turn stopcock to patient *off.* Flush air out through open stopcock with sterile saline. Rebalance and recalibrate transducer and monitor.
Loose connection in line	Check tubing stopcocks. Turn stopcock *off* to patient. Tighten all connections.
Disconnection in line	Turn off stopcock to patient immediately.
Change in patient's position	Reposition transducer's balancing port level with foramen of Monro. Rebalance and recalibrate transducer and monitor.

Damage at the cervical cord level results in the most serious injury. Severe damage at this level causes quadriplegia. Injury at the thoracic level can result in chest, trunk, bowel, bladder, and lower extremity muscle losses. At the lumbar and sacral levels, severe damage can result in paralysis of the lower extremities.

Most of the victims of spinal cord injuries (SCIs) are young males between the ages of 15 and 30 years old. Common causes of SCI include vehicular accidents, injuries from assaults, falls, and sports-related injuries.[10] The most frequent sites of spinal cord injury are the lower cervical (C4 to C7) region and the thorocolumbar (T12, L1, and L2) area.

Injuries may include the loss of voluntary and autonomic motor activity. The location of the injury (i.e., cervical, thoracic, lumbar, or sacral) and the type of spinal cord injury determine which motor and sensory functions are lost. The patient must be carefully assessed for auto-

nomic dysreflexia (Fig 12-15) or spine shock.

Regardless of the level of the injury, the effects of permanent SCI are devastating. Almost every aspect of the patient's and family's life will be changed.[10]

Stabilization of the spinal column is crucial and must be maintained. Permanent stabilization is accomplished by prolonged skeletal traction alone or in conjunction with surgery.[10]

Once the spinal immobilization device is applied, careful skin care must be provided to prevent skin breakdown. This is particularly true in patients who have significant sensory or motor defects. Patients who have a SCI above the thoracic level are at risk for respiratory insufficiency or failure. SCI patients are at risk for lethal dysrhythmias, hypotension, emboli, and thrombophlebitis. Common elimination complications include GI bleeding, paralytic ileus, and urinary stasis.

Cervical Spine Traction

Skeletal traction is an alternative nonsurgical method of treating acute cervical SCIs. Cervical spine traction is an external fixation device (tongs) used to immobilize, reduce, and provide stability to the cervical vertebral column. The goal of treatment is to prevent further damage to the spinal cord and spinal nerves. The tongs are a stainless steel body with two sharp pins at either end. The method of placement and location of the different devices varies but the care is essentially the same.[30]

The length of time a patient stays in traction can vary from hours to weeks, depending on the type and location of the injury.[30] A patient may only be placed in traction long enough to achieve proper alignment and later progress to an alternate immobility device, such as a brace or halo vest.

Skull tongs

If the spinal injury is a stable cervical injury, the treatment of choice is the insertion of tongs into the skull. There are several types of tongs. Traditionally, Crutchfield tongs (Fig. 12-16, *A* and *B*) were widely used, but Gardner-Wells tongs (Fig. 12-16, *C* and *D*) are gaining in popularity.

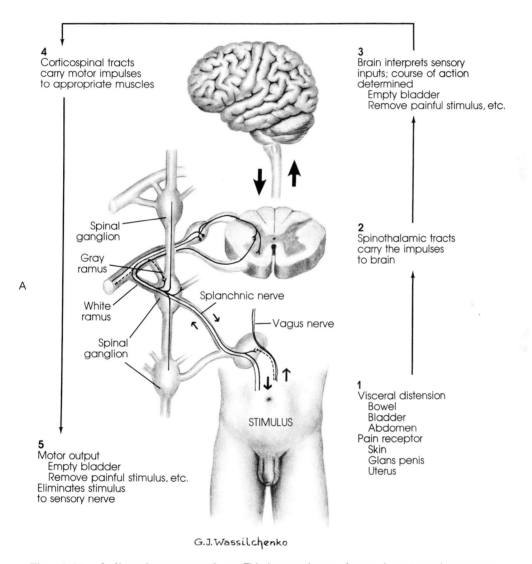

4
Corticospinal tracts
carry motor impulses
to appropriate muscles

3
Brain interprets sensory
inputs; course of action
determined
    Empty bladder
    Remove painful stimulus, etc.

Spinal
ganglion

Gray
ramus

White
ramus

Spinal
ganglion

Splanchnic nerve

Vagus nerve

2
Spinothalamic tracts
carry the impulses
to brain

A

STIMULUS

1
Visceral distension
    Bowel
    Bladder
    Abdomen
Pain receptor
    Skin
    Glans penis
    Uterus

5
Motor output
    Empty bladder
    Remove painful stimulus, etc.
Eliminates stimulus
to sensory nerve

G.J.Wassilchenko

Fig. 12-15   A, Normal response pathway. This is a syndrome of excessive autonomic response occurring in patients with cervical and high thoracic cord lesions. This mass reflex syndrome is triggered when afferent impulses ascend the spinal cord, usually due to an overdistended bladder (or bowel). (From Rudy EB: *Advanced neurological and neurosurgical nursing,* St Louis, 1984, Mosby–Year Book.)

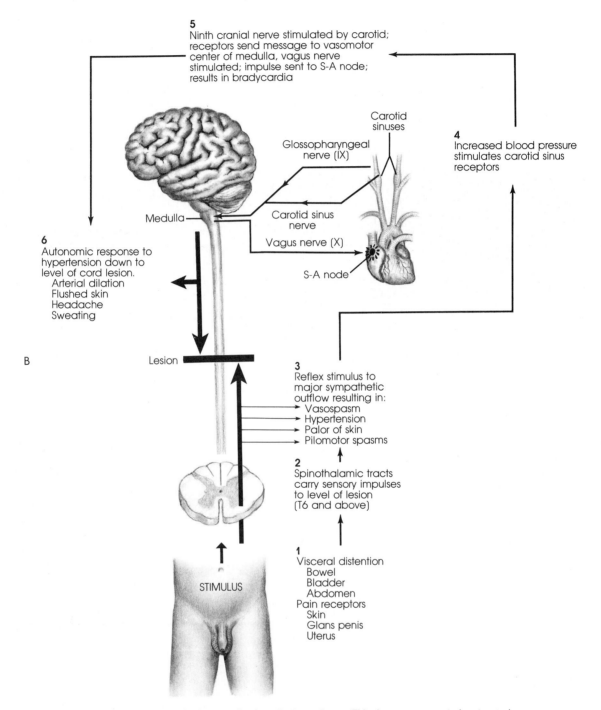

5
Ninth cranial nerve stimulated by carotid;
receptors send message to vasomotor
center of medulla, vagus nerve
stimulated; impulse sent to S-A node;
results in bradycardia

Carotid
sinuses

Glossopharyngeal
nerve (IX)

4
Increased blood pressure
stimulates carotid sinus
receptors

Medulla

Carotid sinus
nerve

Vagus nerve (X)

S-A node

6
Autonomic response to
hypertension down to
level of cord lesion.
   Arterial dilation
   Flushed skin
   Headache
   Sweating

B

Lesion

3
Reflex stimulus to
major sympathetic
outflow resulting in:
   Vasospasm
   Hypertension
   Palor of skin
   Pilomotor spasms

2
Spinothalamic tracts
carry sensory impulses
to level of lesion
(T6 and above)

1
Visceral distention
   Bowel
   Bladder
   Abdomen
Pain receptors
   Skin
   Glans penis
   Uterus

STIMULUS

Fig. 12-15 cont'd   B, Autonomic dysreflexia pathway. This is an exaggerated autonomic response and is a medical emergency that can result in convulsions, CVA, respiratory arrest, or cardiac arrest if untreated.

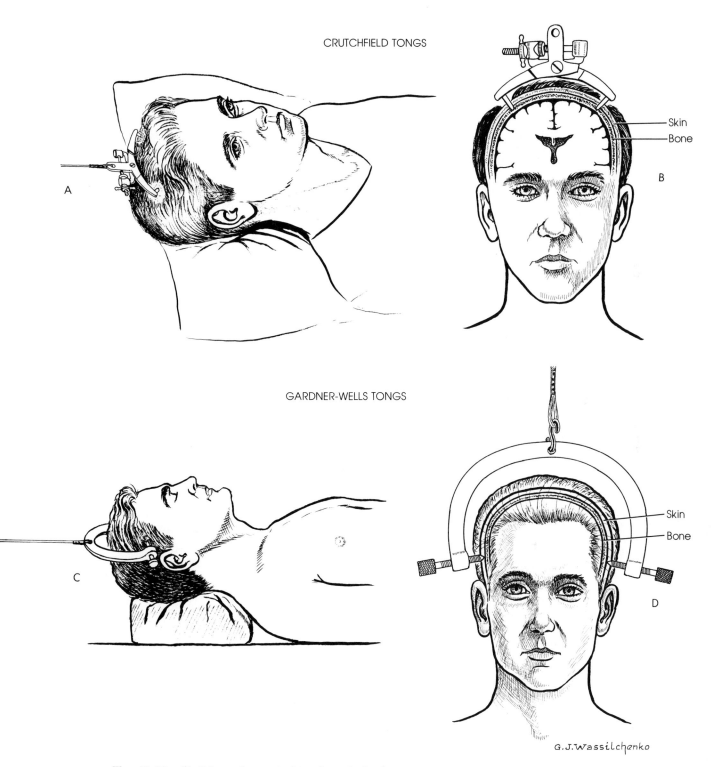

Fig. 12-16 Skull tongs for cervical tractions. **A,** Supine position. **B,** Cross section. **C,** Supine position. **D,** Cross section. (From Rudy EB: *Advanced neurological and neurosurgical nursing,* St Louis, 1984, Mosby–Year Book.)

Halo brace

The halo brace or vest is a form of spinal traction that allows the able patient to ambulate (Fig. 12-17), but the vest may lead to pressure sores and is rather heavy (about 4.5 kg [10 lbs]) and may unbalance the patient.

Sukoff Cervical Traction Transfer Device

The Sukoff board is a travel device designed to provide a safe method for immobilizing cervical spine–injured patients and transporting them for radiological studies. A major advantage of the Sukoff board is that cervical traction is only removed for a brief moment during transfer from the patient's original stabilization device to the travel device. This method of providing continual traction during transportation optimizes patient safety. This transfer device may be used whenever the patient is removed from the primary traction. Transferring the patient on the Sukoff board must always be supervised by a neurosurgeon familiar with the procedure.

Mechanical Beds

The last decade has brought many changes to the hospital environment. Increased technology is seen in all aspects of care, especially in the critical care areas and the rehabilitation setting. To assist the nurse in providing care, mechanical beds have been introduced into the care areas. Compared with the old Foster frames and circoelectric beds, these new beds not only help to position the patient but offer other advantages to the nurse and to the patient. The beds in this section fall into three major categories: rotating beds, low-air beds, and flotation beds (Table 12-5). Each of these beds is used for a distinct purpose and can be helpful in managing the patient with sensory-perceptual alteration.

PEDIATRIC CONSIDERATIONS

The complete pediatric neurological assessment is similar to that of the adult but must be adapted for the age of the child. Mental status, behavior, cerebellar function and coordination, motor function, sensory, as well as cranial nerve function and reflexes, are assessed.[33]

The central nervous system (CNS) of the newborn is not fully mature and develops slowly as the myelinization and maturation of the nervous system continues. The degree of neurological maturation can only be estimated in infants and children up to 2 years of age. The chief methods of assessment are observation and inspection, aided by palpation and passive manipulation of the infant.

Neurological assessment of the child requires knowledge of growth and development. One instrument used to identify potential growth and development problems (toddler to preschool) is the Denver Developmental Screening Test.

Allowing the parent to be present during the pediatric evaluation often puts the child at ease and more natural behavior is exhibited. One should approach the child's parent before beginning the evaluation of the child. The medical

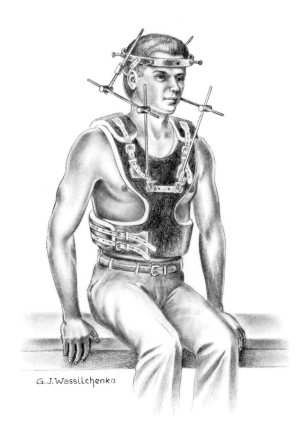

Fig. 12-17   The halo vest for spinal stabilization. (From Rudy EB: *Advanced neurological and neurosurgical nursing,* St Louis, 1984, Mosby–Year Book.)

history is obtained, and the nurse has time to observe the child during activity, feeding, and play.

The nurse should approach the child indirectly; for example, by allowing time for the child to adjust. Talking, holding, or playing with the child before beginning the examination is important. One should leave the child's clothing on as long as possible and take shoes and socks off before the examination and undress as needed; young children especially resist and are negative about being undressed.

The child will be more comfortable if the examiner sits or squats beside the child. It is important to begin the exam with nonthreatening procedures, such as testing motor skills, and to end with examination of head and eyes. Sensory functioning is easier to conduct with the older child but can still be difficult. Children are likely to be fearful of being stuck with pins and feeling hot liquids or icy liquids. It is helpful to involve the child in the testing preparation.

In the newborn, one should observe the level of alertness and response to stimuli. Evaluation of the infant and newborn includes the following: inspecting skin color; lesions; masses; size, shape and condition of head; shape of spinal column; spontaneous movements; tone and pitch of cry; and level of responsiveness. One should assess cranial nerves systematically. The first, second and eighth cranial nerves are difficult to test in the infant (Table 12-6). The twelfth cranial nerve can be checked by pinching the nos-

Skill 12-6   Troubleshooting Cervical Traction[6]

EQUIPMENT AND SUPPLIES

- Stryker frame (if appropriate)
- Two securing straps
- Cervical collar
- Two sandbags

NURSING INTERVENTIONS

1. Monitor baseline motor and sensory level to detect motor and sensory changes caused by interruption of skeletal integrity.
2. Log roll patient at all times to prevent twisting motion of the head, neck, and body that could cause further neurological damage.
3. Check bolts and pins every 4 hours to ensure proper functioning of immobilization devices.
4. Monitor weights; the number of pounds should correspond with written order. Do not add weight without a physician's order.
5. Maintain head in neutral position along axis with cervical alignment. Weights are to be hanging freely at all times. Traction knot should be 2.5 to 5 cm (1 to 2 inches) from pulley at all times to promote proper cervical alignment and traction.
6. Turn Stryker frame as ordered to maintain patient's skin integrity (usually every 2 hours).
7. Monitor body alignment on the frame to promote cervical alignment.
8. Pull patient down (in the supine position only), since patient is at high risk to fall face first through frame when prone. Use the following method:
   - Three people are needed; one person to guide the weights and head and two people to actually pull the patient down.
   - Pull patient down with one fluid motion. Never pull patient up on a frame because of a high potential to disalign bones of the neck and break traction.
   - Apply top of Stryker frame and place forehead and chin strap in place. Strap patient with C-bar and two straps, one at the elbows and one at the wrist. Properly position any additional equipment the patient may have; such as chest tubes and Foley catheter. Ensure monitoring lines clear of moving parts.
   - Turn patient slowly, to avoid orthostatic hypotensive episodes.
   - Check patient's head placement and support from chin and head straps to ensure proper alignment.
   - Provide pin site care at least every 8 hours.

trils, producing a reflex of opening the mouth and raising the tip of the tongue. Cerebellar functioning can be assessed by observing body movements. One can have the child place a finger to the nose, then walk, hop, and stand on one leg. In the toddler, eye-hand coordination movements should be monitored. Motor functioning can be checked by assessing muscle development; that is size, tone, strength, and abnormal involuntary movements, such as rigidity, twitching, or spasticity. Handedness should be observed. Infants and young children generally show no preference. Failure to demonstrate handedness by school age could indicate failure of the brain to develop dominance on one side.

Skill 12-7   Transfer to Sukoff Cervical Traction Device[19]

EQUIPMENT AND SUPPLIES

- Sukoff board with all components
- Stryker frame or stretcher

NURSING INTERVENTIONS

1. Obtain Sukoff board and correct number of weights. Neurosurgeon is present at bedside for transfer.
2. Patient is placed in the prone position on the Stryker frame. The mattress pad may be removed from posterior portion of the frame for larger patients to aid in closing the frame for turning.
3. Place Sukoff board with its pad in place on the patient's back. The bottom of the Stryker frame is applied over the back of the Sukoff board and the patient is turned, as the previously described method for turning Stryker frames.
4. Once supine, the top of the Stryker is removed. The neurosurgeon applies hand traction to the tongs or halo ring and transfers patient to the Sukoff board.
5. During transfer, the nurse assists the physician by removing weights from the Stryker traction, lifting the metal traction bar or the Sukoff frame or positioning the traction rope, as needed. The neurosurgeon will maintain hand traction and prevent any neck motion during the transfer.
6. The patient must be positioned far enough down on the board to ensure that cervical traction is maintained. When the weight bar is resting on the board, there is no cervical traction; therefore the patient must be pulled down.
7. Connect the four straps: one across the chest, one across the shins, and two crisscrossing the chest. They should be snug but not tight. Pad the straps as needed. The patient's arms should be placed inside the straps.
8. The patient is now ready for transfer to a cart for interhospital transport or may be left on the Stryker frame. The Stryker frame may be angled if contrast has been injected and this will be specified by the neurosurgeon. This is done to prevent upward movement of contrast to the vital structures of the brain, which can cause seizure activity.
9. The Sukoff device with the patient secured to it is only sitting on the stretcher. Extra straps are necessary to prevent the frame from falling off the Stryker during transfer.

Skill 12-8   Management of Sukoff Device in Radiology[19]

EQUIPMENT AND SUPPLIES

- Sukoff board with all components
- Stryker frame or stretcher

NURSING INTERVENTIONS

1. Four people use the hand holes on either side of the Sukoff board to transfer the patient slowly in a totally horizontal manner. The neurosurgeon does not need to be present, as traction is maintained at all times by correct use of the board.
2. If there is an extended wait in the radiological department, the straps may be loosened and the patient rolled side-to-side 15 degrees as one would in bed. The four straps are kept on to prevent the patient from falling off the board when they are rolled side-to-side. The straps may be loosened for turning. The straps should be snug for the computed tomography (CT) radiological procedure, this will minimize motion during the study and hence improve image quality.

Table 12-5   Mechanical Beds

Type	Purpose	Principle use	Advantages	Disadvantages	Nursing responsibilities
Rotation beds (Kinetic therapy treatment table, Rota-rest [Fig. 12-18])	To turn patient by a passive mechanical means through an arc of 124 degrees every 3-5 minutes.	Immobilized patients, SCI patients, head injury patients, unconscious patients, poststroke patients, patients with pulmonary complications, and patients with any chronic debilitating neurological disorders.	Continual turning, up to 300 times a day, traction can be used on bed, prevents pressure sores, continual postural drainage—prevents hydrostatic pneumonia and atelectasis, decreases venous stasis, stimulates peristalsis, reduces muscle wasting and contractures, and can be used at home.	Claustraphobia, patients may have pain when turning onto traumatic fractures, may increase agitation, can cause diarrhea, and must rotate patient 16-20 hours a day for positive effect.	Assess patient for pressure areas around padding. Block care to minimize turning off to bed. Check patient's orientation frequently to detect sensory-perceptual changes.
Low-air loss beds (Kinair or Flexicair)	To prevent or treat tissue trauma in high-risk patients.	Patients at high or intermediate risk for the development of skin breakdown, agitated head injuries, patients on bed rest, immobile patients, SCI patients, and patients with poor nutritional status.	A regular size bed (in most cases), segmented cushions to provide different levels of pressure to different parts of the body, able to control bed temperature, and can be deflated for ease of transferring patients.	If not used properly, can cause as much pressure as a regular mattress.	In most models (except Flexicair), pressures must be adjusted each time the patient's position is changed.
Flotation beds (Clinitron)	To create an environment for the human body to float without the inherent problems of flotation: instability, maceration of the skin, and difficulty in positioning the patient	Patients with decubitus ulcers, patients with skin loss because of trauma, postoperatively following a skin flap, and burn patients.	Reduction of constant pressure on skin and bony prominences, decreases friction when moving patient, and by turning the air flow off, the bed becomes firm and allows for positioning of the patient.	Difficult to use with cervical traction, not suitable during the acute phase of SCI, increased insensible fluid losses in patient (may affect electrolytes and fluid balance), and difficult to perform chest physical therapy.	Understand how to turn bed off should cardiopulmonary resuscitation (CPR) be necessary. Accurate intake and output. Follow electrolytes to prevent dehydration.

Table 12-6 Cranial Nerve Assessment for Infants and Children

Cranial Nerve	Test
I, Olfactory	Difficult to test in very young children
II, Optic	Test acuity
III, Oculomotor	Test pupil reflexes
IV, Trochlear	Have child follow toy with eyes, move up, down, and in
V, Trigeminal	Observe jaw movements and sucking
	Test corneal reflex
VI, Abducens	Make noises, note eye movement, and use toys
VII, Facial	Watch face while laughing or crying, facial expressions
	Check wrinkle of forehead
VIII, Acoustic	Make loud sounds—ring bell
	Newborn: startle reflex
	Vestibular: difficult in small children
IX, Glossopharyngeal	Prefers sweet taste to sour taste
X, Vagus	Gag reflex—variable responses test same as adult
XI, Spinal accessory	Look for symmetry of muscles
	After 5 months, look for head lifting when supine
XII, Hypoglossal	Observe tongue movement

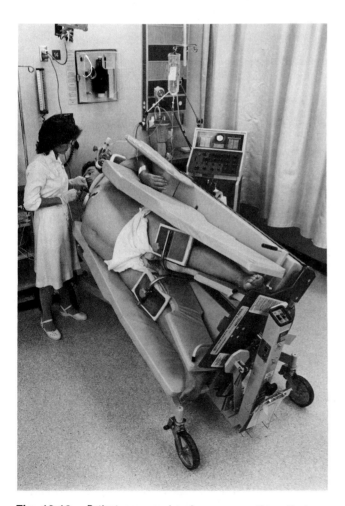

Fig. 12-18 Patient care can be given even as the patient rotates. This patient is being suctioned as he turns. *(Courtesy of Kinetic Concepts, San Antonio, Tex.)*

Sensory functioning is difficult to assess in infants because their threshold to touch, pain, and temperature are higher than children but they have a slower reaction time. Corticospinal pathways are not fully developed in infants: therefore, the spinal reflex mechanisms (deep tendon and plantar) vary during infancy. Exaggerated or absent responses mean little in terms of assessment unless they are asymmetrical or a change has been noted from a previous response. Babinski's response to plantar stimulation is usually elicited in normal infants until about the age of 2. Infants demonstrate a wide variety of primitive reflexes because of the developmental level of their nervous systems. Each reflex and movement is assessed, evaluated, and recorded.[22]

LOC can be assessed by using the Glasgow Coma Scale for Children (Table 12–7). One should observe gross motor skills during initial contact with the child. The time the child needs to adapt to examiner's presence should be noted as well as the child's mood and behavior and general physique and nutritional status. The child can be asked to lie flat and then stand up to observe gait and running, and the muscle groups used. One should try to perform the examination in a playful manner to reassure the child and allow for extra time.[22]

The adolescent neurological examination is not different from the adult neurological evaluation. Adolescents usually suffer head and spinal cord trauma because of their active lifestyles.

Seizures

There are two examples of nonage specific seizures: tonic-clonic and focal motor. Neonates may have seizure activity characterized by a period of sucking, apnea, unresponsiveness, or ridigity. An EEG is necessary to determine if behaviors denote seizure activity.

Children, 1 month to 3 years of age, may exhibit minor motor seizures; that is myoclonic, akinetic spells, or head dropping. These can be caused by metabolic factors, cerebral trauma, or an unknown cause. This group commonly has febrile convulsions. Children older than 3 years of age exhibit petit mal, temporal lobe, and focal seizures.[8]

Treatment and medications vary according to a child's individual response. Often diazepam (Valium) is used for acute treatment. Valproic acid (Depakene) works well with infants and toddlers. Phenobarbitol works well with the older child and Dilantin is used cautiously because of its side effects. Blood levels need to be monitored routinely for therapeutic levels.

Increased Intracranial Pressure[8]

Increased ICP is a complication of injuries and diseases of the brain. In the pediatric population, causative agents vary but treatment modalities are generally the same as that of the adult. In the infant, increased ICP is frequently seen as the result of congenital hydrocephalus or a complication of the birth process itself. Space-occupying lesions, contusions, edema, or hydrocephalus are the most common

Table 12-7 Pediatric Coma Scale*

Response	Score	Over 1 year	Less than 1 year	
Eyes opening	4	Spontaneously	Spontaneously	
	3	To verbal command	To shout	
	2	To pain	To pain	
	1	No response	No response	

Response		Over 1 year	Less than 1 year	
Best motor	6	Obeys		
	5	Localizes pain	Localizes pain	
	4	Flexion withdrawal	Flexion withdrawal	
	3	Flexion—abnormal (decorticate rigidity)	Flexion—abnormal (decorticate rigidity)	
	2	Extension (decerebrate rigidity)	Extension (decerebrate rigidity)	
	1	No response	No response	

Response		Over 5 years	2-5 years	0-23 months
Best verbal	5	Oriented and converses	Appropriate words and phrases	Smiles, coos, cries appropriately
	4	Disoriented and converses	Inappropriate words	Cries
	3	Inappropriate words	Cries and/or screams	Inappropriate crying and/or screaming
	2	Incomprehensible sounds	Grunts	Grunts
	1	No response	No response	No response
Total	3-15			

*Modification of Glasgow Coma Scale: A sum of seven or less is an objective measure of coma. The lower the score, the deeper the coma. (From Whaley LF, Wong DL.: *Nursing care of infants and children*, ed 3, St Louis, 1987, Mosby–Year Book.)

causes for increased ICP. Cerebral edema is often the result of the following pathological conditions: anoxic brain injury, infections (meningitis), and metabolic disorders (Reye's encephalopathy and lead poisoning). Treatment of increased ICP in children using dexamethasone (Decadron) or mannitol does not always have the rapid response needed. Basically, the treatment is to remove the causative agent, decrease ICP, and maintain an adequate CPP. A few pediatric variations exist for monitoring of ICP. In infants, the skull is unable to support the subarachnoid bolt so the choices are routinely an IVC (caution is used because of the small size of the ventricles and the risk of infection) or a type of the following subarachnoid transducers: the epidural sensor, pneumatic sensor, telemetric pressure sensor, or the LADD ICP monitor.[8,10,34]

Clinical manifestations of ICP vary with age. Infants with increased ICP present with full fontanelle, increased head circumference, suture separation, high pitched cry, and delayed or absent motor skills. The child with increased ICP shows headache (often worse in the morning), visual problems, nausea and vomiting, seizures, and papilledema (usually 48 hours after the increase). For all ages, the late signs and symptoms of increased ICP are the same as those of the adult.

Cervical Traction

SCIs in children are rare. Many times these are related to tumors or congenital problems. These problems can often predispose the child to more severe consequences despite less trauma to the spinal cord. Major cord damage as a result of injuries includes compression fractures, frac-

ture-dislocations, burst fractures, stretch rupture, or penetrating transection. The mechanism of a SCI and type of injury sustained varies with the child's age. For example, SCIs in the infant are often related to child abuse or falling. As children grow, injuries involve bicycle riding. In adolescence, SCIs may result from diving accidents and sports. Attempted suicide may also result in a SCI.

As with the adult, the acute SCI should be treated emergently with decompression in whatever fashion is deemed necessary with the type of injury sustained; that is, immobilization and traction (Crutchfield or Cone-Barton tongs), steroid therapy, or a combination of any of the above. Surgery is the final intervention for stabilization.

The child and family will be extremely frightened because of the pain, the separation, and the severity of the injury. Supporting them and supplying information is extremely important and will assist them to determine what their immediate, intermediate, and long-term needs will be.

PSYCHOSOCIAL CONSIDERATIONS

Psychosocial care of the patient with a neurological injury begins on admission. These injuries are generally unexpected and initial support from the nurse can help the family through the initial crisis and realization of the injury. After the acute phase of hospitalization and crisis intervention, the long term consequences of these injuries require an ongoing plan of psychosocial support for the patient and family. The long-term loss of specific neurological functions causes the patient and family to go through a grieving process, like the stages of death and dying. It is essential that support be directed to first helping the patient and family accept the loss; then working toward compensating for it and restructuring a life with significant and often fundamental changes.

Information about the injury and long-term consequences, as well as the appropriate resources for support, should be given to the family. This helps provide a realistic outlook for the patient and hope that a plan to cope with the injury is possible. Discharge from the hospital and returning home can also be a frightening experience. Both patient and family have to face the full impact of a disability in the home environment. Psychosocial support is essential to minimize the transition to home. Follow-up planning and assurance that support will continue through group process is essential for a smooth transition to independence.

PATIENT AND FAMILY TEACHING

Trauma to the brain or spinal cord is one of the most devastating types of impairment to patient and family. The unresponsiveness of the brain-injured patient, the paralysis of the spinal cord-injured patient, the unpredictable outcome, and the possibly long rehabilitative process all contribute to the uncertainty of the family situation.

Communication and emotional support are essential for the patient and family members. Teaching involves answering questions with understandable explanations, explaining equipment, orienting to the ICU, and providing additional information as needed.

It is important when teaching patients to include the family in the educational process. Patients who have suffered a CNS injury require specific information related to their injury. The following are instructions that can apply to any neurologically impaired patient:
1. Take frequent naps.
2. If you feel tired, lie down.
3. Eat balanced meals.
4. AVOID the following hazardous situations:
   - Heavy lifting.
   - Tub bathing.
   - Bending or twisting.
   - Contact sports.
   - Driving until seizure-free.
   - Swimming alone.
   - Drinking alcoholic beverages.
5. Take any medications that are prescribed by your physician.
6. Follow any additional discharge instructions given to you by your physician or nurse.

Brain Injury

Brain injuries occurring from the lack of oxygen, blood, or bruising of the brain, can affect the thinking process and movement and coordination. Sometimes the patient may notice behavior changes that are a result of the injury. When the injury first occurs, it is hard to predict how much damage may be permanent. Whatever improvement will occur is generally within 3 to 12 months from the injury.

Many of the behavior changes accompanying head injury are temporary and will resolve within a few weeks to months; therefore the patient should not make major changes in lifestyle or home. Many of the following may occur:
- Altered thought processes; the patient may feel speeded up or slowed down.
- Difficulty in concentrating; the patient may be unable to read or watch TV for a prolonged time.
- Distracted easily; the patient may be unable to complete tasks.
- Loss of recent memory; the patient may be unable to recall events that happened earlier in the day.
- Changes in temperament; the patient may be more easily frustrated and have less patience.
- Changes in moods and emotions; the patient may laugh or cry more easily.
- Dwelling more on significant past experiences; the patient may talk or think more about a war experience or the accident itself.
- Difficulty in understanding jokes; the patient may not understand punch lines or they may not seem funny.
- Changes in sleeping patterns; the patient may sleep more or less than before.

Recommendations include the following:
1. When the patient first goes home, he/she should have a written schedule of day and evening activities to improve memory, concentration, and thinking processes.
2. For the first 2 weeks, someone should be with the patient at all times.
3. The patient should do the following:
   - Use safety precautions at home to avoid reinjury; remove scatter rugs, use handrails on stairs, pad sharp corners or objects, use a seat belt with shoulder straps when riding in a car, and do not ride motorcycles.
   - Gradually return to normal activities, as prescribed by your doctor. Take short walks and light exercise, but take it easy until the physician authorizes more strenuous physical activity.
   - Resume normal sexual activity at any point during recovery.
   - Ensure that a family member is close during the night. A night light may help to prevent disorientation.

   But:
   - Do not drive or return to work until cleared by doctor.
   - Do not take unprescribed or illegal drugs or drink alcohol.

Seizures

Teach families about seizure management. Family members should know to do the following if a seizure occurs:
- Be alert to prodromal stages of seizures.
- Lower person to floor.

- Remain calm and stay with seizing person.
- Clear area.
- Place some small, flat, soft article under the person's head.
- Insert airway if the person's jaw is not clenched.
- Loosen tight clothing.
- Do not restrain.
- Give CPR if necessary. (Encourage family members to become CPR certified.)
- Turn person on side following seizure.
- Remain with person during and after seizure.
- Reorient as needed.
- If another seizure begins before person regains consciousness, call a physician or rescue squad.

The following are safety precautions for a patient with seizure disorders in the event of a seizure:

- If there is a warning, lie down.
- Wear emergency medical identification.
- Teach friends, family, and coworkers what to do if a seizure occurs.

HOME HEALTH CARE CONSIDERATIONS
Altered Level of Consciousness

It may be necessary to provide home health care for a patient with an altered LOC. This type of patient at home requires constant care. Not only the patient but the family needs support and encouragement. Respite care will probably be required to prevent care giver burnout.

Maintaining a patent airway is of primary importance because of the patient's inability to clear secretions. The following measures are useful:

- Provide aggressive pulmonary toilet.
- Position on the sides and never the back.
- Change position frequently.
- Elevate the head of the bed slightly.

Adequate nutrition must be provided to the patient. Tube feedings, either continuous or intermittent, may be required, so do the following:

- Assess tube placement before beginning intermittent feeding and every 4 hours for continuous feedings.
- Assess residual gastric contents (see Chapter 16).
- Warm tube feeding to room temperature before feeding.
- Maintain head of bed at 30 to 45 degrees during each feeding and at least 1 hour following intermittent feedings, and at all times with continuous feedings.
- If patient has cuffed tracheostomy, keep it inflated during and after feeding.
- Assess for signs of aspiration (i.e., coughing, increased secretions, and cyanosis).

Total parental nutrition may be required for patients who are unable to tolerate tube feedings or who require additional nutrition.

Decreased mobility creates many problems. Measures to reduce complications include the following:

- Aggressive pulmonary toilet.
- Meticulous skin care and frequent turning.

- Passive (and active, if possible) range-of-motion exercises.
- Support stockings.
- Avoiding massage of the legs.

Urinary and bowel elimination are frequent problems for patients with altered LOCs. A catheter for urine and assistance for bowel elimination may be necessary. Eye care will be needed for the unconscious patient to prevent corneal conjunctival injury. Finally, complete personal care of the patient may be necessary.

Seizure Precautions and Care

Once the patient who could potentially have seizures is discharged, certain precautions need to be taken in the home to ensure safety. Foremost is patient and family teaching, including the following steps:

- Encourage the patient to comply with the medical regimen.
- Provide the patient with information about acquiring an emergency alert bracelet or tag.
- Encourage the patient to carry a wallet card identifying him or her as a person who may have seizures.
- Have quick access to mouth gag, padded tongue blade, or airway.

Spinal Cord Injury

The extent of the damage to the spinal cord will in most instances, determine the amount of home health care required. The greater the damage, the more supportive the care. In severe injury, months of rehabilitation will be required before the patient is discharged home.

The patient with SCI may experience ineffective airway clearance. Several techniques are helpful in assisting the patient to maintain a clear airway. A fluid intake of 35 ml/kg per day for adults helps to keep secretions moist so that they can be removed easily. Air humidification is also helpful. Kinetic beds provide automated movement of the patient over a 124 degree range and are helpful in preventing pulmonary secretions. Coughing and deep breathing are vital to the patient with a SCI. The cough reflex may be significantly impaired especially in those patients who have paralysis of the intercostal and abdominal muscles. The patient, nurse, or a family member can assist with a cough maneuver. This technique is a modification of the Heimlich maneuver.

Whether full-time or part-time assistance will be needed depends on the abilities and energies of the patient. Physical therapy, vocational training, and psychological support may also be required.

Active and passive range-of-motion exercises may be required, as well as bowel and bladder care and training (or catheter care). Furthermore, assistance may be needed to perform skin and pressure sores care.

Decisions regarding work or about returning to school (if schooling has been interrupted by the CNS injury) will have to be made. Other decisions will also be made about socialization and all aspects of daily living. Involvement in a support group, such as a local chapter of the National Spinal Cord Injury Association, may be helpful.

Sexual function is an important concern for patients who have experienced an SCI. Many times this concern is not voiced until the patient gets home. The home health care nurse needs to determine the patient's level of concern, knowledge, and physical capabilities. Important areas to assess include neurological functioning, emotional status, attitudes, level of coping, and past experience.

REFERENCES

1. American Association of Neuroscience Nurses: *Core curriculum for neuroscience nursing,* Park Ridge, Ill, 1984, The Association.
2. Aumic KJ: Head trauma guidelines, *RN* 54(4):27, 1991.
3. Bishop BS: Pathologic pupillary signs: self-learning module, part II, *Crit Care Nurse* 11(7):58, 1991.
4. Chapman PA: *Insertion and care of intracranial pressure monitoring devices.* In Ropper AH, Kennedy SK, Zeras NT, editors: *Neurological and neurosurgical intensive care,* Baltimore, 1983, University Park Press.
5. DeLoach P: *Intraventricular catheter master care plan,* Baltimore, 1984, MIEMSS Care Plan Committee.
6. DeLoach P: *Spinal cord injury master care plan,* Baltimore, 1985, MIEMSS Care Plan Committee.
7. Donegan M, Bedford RF, Dacey R: IV lidocaine for prevention of intracranial hypertension, *Anesthesiology,* 61:201, 1979.
8. Gilliam EE: Intracranial hypertension, *Crit Care Nurs Clin North Am* 2(1):21, 1990.
9. Hannon K, Flynn J-B McC, McNeely J: *Neurosensory integration.* In Berger K, Williams M: *Collaborating for optimal health,* Norwalk, CT, 1992, Appleton & Lange.
10. Hughes MC: Critical care nursing for the patient with a spinal cord injury, *Crit Care Nurs Clin North Am* 2(1):33, 1990.
11. Ladd: *Ladd/Steritek ICP monitoring system,* Burlington, Vt.
12. Lehman LB: Intracranial pressure monitoring and treatment: a contemporary view, *Ann Emerg Med* 19(3):295, 1990.
13. Luce JM: Neurologic monitoring, *Respir Care* 30(6):471, 1985.
14. Lucha S: Working with ICP monitors, *RN* 54(4):34, 1991.
15. Martin ML: Pharmacologic therapeutic modalities: phenytoin, dimethyl sulfoxide, and calcium channel blockers, *Crit Care Q* 5(3):72, 1983.
16. MIEMSS Nursing Procedure Committee: *Balancing intraventricular catheters,* Baltimore, 1985, The Institute.
17. MIEMSS Nursing Procedure Committee: *Balancing richmonde screw,* Baltimore, 1985, The Institute.
18. MIEMSS Nursing Procedure Committee: *Care and management of intraventricular catheter drainage system,* Baltimore, 1985, The Institute.
19. MIEMSS Nursing Procedure Committee: *Sukoff cervical traction transfer device,* Baltimore, 1984, The Institute.
20. MIEMSS Montebello Nursing Staff, DeLoach P: *Master care plan for seizures,* Baltimore, 1987, MIEMSS Care Plan Committee.
21. Millar S, Sampson LK, Soulup M: *AACN procedure manual for critical care,* Philadelphia, 1985, WB Saunders.
22. Mitchell P: Decreased adaptive capacity, intracranial: a proposal for a nursing diagnosis. *J Neurosci Nurs* 18:170, 1986.
23. O'Brien K: Managing the seizure patient, *Nursing* 21(1): 63, 1991.
24. Pollack-Lathum C: Intracranial pressure monitoring, Part I, physiologic principles. *Crit Care Nurse* 7(5) 40, 1987.
25. Pollack-Lathum C: Intracranial pressure monitoring, Part II, patient care. *Crit Care Nurse* 7(6) 53, 1987.
26. Radionic: *The cosman ICP tele-sensor,* Burlington, Mass, 1983, Radionics.
27. Ricci MM: *Intracranial pressure monitoring.* In : *AACN procedure manual for critical care,* Philadelphia, 1985, WB Saunders.
28. Ridgeway G: Demystifying tonic-clonic seizures, *Nursing,* 21(11): 63, 1991.
29. Rudy EB, Turner BS, Baun M et al: Endotracheal suctioning with head injury, *Heart Lung* 20(6):667, 1991.
30. Rudy EB: *Advanced neurological and neurosurgical nursing,* St Louis, 1984, Mosby–Year Book.
31. Shepard R and Hotter A: Evaluating an ICP epidural catheter, *Crit Care Nurse* 9(2):74, 1989.
32. Walleck CA: Intracranial hypertension: interventions and outcomes, *Crit Care Nurs Q* 10(1):45, 1987.
33. Walleck CA, Rochon CA: *Neurological assessment.* In Flynn J-B McC, Hackel R: *Technological foundations for nursing,* Norwalk, Conn, 1990, Appleton & Lange.
34. Walleck CA: Neurological considerations in the critical care phase, *Crit Care Nurs Clin N A* 2(3): 357, 1990.
35. Walleck CA: Preventing secondary brain injury, *AACN Clin Issues Crit Care Nurs* 3(1):19, 1992.

CHAPTER 13

Intravenous Fluid Therapy

Objectives

After completing this chapter, the reader will be able to:

- List the purposes of intravenous (IV) therapy.
- Identify the various IV solutions.
- Compare and contrast the complications of IV therapies.
- Formulate nursing diagnoses and patient outcomes.
- Calculate drops per minute for both macrodrop and microdrop tubing sets.
- Regulate IV flow rates based on calculations.
- List factors that affect the flow rate of an IV infusion.
- Describe the process of starting, maintaining, and discontinuing the IV infusion.
- Discuss pediatric considerations for IV therapy.
- Discuss IV use in home health care.

Patients require IV fluids for a wide variety of reasons. These include situations in which patients have an alteration in fluid and electrolyte imbalance related to the following:

- Shock.
- Hemorrhage.
- Burns.
- Excessive vomiting or diarrhea.
- Nasogastric suctioning.
- Nothing-by-mouth (NPO) order.
- Altered level of consciousness (LOC).

Other reasons for IV therapy include the following:

- Provision of a route for IV medications.
- Infusion of high molecular weight fluids.
- Frequently obtained blood specimens.
- Provision of a route for physiological monitoring or artificial cardiac pacing.
- Surgery or emergency.

TYPES OF IV SOLUTIONS

A list of some commonly used IV fluids along with their tonicity (concentration), purposes, and caloric content can be seen in Table 13-1. Caloric content of commonly used IV fluids is low; therefore they are rarely administered to meet total nutritional needs. Infusions that are administered for this purpose are referred to as total parental nutrition (see Chapter 15).

ASSESSMENT

Critically ill patients are at risk for developing fluid and electrolyte imbalances. Therefore nurses should assess a patient's fluid and electrolyte status frequently by the following:

- Assess respiratory status and breath sounds for crackles.
- Obtain patient history.
- Assess patient for signs and symptoms of fluid and electrolyte imbalances (Table 13-2).
- Measure abdominal girth, as well as ankle and wrist circumference.
- Weigh patient daily. A weight change of 0.5 kg(1 lb)/24 hr may indicate fluid imbalance.
- Assess general appearance and mental status.
- Inspect eyes for sunken eyeballs or puffy lids.
- Assess neck veins (see Chapter 6).
- Auscultate heart and lungs.
- Monitor hemodynamic measurements for central venous pressure (CVP), pulmonary artery wedge pressure (PAWP), mean arterial pressure (MAP), cardiac output (CO), and systemic vascular resistance (SVR) (see Chapter 8).
- Assess for orthostatic hypotension.
- Assess skin turgor, condition of mucous membranes, and conjunctivae.
- Review recent fluid intake and losses.
- Review laboratory studies.
- Monitor rate of IV fluids.
- Monitor output.

NURSING DIAGNOSIS

Possible nursing diagnoses for patients requiring IV therapy include the following:

- Fluid volume deficit related to shock.
- Fluid volume excess related to renal failure.
- Potential fluid deficit related to electrolyte imbalances secondary to burn injury.

Table 13-1   Types of Intravenous Solutions*

Solution	Type	Calorie/L	Purpose
Dextrose (%) in water			
2.5 (D2.5/w)	Hypotonic	85	Provides minimal calories and water without electrolytes.
5.0 (D5/w)	Isotonic	170	Provides hydration.
10.0 (D10/w)	Hypertonic	340	Provides calories in small amount of
20.0 (D20/w)	Hypertonic	680	fluid.
50.0 (D50/w)	Hypertonic	1700	Increases blood sugar when adminis-
70.0 (D70/w)	Hypertonic	2380	tered quickly.
Saline (%) (NS)			
0.45 (½ NS)	Hypotonic	0	Provides daily salt and water require-ments.
0.9 (NS)	Isotonic	0	Hypotonic solutions provide hydration.
3.0 (3% NS)	Hypertonic	0	Hypertonic solutions treat severe Na^+
5.0 (5% NS)	Hypertonic	0	deficits.
			Used to treat H^+ imbalances.
Dextrose (%) in saline (%)			
2.5 in 0.45 (D2.5/½ NS)	Isotonic	85	Provides Na^+Cl^- and minimal calories
5.0 in 0.45 (D5/½ NS)	Hypertonic	170	Provides Na^+Cl^- and electrolytes
2.5 in 0.9 (D2.5/NS)		85	Used to treat temporary hypovolemia.
5.0 in 0.9 (D5/NS)	Hypertonic	170	Provides fluids.
10.0 in 0.9 (D10/NS)	Hypertonic	340	
Ringer's solution (Contains Na^+, Cl^-, K^+, and Ca^{++})	Isotonic	9	Supplies K^+ and Ca^{++} in addition to Na^+ and Cl^- Used in extracellular volume depletion.
Ringer's lactate (%) (Contains Na^+, Cl^-, K^+, Ca^{++}, and lac-tate)			
5.0 D/RL	Hypertonic	179	Increases interstitial fluid pressure.
10.0 D/RL	Hypertonic	340	Maintains volume (expander). Supplies blood lactate ions. Used similarly to plasma.
Bulter's solution	Hypotonic	0	Replaces multiple electrolytes. Supplies free water.
Dextran (%)			
10.0 dextran 40 in D5/w	Isotonic	170	Osmotically active. Maintains (expands) blood volume.
10.0 dextran 40 in NS	Isotonic	0	Used to treat shock and hypovolemia.
Hetastarch			
6.0% Hetastarch in 0.9% NS	—	—	Plasma volume expander. Increases plasma colloid osmotic pres-sure.
Solutions containing alcohol			
5.0% alcohol in 5.0% D5/w	Hypertonic	525	Provides calories. Provides sedative effect. Increases feeling of well being. May provide analgesic effect. Diuretic effect. Expands circulating blood volume.

*NSS, normal saline solution; Na^+Cl^-, sodium ion; Na^+, sodium ion; H^+, hydrogen ion; Na^+Cl^-, sodium chloride ion; K^+, potassium ion; Ca^{++}, calcium ion.

Continued.

Table 13-1 Types of Intravenous Solutions —cont'd

Solution	Type	Calorie/L	Purpose
Blood and blood components	—	—	Supports plasma osmotic pressure. Prevents shock. Prevents circulatory collapse. Provides clotting factors.
Protein hydrolysates (Amino acid solutions) Aminosol Travasol	Hypertonic	Calories vary depending on type of solution. Can range from 255 to 1010.	Supplies proteins. Corrects negative nitrogen balance.
Fat emulsions Intralipid (10%) Intralipid (20%)	Isotonic Isotonic	1100 2000	Provides calories. Provides fatty acids. Prevents fatty acids deficiencies. Used in severe nutritional disorders.

Table 13-2 Selected Fluid and Electrolyte Disorders[2,8,11,12,17]

Physiological status	Value	Selected causes	Signs and symptoms	Nursing interventions
Fluid balance Hypovolemia	Blood osmolarity > 295 mOsm. Urine sodium content 20 mEq/L. Specific gravity >1.026. Urine-to-serum osmolality ratio > 2.	Low fluid intake, vomiting, diarrhea, high temperature, burns, massive crushing injuries, perforated peptic ulcer, intestinal obstruction, blood loss, and nasogastric suction.	Dry skin and mucous membranes; decreased skin turgor; tongue furrows; reduced urinary output, increased specific gravity; hard, dry stools; weight loss; lassitude and fatigue; rapid pulse and respirations; hypotension; depressed fontanels in infants; sunken eyeballs in adults; elevated red blood cell count and hemoglobin; and cold extremities; apprehension, disorientation, and unconsciousness.	Provide mouth care and use glycerine swabs and lip balm; measure urine output hourly; weigh daily and measure skin folds; assist with activities of daily living; monitor vital signs every 4 hours or more frequently; monitor laboratory data; keep warm; provide emotional support; assess level of consciousness; encourage fluids if appropriate; and maintain and monitor IV fluids if being administered.
Hypervolemia	Blood osmolarity < 275 mOsm urine specific gravity.	High fluid intake, high salt or sodium bicarbonate intake, renal malfunction, congestive heart failure (CHF), and compensatory response following hemorrhage.	Shortness of breath, dyspnea, rales, and air hunger; bounding pulse and engorged neck veins; reduced temperature; edema; "finger imprinting" on sternum; puffy eye lids; weight gain; decreased red blood cell count, hemoglobin, and hemocrit; early—high blood pressure (BP); late—low BP; increased urine volume; and decreased specific gravity.	Elevate head of bed; administer oxygen through nasal cannula as ordered; encourage coughing and deep breathing; assess vital signs and monitor neck veins; measure and assess temperature; weigh daily; monitor laboratory data; monitor BP; reduce fluid intake; monitor output; and teach patient signs and symptoms of hypervolemia.
Sodium Hyponatremia	Serum sodium < 135 mEq/L. Serum chloride < 96 mEq/L. Urine sodium < 20 mEq/L.	Excessive perspiration, decreased Na^+ intake, gastrointestinal suction, high intake drinking water, vomiting, IV infusions free of electrolytes, diuretic administration, cirrhosis, and nephrosis.	Apprehension, anxiety, and confusion; anorexia and nausea; abdominal cramps; rapid weak pulse; cold, clammy skin; hypotension; convulsions; weakness; scant urine with low specific gravity (1.001-1.003); and circulatory collapse.	Provide emotional support and assess for anxiety; monitor vital signs frequently; keep warm and dry; assist when out of bed; monitor BP; maintain airway; measure urine and monitor specific gravity; monitor IV infusions; limit drinking water; encourage increase of sodium in diet (if appropriate); and teach about sodium intake.

Table 13-2   Selected Fluid and Electrolyte Disorders[2,8,11,12,17]—cont'd

Physiological status	Value	Selected causes	Signs and symptoms	Nursing interventions
Hypernatremia	Serum sodium 147 mEq/L. Serum chloride > 106 mEq/L. Urine sodium chloride < 50 mEq/L	Inadequate water intake, excessive sodium intake, diarrhea, renal failure, and hypothalamic lesions.	Dry, sticky mucous membranes; rough, dry tongue; excessive thirst; firm skin turgor and flushed skin; scant urine with high specific gravity; decreased BP; convulsions; elevated temperature; edema; and pulmonary congestion.	Teach and assist with good mouth care; assess mouth; supply fluids as needed; provide skin care; monitor urine output and measure specific gravity; monitor intake; monitor IVs (if appropriate); maintain airways; monitor vital signs; and keep warm and dry.
Potassium				
Hypokalemia	Serum potassium < 4 mEq/L	Diarrhea, intestinal disease, vomiting, stress, physical insult, burns, diuretic administration, sodium wasting, and kidney diseases.	Weak, faint pulse; falling blood pressure; malaise; abdominal distention; few stools; anorexia; nausea and vomiting; soft, flabby muscles; depressed ST segment on ECG; prolonged P-R interval; flattened or inverted T wave, first and second degree block, atrial flutter, premature atrial contractions (PACs), premature ventricular contraction (PVCs), and prominent U wave on ECG; shallow respirations (in severe deficits); muscle cramps; and predisposition to digitalis toxicity.	Monitor vital signs; assist with activities of daily living (ADLs); provide favorite foods; administer antiemetic drugs as ordered; protect when out of bed; evaluate ECG; observe for symptoms of digitalis toxicity; monitor laboratory values; and teach about foods high in potassium and encourage ingestion of high potassium foods.
Hyperkalemia	Serum potassium > 5.6 mEq/L.	Burns, crushing injuries, kidney disease, excessive infusion of potassium, adrenal insufficiency, and metabolic acidosis.	Nausea, intestinal colic, vomiting, anorexia, and diarrhea; irritability; reduced memory; generalized muscle weakness; easy fatigability; scant or no urine; weak, irregular pulse; ventricular fibrillations; shallow respirations (in severe deficits); tall T waves on ECG with short QT interval; and widening of the QRS complex.	Administer medications as ordered; assist with ADLs; protect when out of bed; measure urine; monitor vital signs; and monitor laboratory values.
Calcium				
Hypocalcemia	Serum calcium < 4.5 mEq/L.	Sprue, excessive infusion of citrated blood, peritonitis, hypoparathyroidism, diarrhea, rapid or overcorrection of acidosis, magnesium excess, and lack of vitamin D.	Tingling in fingertips; numbness in extremities; abdominal cramps; tetany; convulsions; carpopedal spasm; presence of Chvostek's sign; and prolonged QT interval.	Medicate according to physician's orders; maintain airways, protect from injury, and notify physician of abnormal signs and symptoms; and monitor laboratory values.
Hypercalcemia	Serum calcium > 5.8 mEq/L	Prolonged bedrest, hyperparathyroidism, calcium producing lung tumor, excessive vitamin D intake, excessive milk intake, excessive "hard" water intake, sarcoidosis, and bone cancer.	Flank pain; kidney stones; nausea and vomiting; anorexia; constipation; stupor and coma; deep bone pain; weight loss; increased excretion of calcium in urine; kidney stones; decreased heart rate; shortened QT interval; and shortened ST segment.	Support and assist in ADLs daily living; assess; medicate as ordered; strain all urinary output; record output; maintain airway and protect from injury; monitor LOC; monitor laboratory data; and notify physician of any sudden or unexpected changes.

Continued.

Table 13-2   Selected Fluid and Electrolyte Disorders[2,8,11,12,17]—cont'd

Physiological status	Value	Selected causes	Signs and symptoms	Nursing interventions
Chloride				
Hypochloremia	Serum chloride < 95 mEq/L	Diuretic therapy, hyponatremia, metabolic alkalosis, bicarbonate gain, Addison's disease, gastric suctioning, vomiting, excessive diaphoresis, diabetic acidosis, severe diarrhea, and burns.	Decreased BP; hyperexcitablity; tetany; tremors; and shallow breathing.	Assess; administer medications according to physician's orders; and monitor laboratory values.
Hyperchloremia	Serum chloride > 105 mEq/L	Dehydration, head injury, hyperventilation, cancer of stomach, eclampsia, and cardiac decompensation	Weakness; lethargy; and deep, rapid respirations.	Monitor daily weights; measure input and output; and restrict sodium intake.
Phosphates				
Hypophosphatemia	Serum phosphate < 2.5 mg/dl	Inadequate intake, antacid therapy, diarrhea, hyperparathyroidism, glycosuria, diuretics, insulin administration, acute respiratory alkalosis, and catecholamine administration.	Weakness; respiratory failure; cardiomyopathy; osteomalacia; obtundation; and seizures and coma.	Assess status; evaluate intake and output; administer medication according to physician's orders; check medication orders for insulin; and monitor laboratory data.
Hyperphosphatemia	Serum phosphate > 4.5 mg/dl	Decreased glomerular filtration rate (GFR), hypoparathyroidism, acromegaly, thyrotoxicosis, cytotoxic drugs, laxative abuse, and phosphate enemas.	Tetany, hypotension, and cardiac arrest.	Patient history regarding laxative and enema use; monitor vital signs; monitor intake and output; assess status; and monitor laboratory data.
Magnesium				
Hypomagnesemia	Serum magnesem < 1.5 mEq/L	Chronic alcoholism, vomiting, diarrhea, cirrhosis, impaired intestinal absorption, enterostomy drainage, severe renal disease, ingestion of diuretics, pancreatic insufficiency, hypercalcemia, hyperaldosteronism, glycosuria, and hyperthyroidism.	Disorientation, and hallucinations; hypertension; tremors; tetany; hyperactive deep reflexes ; convulsions; rapid pulse rate; and elevated BP.	Assess and reorient (if appropriate); monitor vital signs; maintain airway and administer medications as ordered; and assess laboratory values.
Hypermagnesemia	Serum magnesem > 2.5 mEq/L	Renal failure, acidosis, tissue trauma, administration of magnesium salts or antacids, purgatives or enemas, administration of lithium, and ingestion of "hard" water.	Rarely symptomatic except at very high levels—drowsiness, coma, muscle weakness, and skin irritation.	Assess and maintain airway; assist with ADL; provide skin care; keep warm and dry; and turn frequently.

PATIENT OUTCOMES

The following are sample expected outcomes for patients requiring IV fluid therapy.

Patient evidences:

- Weight change of less than 0.5 kg(1 lb)/24 hr.
- Blood pressure and pulse rate within normal limits for the patient.
- CVP 0 to 6 mm Hg; PAWP, 6 to 15 mm Hg.
- ECG normal for patient.
- MAP, 70 to 90 mm Hg.
- Respiratory rate, 12 to 20 breaths/min.
- Urine volume ideally between 600 to 1600 ml/24 hr or in accordance with intake ($\geq$ 30 ml/hr).
- Moist mucous membranes and normal skin turgor.
- Serum electrolyte levels within normal ranges.
- Urine specific gravity, 1.003 to 1.030.
- Tendon and muscular strength normal for patients (i.e., absence of muscle cramping).

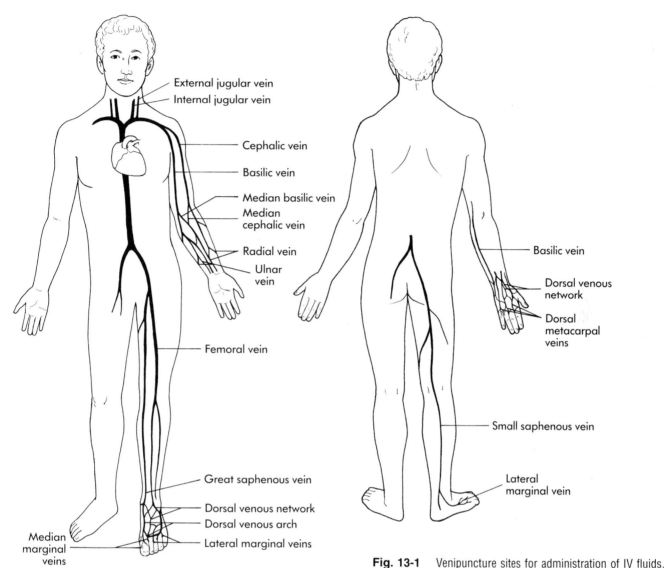

Labels on front figure:
External jugular vein
Internal jugular vein
Cephalic vein
Basilic vein
Median basilic vein
Median cephalic vein
Radial vein
Ulnar vein
Femoral vein
Great saphenous vein
Dorsal venous network
Dorsal venous arch
Lateral marginal veins
Median marginal veins

Labels on back figure:
Basilic vein
Dorsal venous network
Dorsal metacarpal veins
Small saphenous vein
Lateral marginal vein

Fig. 13-1 Venipuncture sites for administration of IV fluids.

SITES FOR IV INFUSIONS

The most common sites for IV placement can be found on Fig. 13-1. Additionally, there are many factors to be considered when selecting an IV site. These include the following:

- Accessibility of the vein.
- Condition of the vein.
- Size of the vein.
- Purpose of the infusion.
- Condition of the surrounding skin.
- Condition of the patient.
- Patient's preference.
- Age of the patient.
- Amount and type of infusion.
- Duration of the infusion.

Cannulation of Central Veins

The most commonly cannulated central vein is the subclavian. It is used for rapid administration of large amounts of fluids, for hypertonic solutions, and for the measurement of central venous pressure. (See Chapter 8 for more information on this topic.) A relatively new type of central venous access is now available. This is known as the peripherally inserted central catheter (PICC). The PICC line is a Silastic IV catheter that is primarily inserted into the basilic or cephalic veins through the antecubital space and then advanced into the superior vena cava to serve as a central line. This type of catheter may be inserted at the bedside by specially trained nurses.

The superior vena cava placement is recommended for the infusion of total parental nutrition (TPN) or any irritating agent. PICCs are useful for those patients who require long term IV therapy. Complications from the PICC are fewer in number and usually less severe than with conventional IVs. Insertion complications include the following: bleeding and compartment syndrome, tendon or nerve damage, dysrhythmias, chest pain, respiratory distress, malposition of the catheter, and embolism. Complications following insertion include phlebitis, sepsis, air embolism, and pulmonary embolism.

Arterial Line

An arterial line is placed to measure arterial pressures. Arterial lines are presented in Chapter 8.

Skill 13-1 Venipuncture

EQUIPMENT AND SUPPLIES

- IV fluid as ordered by physician
- IV tubing with rate-control device or volume infusion pump, if needed
- Good lighting
- Alcohol sponges or other antimicrobial cleansing wipe
- Syringe and appropriate needles or catheters
- 2 × 2 or 4 × 4 gauze pads (sterile and unsterile)
- Tourniquet or blood pressure cuff
- Tape
- Arm board (optional)
- IV pole
- Sterile needles and catheters in a variety of gauges
- Time tape
- Filter (optional)
- Heparin flush (if using intermittent infusion device)
- Rubber gloves
- Landry vein light venoscope, if needed

NURSING INTERVENTIONS

1. Organize equipment and open sterile packages.
2. Prepare the IV solution by doing the following:
   - Read label.
   - Note clarity of solution, check sterility, and note expiration date.
   - Attach tubing.
   - Gently rotate bag (if medication is added to mix).
   - Run solution through tubing to clear air. (If Y-tubing is to be used, attach solutions and clear both lines of air. If volume control set is used, fill with the prescribed amount of solution and clear line of air.)
   - Fasten the clamp.
   - Attach needle or catheter. When using IV bottles, break metal cap and remove both metal and rubber diaphragms. Insert tubing into largest opening.
3. Choose site (i.e., a fairly large vein in a convenient site). If using the Landry venoscope, locate vein. Adjust lighting. Larger veins should be used when hypertonic or irritating solutions are to be infused since these solutions often produce inflammatory responses in the vein. Some IV solutions cannot be infused safely through the peripheral veins because of their hypertonicity. In such cases a central vein, usually the superior vena cava or the subclavian, is used. The blood flow through these great veins is large enough to dilute hypertonic solutions and prevent pain, irritation, and phlebitis commonly encountered with use of peripheral veins. Central venous lines are also used for the following: central venous monitoring, rapid fluid infusion, as an alternative when peripheral veins are unusable and for greater patient comfort and mobility.
4. Apply tourniquet or BP cuff (inflated to a pressure setting of 100 mm Hg) above the site to distend the veins. The site can be patted lightly to make veins more visible. Do not leave tourniquet in place for more than 5 minutes. If using Landry venoscope, tighten strap.
5. Wear gloves and protective eyewear.
6. Ask patient to open and close the hand several times (if able) to further distend the vein. Lightly palpate the vein. Distended veins feel like flexible, hollow tubes (Fig. 13-2). If the vein feels hard or ropelike, do not use but choose another vein.
7. Support the IV site with the nondominant hand and use the thumb of the nondominant hand to stretch the skin and anchor the vein.
8. Swab the skin (for at least 1 minute) with a quick drying antiseptic. Alcohol is a cold solution and may cause local vasoconstriction because of the skin's reaction to the rapid temperature change. Betadine is frequently used. Once skin has been cleansed, do not touch the site. If the skin is touched to relocate the vein, it must be re-cleansed. (Fig. 13-3).
9. Hold the needle or catheter in the dominant hand. Point the needle or catheter in the direction of the course of the vein at the proposed site of entry. The bevel of the needle should be facing upward during venipuncture. When a large needle is introduced into a small vein, the bevel may be downward to prevent puncturing the posterior wall of the vein when the tourniquet is removed. Most short-term IV infusions started on children use a scalp vein or butterfly. For long-term therapy, a flexible catheter is used. When using an over-the-needle catheter, inspect the catheter tip. Do not use if it is not smooth and intact.
10. The needle should be held at an angle slightly lower than 45 degrees and inserted into the skin adjacent to the vein.
11. Depress the needle so that it is almost flush with the skin. Move the tip of the needle directly above the vein. If veins roll easily insert needle at a section of vein where it bifurcates.
12. Slowly insert the needle into the vein. A backflow (flashback) of blood into the tubing or syringe will indicate satisfactory entry. If using a teflon catheter-inside-needle, do not allow the plastic catheter to touch the skin. Thread the catheter into the vein while holding the metal needle portion in a secure position. If resistance is met, release the tourniquet and remove both portions of the set (i.e., the metal needle and the catheter).
13. When blood appears, carefully advance needle or catheter until it lies well within the vein.
    For the following catheter-over-the-needle:
    - Stabilize needle by holding hub with nondominant hand, carefully advance catheter until it lies well within the vein to ensure that the teflon section lies well within the vein.
    - Place 2 x 2 gauze pad under end of catheter to catch blood.
    - Remove needle from catheter, while applying gentle pressure above the catheter to prevent blood from flowing out.
    - Never reinsert the metal stylet back into the teflon portion of the catheter. This could damage the catheter and cause an embolism.
    - Connect primed tubing.
    - Release the tourniquet or Landry venoscope strap.
    - Slowly begin flow of IV fluid.
      For the following catheter-through-the-needle:
    - Stabilize needle by holding hub and advance catheter by applying pressure through plastic jacket.
    - Engage needle hub into catheter hub.
    - Withdraw needle from vein until about 2.5 to 5 cm (1 to 2 inches) of catheter are showing.
    - Remove catheter jacket.
    - Remove control plug and stylet.
    - Connect primed IV tubing.
    - Release tourniquet or Landry venoscope strap.
    - Initiate flow.
    - Secure needle guard over point of needle.
14. Adjust the clamp and begin the IV solution flow.

Skill 13-1   Venipuncture—cont'd

15. Check the solution to ensure that it is flowing freely. Assess for infiltration. Screw clamps or other type of speed regulator should be placed out of reach of children, if they open it they can suffer from speed shock or circulatory overload.
16. Apply topical antimicrobial ointment at catheter insertion site (if this is agency policy).
17. Secure the needle or catheter with tape. A small gauze pad may be placed under the hub of the needle if necessary. A small sterile dressing (i.e., 2 × 2 gauze pad) can be placed over the site. If polyurethane adhesive dressing is used, apply according to manufacturer's directions.

18. To minimize movement of the needle in the vein, loop tubing and tape near the venipuncture site.
19. An arm site can then be immobilized on an arm board. Label a piece of tape indicating the vein path, type and size of needle or catheter, and date, time, and initials of person starting the IV. Attach to IV dressing.
20. Adjust the flow rate.
21. Remain with patient for several minutes to monitor flow. Position patient comfortably.

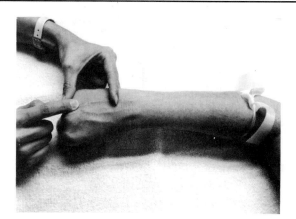

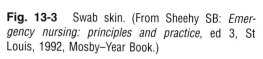

Fig. 13-2   Palpate the vein. (From Perry AG, Potter PA: *Clinical nursing skills and techniques,* ed 2, St Louis, 1990, Mosby–Year Book.)

Fig. 13-3   Swab skin. (From Sheehy SB: *Emergency nursing: principles and practice,* ed 3, St Louis, 1992, Mosby–Year Book.)

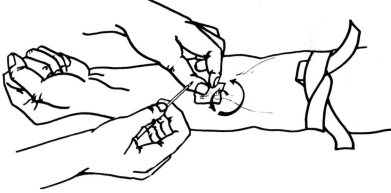

Intraosseous Infusion

Intraosseous infusion is the infusion of fluids, blood, or drugs directly into the bone marrow cavity. The intraosseous route has been shown to be clinically equivalent to the IV route in terms of absorption time and drug effectiveness.[10]

Intraosseous infusions are used during emergency situations when IV access is not easily obtained.

There are few contraindications for intraosseous infusion. These include the presence of bone disorders, such as osteopetrosis, osteogenesis imperfecta, or an ipsilateral fracture of the extremity. The risk of infection is increased when the needle is introduced through an area affected by cellulitis or an infected burn.[4,14]

The site of choice is the anterior medial aspect of the

tibia. An alternate choice is the midanterior, distal one-third of the femur.

The most common complication associated with intraosseous infusions is extravasation of fluid and medication into the subcutaneous tissue.[14] The complication causing the most concern is osteomyelitis. This complication is related to long-term administration of intraosseous infusion. Localized cellulitis and the formation of subcutaneous abscesses are also complications.

Cutdown

A cutdown is a surgical procedure performed when peripheral veins cannot be found or are not adequate. Cutdowns are usually performed at the patient's bedside in emergency situations by the physician.

Skill 13-2 Inserting a Heparin Lock (or Intermittent Infusion Device or Male Plug Adaptor)

▼

EQUIPMENT AND SUPPLIES

- See equipment and supplies for Skill 13-1
- Heparin lock or intermittent infusion device
- Dilute heparin solution or NSS

NURSING INTERVENTIONS

Before inserting heparin lock, inject dilute heparin solution to fill tubing and needle. This removes air from the tubing preventing formation of air embolus.

1. Open intermittent infusion device.
2. Prime with heparin or normal saline.
3. Follow Skill 13-1, steps 2 to 12 for venipuncture (if an IV solution is to be administered).
4. Insert device into catheter.
5. Flush with 2 ml of flush solution to prevent clot formation.
6. Apply dressing. Write time, date, and initials.

REGULATING AND MONITORING IV SOLUTION FLOW

Regulating and monitoring the IV infusion is the nurse's responsibility. The amount and rate of administration are determined by the physician based on the patient's needs.[5]

The most accurate way to regulate the IV flow is to calculate the flow rate. The rate is calculated on the basis of drops per minute and size of the drop. The drop factor is the number of drops necessary to deliver one ml of solution to the patient. The drop factor is usually found on the package containing the tubing (see box).

IV Push or Bolus

Many times medical intervention is aimed at achieving and maintaining therapeutic plasma drug concentrations as quickly as possible to provide relief of symptoms or preserve and support vital organ function. To do this, a high concentration of medication may be administered by bolus.

The IV push or IV bolus is a rapid method of administering medications intravenously. An IV bolus is most commonly used in the following situations:

- During emergency situations.
- When the patient is critically unstable.
- When administering IV medications that cannot be diluted (e.g., many chemotherapy drugs, Dilantin, digoxin, Hyperstat, Lasix, and Valium).
- When a peak drug level in the blood is required.
- When an alternate route for drug administration is essential.

The dosage of medications given by IV bolus may need to be adjusted on the basis of several of the following factors:

- Body weight.
- Age (i.e., young or elderly).
- Selected route.

Skill 13-3 Regulating the IV Solution Flow

▼

NURSING INTERVENTIONS

1. Check doctor's order for flow rate.
2. Calculate the drop rate per minute (see the box below).
3. Determine the present flow rate by counting the number of drops per minute, using the second hand of a watch held up to the drip chamber. If infusions are potentially toxic, the flow rate should be timed for one full minute, if not, time for 15 seconds and multiply by 4.
4. If infusion is too slow, speed up; if too fast, slow down.
5. Recount.

Skill 13-4 Maintaining Arterial Line Patency

▼

NURSING INTERVENTIONS

1. Check pressure bag frequently.
2. Ensure constant reading of 150 to 300 mm Hg.
3. Maintain a continuous or hourly heparin flush on arterial lines used for blood pressure monitoring.

▼

Calculation of Drop Rate

STEP 1
$$\frac{\text{Total amount of solution}}{\text{Number of hours}} = \text{Number of ml/hr}$$

STEP 2
$$\frac{\text{Ml/hr}}{60} = \text{Number of ml/min}$$

STEP 3 Ml/min × number of drops/ml = Number of drops/min

Example A: Macroset
IV order: 2000 ml D5/W to infuse over 16 hours
Drop factor: 10 drops/ml

Step 1: 2000/16 = 125 ml/hr
Step 2: 125/60 = 2.08 ml/min
Step 3: 10 × 2.08 = 20.08 drops/min
(round to 20 or 21)

Example B: Microset

IV order: 750 ml D5/NSS to infuse over 16 hours
Drop factor: 60 drops/ml

Step 1: 750/16 =41.6/min
Step 2: 41.6/60 = 0.78 ml/min
Step 3: 60 × 0.69 = 46.8 drops/min
(round to 46 or 47)

- Patient's expected response.

IV push medications can be given directly by venipuncture through a needle or by using the ports on the IV tubing or on a heparin lock.

Skill 13-5 IV Push or IV Bolus

EQUIPMENT AND SUPPLIES

- 2 syringes filled with 3 to 5 ml sterile normal saline solution
- Alcohol wipes
- Prefilled syringe with medication

NURSING INTERVENTIONS

The nursing interventions listed here will identify the steps for administering an IV bolus medication through an existing IV site.

1. Prepare the prescribed medication using the appropriate amount of diluent as identified by the package insert.
2. Determine if the drug is compatible with the primary IV solution.
3. Inspect the venipuncture site to determine that the infusion is patent and has not infiltrated or caused a phlebitis. To check for blood return, twist tubing tightly around your finger and release, creating a vacuum effect. Observe for blood return. If either has occurred, stop the present infusion and restart IV.
4. If the IV solution is incompatible with the medication, clamp off the IV flow and flush the line between the medication port and the patient with 3 to 5 ml sterile normal saline after drawing back to check for blood back flow.
5. Cleanse the injection port closest to the needle on the IV tubing with an alcohol swab and allow to dry.
6. Hold medication port firmly with the nondominant hand and insert the medication syringe into the port.
7. Inject the medication at the designated rate. NOTE: Check agency policy to determine if compatible IV is to be clamped or to remain open. Use a watch with a second hand to time all IV bolus medications.
8. Remove syringe and needle when drug administration is completed. If drug is incompatible with the IV solution, flush line with 3 to 5 ml of sterile saline solution.
9. Unclamp tubing; readjust flow rate.
10. If the medication is to be administered through a heparin lock, use the following steps:
    - Swab with alcohol wipe.
    - If medication is incompatible with heparin, insert needle with syringe of sterile saline into the port.
    - Aspirate to determine patency.
    - Flush the heparin lock and remove.
    - Insert needle with medication syringe into port and inject medication at the designated rate.
    - Remove needle and syringe from port.
    - For incompatible medication, flush with saline.
    - Instill heparin into heparin lock.

Table 13-3 Selected Complications of IV Infusion

Type of complication	Cause	Signs and symptoms	Nursing interventions
Infiltration	Needle or catheter displacement	Slow or stopped flow rate; pain; swelling; coldness; palor of area; no blood return when IV bag hung below needle; and tissue necrosis.	Discontinue infusion; remove needle; apply warm, moist towels to affected area; and restart IV in another location.
Phlebitis	Inflammation of vein related to chemical irritation; mechanical irritation by venipuncture, infection, or allergic reaction	Pain, redness, tenderness, and heat along affected vein; sluggish flow rate; and edema.	Same as above.
Thrombophlebitis	Inflammation of vein and subsequent thrombosis	Pain, redness, tenderness, and heat along affected vein; swelling around affected vein; and cord-like vein.	Same as for infiltration.
Circulatory overload	Delivery of fluid in excess	Increased venous pressure; congestive heart failure (CHF); shortness of breath (SOB); pulmonary edema; cough, chest pain, tachycardia, cyanosis, rales; anxiety; dilated neck veins; and wide variance between input and output.	Reduce flow and keep vein open; monitor vital signs; notify physician; raise head of bed; and administer oxygen and medications as ordered.
Pyogenic reaction	Pathogens present in tubing or solution	High temperature; chills; headache; nausea and vomiting; and circulatory collapse.	Discontinue infusion; monitor vital signs; send IV solution to laboratory; do not administer solutions that are cloudy or if there is a question about their sterility; and restart infusion.

Continued.

Table 13-3   Selected Complications of IV Infusion—cont'd

Type of complication	Cause	Signs and symptoms	Nursing interventions
Air embolism	Air enters circulatory system through bubbles in the tubing or infusion running out	Cyanosis; pain; SOB; low BP; tachycardia; rise in venous pressure; and unconsciousness.	Stop flow and check for leaks or air in tubing; turn patient on left side and lower head of bed; if air has entered the heart chambers, this position may keep air on the right side of the heart; the pulmonary artery might absorb the small air bubbles; monitor vital signs; and administer oxygen.
Speed shock	Solution infusing at too fast a rate or improper administration of bolus infusions	Pounding headache; hypertension; potential loss of consciousness; rapid pulse; anxiety; chills; dyspnea; flushed face; shock; and cardiac arrest.	Slow infusion; monitor vital signs; and monitor LOC.
Blood loss	Tubing becoming disconnected and allows a backflow of blood	Usually few signs and symptoms.	Clamp tubing; remove needle; monitor vital signs; restart IV (as needed); reassure patient; and change bedding as needed.
Electrolyte imbalance	Too rapid infusion of electrolyte solution or failure to provide electrolytes	See Table 13-2.	Careful calculation and monitoring of drip rate; monitor electrolyte level on laboratory studies; careful checking of IV orders; observation of symptoms; slow drip; and monitor vital signs.
Catheter embolism	Broken catheter	Discomfort along vein in which the catheter is lodged; hypotension; rise in CVP; weak rapid pulse; cyanosis; and loss of consciousness.	Discontinue IV and apply tourniquet above site.
Infection of venipuncture site	Poor aseptic technique	Swelling; soreness; redness; and foul-smelling discharge.	Discontinue IV and remove needle; send IV equipment to laboratory for bacterial analysis; culture drainage; clean site with antimicrobic ointment and cover with sterile dressing; and restart IV at another site.

COMPLICATIONS OF IV THERAPY

Administration of IV fluids is not free of the threat of complications. Patients receiving IV infusions should be closely monitored during the procedure. Table 13-3 lists selected complications.

IV SITE CARE

The area surrounding the venipuncture site is mechanically cleansed with a povidone-iodine solution or antimicrobial solution. This allows for inspection of the site and reduces the chance for infection.

THROMBOLYTIC THERAPY

Thrombolytic therapy is used in the treatment of a new acute myocardial infarction (AMI). Patients receiving a thrombolytic agent within 1 hour of symptom onset showed a 47% reduction for in-hospital mortality.[1]

The goals of thrombolytic therapy include improving coronary artery perfusion, myocardial oxygenation, left ventricular function, and cardiac output; limiting the zones of myocardial ischemia; reducing dysrhythmias associated with myocardial ischemia; and decreasing mortality.

Careful screening of patients is necessary before the ad-

Skill 13-6   IV Site Care

EQUIPMENT AND SUPPLIES

- Povidone-iodine swab or sterile cotton tipped applicators
- Povidone-iodine ointment
- 2 × 2 sterile gauze pads
- Tape or transparent occlusive dressing.

NURSING INTERVENTIONS

1. Remove tape and dressing from insertion site. Assess site for redness, tenderness, or swelling. If observed, discontinue IV.
2. Cleanse puncture site with antimicrobial solution in a circular fashion for 1 minute and allow to dry.
3. Apply antimicrobial ointment (according to agency policy) to needle or catheter site.
4. Apply sterile 2 × 2 gauze pad and tape in place. NOTE: Dressing should be airtight. Transparent occlusive dressing may be applied instead of gauze pad.

ministration of thrombolytic therapy. This type of therapy is indicated when patients present with chest pain, lasting at least 30 minutes unrelieved by nitroglycerin[3,6,7]; when there is a family history of AMIs or coronary artery disease; and when a 12-lead ECG documents an AMI. Contraindications for thrombolytic therapy include recent major surgery, cerebrovascular accident, intracranial neoplasm, recent trauma, cardiopulmonary resuscitation (CPR), gastrointestinal bleeding, pregnancy, uncontrolled hypertension, high likelihood of left heart thrombus, age greater than 75 years, liver dysfunction, bleeding abnormalities, pericarditis, and previous transmural infarct in the actual ischemic region.[3,9,16] The major complication of thrombolytic therapy is bleeding.

Thrombolytic agents available for use in the United States include streptokinase, urokinase, tissue plasminogen activator (TPA), and anisylated plasminogen streptokinase activator complex (APSAC).[1,16] Each of these agents requires specific procedures for safe and accurate administration (Table 13-4). The following precautions need to be taken when administering thrombolytic therapy[1,10]:

- Avoid all invasive procedures after beginning treatment.
- Avoid taking blood pressure in the lower extremities.
- Avoid unnecessary handling and moving of patient.
- Do not give any intramuscular or IV drugs for 24 hours after terminating treatment.
- Do not administer anticoagulants following TPA administration. (Check agency policy.)
- Do not administer antiplatelet agents (i.e., aspirin, dipyridamole [Persantine], or sulfinpyrazone [Anturane].

DISCONTINUING THE IV INFUSION

The IV infusion is discontinued when the patient no longer needs it or if a complication related to the infusion occurs. An IV may be terminated by the nurse without an order, if the IV is causing a complication.

PEDIATRIC CONSIDERATIONS

Generally, the smallest IV bottle or bag that will last for 24 hours is used. Rate of infusion may vary from 2 to 10 ml/kg/hr. A volume control chamber with a microdrip should be used to decrease the chance of fluid overload and should not be filled with more than two hours worth of solution.

Tongue blades can be used to immobilize the arm or leg of the newborn. Sandbags placed on either side of the head can be used to immobilize the head for babies with scalp

Table 13-4   Thrombolytic Agents[12,15]

Drug and Route	Administration and Dose	Adverse Effects
Streptokinase (SK)		
Continuous infusion IV IC†	1.5 million IU* over 30-60 min 20,000 IU bolus 2000 IU/min for 60 min to total of 140,000 IU	Allergic reactions, fever, drug rash, hypotension, inappropriate bleeding, bruising, stroke
Urokinase (UK)		
IV Bolus IC	750,000–3 million IU as a bolus or over 30-60 min 4000-8000 U/min	Bleeding complications
Tissue Plasminogen Activator (TPA)		
Continuous infusion IV	First Hour: 6-10 mg bolus and 50-54 mg/hr drip Second Hour: 20 mg/hr Third Hour: 20 mg/hr Total: 100 mg over 3 hrs	Bleeding complications
Anisoylated Plasminogen Streptokinase Activator Complex (ASPAC)		
IV bolus	30 U over 5 min	Allergic reactions Hypotension

*International units.
†Intracoronary units.

Skill 13-7 Administering Thrombolytic Agents

EQUIPMENT AND SUPPLIES

- 4 infusion pumps
- Double cannula needles
- Doppler
- IV poles

NURSING INTERVENTIONS

1. Obtain baseline hematocrit, hemoglobin, platelet count, and clotting studies.
2. Explain benefits and risks to patient.
3. Monitor 12-lead ECG. Obtain history and complete assessment. Confirm that patient meets inclusion criteria, and establish continuous cardiac monitoring.
4. Complete all invasive monitoring procedures before initiation of treatment since patient may have a tendency to bleed after treatment.
5. Start a minimum of three IV lines: one for nitrates, one for thrombolytic medications, and one for heparin. Other lines may be started for antidysrhythmics and narcotics as needed. Do not add other medications to IV lines containing thrombolytic drugs. Use double cannula needles, if available.
6. Establish perfusion baseline by auscultating all peripheral pulses with a Doppler stethoscope. Check and document color, temperature, and sensitivities in all extremities.
7. Reconstitute thrombolic agent following manufacturer's instructions.
8. Check physician's order for doses and infusion rates with another registered nurse.
9. Put the total dose the patient is to receive into one IV bag. Do not use tubing with an inline filter since some filters can remove up to 47% of the drug.
10. Prime IV tubing with medication, not the IV fluid; otherwise the dosing for about the first 20 ml will be without the drug. Extra caution must be taken not to waste even one drop of medication.
11. Withdraw any air bubbles from tubing through the medication addition port with a syringe and then return any solution obtained back into the IV bag.
12. Withdraw the bolus of drug from the IV bag and administer through the medication administration port, clamping off tubing from above.
13. Attach infusion line to infusion pump.
14. Maintain the involved extremity in straight alignment to prevent bleeding from infusion site.
15. Monitor vital signs, cardiac output, and ECG every 15 minutes. Inspect the skin for petechiae, subcutaneous bleeding, or bruising, and IV site for bleeding or hematoma formation. Monitor pulses, color, temperature, and sensitivities in extremities. Allow no unnecessary arterial or venous punctures.
16. Use a flow sheet to monitor partial thromboplastin time (PTT), prothrombin time (PT), and hemoglobin and hemocrit counts.
17. Every hour, monitor for signs of gastrointestinal bleeding, test all emesis, stool, urine and nasogastric aspirate; perform neurological checks.
18. If giving streptokinase or APSAC, assess for allergic reaction.
19. When the drug administration is completed, flush the remaining dose of the drug from the tubing into the patient by injecting normal saline solution. Be sure to maintain the prescribed rate.
20. Continue to monitor as previously listed.
21. Record data, including documentation of IV puncture sites and the occurrence of the clinical markers of reperfusion, such as sudden reduction of chest pain, reduction of ST segment elevation, and the occurrence of reperfusion related dysrhythmias (i.e., sinus bradycardia, heart block, ventricular tachycardia or fibrillation, or frequent premature ventricular contractions [PVCs]).

Skill 13-8 Discontinuing the Peripheral IV Infusion

EQUIPMENT AND SUPPLIES

- Alcohol wipe, 2 × 2 gauze pads, and tape
- Gloves
- Bandaids

NURSING INTERVENTIONS

1. Clamp the tubing leading from the infusion. Wear gloves.
2. Loosen all the tape at the venipuncture site.
3. Hold sterile gauze or alcohol wipe over the venipuncture site without applying pressure. (Alcohol may sting or interfere with coagulation at the site.)
4. Withdraw the needle or catheter slowly in the same angle that it was inserted and check that it is intact. NOTE: Check catheter tip for intactness and assess site.
5. Apply pressure to the site for 2 to 3 minutes to prevent blood leakage into the site.
6. Apply small dressing or Bandaid.
7. Assist patient into comfortable position.
8. Note amount of IV solution infused and amount remaining.
9. Discard administration set and IV bag, dispose of needle according to universal precautions, and remove IV pole.

veins. Since the appearance of a scalp vein IV can be frightening, parents should know why the scalp vein site was chosen. The umbilical vein can be used in newborns.

Although umbilical catheterization provides ease of route, it has many hazards including thrombosis, embolism, vasospasm, vascular perforation, infection, and hemorrhage.

Small children may have IVs started in a superficial vein in the wrist, arm, hand, or foot since these are the easily immobilized sites.

Children may not be old enough to comprehend the purpose of the IV or what is happening. They may be fearful and fretful. Occasionally a sedative is ordered for young children who are receiving an IV by a scalp vein, because they may be agitated. This may be done since crying tends to increase resistance in the vein and impedes IV flow. If possible, a nurse or preferably the child's parent can remain with the child to provide comfort. If the child is old enough, an explanation of what will be done should be provided at a level that the child can understand.

To start the IV infusion, the infant or child may need to be restrained. Once the needle is taped in place and protected from becoming dislodged by immobilizing the extremity; a plastic or paper cup can be taped securely over the needle site for further protection.

PATIENT TEACHING

Teaching should begin early before insertion of catheters or needles, if possible. The teaching program should be divided into a series of small, manageable steps. After each step is mastered, the next can be added with the patient repeating the previous steps. Printed materials and a written copy of the procedure should be given to the patient and to the support person. Samples of the equipment and supplies should be given to the patient for practice handling. Additionally, the teaching program should include the hazards of the procedure and the complications. The basic understanding of sanitary practices used at the home by the patient or caregiver needs to be assessed. The nurse should also observe the patient's or caregiver's technique of changing the IV dressing and performing site care.[13]

HOME HEALTH CARE CONSIDERATIONS

Patients are being discharged from the hospital earlier and many procedures that were once carried out in the hospital are being performed at home.

Safe, effective, and less costly administration of IV therapy is now commonly being performed in patients' homes. This trend has emerged and will continue to expand in efforts not only to help stem the rising costs of health care, but also to promote the home environment as integral in the healing process. Home IV therapy generally involves intermittent administrations, such as antibiotics that do not necessarily need 24-hour hospitalizations. Specific criteria determine patient selection. These criteria include the following:

- Medical stability.
- Emotional stability.
- Patient's life-style.
- Intellectual ability.
- Visual activity.
- Manual dexterity.
- Family or friend to assume responsibility or to serve as a backup.
- Home setting equipped with clean dry storage, refrigeration, sufficient space, privacy, equipment, and safety features.
- Written medical order is needed to institute this procedure.

Home IV infusion policies differ among agencies depending on certain factors. One factor is the availability of trained and knowledgeable registered nurses who have excellent IV therapy skills and can adapt these skills to the home health care setting. Another may be the availability of services that can be provided. Agencies providing IV therapy services must consider 24-hour coverage for handling late-night emergency calls. Calls may involve infiltration of a peripheral site or an IV pump malfunction.[13]

Home IV therapy requires extra precautions to assure patient safety. At least two people should check the infusion pump's setting to be sure it is programmed correctly. Additionally, when the pump setting is to be changed, at least two people should confirm the change.

The initial dose of IV therapy is usually administered in the acute care setting. Any untoward reaction may show on this first dose and therapy adjusted accordingly. The course may be completed in the home with the physician's approval and the patient's or caregiver's consent.[13]

In the home health care setting, it is the registered nurse who is responsible for initiating and changing peripheral IV therapy sites. Patients who have implanted central access devices will be given instruction on how to maintain the catheter if, and when, they can learn to self-administer their care. A caregiver must be present as well to assume responsibility for monitoring the course of therapy and to receive the necessary training to assist with home health care.[13]

Check to be sure that insurance counseling has been provided and determine if third party payers will reimburse the patient for home IV therapy. The nurse may also need to assist the patient in finding and comparing the costs of material provided by the various vendors.[13]

Standards of care for the home patient should parallel those determined by the National Intravenous Therapy Association (NITA) and the Centers for Disease Control.

Safety features regarding others in the home need to be established as well. For example, equipment and supplies must be stored away from children and safe methods for disposing of used supplies must be instituted.

There are several advantages to home IV therapy. These include the following features:

- Less expense.
- Allows the patient to be home with family.
- Allows the patient to resume usual activities between treatments.
- Hazards of hospitalization are minimized.
- Allows the patient more control over care.

A patient on home infusion therapy will also need frequent monitoring and assessment during the course of therapy regardless if the nurse is present for part or all of the infusion period. The patient and caregiver can be taught how to maintain the IV and keep a record of intake and output.[13]

REFERENCES

1. Belle-Isle C: Patient selection and administration of trombolytic therapy, *J Emer Nurs* 15(2):155, 1989.
2. Corbett JV: *Laboratory test and diagnostic procedures with nursing diagnoses,* ed 2, Norwalk, Conn, 1987, Appleton & Lange.
3. Daly EK: Clinical management of patients receiving thrombolytic therapy, *Heart Lung* 20(5):552, 1991.
4. Fiser DH: Intraosseous infusion, *N Engl J Med,* 322(22):1579, 1990.
5. Flynn J-B McC: *Administration of intravenous infusions.* In Flynn J-B McC, Hackel R: *Technological Foundations of Nursing,* Norwalk, Conn, 1990, Appleton & Lange.
6. Grigg JC, Stromberg RM: Immediate emergency department intervention in acute myocardial infarction, *Top Emerg Med* 12(4):19, 1991.

7. Gurwitz J, Goldberg RJ, and Gore: Coronary thrombolysis for the elderly? *JAMA* 265(13):1720, 1991.

8. Kinney MR, Packa DR, Dunbar SB: *AACNs critical reference for critical care nursing,* ed 2 New York, 1989, McGraw-Hill.

9. Kline EM: Comparison of thrombolytic agents: mechanisms of action. *Crit Care Nurs Q,* 12(2):1, 1989.

10. Manley L, Haley K, Dick M: Intraosseous infusion: rapid vascular access for critically ill or injured infants and children, *J Emerg Nurs* 14(2), 63, 1988.

11. Mathewson M: Intravenous therapy, *Crit Care Nurse,* 9(2):21, 1989.

12. Metheny NM, Snively WD: *Nurses' handbook of fluid balance,* ed 4, Philadelphia, 1983, JB Lippincott.

13. Monzon E: *Home care considerations.* In Flynn J-B McC, Hackel R, *Technological foundations of nursing,* Norwalk, Conn: 1990, Appleton & Lange.

14. Ponaman ML, White L: *Intraosseous infusions.* In Levin DL, Morriss FC: *Essentials of pediatric intensive care,* St Louis, 1990, Quality Medical.

15. Topol E, Wilson VE: Pivotal role of early unsustained infarct vessel patency in patients with acute myocardial infarction, *Heart Lung* 19(6):583, 1990.

16. *Spartanburg General Hospital policy book on IV therapy administration: part 1, NITA* 9(4):267, 1989.

17. Valle BK, Lemburg L: Update on thrombolytic therapy in acute myocardial infarction, *Heart Lung* 20(5):526, 1991.

CHAPTER 14

Blood and Blood-Component Administration

Objectives

After completing this chapter, the reader will be able to:

- List the uses of blood therapy.
- Describe the types of blood, blood components, and blood substitutes.
- State the reasons for blood transfusions.
- Describe the Rh factor.
- Describe the major types of blood transfusions.
- Describe transfusion reactions and appropriate nursing interventions.
- Compare and contrast types of transfusions.

Blood accounts for about 8% of total body weight.[22] The blood volume is composed of two main components: cellular components consisting of red blood cells (RBC), white blood cells (WBC), and platelets; and a liquid component, which is plasma. Approximately 45% of the total blood volume is made up of cellular components and 55% is plasma. Normal blood volume is 5 to 6 liters.[22]

Clear indications for the administration of blood must be present because transfusions have the potential to cause severe, dangerous, and sometimes life-threatening reactions. Therefore the potential benefits must be weighed against known risks before administering blood or blood components.

The administration of blood and blood components is one of the integral parts in the treatment of critically ill patients.[12] It is one of the tasks that nurses perform in conjunction with physicians. Generally, the physician assesses the need, determines the type of transfusion, and orders the blood or blood component. The nurse assesses the patient, verifies that the blood or blood component is the correct type, adds the blood to the intravenous (IV) infusion (according to agency policy), and monitors the patient.

Persons of some religions and cultural groups will not accept transfusion blood or blood components. Jehovah's Witnesses are an example of a religious group who will not allow transfusions. However, in emergencies, they may accept plasma expanders and intramuscular iron substances. This must be assessed and validated with the patient. These patients may also be considered for blood-substitute products.

Patients who do not wish to receive blood because of personal beliefs should be asked to sign a form refusing transfused blood or blood components. A medical alert stating the refusal of blood and blood products must be taped to the front of the chart. If the physician has ordered blood or if surgery is pending, the physician must be notified of the patient's beliefs.

TYPES OF BLOOD AND BLOOD COMPONENTS

There is a variety of blood and blood-component types. Blood and blood products are ordered and administered based on specific patient needs (Table 14-1).

BLOOD GROUPS

Blood typing depends on the type of antigens *(agglutinogens)* present on RBC membranes and the type of antibodies *(agglutinins)* in the plasma.[26]

The possible blood groups in the ABO system are A, B, O, and AB (Tables 14-2). It is not acceptable to transfuse A, B, or AB blood to persons whose red cells are not of the same type, since their plasma will contain incompatible antibodies. In extreme emergencies, persons with types A, B, or AB, may receive type O blood shown not to have an anti-A or anti-B titer higher than 1:50 (Group O "low titer").[27] If an individual is inadvertently transfused with an incompatible blood type, antibodies in the plasma agglutinate or hemolyze the donor's red cells.

Traditionally, individuals with type O blood are frequently called *universal donors,* and those with type AB blood are known as *universal recipients.* These terms may be misleading and potentially dangerous, since there are a host of other incompatible erythrocyte antigens besides those of the ABO classification.[2]

Table 14-1   Blood and Blood Components[*]

Product	Composition	Volumes	Indications	Storage life
Whole blood	RBCs, plasma, platelets, proteins, and preservatives (citrate phosphate dextrose [CPD] or acid-citrate-dextrose [ACD])	500 ml total 200 ml RBCs 300 ml plasma	Rarely used Hemorrhage Burns Extensive trauma Severe anemia Hypoxia Volume deficit	21 days at 4° C (39° F)
Packed RBCs	Whole blood with 80% of plasma removed	250 ml total 200 ml RBCs 50 ml plasma	Anemia Renal impairment Infants, children, and the elderly Severe bleeding	21 days when stored fresh
Leukocyte-poor RBCs	RBCs; plasma; no leukocytes	200-300 ml	Persons susceptible to febrile reactions Renal transplants Dialysis liver disease	Varies
Washed RBCs (WRCs)	RBCs, fewer WBCs, platelets, and plasma than packed cells	200-300 ml total 200 ml RBCs 50 ml saline	Paroxysmal nocturnal hemoglobinuria Antibodies to immunoglobulin A (IgA) or immunoglobulin B (IgB) Hyperkalemia Neonates Transplant patients Open-heart surgery	24 hours after washing
Deglyceralized RBCs	RBCs preserved with glycerol, frozen; washed later to remove glycerol	200-300 ml total 200 ml RBCs 50 ml saline	Paroxysmal nocturnal hemoglobinuria Antibodies to IgA or IgB Hyperkalemia Neonates Transplant patients Open-heart surgery Intrauterine transfusion	Up to 3 years Limited shelf life after thawing, (i.e., 24 hours)
Fresh whole blood (FWB)	RBCs; plasma; clotting factors	500 ml	Rarely used Bleeding disorders Used when stored whole blood is unavailable	Immediate use
Fresh pooled plasma	All coagulation factors plus 400 mg of fibrinogen	200-300 ml	Burns Shock Trauma	6 hours after collection; 12 months if frozen at −18° C (−4° F)
Fresh frozen plasma (FFP)	Fluid portion of blood after centrifuging	200-250 ml (amount will be written on unit)	Burns Shock Trauma	12 months when frozen
Random platelets	Platelet sediment	30-60 ml unit	Hypocoagulation Decrease in platelets Thrombocytopenia platelet destruction Extra corporeal circulation Massive transfusions	Few hours to 3 days (at room temperature)

[*]Refs 1, 6, 10, 16, 18, 22, 25
Volumes may vary from blood bank to blood bank. Inquire at agency blood bank.

Table 14-1 Blood and Blood Components —cont'd

Product	Composition	Volumes	Indications	Storage life
Single-donor platelets	Platelet concentrate	300 ml	(See random platelets)	5 days at 24° C
Cryoprecipitate	Clotting factor VIII, XIII, and fibrinogen recovered from FFP	20-30 ml	Lack of clotting factor VIII Classic hemophilia (A) Replace fibrinogen	Months if frozen
Granulocytes	WBCs	200-300 ml	Granulocytopenia Severe infections in immuno-suppressed patient	24 hours
Albumin	Plasma protein	50-100 ml	Shock Burns	3 years at room temperature; 5 years if frozen
Albumin 25%	(25% Albumin + 75% NS)	50 ml = 12.5 gm 100 ml = 25.0 gm	Intestinal obstruction Plasma losing conditions	
Albumin 5% (Buminate)	(95% NS + 5% Albumin)	50-500 ml	Hypoalbuminemia	
Gamma globulin (Administered intramuscularly)	Gamma globulin	1-100 ml, depending on type	Agammaglobulinemia Hypogammaglobulinemia Increase antibodies	
Coagulation factors	Plasma proteins		Hemophilia Clotting dyscrasias	1 year if frozen

Table 14-2 Blood Groups

Blood type	Percent of population	Antigen agglutinogen	Antibody (agglutinins)	Incompatible donor	Preferred donor	Permissible donor
A	41	A	Anti-B	B and AB	A	O
B	9	B	Anti-A	A and AB	B	O
AB	3	A and B	Neither anti-A nor anti-B	None	AB	A, B, and O
O	47	None	Both anti-A and anti-B	A, B, and AB	O	None

Rh System

Another system of important antigens is the Rh system. This system is extremely complex, and aspects of its genetics, nomenclature, and antigenic interactions are controversial. Basically, if Rh factors (antigen D) are present on the red cell membranes, the blood is classified as Rh positive. Approximately 85% of the population is Rh positive. Conversely, red blood cells without these antigens are classified as Rh negative. As in the case of agglutinogens A and B, the presence or absence of an Rh agglutinogen is an inherited trait.

Individuals with Rh-negative blood develop anti-Rh antibodies if they are sensitized to the Rh-positive factor either from transfusion of Rh-positive blood or by transplacental exchange of red blood cells from an Rh-positive fetus to an Rh-negative mother. If introduction of the Rh-positive cells to Rh-negative persons occur, they become sensitized to the Rh-positive cells. Should sensitized persons inadvertently receive a second transfusion of Rh-positive blood, a transfusion reaction will occur.

HLA System

The human leukocyte antigen (HLA) system includes a group of antigens found on the membranes of all nucleated cells of the body.[27] The antigens in the HLA system are second in importance only to the ABO antigens in regard to organ transplantation, since immunological recognition of the differences in the HLA antigens is most likely the first step in organ rejection. This blood system is frequently used for tissue typing, platelet transfusion, and parentage tests.

Typing and Crossmatching Blood

Recipient typing is performed to determine the major ABO blood group and Rh factor. Some agencies also do a minor crossmatch testing of the recipient's RBCs against the donor's serum.

In addition to antigen-antibody typing and crossmatching, platelet and leukocyte antigenic factors involving the HLA can be analyzed.

ASSESSMENT

Before receiving blood or blood components, the patient should undergo a thorough assessment. An array of disorders can affect the hematological system. Therefore accurate assessment findings are of critical importance (see Skill 14-1).

NURSING DIAGNOSIS

Sample nursing diagnoses for the patient requiring blood or blood components include:
- High risk for injury related to transfusion.
- Deficit in blood volume related to hemorrhage.
- High risk for injury related to chest tube insertion.
- High risk for decrease in urinary elimination related to decreased renal perfusion.
- Anxiety related to transfusion (and trauma, if present).
- Knowledge deficit related to transfusion procedure.

Skill 14-1   Assessing the Blood or Blood-Component Recipient

▼ ....

NURSING INTERVENTIONS

1. Obtain transfusion history.
2. Assess airway.
3. Observe skin for rashes, hives, or reddened areas. Inspect eyes for jaundice. Note any rhinitis.
4. Palpate neck for lymph nodes.
5. Auscultate lungs, assessing breathing patterns and skin color.
6. Auscultate heart for gallop rhythm.
7. Monitor ECG and vital signs (i.e., temperature, pulse, respirations, and blood pressure).
8. Monitor urinary output for amount and hematuria.
9. If patient is conscious, monitor for signs of hypoxemia (i.e., level of consciousness, confusion, anxiety, or restlessness).
10. Assess needle, catheter, wound, and surgical sites for bleeding. Observe for petechiae and ecchymosis.

PATIENT OUTCOMES

The following are possible expected outcomes for patients receiving blood or blood components.

Patient evidences:
- Cardiac rate and rhythm within normal limits, 60 to 100 beats/min.
- Respirations, 12 to 20 breaths/min (symmetrical and bilateral).
- Blood pressure stable within $^{100}\!/\!_{60}$ to $^{140}\!/\!_{90}$ or within normal patient limits.
- Blood potassium level within normal limits after transfusion, 3.5 to 5.0 mEg/L.
- Temperature of 36° to 38° C (97° to 100.5 ° F).
- Arterial blood pressure within ±10 mm Hg of pretransfusion levels.
- Hemoglobin and hematocrit levels within the designated normal limits.
- Urine output of at least 0.5 ml/kg/hr and urine specific gravity of 1.003 to 1.030.
- Ability to identify factors in the environment that are causing anxiety.
- Ability to briefly state purpose of procedure.

TYPES OF BLOOD TRANSFUSIONS

There are a variety of blood transfusions. The most common is known as an *indirect transfusion*. This type of transfusion uses a volunteer random donor who provides blood to be given as whole blood or as blood components to a compatible recipient. Types of indirect transfusions include whole blood, packed red blood cells (PRBCs), plasma, platelets, cryoprecipitate, and albumin.

Therapeutic plasma exchange (TPE) is a technique where blood is withdrawn from a patient and separated into plasma and formed elements (RBCs, WBCs, and platelets) either by centrifugation or by microporous membrane filtration. The plasma is then discarded, and the formed elements are mixed with a plasma replacement and returned to the patient. The choice of this plasma replacement is extremely important. Crystalloid solutions (i.e., saline or Ringer's lactate) can produce severe hypotension. They can be used however if only 1 or 2 liters are received. If a 4-liter replacement is needed, a colloid solution, such as 5% albumin, should be used.

TPE is used to remove unwanted substances, such as toxins, metabolic wastes, and plasma constituents linked to disease. TPE benefits patients with immune-related disorders, such as systemic lupus erythematosis, rheumatoid arthritis, and glomerulonephritis. It is also used for individuals with neuromuscular conditions, such as myasthenia gravis and Guillain-Barré syndrome.

Fluid balance, clotting mechanisms, and basic immunological functions can be altered severely by plasma exchange. There is a risk of morbidity and mortality with this procedure. Informed consent should be obtained before TPE is begun. Further, only trained professionals should perform TPE procedures.

Autotransfusion is the collection, filtration, and reinfu-

EQUIPMENT AND SUPPLIES

- IV solution, as ordered by physician. Small bag amount of solution can be used if the patient is at risk for circulatory overload.

  NOTE: Avoid solutions containing dextrose because they cause hemolysis of RBCs. Solutions containing calcium, such as Ringer's lactate, should also be avoided because they may cause clotting of the blood to be transfused.
- Blood or blood components
- IV tubing with appropriate drip chamber with filter
- Straight or Y-tubing with in-line filter, as required
- Alcohol sponges
- Syringes as needed
- 2 × 2 and 4 × 4 (sterile and unsterile) gauze pads
- Tourniquet
- Tape
- Armboard (optional)
- IV pole
- Sterile needles
- Signed informed consent
- Gloves and protective eyewear
- *Additional equipment as needed:* blood warming device and autoinfusion device and equipment

NURSING INTERVENTIONS

1. Check chart for order and signed consent. Parents may sign for children, unconscious patients, or incapacitated patients.
2. Ensure that patient has IV catheter with adapter plug inserted or IV line with extension tubing.
3. If the existing needle or catheter is smaller than an 20 gauge, a larger one must be inserted. This allows for ease of blood flow and reduces destruction of RBCs.
4. If blood is to be administered through the subclavian vein, check agency policy for procedures. Administration of cold blood through the subclavian vein may result in shock, hypothermia, or cardiac standstill.
5. Monitor and document patient's baseline temperature, pulse, respirations, and blood pressure. Assess and document these several times during the first 15 minutes of transfusion, since most hemolytic reactions occur during this time.
6. Obtain blood components from blood bank, one unit at a time, unless patient is receiving more than one unit. Blood must be kept in a monitored environment where the temperature stays between 1° and 6° C (34° and 36° F) to maintain its quality. Blood should not be requested until it is ready to be used. Blood and packed cells are generally administered cold, unless otherwise indicated.
7. Infuse the blood within 4 hours. If the infusion will exceed this time limit, it should be divided into small units by the blood bank.
8. Check expiration date. Note any abnormal color, extraneous material, clumping, or other unusual findings. If blood or blood components are outdated, do not use them.
9. Check the compatibility tag attached to the blood bag and the information printed on the bag itself to verify that the ABO, Rh, and unit number match (Fig. 14-1).
10. Check the patient's ABO group and Rh type. Match to the blood bag and tag.
11. Check the doctor's order against blood or blood product. If any discrepancies are found, report them to the blood bank immediately.
12. Another nurse should independently verify all information to reduce chances of error. If there are any discrepancies, the blood or blood product should be returned to the laboratory.
13. Ask patient to state full name (if able). Check identification number of wristband.
14. Obtain a blood-administration tubing set. Close the clamps and attach a bag of normal saline to one end of the Y tubing.
15. If required, add a filter to the other Y connection. The filter that comes with the blood set has a pore size of 170 to 180 micrometers (μm) and is generally used to infuse 2 to 4 units. It is discarded when filled with blood and debris (such as glass, rubber, metal, molds, bacteria, and drug precipitates).
16. Use a microaggregate filter for the administration of 5 to 10 units of blood and for patients with compromised pulmonary function, total body replacement (in 24 hours), and a history of febrile reactions.
17. Open clamp to saline, prime all tubing and filter, and reclose clamp. Don rubber gloves. Obtain blood and pull back blood bag cap to expose port. Insert spike above filter into the bag port with a twisting motion. Maintain sterility. Be careful not to puncture bag. NOTE: Sometimes saline is added to blood bag to reduce viscosity. This is true with packed cells when rapid administration is desired.
18. Squeeze the drip chamber and ensure that the ball in the tubing is free floating. Fill the drip chamber as high as possible while still permitting the blood to drop. Blood that drops far down into the drip chamber will increase the chance of RBC destruction.
19. Disconnect patient's other IV fluids from extension tubing and attach blood-set tubing. Open roller clamp and flush extension tubing with the saline (Fig. 14-2).
20. Close clamp to bag of saline and open clamp to blood, allowing blood to flow through saline-primed filter.
21. Adjust the flow using the roller clamp. If the patient is a child, move tubing out of reach so the child cannot play with it. In most instances the physician orders the flow rate depending on the patient's needs and the viscosity of the blood or blood components. The drip rate depends on the size of the tubing (read manufacturer's label), the amount to be infused, the condition and age of the patient, and reaction to the blood (Table 14-4).
22. Administer blood initially at a slow rate (1 ml/kg of body weight/hr) for the first 15 minutes so that any adverse reactions can be noted at once. If patient has no adverse reaction during the first 15 minutes, increase the rate (Table 14-4).
23. Infuse 1 unit of packed RBCs in 1½ to 2 hours for most patients. Patients who have a history of congestive heart failure or fluid overload require infusions given over a longer period of time, up to 4 hours.
24. Use blankets to keep patient warm during the transfusion. For some patients a blood warmer may be required.
25. Remain with patient and observe for signs of transfusion reactions. If signs of reaction appear, stop blood by closing clamp and releasing clamp to saline. Take and record vital signs and notify physician. Return blood with tubing to laboratory.
26. After completion of the ordered transfusion fluids, flush the tubing with normal saline and disconnect at extension tubing site.
27. Reconnect or discontinue previous IV, as ordered.
28. Take and record vital signs. Note presence or absence of signs of blood transfusion reaction.
29. Discard tubing and blood bag or return to laboratory according to agency policy.
30. Wash hands carefully.
31. Draw posttransfusion hemoglobin and hematocrit 1 hour after transfusion has been completed, as ordered.
32. Document each administration of blood, blood components, or expanders. Retain copies of blood-transfusion documents on the patient's chart and in the blood bank.

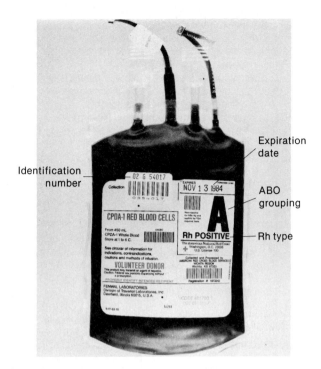

Fig. 14-1 Blood product identification. (From LaRocca JC, Otto SE: *Pocket guide to intravenous therapy,* St Louis, 1989, Mosby–Year Book.)

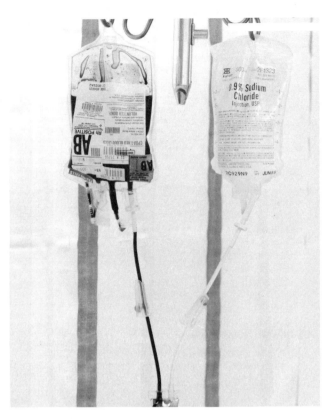

Fig. 14-2 Y-tubing for blood administration with normal saline. (From Perry AG, Potter PA: *Clinical nursing skills and techniques,* St Louis, 1986, Mosby–Year Book.)

Table 14-3 Needle Sizes for Blood and Blood-Product Administration

Blood/component		Age group	Needle gauge
Whole blood	Usual administration	Adult/adolescent	18-20
		Infant/child	22
	Rapid administration	Adult/adolescent	14-18
		Infant/child	18-20
RBCs	Usual administration	Adult/adolescent	18-20
		Infant/child	19-21
	Rapid administration	Adult/adolescent	14-18
		Infant/child	16-18
Platelets, plasma, cryoprecipate, clotting factors; albumin; plasma protein fraction (PPF); plasmanate		Adult/adolescent	20-22
		Infant/child	22-24

sion of a person's own blood.[9] Autotransfusion is used for the following:

- Blood replacement after traumatic injuries, such as hemothorax or open-heart surgery.
- Patients who have rare antibodies.
- Bone marrow transplants.
- Patients who object to blood transfusions from others because of religious beliefs.

Autotransfusion has become a valuable technique in major procedures and in a massively hemorrhaging patient when large volumes of blood can be recovered.

Autotransfusion should not be used if the individual has a cancerous lesion in the area of the hemorrhage, if the blood is contaminated with gastrointestinal secretions, or if the wounds are more than 6 hours old. The benefits of autotransfusion in emergency situations gives it some important advantages over other types of transfusions. Risks of technical errors in typing and crossmatching are eliminated. It provides compatible blood quickly, since it avoids time-consuming typing and crossing procedures.[17] Autotransfusion eliminates the transmission of diseases such as hepatitis, malaria, AIDS, and other blood-borne disorders. This blood has normal body temperature, pH, and nearly normal clotting factors.[10] In addition, it has high oxygen-carrying capacity. Autotransfusion may provide cost savings because it reduces the cost of blood for the patient.

Table 14-4   Rates of Infusion

Blood product	Age group	Rate of administration*
Whole blood	Adults/adolescents	2-3 hours; no more than 4 hours
	Infants/children	Ml/hr; rate based on weight
PRBCs	Adults/adolescents	1½ -2 hours; no more than 3-4 hours
	Infants/children	Ml/hr based on weight
WBCs (Leukocytes)	Adults/adolescents	As ordered
	Infants/children	As ordered
Fresh frozen plasma (FFP)	Adults/adolescents	15-20 minutes when given for clotting factors; 1-2 hours when given for other reasons
	Infants/children	Quickly when given for clotting factors; up to 4 hours when given for other reasons
Platelets	Adults/adolescents	As rapidly as patient can tolerate regardless of age
	Infants/children	Same as for adults
Albumen 25%; 12.5 gm	Adults/adolescents	Infuse within 1 hour
Albumen 5%; 12.5 gm	Infants/children	Rapidly for shock; 5-10 ml/min for hypoproteinemia (less rapidly in neonates)
PPF; volume varies according to scheduled dose	Adults/adolescents	Infuse no more than 10 drops/min
	Infants/children	5-10 ml/min (less for small children and infants)
Factor VIII (Cryoprecipitate)	Adults/adolescents	As fast as tolerated to a maximum of 6 ml/min
	Infants/children	10-20 ml/3 min via drip; 1 ml/min IV push
Factor IX	Adults/adolescents	Same as factor VIII
	Infants/children	One vial over 5-10 minutes; do not push

*Rates listed are standard. Other rates may be necessary based on the patient's condition. If rate is slow because patient has unstable cardiac function, chronic severe anemia, congestive heart failure, or is very small, request blood bank to split unit.

Autotransfusion may be acceptable to some Jehovah's Witnesses.

Autotransfusion after trauma or surgery is used anytime the patient had or is going to have blood loss of 1000 to 4000 ml. Reinfusion is begun when all blood has been evacuated from the site, when immediate transfusion is necessary, or when the collection bag is full.

Complications of autotransfusion include coagulation, hemolysis, coagulopathies, microemboli or air emboli, sepsis, citrate toxicity, and deficiencies in factor V, VIII, and fibrinogen.

Intrauterine transfusion is performed on a fetus when the level of maternal antibodies against the fetal red blood cells is high enough to produce a fatal anemia. In this type of transfusion, a needle is passed with radiographic monitoring through the mother's abdomen and uterine wall into the fetal abdomen.

Exchange transfusion, originally used to treat hemolytic disease of the newborn, has recently been used to treat a wide variety of life-threatening conditions affecting newborns, such as respiratory distress, disseminated intravascular coagulation (DIC), and sepsis. This method is also used to treat hyperbilirubinemia related to fetal-maternal blood group incompatibility.

The objectives of exchange transfusions are the removal of the sensitized cells and replacement with compatible RBCs, reduction of intravascular volume removal of bilirubin, replacement of bound albumin with unbound albumin, and removal of maternal antibodies.

Risks associated with exchange transfusions are provided in the box on p. 331.

Skill 14-3   Administration of Cryoprecipitate

EQUIPMENT AND SUPPLIES

- Cryoprecipitate tubing
- Sterile saline for injection
- 10- and 35-ml plastic syringes
- 23- and 25-gauge scalp vein set

NURSING INTERVENTIONS

1. Follow steps 1 to 14 in Skill 14-2. A separate IV line with special cryoprecipitate tubing is used, and venipuncture is made with 23- or 25-gauge needle to reduce risk of bleeding.
2. Spike cryoprecipitate with cryoprecipitate infusion set or draw up commercially prepared clotting factor solution with filter needle after diluting with special sterile diluent. Sterile water should not be used for diluting commercially prepared solutions, since it is not isotonic and can cause hemolysis.
3. Close all clamps on cryoprecipitate set.
4. Attach 35-ml syringe to female port above the Y-connection on cryoprecipitate. Use a plastic syringe, since clotting factor VIII may bind to surface of glass.
5. Open clamp from cryoprecipitate; draw into syringe. Close clamp.
6. Open clamp on tubing. Fill tubing with cryoprecipitate.
7. Attach tubing to patient's IV access.
8. Administer cryoprecipitate at a rate of about 10 ml/min.
9. Remove 35-ml syringe and replace with 10-ml syringe filled with sterile saline. Flush tubing and needle to assure that patient gets all cryoprecipitate.

Skill 14-4 Collection of Blood for Autotransfusion

EQUIPMENT AND SUPPLIES*

- 1900-ml rigid plastic canister
- Chest tube with suction tubing
- Sterile collection and infusion liner for autotransfusion
- Microemboli blood-filter tubing
- 500-ml bottle of anticoagulant (CPD or ACD)
- Heparin, 30,000 to 60,000 units
- IV tubing with burette
- IV pole
- Tape
- 4 × 4 gauze pads
- Hemostats or other clamps
- Sterile gloves
- Povidone-iodine or other cleansing solution
- Low-pressure suction

NURSING INTERVENTIONS (Figs. 14-3 and 14-4)

1. Follow manufacturer's instructions for setting up the autotransfusion set.
2. Place sterile liner inside the canister and snap lid on tightly so that air cannot leak in. Avoid contamination of the sterile spaces.

3. Connect tubing on liner lid to suction apparatus using sterile spacer joined to the canister tee. (If not available, use any suction source.)
4. Attach chest drainage tubing to top port of liner lid.
5. Open anticoagulant solution (either acid-citrate-dextrose (ACD) or citrate-phosphate-dextrose (CPD). CPD is less acidotic and less of it is needed so it is the most commonly used). Using sterile technique, attach IV burette. Flush and fill the set; hang on IV pole. Prime burette. Prime liner with 20 to 25 ml anticoagulant solution.
6. Attach the flushed IV line of anticoagulant solution to the anticoagulant connector. Set drip rate so that 25 to 70 ml of anticoagulant solution mixes with every 500 ml of blood collected.
7. Connect the patient's clamped chest tube to the autotransfusion site and apply 2.5 cm (1-inch) tape around the connection points.
8. Release the clamp on the tubing.
9. Check the proper functioning of the system. Turn on suction to 10 to 30 mm Hg.
10. Monitor patient's condition throughout the procedure.
11. When the accumulation of shed blood is completed, clamp chest tube.

*May vary with type of system.

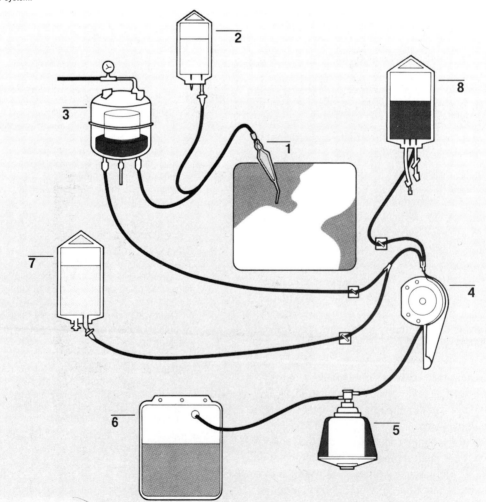

Fig. 14-3 Cell Saver method of recovering and collecting autologous blood for transfusion. *1,* Suction from patient. *2,* Anticoagulant. *3,* Collection reservoir. *4,* Pump. *5,* Centrifuge bowl. *6,* Waste bag. *7,* Sterile saline solution. *8,* Reinfusion bag. *(Courtesy Haemonetics Corp, Braintree, Mass.)*

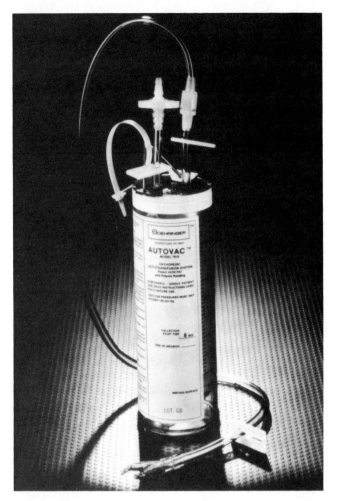

Fig. 14-4 AUTOVAC R postoperative orthopedic autotransfusion system. *(Courtesy Boehringer Laboratories, Norristown, Pa.)*

Skill 14-5 Administering the Autotransfusion

NURSING INTERVENTIONS

1. Clamp the patient line near the distal end of the tubing to prevent pneumothorax.
2. Disconnect the patient's chest drainage line and anticoagulant connector from the patient port on the liner lid.
3. Disconnect the tubing connector on the liner lid and sterile spacer on the canister tee.
4. Remove and discard liner. Never reuse the liner. Reline canister and reattach if further blood is to be collected. Use new filter.
5. Remove the liner from the canister. Squeeze out the air. Clamp liner-lid tubing. Cap port on lid.
6. To begin infusion, remove cap at bottom of liner and insert a 40-micron microemboli blood filter. Prime the tubing (40-micron in-line filter reduces the risk of microemboli and pulmonary insufficiency). After 6 liters of blood have been infused, significant hemolysis tends to occur and a platelet transfusion may be required at this time.
7. Infuse. Rate depends on patient's condition and doctor's orders.
8. If continuing, insert new liner assembly into canister. Connect suction and patient lines to continue blood collection.
9. Carefully monitor coagulation and blood culture studies. After 6 liters of blood are infused, a platelet infusion should be administered to counteract hemolysis. If the platelet count drops to 80,000 or below, FFP may be needed.
10. Record the following data:
    - What time procedure was begun and ended.
    - Size and location of chest tube.
    - How the procedure was tolerated.
    - Temperature, pulse, respiration, and blood pressure.
    - Volume of blood collected and transfused.
    - Type and amount of citrating used.
    - Type and amount of anticoagulant used.
    - Adverse reactions, including potassium intoxication, sepsis, emboli, and vascular trauma.

Complications of Exchange Transfusions

Vascular	Embolization, thrombosis, necrotizing, enterocolitis, and aortic perforation.
Cardiac	Dysrhythmias, volume overload or underload, and cardiac arrest.
Neurological	Reproducible decrease in intracranial pressure during withdrawal of blood and increased intracranial pressure during blood infusion may cause intracranial hemorrhage.
Electrolyte	Hypernatremia, hyperkalemia, acidosis, and alkalosis after exchange.
Clotting	Thrombocytopenia, overheparinization, and bleeding.
Infection	Bacteremia, viral hepatitis, and human immunodeficiency virus (HIV).
Other	Hemolysis from old donor blood or from mechanical or thermal injury, perforations of vessels and viscera, hypoglycemia (from induced insulin release), hypothermia, and hepatic necrosis.

Extracorporeal transfusion is the type of transfusion given to individuals undergoing heart surgery. A cardiopulmonary bypass machine is used for this transfusion. Blood is usually heparinized in the machine before administration to the patient rather than citrated, to prevent citrate toxicosis.

TRANSFUSION REACTIONS

Transfusion reactions can occur from a single or massive transfusion of blood or blood components (Table 14-5). Approximately 5% of all transfusions are associated with some type of adverse reaction.

Most transfusion reactions occur during a transfusion, especially during the first 15 minutes or shortly thereafter. Viral infections, however, may take as long as 6 months to become symptomatic.

Transfusion reactions require early recognition and prompt nursing actions to prevent further complications. This is especially true when blood is being administered to

Table 14-5   Transfusion Reactions and Nursing Actions*

Type of reaction/signs and symptoms	Cause	Nursing interventions	To minimize risk
Febrile, nonhemolytic Chills; fever; flushing; chest pain; back pain; malaise; hypotension; tachycardia; headache dyspnea; confusion; nausea; vomiting.	Antibody-antigen reaction involving leukocytes; platelets or plasma proteins.	Stop transfusion. Keep vein open. Monitor vital signs every 15 minutes. Monitor temperature at least every hour and begin cooling procedures as indicated (tepid baths, cool sponges, alcohol rubs, or hypothermia blankets). Administer medications as ordered.	Use saline washed RBCs. Administer antipyretic medications with blood.
Allergic Chills; no fever; urticaria; pruritis; nausea; vomiting; anxiety; headache; nasal congestion; wheezing; severe dyspnea; laryngeal edema; circulatory collapse (generally innocuous).	Cause is unknown, but probably results from allergens in the donor blood with antibodies in the recipient's blood.	Slow transfusion to keep vein open. Notify physician and blood bank. Monitor and record vital signs at least hourly. Administer oral antihistamines, epinephrine, or steroid medications, as ordered by physician.	Ask if person reacted allergically to previous transfusions or check history on patient's chart.
Circulatory overload Cough; hemoptysis; chest pain; dyspnea; engorged neck veins; tachycardia; S gallop, cyanosis; frothy sputum; rales; anxiety.	Rate of infusion or volume exceeds the circulatory system's capacity.	See hemolytic reaction. Administer cardiac drugs as ordered. Prepare for phlebotomy or rotating tourniquets. Elevate head of bed. Support patient. Administer oxygen as ordered by physician.	Use PRCs. Infuse at slow rate for those at risk or split the unit. Keep patient sitting up. Administer diuretic (as ordered) when transfusion is begun.
Acute hemolytic Chills; fever; dyspnea; chest, abdominal, or back pain; extreme anxiety; headache; nausea; vomiting feelings of coldness; tachycardia; cyanosis; hemoglobinuria; oliguria; anuria; jaundice; hypotension; circulatory collapse; DIC (potentially life threatening).	ABO or Rh incompatibility or improper storage.	Discontinue blood flow. Notify physician and laboratory. Return blood and fresh sample to the lab. Keep vein open with NS, until a new venipuncture can be made. Start intake and output record. Insert Foley catheter to monitor hourly urine output. Provide emotional support. Monitor vital signs and other symptoms. Keep patient comfortable. Document reaction.	Triple check patient's identification bracelet and blood type. Cross-check above with blood. Have another nurse check as well. Begin transfusion slowly. Remain with patient for first 20 minutes of transfusion.
Delayed hemolytic Decreased hemoglobin level; possible persistent low-grade fever.	Incompatability of RBC antigens other than ABO group.	Notify physician and blood bank.	Monitor closely.
Gram-negative reaction Chills; fever; abdominal and extremity pain; hypotension; vomiting; bloody diarrhea; shock; tachycardia; death.	Transfusions of blood contaminated by gram-negative bacteria; grows in cold temperature and releases endotoxins	See hemolytic and febrile reactions.	Use air-free, touch-free methods to collect blood. Maintain strict storage control. Use strict aseptic technique when warming blood for transfusion. Change the filter and tubing and blood at least every 4 hours.
Embolism Chest pain; dyspnea; cyanosis; cough; tachycardia; anxiety; death.	Air in the transfusion system.	See circulatory overload *but* instead of cardiac drugs administer morphine sulfate to relieve pain as ordered by physician. Place patient on left side in a headdown position.	Expel all air from tube.

*Refs 1, 11, 18, 23, 25, 32, 33, 34.

Table 14-5   Transfusion Reactions and Nursing Actions—cont'd

Type of reaction/signs and symptoms	Cause	Nursing interventions	To minimize risk
Infectious diseases Vary depending on the organism or parasite; onset also varies depending on organism but are generally delayed.	Introduction of viable organism or parasites from the donor's blood to the recipient. Diseases include hepatitis, HIV, syphilis, malaria and cytomegalovirus.	Careful follow-up history. Notify physician and blood bank. Supportive nursing actions, based on symptoms. Nurses are at risk for infections with these diseases. Special caution must be observed when handling blood specimens and items contaminated with blood. Needles are not broken, cut, or recapped.	Careful donor assessment.
Pulmonary Rapid onset; anxiety; cough; cyanosis; bilateral pulmonary infiltrates; hypoxia; respiratory distress; adult respiratory distress syndrome (ARDS); death.	Microaggregates embolize pulmonary vasculature; blocked capillary blood flow; WBC antibodies†; donor leukoagglutinins†; response to complement activation.†	Stop transfusion. Administer oxygen. Monitor vital signs and pulmonary artery wedge pressure (PAWP).	Transfuse with saline-washed RBCs, leukocyte-poor cells, or frozen RBCs. Use microaggregate filtration.
Anaphylactic reactions Flushing; bronchospasm; substernal pain; laryngeal edema; gastrointestinal distress; vomiting; diarrhea; collapse; death.	Idiosyncratic reaction in patients with antibodies against IgA.	Discontinue blood flow. Notify physician and blood bank. Keep vein open with NS. If further transfusions are required, frozen washed cells or blood from donors lacking IgA are products of choice. A file of these persons has been established by the American Association of Blood Banks Rare Donor File. Administer epinephrine (as ordered). Start intake and output. Insert Foley catheter. Monitor hourly urine. Monitor vital signs every 15 minutes. Document.	Careful assessment of donor and recipient. Use frozen, washed cells.
Hypothermia Chills; decreased body temperature; irregular heart rate; potential cardiac arrest.	Administration of large amount of cold blood.	Monitor temperature. Call physician. Keep patient warm. Document.	Allow blood to warm for 15 to 30 minutes. Use electric warming device.

†Cause not clearly established

persons who are unable to communicate untoward physical responses to the transfusion, such as in the following kinds of patients:

- Confused.
- Heavily sedated.
- Anesthetized.
- Unconscious.
- Very young.

It is the nurse's responsibility to observe, assess, and document the response of patients who are receiving blood or blood products. If an adverse reaction occurs, the transfusion should be stopped immediately and the physician should be notified.

The following steps can be taken to help avoid transfusion reactions:

- Check physician's orders carefully. The order must be: written, signed, dated, and specific (i.e., transfuse two units of packed red cells).
- Fill out requisition form completely and correctly.
- Check order and requisition form with another nurse.
- Draw blood sample from patient and send blood to lab to be typed and crossmatched.
- When obtaining blood from lab (refer to your agency policies for the procedure), match the name, room number, and patient identification number on the blood bag tag with the requisition form.

- Match the patient's identification number, ABO and Rh groups, unit, blood donor number, blood groups, and the expiration date.
- With another nurse assisting to ensure accuracy, match the patient's blood type with the blood type indicated on the blood bag and blood bag tag. Compare for the following:

    Patient's name and identification number.
    Number on blood bag label.
    ABO and Rh groups.
    Expiration date.
- If all data match, begin transfusion.
- Monitor patient closely.

MASSIVE TRANSFUSIONS

Many times in critical care the patient receives massive transfusions (infusion of blood approaching or exceeding replacement of the recipient's total blood volume in a 24-hour period).[3] This may occur unexpectedly, in a surgical or medical emergency, and/or in a planned situation, such as open-heart surgery or neonatal exchange transfusion.

Graded Response to Blood Loss

Shock results when there is a decrease in intravascular fluid volume, venous return to the heart, myocardial contractility, or when capacitance vessels are dilated.[28] The American College of Surgeons has classified shock into four stages based on blood loss[5] (Table 14-6). The box on p. 335 outlines an infusion protocol for profound shock.

Many adverse complications can result from massive transfusions (Table 14-7). In addition to complications from massive blood transfusions, complications may result from massive infusions of albumin.

Skill 14-6   Transfusion Reaction Protocol

NURSING INTERVENTIONS

1. Stop transfusion by closing clamps immediately.
2. Wash hands.
3. Disconnect the blood using sterile technique. Carefully detach needle and discard using universal precautions.
4. Cap tubing with new sterile needle.
5. Run normal saline at slow rate to keep vein open.
6. Monitor temperature, pulse, respiration, and blood pressure.
7. Examine label on blood containers and all related documents to detect if error has occurred in identifying the patient or the blood.
8. Notify physician.
9. Administer medications as per physician's order (if order is telephone order, have another nurse listen on another phone line to validate order). Check agency policy for any other requirements.
10. Fill out blood reaction forms.
11. Draw blood specimen and send to laboratory.
12. Return the blood or component, tubing, and sterile needle to the laboratory.
13. Obtain urine specimen as soon as possible and send to laboratory.
14. Begin 24-hour urine collection.
15. Document the following:
    - Signs and symptoms of reaction.
    - Temperature, pressure, respiration, and blood pressure.
    - Time and name of physician notified.
    - Any medications administered.
    - Amount of blood infused.
    - Amount remaining.
    - Any other findings about blood or component infused.
16. Continue to monitor.
17. Draw second blood specimen 5 to 7 hours after reaction (according to agency policy) and send to laboratory.
18. Send urine specimen to laboratory 5 to 7 hours after reaction.

Table 14-6   Estimated Fluid and Blood Loss

	Blood loss (ml) (volume)	Blood pressure*	Pulse pressure	Resp rate	Pulse	Urine output	Fluid replacement
Class I	Up to 750 ml (up to 15%)	118/82	NC	14-20	72-84	Greater than 30 ml/hr	Crystalloid
Class II	750-1500 ml (15%-30%)	110/80	Decreased	20-30	Above 100	20-30 ml/hr	Crystalloid
Class III	1500-2000 ml (30%-40%)	Decreased 70-90/50-60	Decreased	30-40	Above 120	5-15 ml/hr	Crystalloid plus colloid (blood)
Class IV	2000 or more (40% or more)	Severely decreased 50-60 systolic	Decreased	>35	Above 140	Less than 5 ml/hr	Crystalloid plus colloid

*NC, normal/no change.

▼ **Infusion Protocol for Profound Shock**[7,19,30]

1. Type and crossmatch for 6 to 10 units of PRCs.
2. Estimate blood loss for a 70-kg (154 lbs) man (5000 ml).
3. Give crossmatched packed cells whenever possible. If not available, administer grouped packed cells. If not available, administer O+ packed cells or deglycerized cells.
   - If patient has a loss of over 1500 to 2000 ml, begin colloid infusion of 5% Albumin or Hydroxyl starch and start infusion with a balanced salt solution.

- Give 500 ml of plasma substitute or 1000 ml of balanced salt solution after each unit of packed cells.
- Administer 2 units fresh frozen plasma after 5000 ml has been administered. Repeat after each 5000 ml infusion.
- Infuse 6 units of platelets after each 10,000 ml has been infused. Repeat every 10,000 ml.

4. Monitor hematocrit, hemoglobin, and serum potassium levels, and blood gases every 10,000 ml infusion.

Table 14-7   Adverse Reactions to Massive Transfusions and Nursing Interventions

Type of reaction/signs and symptoms	Cause	Nursing interventions	To minimize risk
Citrate toxicosis (Hypocalcemia)			
Muscular twitching and spasms; tingling in fingers; tetany; carpopedal tetany; respiratory arrest; ECG shows prolongation of the QT interval; hypotension; convulsions; cardiac arrest.	Occurs from the citrate present in the anticoagulant-preservative solution binding with serum calcium. It occurs from too-rapid transfusion, too-massive transfusion, and in patients with liver or kidney disease (rare).	As in hemolytic reactions. Infuse blood slowly. IV administration of calcium gluconate or calcium chloride (as ordered by physician) to prevent or neutralize the toxic effect.	Administer blood at a slower rate. Administer blood carefully to patients with renal and liver diseases.
Electrolyte imbalance (Hyperkalemia)			
Nausea; diarrhea; oliguria; anuria; muscle weakness; flacid paralysis; serum K increases; bradycardia; cardiac arrest.	Results from the release of potassium into the plasma from red blood cell lysis.	As in hemolytic reactions. Use fresh blood or PRBCs. Administer drugs to reduce serum potassium (as ordered by physician).	Administer packed RBCs. Administer FFP. Administer blood stored for less than 7 days.
Dilutional coagulopathy			
Excessive wound or needle site bleeding; hyponatremia; DIC; shock.	Massive transfusions. Depletion of coagilation proteins and platelets.	Notify physician; keep vein open. Monitor vital signs. Follow protocol for massive transfusions according to agency policy.	Administer 2 units FFP or platelets for every 10 units packed RBCs and plasma protein fraction administered (according to physician's order or agency policy.
Chemical toxicity (Lactic acid, Ammonia)			
Impaired cardiac function; decreased blood pressure; forgetfulness; confusion; shock; elevated serum ammonia level.	Massive transfusion of older whole blood.	As for hemolytic reactions.	Avoid use of older blood for massive transfusions.
Hypothermia (See Table 14-6)			
Increased oxygen affinity			
Depressed respirations.	A decreased level of 2,3-diphosphoglycerate (DPG) in stored blood results in an increase in the blood's hemoglobin affinity. When this occurs, blood remains in circulation and does not reach the tissues, resulting in hypoxia.	Monitor vital signs. Notify physician. Monitor blood gases. Provide respiratory support as needed.	Use only RBCs or fresh blood, if possible.
Microembolization			
Pulmonary dysfunction; adult respiratory distress syndrome (ARDS); brain and renal dysfunction.	Occurs from the development of microaggregates in stored blood.	Monitor vital signs. Assess carefully for transfusion reaction. Provide respiratory support, if needed.	Use fresh blood if possible. Use microaggregate filter with 20 to 40 micron openings.

*Refs 7, 8, 13, 19, 21, 24, 29, 31.

Continued.

Table 14-7 Adverse Reactions to Massive Transfusions and Nursing Interventions—cont'd

Type of reaction/signs and symptoms	Cause	Nursing interventions	To minimize risk
Denatural plasma proteins Bleeding disorders; DIC; impaired glomerular filtration; impaired pulmonary function.	Unclear at this time.	Monitor vital signs. Notify physician. Provide respiratory assistance, if needed.	Minimize blood use, if possible.
Interdonor incompatibility (Immune hemolysis) Red blood cell hemolysis; anxiety; pain at infusion; fever; hypotension; tachycardia; diffuse bleeding tendency; hemoglobinuria.	Occurs from massive transfusion from multiple donors.	Monitor vital signs. Notify physician.	Attempt to use one donor blood; do not use universal donor blood, if possible. Crossmatch all blood.
Vasoactive substances Hypotension; pulmonary impairment.	Results from both serotonin from platelet breakdown and activated factor XII in stored blood.	Monitor vital signs. Notify physician. Provide respiratory support, if needed.	Use fresh blood, if possible.
Graft versus host syndrome Fever; rash; hepatitis; severe diarrhea; bone marrow suppression; infection; lymphadenopathy; enlarged liver; hemolytic anemia; pancytopenia.	Most likely to occur with white blood cell or platelet transfusion.	Stop transfusion. Monitor vital signs. Notify physician. Monitor lab data. Assess patient.	Minimize transfusions, if possible.

TRANSFUSION DEVICES

There are support devices that are used for facilitating the administration of blood. These devices include positive pressure infusers, blood warmers, and mechanical infusion devices.

Pressure bags or infusers are designed to increase the flow rate of the blood or blood product. They are frequently used with viscous blood components or when rapid blood administration is needed. The pressure cuff is the most commonly used device.

Mechanical infusion pumps facilitate the administration of solutions at controlled rates.

Mechanical infusion devices are especially useful when blood is to be administered at a very slow rate.

Large volumes of rapidly infused cold blood can lower the temperature of the sinoatrial (SA) node to 30° C (86° F) or below, causing ventricular dysrhythmias. To reduce the chance of cardiac problems, metabolic acidosis or possible death, blood warming devices are used when large amounts of blood are to be infused in a short amount of time. A warmed blood infusion is also indicated for patients with cold agglutinins syndrome, a condition associated with cold antibodies. Exchange transfusions in neonates and children receiving rapid or massive transfusions must always be warmed.

PEDIATRIC CONSIDERATIONS

Infants and children may require transfusions of blood or blood components when critically ill. Transfusion of blood and blood products to infants and children requires accurate and precise monitoring because of the small volumes that are needed, the adjusted hematocrits, and the narrow acceptable ranges of pH and electrolytes. Blood-component therapy is the preferred method of transfusion. This method minimizes the chances of circulatory overload and of the introduction of antigens that are in the serum. Because of the high susceptibility of neonates for transfusion reactions, they are given washed red blood cells.

Infants and children cannot receive massive amounts of blood over short periods of time (except under dire, life-threatening conditions). Blood for pediatric transfusion is, therefore, generally divided into smaller units (aliquots) in the blood bank. This is because blood should not be left unrefrigerated for more than 4 hours.

Volume-control devices may be used to measure volumes precisely and to prevent circulatory overload. Blood or blood components ordered for infants and children are usually made in terms of ml/kg of body weight. In general the flow rate for neonatal infusion is less than 10 ml/hr.[16]

Vascular access is often difficult in newborns. The umbilical artery may be cannulated. In older infants a 23- or 25-gauge needle or a 22-gauge catheter can be used. Constant-rate syringe-delivery systems have been shown to be effective with these smaller gauge needles and catheters.[4]

The pulmonary vascular system in neonates is hypertensive and the lumens of vessels are undeveloped. Their reticuloendothelial systems (RESs) are also not fully developed. Lungs are not able to clear debris. All of these physiological factors indicate that microaggregate filtration of blood is necessary. Filters are used for all blood and blood components, but the type of filter for pediatric use is controversial. Some clinicians believe that the 170- to 200-micron clot screen is appropriate for most neonatal transfusions. Others argue that microaggregate filtration in infants is unwarranted since most red blood cell products are fresh, frozen, or washed.[15] Such filters may produce hemolysis of transfused cells when negative filtrations and older blood products are used.[14] Still other physicians argue that filters of 170 μm allow the passage of red blood cells and microaggregates of 150 μm in size. Such microaggregates may result in respiratory insufficiency or embolize the pulmonary circulation. These physicians recommend the use of millipore filters or double filters.

PSYCHOSOCIAL CONSIDERATIONS

A number of physical conditions may result in a need for transfusion therapy. Each of these conditions is accompanied by diverse psychological concerns. The patient requiring administration of blood products may experience pain and may need assistance in managing its psychological consequences. A patient may be subject to considerable fatigue and attendant feelings of apathy, malaise, and irritability. Patients may face life-style changes and many will have concern about the viral safety of blood products and the cost of ongoing care (if it is needed). Nurses should support patient and family coping efforts and should make available community resources (e.g., referral to a genetic counselor) for concerns requiring special expertise.

PATIENT TEACHING

The patient's understanding of the procedure should be assessed. Discussion with the patient should cover the complete sequence of events, including the crossmatch, IV line, and activity limitations, if any. To minimize the risks of component therapy, the patient and family should be taught the signs and symptoms that may be associated with a complication of blood component therapy. If explained too graphically, the patient may have symptoms of a reaction before the transfusion is even begun. The patient should be asked to report any "different" sensations after the transfusion has been initiated. When the patient is a young child or disoriented adult, the family can be instructed and asked to observe for any signs of an untoward reaction. The informed patient and family can aid in the early detection of problems.

HOME HEALTH CARE CONSIDERATIONS

Because of the national trend for home health care, the frequency of blood transfusions in the home is increasing. Nursing agencies in several states are now administering blood and blood components in the home. Home transfusions are not appropriate for all patients because of the inherent risk of transfusion reactions with adverse reactions occurring in about 5% of all recipients.[2] Patients who receive blood at home must be homebound (i.e., unable to

drive or leave home without assistance).

Patients who receive transfusions as a home-care procedure have a wide variety of medical diagnoses. Some patients receive blood as a component of oncology treatment, whereas others receive blood or blood component therapy as palliative treatment. Other patients who commonly receive blood transfusions at home are those who have blood dyscrasias or are immunosuppressed because of medications or acquired immune deficiency syndrome (AIDS). All patients who receive transfusions at home should be alert, cooperative, and capable of reporting to caregivers the signs of transfusion reaction.

Written criteria are essential for the home health agency to determine patient eligibility. General and specific therapy guidelines should establish standards for patient and agency safety. Guidelines should consider the patient's physical limitations, mental status, disease, condition, symptoms, blood studies, and history of transfusion reactions. Benadryl and epinepherine should be readily available in the home in the event of a transfusion reaction.

In-home transfusion therapy should be performed by a physician or a registered nurse under the direction of a physician in accordance with federal, state, and local regulations and the standards[3] of the American Association of Blood Banks, in addition to the home health care agency policies.

State regulations differ from state to state. Some states prohibit the administration of blood or blood components without the attendance of a physician. Other states allow registered nurses to administer blood transfusions in the home. Health care agencies also vary in their criteria for determining eligibility for home transfusions. Some agencies (e.g., Group Health Cooperative) require that the patient live within an area where there is an advanced cardiac life support (ACLS) system in case of a potentially lethal transfusion reaction. Other agencies require that the patient must have had at least one blood transfusion in the past.

Blood and blood components are obtained with the approval of local blood banks in accordance with their policies. Additionally, most blood banks require a written physician's order before the release of the blood or blood component. A blood sample should be drawn from the patient for type and crossmatch 24 to 48 hours before the transfusion, labeled at the bedside, signed by the person who obtained it, and delivered to the blood bank. An armband should be placed on the patient's wrist at the time the blood is drawn.

Before the release of the blood or blood component from the blood bank, each unit should be carefully checked by the nurse and the blood bank personnel against the blood (or blood component) requisition for the patient's name, identification number(s), ABO and Rh types, product unit number, color, general appearance, and expiration date. After this verification, documentation should be completed on the appropriate forms and signed by the nurse and the blood bank personnel.

Before the administration of blood or blood components, the nurse or the physician should provide the patient with the necessary information regarding the transfusion procedure and the need for the transfusion. The physician is also responsible for obtaining the signed informed consent. This consent should also contain a statement about home administration. For example, "I understand the additional risk involved in the administration of the blood or blood component in the home, including life-threatening complications and that in the event a complication would occur, immediate treatment of the complication will be limited because of available resources." The informed consent should be signed by the nurse, the patient, the physician, and a witness.

Once the blood or blood component is procured from the blood bank, it is usually transported to the patient's home is a special insulated bag by the nurse. Timing is of critical importance when blood is being transfused in the home setting. The time gap between the actual delivery of the unit of blood and its hanging has to be kept to a bare minimum. The registered nurse must be present when the unit arrives, or the unit may be transported by the nurse in a special quality-controlled bag filled with wet ice.[20]

Before infusion begins the physician's orders should again be checked in reference to the blood or blood component, number of units, duration, infusion rate, and any other related orders. The procedure to be followed is found earlier in this chapter.

The nurse will need to have excellent venous-access skills, as well as knowledge of side effects and reactions to blood transfusions. The nurse must also be able to recognize signs of a transfusion reaction.

The proper procedure for correctly identifying the unit and the person to receive it is perhaps the most critical step in the home-transfusion process. Without the comfort of carrying out the procedure in a setting where emergencies can be handled, an oversight can potentially be fatal. Safety is of prime importance when administering blood transfusions in the home and should be the principle to govern the nurse's every step in this procedure.

At the home the nurse should identify the patient by asking, "What is your name?" and by checking the patient's armband (if worn). Before administration, each unit of blood or blood product should be checked for the patient's name, ABO and Rh compatibility, product number, and expiration date. If any discrepancy is found the blood bank must be notified and the transfusion must not be administered until the difficulty has been found and corrected.[20]

Detailed documentation of nurse and patient activity at 15-minute intervals will not only provide a history of the transfusion procedure but may also serve as a barometer for subtle changes. Constant assessment of the patient is of prime importance during this procedure.

Patient and caregiver teaching includes providing information about signs and symptoms of transfusion reactions. The nurse will instruct the patient or caregiver about reaction indications that could occur after the nurse has left, and the proper persons to notify in such a case.

Once the administration is completed, the IV is discontinued and the blood bags and tubing are returned to the blood bank. All equipment used in the transfusion procedure should be disposable and discarded appropriately in sealed plastic bags. "Universal Precautions" as defined by the Centers for Disease Control (CDC) is a factor that must also be considered when handling blood products, with the nurse adhering to these specified guidelines.

If acute hemolytic, febrile, nonhemolytic, circulatory, or pulmonary overload transfusion reactions are observed, the blood transfusion should be terminated immediately. Protocols for reactions should be followed in the home. An example of one such protocol follows:

- Stop infusion.
- Maintain patient IV with 0.9% NS.
- Assess patient's condition.
- Monitor temperature, pulse, respiration, and blood pressure.
- Monitor cardiopulmonary status and neurological status.
- Administer medications according to protocol (e.g., epinephrine or Benadryl).
- Check blood or blood component label, documents, and patient armband.
- Notify physician.
- Monitor patient until signs and symptoms subside or until patient is transferred to an acute care setting.
- Notify blood bank of reaction.
- Send specimens of blood, blood/product container, administration set, and IV solution to blood bank.
- Document.

Protocols for delayed reactions should also be followed. For example, the patient should be assessed 1 week after the transfusion for signs and symptoms of an antigen-antibody reaction, such as low-grade fever, hemoglobinuria, drop in hemoglobin, and jaundice.

REFERENCES

1. American Association of Blood Banks: *Blood transfusion therapy,* Arlington, Virginia, 1987, The Association.
2. American Association of Blood Banks: Blood transfusions, *Am J Nurs* 89(4):486, 1989.
3. American Association of Blood Banks: *Standards for blood banks and transfusion services,* ed 13, Arlington, Virginia, 1989, The Association.
4. American Association of Blood Banks: *Technical manual,* ed 9, Arlington, Virginia, 1985, The Association.
5. American College of Surgeons, *Committee on trauma: advanced trauma life support course for physicians,* Chicago, 1984, American College of Surgeons.
6. Bullock BL, Rosendahl PB: *Pathophysiology,* ed 3, Philadelphia, 1992, JB Lippincott.
7. Cerra FB: *Manual of critical care,* St Louis, 1987, Mosby–Year Book.
8. Collins JA, Knudson MM: Metabolic effects of massive transfusion. In Rossi ED, Simon TL, Moss GS: *Principles of transfusion medicine,* Baltimore, 1991, Williams and Wilkins.
9. Drago SS: Banking your own blood, *Am J Nurs* 92(3):61, 1992.
10. Folkes ME: Transfusion therapy in critical care nursing, *Crit Care Nurse* 13(2):15, 1990.

11. Gloe D: Common reactions to transfusions, *Heart Lung* 20(5):506, 1991.

12. Holland PB, Schmidt PJ, editors: *Standards for blood banks and transfusion services,* ed 12, Arlington, Virginia, 1987, The American Association of Blood Banks.

13. Kirklin JK, Lell WA, Kouchoukos NT: Hydroxyethyl starch versus albumin for colloid infusion following cardiopulmonary bypass in patients undergoing myocardial revascularization, *Ann Thoracic Surg* 37(1):40, 1984.

14. Levin DL, Morriss FC editors: *Essentials of pediatric intensive care,* St Louis 1990, Mosby–Year Book.

15. Longhurst DM, Gooch WM, Castillo RA: In vitro evaluation of a pediatric microaggregate blood filter, *Transfusion* 23:170, 1983.

16. Luban NLC editor: *Transfusion therapy in infants and children,* Baltimore, 1991, Johns Hopkins University Press.

17. Martin E, Harris A, Johnson W et al: Autotransfusion systems, *Crit Care Nurse* 9(7):465, 1989.

18. Maxwell M, Kleeman C, editors: *Clinical disorders of fluid and electrolyte metabolism,* ed 4, New York, 1987, McGraw-Hill.

19. McMillan MA: The use of blood and blood products in surgical and critically ill patients. In Cerra FB: Manual of critical care, St Louis, 1987, Mosby–Year Book.

20. McVan VW: The role of the nurse in home transfusion. In Snyder EL and Menitove JE editors: *Home transfusion therapy,* Arlington, Virginia, 1987, The American Association of Blood Banks.

21. Messmer K: Plasma substitutes. In Tinker J and Rapior M editors: *Care of the critically ill patient,* New York, 1983, Springer-Verlag.

22. Moggio RA, Rha CC, Sombert ED et al: Hemodynamic comparison of albumins and hydroxyethyl starch in postoperative cardiac surgery patients, *Crit Care Med* 11(12):943,1983.

23. Perkins SB, Kennally KM: The hidden danger of internal hemorrhage, *Nursing '89* 19(7):34, 1989.

24. Querin JJ, Stahl LD: 12 simple sensible steps for successful blood transfusions, *Nursing '90* 20(10):73, 1990.

25. Rackow EC, Falk JL: Colloid and crystalloid fluid resuscitation. In Shoemaker WC: *Textbook of critical care,* ed 2, Philadelphia, 1989, WB Saunders.

26. Rossi EC, Simon TL, Moss GS: *Principles of transfusion medicine,* Baltimore, 1991, Williams and Wilkins.

27. Schiffer CA, Keller C, Dutcher JP et al: Potential HLA-matched platelet donor availability for alloimmunized patients, *Transfusion* 23:286, 1983.

28. Sommers MS: Fluid resuscitation following multiple trauma, *Crit Care Nurse* 10(10):74, 1990.

29. Schwab W, Shayne JP, Turner J: Immediate trauma resuscitation with type O uncross-matched blood: a two-year prospective experience, *J Trauma* 26(10):897, 1986.

30. Simon TL: Platelet transfusion therapy. In Rossi EC, Simon TL, Moss GS: *Principles of transfusion medicine,* Baltimore, 1991, Williams and Wilkins.

31. Unkle D, Smejkal R, Snyder R et al: Blood antibodies and uncrossmatched type O blood, *Heart Lung* 20(3):284, 1991.

32. Weeks D: Washing the blood, *RN* 54(5):60, 1991.

33. Wilson JD, Braunwald KJ, Petersdorf RG et al: *Harrison's principles of internal medicine,* ed 12, New York, 1991, McGraw-Hill.

34. Winick NJ: Blood product transfusion. In Levin D, Morriss FC: *Essentials of pediatric intensive care,* St Louis, 1990, Quality Medical Publishing.

Total Parenteral Nutrition

Objectives:

After completing this chapter, the reader will be able to:

- Discuss how total parenteral nutrition (TPN) provides the nutritional requirements for the critical care patient.
- Identify the types of patients who may require TPN therapy.
- Describe the methods by which parenteral nutrition may be administered.
- List the nutritive components and additives of parenteral nutrition solutions.
- Describe the assessment for potential complications and nutrient deficiencies associated with TPN.
- Formulate the nursing diagnoses and patient outcomes applicable to patients requiring TPN.
- Discuss current controversies in central venous catheter care.
- Describe the skills required to regulate and maintain a TPN infusion within the acute care setting.
- Specify the possible psychosocial responses and teaching needs of patients receiving long-term TPN.
- Differentiate between pediatric and adult TPN patient care requirements and precautions.
- Describe the skills required to administer TPN therapy within the home health care setting.

Total parenteral nutrition (TPN) or hyperalimentation is the intravenous administration of varying combinations of hypertonic glucose, amino acids, lipids, electrolytes, vitamins, and trace elements. TPN formulas are nutritionally complete and meet the total nutrient needs of the patient when enteral feeding is either impossible or inadequate.

METABOLISM AND NUTRITIONAL REQUIREMENTS IN STARVATION AND STRESS

The human body is in a constant state of flux. Tissues are continuously anabolized (synthesized) and catabolized (broken down). These processes require energy. Many factors prevent the critically ill patient from meeting energy requirements. These include the following:

- Increased or altered energy requirements.
- Altered use of nutrients.
- Possible gastrointestinal disease.
- Anorexia or inability to eat.

A critically ill patient may be exposed to stress in the form of sepsis, a major burn, multiple organ system failure, a traumatic injury, surgery, or respiratory compromise. These stressors are more damaging than starvation because protein becomes a more significant energy substrate. During stress, the metabolic rate increases and hyperglycemia exists. Fat deposits are not tapped in early or mild stress, and protein use occurs. This protein is derived from lean body mass and eventually from the viscera. Peripheral muscle supplies of the branched-chain amino acids (BCAA) are converted to energy. The critically ill patient subjected to stress may display the following characteristics[21]:

- Hyperglycemia.
- Hypermetabolism.
- Hypercatabolism with negative nitrogen balance.
- Altered energy substrate use.
- Increased use of the BCAA.

The critically ill patient may also have protein loss through draining wounds, exudate, and wound healing. Protein deficiency retards vascularization, lymphatic formation, fibroblastic proliferation, collagen synthesis, and tissue building. This leads to susceptibility to infection, delayed wound healing, and prolonged hospitalization and convalescence from illness. Loss of more than one third of total body protein during stress or prolonged starvation is fatal. Table 15-1 shows the substrate requirements in starvation and stress for the critically ill patient. A stress level of 1 might apply to elective surgery, 2 to multiple trauma, and 3 to sepsis.

Usually the energy requirements of a patient are estimated to be in the range of between 30 to 35 kcal/kg body weight/24 hrs, or between 2000 to 2500 kcal/24 hr.[23] Burn patients may require over 4000 kcal/24 hr because of hypermetabolism related to evaporative heat loss and accelerated protein synthesis and turnover. The standard intravenous solution, 1000 ml 5% dextrose with electrolytes and

Table 15-1 Estimated Substrate Requirements

	Stress level			
	Starvation	2 (Low)	3 (Early)	3 (Late)
Nonprotein calorie-nitrogen ratio (kcal/gmN)	150/1	100/1	100/1	80/1
Amino acids* (gm/kg/24 hr)	1	1.5	2	2.0 to 2.5
Total nonprotein calories (kcal/kg/24 hr)	25	25	30	35
Total calories (kcal/kg/24 hr)	28	32	40	50
Fractional requirements of total daily caloric load				
Amino acids (%)	15	20	25	30
Glucose (%)	60	50	40	70
Fat† (%)	25	30	35	‡

*For currently available amino acid formulas, the amount will vary somewhat with the brand of amino acid supplement used.
†For commercially available intravenous fat preparations composed primarily of long-chain triglycerides.
‡Hypertriglyceridemia present.
From Cerra FB: *Manual of critical care,* St Louis, 1987, Mosby–Year Book.

water, contains approximately 170 kcal. The postoperative patient typically receives about 500 kcal/24 hr in the form of 3 liters of 5% dextrose. If a typical patient requires 2000 kcal/24 hr, theoretically about 12 liters of 5% dextrose would be needed. This amount is not likely to be administered because of the danger of circulatory overload.

INDICATIONS FOR TOTAL PARENTERAL NUTRITION THERAPY[1]
Clinical Situations Where TPN Should Be a Part of Routine Care

Severe catabolism with or without malnutrition when the gastrointestinal (GI) tract is not usable within 5 to 7 days. Such patients would include those with greater than 50% body surface area (BSA) burns, multisystem trauma, extensive surgery, and sepsis. In these patients, body mass losses can be significant in 7 to 10 days. These patients should have early aggressive nutritional support within 1 to 3 days.

Severe malnutrition caused by a nonfunctional GI tract. Such patients would need early TPN within 1 to 3 days. A patient who is normally nourished or only mildly malnourished would not need to receive TPN as long as GI tract function is expected to occur within 5 to 7 days.

Inability to absorb nutrients through the GI tract. This includes those with diseases of the small intestine, radiation enteritis, severe diarrhea, intractable vomiting, and massive small bowel resection. Patients who have had 80% to 90% of their small bowels resected will need to go on long-term home TPN.

High-dose chemotherapy, bone marrow transplantation, and radiation. These therapies result in severe illness for 3 to 6 weeks where patients are often unable to eat because of ulcerative stomatitis, nausea, vomiting, and diarrhea. Provision of TPN may prevent premature death.

Moderate to severe pancreatitis. Patients should receive TPN if they need bowel rest and nasogastric decompression for more than 5 to 7 days.

Clinical Situations Where TPN Usually Would Be Helpful

Enterocutaneous fistula. TPN can provide for bowel rest and clinical stabilization so that the patient is ready for surgery or the fistula is able to heal spontaneously.

Inflammatory bowel disease. Two to four weeks of TPN can provide for bowel rest so that surgical intervention may be avoided.

Inflammatory adhesions with small bowel obstruction. Four to six weeks of TPN with bowel rest can allow adhesions to soften and in some cases the obstruction to resolve.

Hyperemesis gravidarum. If nausea and vomiting persists for greater than 5 to 7 days, TPN may need to be instituted to protect both the mother and fetus.

Intensive cancer chemotherapy. TPN has allowed more intensive chemotherapy, in spite of anorexia. The normal nutritional status promotes a sense of well-being in the patient.

Situations where adequate enteral nutrition cannot be established within a 7- to 10-day period of hospitalization. To prevent malnutrition, TPN may be given to supplement enteral feedings.

Moderate stress. TPN should be provided to patients with moderate trauma, 30% to 50% BSA burns, neurological trauma, and other similar moderate stress when an enteral diet cannot be begun for over 7 to 10 days.

Major surgery. If an adequate enteral diet is not expected to be resumed within 7 to 10 days, TPN should be considered beginning at 48 hours and continued until enteral nutrition is achieved.

Moderate malnourishment in a patient who will be requiring intensive medical or surgical intervention. Before a major surgical procedure or initiation of aggressive medical management, a malnourished patient may be given a 7- to 10-day course of TPN that may then be continued through the stressful period.

Clinical Situations Where TPN Is of Limited Value

Proven or suspected untreatable disease state. Little benefit is derived from providing TPN for patients with extremely poor quality of life with no hope for improvement. This would include patients with widely metastic malignancies with no known effective therapy.

Minimal stress and trauma in the well-nourished patient when the GI tract is usable within a 10-day period. This would include patients with limited soft tissue injury, those with mild acute pancreatitis, and burn injuries of less than 20% BSA.

Immediate postoperative or poststress period. If a patient is otherwise well-nourished, the GI tract will recover within 7 to 10 days and the patient will not need TPN.

Clinical Situations Where TPN Should Not Be Used

When the sole dependence on TPN is anticipated to be less than 5 days.

When the risks of TPN are judged to exceed the potential benefits.

Presence of a functional and usable GI tract capable of absorption of adequate nutrients. Enteral feeding should always be used in preference to TPN.

A prognosis that does not warrant aggressive nutritional support. This would include patients who are imminently terminally ill or those with irreversible coma, unless they are being prepared for organ donation.

When an urgent operation should not be delayed to start the patient on TPN. Even when a malnourished patient needs TPN to prepare for surgery, certain surgeries, such as drainage of deep abscesses and acute abdominal catastrophes should not be delayed for TPN.

When aggressive nutritional support is not desired by the patient or legal guardian and when such action is in accordance with hospital policy and existing law.

ADMINISTRATION OF TOTAL PARENTERAL NUTRITION

TPN solutions have very high osmolarities because they contain from 25% to 35% dextrose/L. When mixed with amino acids and other additives, they have a final osmolarity of 1700 to 2200 μmol/L.[6] These concentrated solutions must be administered by the central venous route into a wide-diameter, high-flow vessel to reduce the threat of venous irritation and/or chemical phlebitis. Usually the catheter is inserted into the right subclavian or internal jugular vein and threaded into the superior vena cava, just outside the right atrium (Fig. 15-1). Other veins used for central venous (CV) insertion sites include the external jugular, cephalic, and basilic. The femoral and brachial veins may also be used but are rarely used. Occasionally a catheter-tip location other than the superior vena cava is used. These locations include the innominate vein, the intrathoracic subclavian vein, and occasionally the right atrium for Silastic catheters only.

Central Venous Access Devices

Central venous access devices (VADs) may be divided into short-term and long-term use devices (Table 15-2). The short-term VADs are commonly inserted by a percutaneous venipuncture using the modified Seldinger (guide wire) technique. They are secured by sutures. Short-term VADs are made from rigid materials that make them easier to insert, such as polyvinyl chloride (PVC) or polyurethane. These catheters can cause damage to the intima of the cannulated vein, leading to thrombus formation. Catheters made from polyurethane have been found to be less thrombogenic.

Central VADs designed for long-term use are divided into central venous tunneled catheters, peripherally inserted central catheters (PICCs), and implanted venous ac-

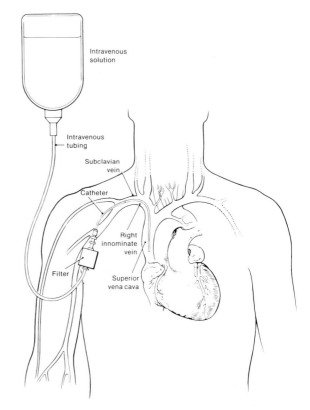

Fig. 15-1 Administration of total parenteral nutrition showing catheter placed directly into subclavian vein and threaded into innominate vein and superior vena cava. (From Phipps WJ, Long BC, Woods NF: *Medical-surgical nursing: concepts and clinical practice,* ed 2, St Louis, 1983, Mosby–Year Book.)

cess ports. The long-term VADs are made of a more flexible silicone rubber (Silastic). This product is the most biocompatible substance available and so causes the least damage to veins.[3]

Peripheral Parenteral Nutrition

Peripheral parenteral nutrition (PPN) is the administration of varying amounts of amino acids, glucose, lipids, electrolytes, vitamins, and trace elements through a peripheral vein. This form of nutrition is used when it is not possible or necessary to insert a subclavian vein catheter. Frequently PPN is used for patients receiving suboptimal oral nutrition or for short-term requirements when a period of starvation is unpredictable.

To prevent thrombophlebitis of the small peripheral vessels where blood flow is much slower, osmolarity of PPN solutions must be kept to a minimum. Infusion sites must be rotated every 24 to 48 hours. Solutions with osmolarities greater than 300 mOsm/L are considered to be hypertonic and are irritating to veins. Phlebitis will occur if the infusate is greater than 500 mOsm or if the potassium concentration is above 60 mEq/L. The final concentration of glucose for peripheral delivery should not exceed 10% to 12.5%.[12] Because dextrose has such a high osmolarity, it has been found that adding lipids to the PPN solution can

Table 15-2 Central venous access devices (VAD)

Description	Flushing requirements	Nursing considerations
Short-Term Central Venous Access Devices		
Short-term single-lumen catheter Made of polyvinylchloride (PVC) or polyurethane Useful for central venous pressure (CVP) monitoring Used for emergency access For patient who needs only a one-lumen IV access	SASH Procedure (**S**aline, **A**dminister infusion, **S**aline, **H**eparin): 1. Flush line with 10 ml normal saline (NS) to establish patency. 2. Administer medication/solution infusion. 3. Flush line with 10 ml NS upon completion of infusion. 4. Follow with 1 ml heparin solution. The concentration of heparin most often used for short and long-term catheters is 100 units/ml.	Catheter needs to be changed every 7 days (sooner if placed during emergency or left in longer if used for TPN only and placed in operating room). Assess frequently for clot formation and signs of infection. Designate each lumen for a separate task, such as TPN administration or blood drawing. Label lumens to prevent confusion.
Short-term multilumen catheter Made of PVC or polyurethane Used for patients who require multiple infusions Short-term central venous access Used from a few days to 4 weeks	Many institutions are now using only 10 units/ml, especially with pediatric patients. The amount of heparin should be about equal to the filling volume of the catheter. No flushing is needed if the line has a continuous infusion. Flush once a day with heparin solution for lines not in use.	Administer TPN in the most distal lumen of multilumen catheter. Change transparent occlusive dressing every 5 days, gauze dressing every 48-72 hours, and if catheter is used for TPN, change dressing every 72 hours. Change administration tubing every 72 hours; if used for TPN, change every 48-72 hours. Change injection caps every 72 hours.
Pulmonary artery catheters/Swan-Ganz catheters Used for physiological monitoring and cardiac pacing		
Groshong CV catheter Made of silicone rubber Come with from 1 to 3 lumens Has closed end with pressure-sensitive three-position valve Retrograde blood flow, air embolism and catheter occlusion are greatly reduced Heparin is not needed to flush Groshong CV catheter	*Inject 5 ml NS:* After administering fluids or medication Following each injection-cap change Every 7 days if catheter is not in use *Inject 10 ml NS:* After aspirating or transfusing blood If you see blood reflux in the tubing *Inject 20 ml NS:* Before aspirating a blood specimen following an infusion of TPN	
Long-Term Central Venous Access Devices		
Central Venous Tunneled Catheters		
Hickman catheter Silicone rubber Useful in home therapy Has dacron cuff and clamps	1. Flush catheter before use with 10 ml NS to establish patency. 2. Administer infusion. 3. After infusion, flush catheter with 10 ml NS. 4. Follow with 2 ml heparin solution. 5. When line is not in use, flush with 2 ml heparin solution every week.	
Broviac catheter Silicone rubber Smaller lumen than Hickman catheter Useful in elderly and in pediatrics		Observe catheters frequently for kinks and tears. Keep gauze or transparent occlusive dressing over exit site at all times. Change the transparent occlusive dressings every 5 days.
Hickman/Broviac catheter Hickman and Broviac catheters in one catheter Used for multiple infusions		Change the gauze dressings every 48-72 hours. Change injections caps every 72 hours. Leave catheters in indefinitely, but observe for signs of infection.
Peripherally Inserted Central Catheter (PICC)		
Long-line catheter Silicone rubber Smaller lumen size Used for patients with poor central access Inexpensive placement since easily inserted at bedside May be inserted by nurses in some states	1. Flush line with 10 ml NS. 2. Administer infusion. 3. After infusion, flush catheter with 10 ml NS. 4. Follow with 1 ml heparin solution. 5. For patients who cannot tolerate heparin, 5-10 ml of NS can be substituted for the heparin.	
Implanted Venous Access Ports		
Med-i-Port ***Port-A-Cath*** ***Infuse-A-Port*** ***Groshong*** Silastic catheter connected to metal or plastic port implanted like a pacemaker Port contains thick, self-sealing silicone septum	1. Flush port system before use with 10 ml NS to establish patency. 2. Administer infusion. 3. After infusion is complete, flush with 10 ml NS. 4. Follow with 3 ml heparin solution. 5. When not in use, flush every 4 weeks with 5-10 ml NS followed by 3 ml heparin solution to help prevent clot formation.	No dressing is required when catheter is not in use. Once accessed with Huber needle, cover with transparent dressing. Change dressing and needle every 5-7 days.

provide a concentrated calorie source without increasing the osmolarity of the solution. Using fats, dextrose, and proteins, a maximum energy supply of 2500 kcal/24 hrs can be delivered through PPN.

Protein-Sparing Therapy

Protein-sparing therapy is the peripheral administration of amino acids, vitamins, minerals, and electrolytes. The goal of this therapy is preservation of skeletal mass, prevention of muscle breakdown, and improvement of the metabolic response to postoperative infections. This solution provides few calories, decreases insulin levels, and mobilizes the body's own fat for energy.

Cyclic Total Parenteral Nutrition

Cyclic TPN is the technique of administering TPN at intermittent intervals rather than continuously over the full 24-hour period. Typically a patient would receive cyclic TPN at night over 10 to 16 hours. The regimen might begin in the evening as follows: 80 ml/hr for 1 hour; 150 ml/hr for 14 hours; 40 ml/hr for 2 hours; off for 7 hours.[7] The TPN is slowed for the last hour or two to prevent rebound hypoglycemia. Most home TPN patients' infusions are cycled. This provides for greater mobility for both home and hospitalized patients. If the patient has a single-lumen Hickman catheter used during the day for the administration of antibiotics, analgesics, and chemotherapy, cyclic TPN will enable the patient to receive the required amount of TPN that is needed. It is thought to have physiological advantages over continuous TPN because it more closely simulates the normal pattern of eating and fasting. One problem occurring in home care cyclic TPN patients is that 12- and 18-hour infusions increase daily urinary calcium excretion so that patients will need to be observed for a negative calcium balance.[22]

Total Nutrient Admixtures

Total nutrient admixture (TNA) is a system where lipids, amino acids, glucose, electrolytes, and trace minerals are mixed in one flexible container. It is know commercially as the All-In-One TPN mixing system or the 3-in-1 admixture system.

Disadvantages of TNAs include the following:
- Rapid microbial growth in lipid solutions and the net effect of adding various dextrose concentrations, different types of amino acids, and the wide range of electrolyte concentrations to lipid emulsions.
- The risk of an unstable emulsion, where oil droplets float to the top of the solution, create a risk of fat embolism.
- The opacity of the solution eliminates the ability to visually check for suspended particles, fine precipitates, or microbial growth.
- Known to cause Hickman catheter occlusions.

The following guidleines are recommended when administering TNA systems[5]:
- The final admixture can be refrigerated up to 48 hours before being used.

- During administration, a container may remain hanging for up to 24 hours.
- Lipid particles are too large for a 0.22 μm end-line filter, so a 1.2 μm filter that has a Luer-Lok to the catheter can be substituted.
- Volumetric rather than peristaltic infusion pumps must be used for delivery of the solution; accurate delivery of the infusion should be verified without total reliance on the pump.

PARENTERAL NUTRITION SOLUTIONS AND ADDITIVES
Dextrose

Most parenteral nutrition solutions contain between 5% and 35% dextrose to deliver from 170 to 1190 calories/L (Table 15-3). In a standard TPN solution, 500 ml of 50% dextrose might be combined with 500 ml amino acids plus vitamins, electrolytes, and trace elements to compose a final TPN solution of slightly more than 1000 ml. The final concentration of the dextrose, 25%, will then be more dilute as expressed per liter. A third component that might be added is 500 to 1000 ml of lipid solution that would then bring the volume of the TPN solution up to 1500 to 2000 ml. It is the final osmolarity of the solution and balance of nutrients that will determine where, how fast, and to whom it will be infused. Stressed hospitalized patients should not receive more than 5 mg glucose/kg/min or hyperosmolar, hyperglycemic nonketotic dehydration (HHND) may occur. Respiratory changes, liver abnormalities, hypophosphatemia, and hypomagnesemia may also result from excessive dextrose administration.

Proteins

Proteins in TPN solutions are provided in the form of crystalline L-amino acid solutions. There are more than 20 amino acid products to choose from, with substantial differences in solution composition, concentrations, indications, and price. A few of the products are listed in Table 15-4. Standard base solutions for TPN usually contain 500 ml of 8.5% or 10% amino acids that will be mixed with 500 ml dextrose to provide a final solution of 4.25% to 5%

Table 15-3   Parenteral Nutrition Additives: Dextrose

Additive	Final concentration/L (%)	gm/L	Kcal/L	Osmolarity (mOsm/L)
Dextrose 10% 500 ml	5	50	170	250
Dextrose 20% 500 ml	10	100	340	500
Dextrose 30% 500 ml	15	150	510	750
Dextrose 50% 500 ml	25	250	850	1250
Dextrose 70% 500 ml	35	350	1190	1750

To determine calories per liter: Volume of solution × (% of dextrose) × 3.4 kcal/gm
Examples: 500 ml × 50% × 3.4 = 850 kcal/L
1000 ml × 25% × 3.4 = 850 kcal/L

Table 15-4   Parenteral Nutrition Additives: Amino Acid Solutions[7]

Utilization example	Formula (% solution)
Protein restriction	FreAmine III 3%
Renal failure	Aminosyn-RF 5.2%
Renal failure	Nephramine 5.4%
PPN	Travasol 5.5%
Low-birth weight infants	Trophamine 6%
Sepsis/trauma	FreAmine HBC, 6.9%
Hepatic encephalopathy	HepatAmine 8%
Standard base solution	Novamine 8.5%
Standard base solution	FreAmine III 10%

To determine grams of protein per liter:
Volume of amino acid solution × (% protein) = gm protein/L
    Example:
        500 ml × 8% = 40 gm/L
        500 ml of an 8% amino acid solution provides 40 gm protein in a 1 L bag.
        40 gm/L × 2.5 L/24 hr = 100 gm/24 hr
        A patient receiving 2.5 L/24 hr would receive 100 gm protein in 24 hours.
        gm protein ÷ 6.25 = gm nitrogen
        The amount of protein divided by 6.25 equals the grams of nitrogen.

amino acids. The amino acid solutions used for PPN have a lower concentration, ranging from a final concentration of 2.5% to 5%. Modified solutions can be prepared using the general-purpose amino acid solutions to make TPN that contains one half the protein concentration of the standard TPN solutions. These are used for patients who require protein restriction, such as patients with liver disease, renal disease, or a history of protein intolerance.[6] Specialized disease-specific amino acid solutions have also been developed for use in certain types of patients.

With a patient in renal failure, a slow TPN infusion with a high calorie to nitrogen ratio is needed so that endogenous urea production is reduced. For patients in stable or worsening acute renal failure who are not being dialyzed, essential amino acids (EAA) solutions are indicated.

Patients with liver failure and encephalopathy have alterations in blood amino acid profiles, increased aromatic amino acids (AAA), and decreased BCAA. If these patients are given the standard amino acid solutions, their encephalopathy may become worse. A special amino acid formula has been developed for their use (HepatAmine, 8.0%) that is enriched with BCAA and deficient in AAA.

The use of infusions enriched with BCAA, such as FreAmine HBC, 6.9%, has been recommended for patients with sepsis or trauma. Energy and protein metabolism is affected and muscle catabolism occurs. This metabolic response to injury increases the oxidation of BCAA by the skeletal muscle, thereby lowering the serum levels of this amino acid.[23] When BCAA-enriched TPN solutions are

provided to septic and trauma patients, they have decreased skeletal muscle breakdown, a greater rate of protein synthesis, normalized amino acid profiles, and an earlier improvement in nitrogen balance.[11]

Lipids

Lipid emulsions come in 10% (1.1 calories/ml) and 20% (2.2 calories/ml) concentrations and 500 ml volumes. They are derived from soybean or safflower oil. Purified egg lecithin phosphatides are used to emulsify the fat. The emulsions are made isotonic by the addition of glycerol so that their osmolarities range from 270 to 340 mOsm/L.[6] The usual dose of IV fat to prevent an essential fatty acid deficiency is 4% of a patient's total calories per week.[23] Essential fatty acids promote platelet function, wound healing, prostaglandin synthesis, and immunocompetence. They also help to preserve the integrity of skin, hair, and nerves.

It is especially advantageous for certain groups of patients to receive some of their daily calories through fats. These patients include those who have the following:
- Surgery or trauma.
- Pulmonary insufficiency.
- Hyperglycemia.

Water

Water must be provided to keep up with urine output and replace other losses from tubes, catheters, and drains, along with increased insensible losses resulting from increased temperature. The normal requirements for water in adults is 1 ml/cal infused or 35 ml/kg.[27] Infants need 1.5 ml/calories infused.

Electrolytes

Electrolytes are added to a TPN solution depending on individual patient requirements. Electrolytes will be needed in larger amounts for patients who are in an anabolic (tissue growth) phase. Serum values are monitored regularly to ensure that patients are receiving the appropriate amount. The commercial amino acids have varying amounts of chloride and acetate salts that must be considered for total daily requirements.

Vitamins and Trace Elements

Supplemental vitamins may be required, especially vitamin C for collagen synthesis and wound repair.

Trace elements are present in human tissue in minute amounts. They participate in protein and nucleic acid synthesis, nerve conduction, muscle contraction, membrane transport, and mitochondrial function. Patients should be observed for trace element deficiencies so that larger individual doses of each trace element may be prescribed as necessary.

Medications

There are a number of medications that can be added directly to TPN solutions. Some of them are controversial.

Except for these few drugs, protocols do not allow the adding of drugs to TPN solutions or piggybacking them into the TPN line. With the advent of multilumen catheters, drugs are now being administered through a separate lumen to prevent mixing of the drug and nutrient solution. Even this practice is avoided, though, where possible and used only with certain patients, such as those who have poor venous access or need to receive chemotherapy (e.g., 5-fluorouracil) without interruption of IV nutrition support. The following medications and solutions are added directly to the TPN solution in some institutions: albumin, aminophylline, antibiotics, cimetidine hydrochloride (Tagamet), heparin, hydrochloric acid, hydrocortisone, insulin, meto-clopramide (Reglan), morphine, and ranitidine hydrochloride (Zantac).

ASSESSMENT

When assessing the patient receiving TPN, the critical care nurse will need to be especially alert for the signs and symptoms listed in Table 15-5 that indicate complications of TPN therapy. Components of the nutritional assessment are discussed in Chapter 16. When performing a physical assessment, it is important to assess for symptoms of nutrient deficiency, especially in the long-term TPN patient being cared for in the home. Table 15-6 lists some clinical signs to look for when assessing for malnutrition.

Text continued on p. 352

Table 15-5 Complications of Total Parenteral Nutrition Therapy

Complication	Signs and symptoms	Nursing interventions
Technical complications		
Pneumothorax, hydrothorax, or hemothorax	Sharp chest pain and dyspnea Decreased breath sounds on side of catheter Crepitus Shock Cyanosis Resonance to percussion	Stop infusion and get chest x-ray as ordered by physician. Monitor vital signs. Provide support to patient. Assist with aspiration or chest tube insertion. Assist with removal of catheter and replacement.
Arterial laceration	Pulsating bright red blood fills syringe Rapidly increasing hematoma Tracheal compression with respiratory distress if severe	Notify physician. Apply direct pressure to artery for 15 min. Monitor vital signs. Provide respiratory support.
Myocardial perforation (causes accumulation of blood in pericardial sac)	Cyanosis Dyspnea Decreased blood pressure Rapid, weak pulse	Notify physician. Provide respiratory support. Monitor vital signs for shock. Chest x-ray, as ordered. Assist with catheter removal and pericardiocentesis to remove blood.
Catheter tip against atrium or ventricle	Cardiac dysrhythmias	Monitor for life-threatening dysrhythmias. Obtain code cart and defibrillation equipment. Assist physician in repositioning of catheter.
Air embolism	Chest pain Dyspnea Tachypnea Tachycardia Cyanosis Apprehension Shock "Mill-wheel churning" sound over anterior precordium	Turn patient to left side in Trendelenburg position to raise right heart, forcing air out of pulmonary artery. Take vital signs. Provide respiratory support. Ensure tight connections. Have patient perform Valsalva maneuver when catheter is open to air.
Catheter embolism	Cardiac dysrhythmias Chest pain Increased central venous pressure	Chest x-ray, as ordered. Prepare for transvenous retrieval with guide-wire snare. Cardiac monitoring.
Venous thrombosis (as a result of trauma or irritation of vessel intima from hyperosmolar solution)	Edema and pain of neck, shoulder, and arm Leaking of infusate around catheter	Remove catheter, culture tip, and provide anticoagulant therapy, as ordered.

From Bruce NP: *Administration of total parenteral nutrition.* In Flynn, J-BMcC, Hackel R, editors: *Technological foundations of nursing*, Norwalk, Conn, 1990, Appleton & Lange.

Table 15-5   Complications of Total Parenteral Nutrition Therapy—cont'd

Complication	Signs and symptoms	Nursing interventions
Technical complications—cont'd		
Infiltration and phlebitis	Inflammation, swelling at insertion site	Inspect site for redness and swelling. Remove catheter, as ordered. Apply heat to area.
Brachial plexus or phrenic nerve injury	Numbness Tingling Pain shooting down arm Paralysis	Remove catheter, as ordered. Provide support.
Thoracic duct injury	Symptoms on left side White, milky drainage at insertion site	
Blockage of TPN infusion caused by clot at catheter tip, kinks in line, or tip against atrium wall	Infusion pump unable to deliver fluid	Check tubing for kinks. Reposition patient. Remove dressing and check for kinks at entry site. If permissible, irrigate catheter at hub.
Hickman and Broviac catheter problems Tear in catheter's external portion		For tear less than 2.5 cm (1 inch) from chest wall, clamp catheter, notify physician, and plan for catheter replacement. If tear occurs more than 2.5 cm (1 inch) from chest wall, flush catheter with heparin solution, notify physician, and obtain Hickman catheter repair kit. Avoid using clamps with prongs or teeth. Protect clamped portions with piece of tape.
Difficulty aspirating blood due to catheter tip against atrium wall or fibrinous sheath around catheter tip		Flush with heparinized saline. Have patient change position, raise arms, take a deep breath, or cough. Lower patient's head and chest.
Clot or other blockage in catheter		Irrigate blocked catheter if directed.
Metabolic complications		
Hyperglycemia	Thirst, malaise Dry mouth Flushed skin Nausea or vomiting Polyuria	Insulin drip or insulin added to TPN solution, as ordered. Infuse at constant rate with infusion pump. Test urine for sugar and acetone every 6 hr. Monitor serum glucose until stable, then 2 to 3 times per week. Prevent kinks and interruptions.
Rebound hypoglycemia	Headache Drowsiness Diaphoresis Dizziness Tremor Tachycardia Muscle twitching Seizures	Give one ampule $D_{50}W$ IV for dangerously low blood sugar, as ordered. Taper TPN decrease over at least 2-day period. If sudden need for discontinuation, give $D_{10}W$.
Hyperosmolar, hyperglycemic nonketotic coma	Urine output 800-900 ml in 1-2 hrs Confusion Lethargy Seizures	Stop TPN solution, as ordered. Give IV insulin in small amounts. Give large volumes of hypoosmolar solutions, such as .45% NaCl. Monitor sugar and acetone. Measure intake and output and serum glucose and osmolality.

Continued.

Table 15-5   Complications of Total Parenteral Nutrition Therapy—cont'd

Complication	Signs and symptoms	Nursing interventions
Metabolic complications—cont'd		
Protein intolerances		
Sensitivity to infused amino acids resulting from rapid infusion of protein	Nausea, vomiting Diarrhea Cholestatic jaundice	Reduce rate of infusion, as ordered.
Hyperchloremic metabolic acidosis, caused by amino acid solutions with high chloride	Nausea, malaise Dizziness Disorientation Dehydration	Administer sodium bicarbonate, as ordered. Reduce concentration of protein source. Monitor serum electrolytes. Observe for rise in chloride and drop in carbon dioxide.
Hyperammonemia caused by diminished ability to handle protein load		Provide low-dose arginine administration, as ordered.
Electrolyte imbalances		
Hyperkalemia	Peaked T waves Dysrhythmias Possible arrest Nausea, vomiting Muscle weakness	Treat imbalances, as ordered Monitor serum levels every 1-3 days. Assess behavior and symptoms of imbalance. Use only appropriate additives. Encourage exercises and early ambulation to prevent excess potassium loss.
Hypokalemia	Low amplitude T wave Muscle weakness Confusion	
Hypermagnesemia	Hypertension Nausea, vomiting Muscle weakness	
Hypomagnesemia	Cramps, confusion Muscle weakness	
Hypercalcemia	Mental confusion Anorexia, nausea Vomiting, lethargy Constipation	
Hypocalcemia	Tetany, cramps Clotting problems Laryngeal stridor	
Hyperphosphatemia	Soft tissue calcification resulting in renal damage	
Hypophosphatemia	Perioral numbness Respiratory difficulty	
Essential fatty acid deficiency	Dry, scaly skin Eczematous rash Sparse hair Thrombocytopenia Poor wound healing Fatty degeneration of the liver	Evaluate serum triglyceride levels on laboratory forms. Infuse 4% to 10% of total caloric intake as IV fat or give unsaturated oil orally or to skin, as ordered.
Trace element deficiences		
Zinc	Dermatitis Hair loss Impaired wound healing, Diarrhea	Monitor weekly serum copper and zinc levels. Add IV trace elements to TPN, as ordered.
Copper	Anemia unresponsive to iron Neutropenia	
Liver toxicity (resulting from huge doses of dextrose)	Liver tenderness Elevated liver function tests	Evaluate weekly liver function tests.

Table 15-5   Complications of Total Parenteral Nutrition Therapy—cont'd

Complication	Signs and symptoms	Nursing interventions
Allergic reaction to amino acids, peptides, or fats	Headache Fever Chills Nausea Vomiting Rash Abdominal pain Hypotension Tachycardia	Change infusion to $D_{10}W$, as ordered Take vital signs every 4 hours. Ask patient to report changes and problems.
Allergic reactions to fat emulsions	Dyspnea Cyanosis Headache Nausea Vomiting Flushing Pain in back and chest	Discontinue infusion and notify physician. Monitor vital signs.
Incompatibility of additives	Precipitate in bottle Clotting of TPN catheter Allergic reactions	Return bottle to pharmacy. Treat symptoms, as ordered. Monitor vital signs. Have pharmacist check all orders.
Hypervolemia	Increase in blood pressure, pulse, and respiratory rate Crackles in lung fields Dependent edema Distended neck veins	Treat symptoms, as ordered. Adjust daily requirements, as ordered. Monitor vital signs. Assess respiratory status. Weigh daily. Check neck veins. Record intake and output.
Hypovolemia	Decreased blood pressure Increased pulse rate Orthostatic blood pressure changes Flat neck veins Dry mucous membranes Mental status changes	Administer increased fluids, as ordered. Monitor vital signs.
Excessive weight gain	Gain of weight more than (0.5 kg [1 lb]/24 hr) Signs of fluid weight gain	Evaluate daily weights. Encourage active exercise to promote gain of lean body mass instead of fatty tissue. Monitor total protein and albumin levels.
Septic complications		
Catheter-related sepsis (bacteria and toxins in blood) Bacteremia	Chills Fever Leukocytosis Hypotension Tachycardia Increase in respiration New, sudden onset glycosuria Change in level of consciousness	Discontinue TPN infusion and get blood cultures, as ordered. Rule out other sources of infection before catheter is removed. Send catheter tip for culture. Establish TPN team and protocol. Monitor vital signs every 4 hours. Monitor sugar and acetone every 6 hrs. Evaluate white blood cell count biweekly or weekly, as ordered. Observe for signs of septic shock.
Candidemia		Remove catheter. Culture tip. Give amphotericin B, as ordered.
Catheter entrance site infection	Swelling Purulent drainage	Culture and remove catheter, as ordered. Change dressing every 72 hrs with sterile technique. Inspect site for redness and drainage. Use povidone-iodine as scrub and ointment. Use clean-to-dirty technique when prepping skin. Ensure occlusive dressing.

Continued.

Table 15-5 Complications of Total Parenteral Nutrition Therapy—cont'd

Complication	Signs and symptoms	Nursing interventions
Septic complications—cont'd		
Solution-related sepsis	Dramatic temperature spike	Change entire IV system and bottle. Return solution to pharmacy. Send solution samples for culture, as ordered. Monitor vital signs. Observe for septic shock. Always inspect bottle for foreign objects and expiration date. Mix solutions in aseptic mixing room with laminar flow hood. Change solution at least every 24 hrs. Change tubing every 48-72 hrs. Use line only for TPN. Use Leur-Lok connecting joints. Use micropore filters.
Septic thrombosis (caused by catheter)	Swelling of arm and neck on catheter side Pain Fever	Remove catheter, as ordered. Monitor vital signs. Provide anticoagulants and high doses of antibiotics, as ordered. Observe for embolism.
Psychological and knowledge deficit complications		
Depression related to illness and requiring TPN	Silences Crying Avoidance behavior Withdrawal	Ask patient to ventilate feelings. Have patient ambulate with battery infusion pump. Explain procedures and changes to be expected. Promote maximum independence.
Anxiety related to insufficient knowledge of TPN	Refusal of treatments Nervousness Crying Confusion	Assess patient and family levels of anxiety and knowledge. Provide for diversional activities. Provide patient and family teaching. Explain rationale for TPN therapy. Administer comfort measures. Support and encourage patient and family.
Knowledge deficit of TPN	Frequent questions Fear Lack of self-care	Explain to patient what will be experienced during procedures. Instruct patient on signs and symptoms of potential problems that should be reported. Encourage patient to participate in own care.
Decreased oral intake complications		
Physical problems related to a lack of oral intake	Parotitis Dry tongue, throat, and mouth Oral lesions Dental deterioration Physical unpleasantness resulting from absence of taste	Provide mouthwashes, rinses with beverages, flavored lip balm, and hard candies. Give consistent mouth care. Teach patient to make observations and provide own mouth care.
Psychological problems related to lack of oral intake	Anxiety, fear Olfactory and gustatory hallucinations Hunger sensations Confusion over whether proper nutrition is being received Oral cravings Feelings of exclusion from social activities	Assure the patient that hunger sensations are normal and can occur. Provide the patient with thorough explanations and emotional support. Patient should be included in social activities even though others will be eating food.

Table 15-6 Nursing Physical Assessment for Nutrient Deficiencies[17,21]

Clinical sign	Nutrient deficiency	Clinical sign	Nutrient deficiency
Integumentary		**Sensory**	
Skin		Eyes	
Dry and scaly	Essential fatty acids	Pale conjunctivae due to anemia	Iron, folic acid, Vitamin B$_{12}$, copper, and Vitamin E (in premature infants)
Dermatitis	Zinc		
Plaques around hair follicles	Vitamin A	Corneal arcus (white ring around eye) and xanthelasma (small yellowish lumps around eyes)	Hyperlipidemia
Petechiae and ecchymoses (excessive bruising)	Vitamins K and C	Red membranes, conjunctival dryness, corneal dullness, Bitot's spots (foamy spots on whites of eye)	Vitamin A
Peeling skin on vulva or scrotum	Vitamin B$_2$		
Nails		**Neurological**	
Thin, spoon-shaped, brittle, and ridged	Iron	Lethargy	Protein calories
Hair		Motor weakness, paresthesia, sensory loss, and confusion	Vitamin B$_1$ (thiamine)
Thin, brittle, alopecia, lackluster, easily plucked, and dyspigmented.	Protein calories	**Circulatory**	
		Anemia or neutropenia	Copper
Lips		Edema	Protein
Angular stomatitis (inflammation at corners of mouth)	Vitamin B$_2$ (riboflavin)	Pallor and tachycardia due to anemia	
Cracked, reddened; vertical crack in lower lip	Vitamin B$_2$ Vitamin B$_6$ (pyridoxine)	Beriberi (congestive heart failure, enlarged heart)	Vitamin B$_1$
Tongue		**Musculoskeletal**	
Glossitis (inflammation of tongue)	Vitamin B$_6$, B$_2$, and B$_3$ (niacin)	Thigh tenderness	Selenium
Magenta color	Vitamin B$_2$	Calf muscle tenderness	Thiamin
Fissures	Vitamin B$_3$	Swollen joints	Vitamins C and D
Gums		Scurvy (hemorrhages and tenderness)	Vitamin C
Spongy and bleed easily	Vitamin C	Skeletal lesions	Copper
Teeth		Muscle wasting	Protein calories
Dental caries and mottled enamel	Fluoride	Rickets (bowed legs)	Vitamin D
		Gastrointestinal	
		Hepatosplenomegaly (enlarged liver and spleen)	Protein calories
		Endocrine	
		Thyroid enlargement	Iodine

NURSING DIAGNOSIS

Sample nursing diagnoses for patients requiring TPN include the following:

- High risk for nutritional deficit related to diarrhea secondary to GI intolerance of enteral feeding.
- Impaired GI motility related to ileus secondary to acute burn injuries.
- High risk for infection related to catheter sepsis secondary to central TPN.
- Disturbance in gustatory perception related to lack of oral intake.
- Impaired swallowing related to tumor obstruction secondary to throat cancer.
- High risk for trace mineral deficiencies related to chronic dependence on home parenteral nutrition.
- High risk for allergic response related to administration of fat emulsion.
- Knowledge deficit of procedures needed to administer home parenteral nutrition.

PATIENT OUTCOMES

The following are possible outcomes for patients receiving TPN.

Patient evidences:

- Lungs clear to bases on auscultation.
- Respiratory rate of 12 to 20 breaths/min (or appropriate for patient).
- Strong, regular pulse ranging from 60 to 100 beats/min.
- Mean arterial blood pressure ranging from 70 to 90 mm Hg.
- Negative blood and intravenous catheter cultures.
- White blood cell count of <11,000 µl.
- Electrolyte values within normal limits (WNL).
- Balanced fluid intake and output.
- Weight change of 0.5 kg (1 lb) or less/24 hr.
- Temperature of 36° to 38° C (97° to 100.5° F).
- Adequate glucose metabolism with blood glucose below 200 mg/dl and urine glucose < 3+.
- Liver function tests WNL.
- Serum triglyceride levels WNL.
- Nitrogen balance.
- Serum albumin 3.5 to 5.5 g/dl.
- Retinol-binding protein 40 to 50 µg/ml.
- Thyroxine-binding prealbumin 200 to 300 µg/ml.

CONTROVERSIES IN CENTRAL VENOUS CATHETER CARE

Over the past few years many controversial issues have arisen about the care of the central venous catheter in parenteral nutrition. The following methods of care can be recommended:

- *Dressing change materials.* Using a transparent, semipermeable, polyurethane film dressing, such as Op-Site, rather than the traditional gauze and tape is extremely advantageous.[15,26,32]
- *Frequency of dressing changes.* Most protocols for

TPN dressing changes with traditional gauze and tape require three dressing changes a week. Although transparent dressings can remain intact without needing to be changed for 7 to 10 days, the longer they are left on, the greater the chance of getting colonized catheters. For those used for TPN, dressing changes should be every 72 hours or twice per week and as required (prn) when wet, dirty, or nonocclusive.[15,24]

- *Use of acetone-alcohol solution.* This solution has been widely used as a skin defatter in preparation for catheter insertion and for dressing changes. It is used to remove microorganisms that harbor in lipids on the surface of the skin. Some researchers claim that acetone seems to increase pain and inflammation at catheter insertion sites and that it does not impact on overall infection rates.
- *Use of antibiotic ointment at insertion site.* Studies support the use of antibiotic ointments under either gauze or transparent dressings.[15] Iodophor ointment, because of its antibacterial and antifungal properties, is the most commonly used in TPN dressing change protocols.[24]
- *Cleansing of catheter hub connection sites.* Infecting organisms gain entry through line connections. Therefore, it is recommended that when tubing is changed, the connection of the catheter hub and extension tubing should be cleaned with a povidone-iodine solution and allowed to dry before it is disconnected.[15] New connection shields can be purchased containing a povidone-iodine–impregnated foam.
- *Tubing changes.* It is recommended that all TPN administration tubing, filters, and extension sets be changed every 48-72 hours. Tubing changes should be coordinated with the time to hang a new bag of solution, such as with the first new bottle of the day.

REGULATING AND MAINTAINING THE TOTAL PARENTERAL NUTRITION INFUSION

During the first few days of intravenous feeding, the volume and concentration of solutions may be increased gradually according to fluid and glucose tolerance. The pancreas will respond by increasing insulin production. The TPN rate that can be tolerated is determined by the concentration of the solution and the patient's clinical status. An example of a typical TPN base solution (dextrose 50%/500 ml plus amino acids 8.5%/500 ml and additives) can be administered as follows:

- *Day 1*—rate of 42 ml/hr × 24 hr = total of 1008 ml. The remainder of the patient's daily fluid requirements should be given through the peripheral venous route. The patient's urine is checked for sugar and acetone four times daily and serum glucose is evaluated every 12 hours. If the blood glucose is below 200 mg% and the urine glucose less than 3+, the rate of administration is increased.
- *Day 2*—rate of 85 ml/hr × 24 hr = total of 2040 ml. The standard TPN formulation is based on delivery of

2 L/24 hr. If a patient still has glucosuria, 10 units of regular insulin may need to be added to the TPN solution as a starting dose and then regulated by the patient's blood glucose and medical condition.

- *Day 3*—rate of 125 ml/hr × 24 hr = total of 3000 ml. For patients with high fluid requirements, the dextrose concentration can be reduced to 10% or 15% to avoid excess calories.

Patients who require large amounts of calories and fluids, such as those with massive trauma and burns, are immediately started on a very high (3300) calorie TPN infusion. Therefore, large doses of insulin may be needed.

The PPN solutions are delivered initially at higher intravenous flow rates (e.g., 125 ml/hr). If a hypertonic solution falls behind schedule, it should not be speeded up to catch up. Rapid onset of hyperglycemia results if the prescribed rate of dextrose is exceeded. If the infusion is to be interrupted for a long period of time, 10% dextrose should be infused until TPN can be restarted.

Stress and injury provoke hormonal changes that provide substrates for energy, leading to a hyperglycemic condition. Rather than add insulin to the TPN solution, such patients should have a separate, continuous insulin infusion (CII). This prevents the need for frequent changing of TPN solutions and wastage. In critical care units, unstable patients will have CII requirements. The infusion may be run concurrently with the TPN solution through a Y-connector or multilumen catheter. The CII rate should be titrated to attempt to keep the serum glucose (SG) in the range of 120 to 250 mg/dl with no glycosuria. CII rates are usually administered as follows:[28]

For SG 200 to 300 mg/dl, administer 2 U insulin/hr.
For SG 300 to 400 mg/dl, administer 3 to 4 U insulin/hr.
For SG >400 mg/dl, administer 4 to 5 U insulin/hr.

TPN solutions are kept refrigerated until used to decrease bacterial growth. The nurse verifies the solution label with the prescribed order and checks the expiration date and time. The pharmacist will usually number the containers so that the nurse will know which solution to administer next. The solution container should be inspected for cracks or punctures. Then the solution should be examined for clarity to prevent infusion of possible contaminants or precipitates.

A catheter used for TPN infusion should not be violated by measuring central venous pressures, withdrawing blood, or delivering piggyback medications. The only exception to the violation of the tubing system is made for the administration of fat emulsions or insulin through a Y-site. Multilumen catheters are now being used to administer TPN under special highly monitored situations. If during an emergency a TPN line must be used, the medications or extra fluids should be piggybacked into the TPN line upstream of the final filter. If a catheter becomes contaminated through use during a resuscitation effort, it must be replaced as soon as possible or within 24 hours.

Because they trap particulates, bacteria, fungi, and air, filters should be used with TPN solutions. Some hospitals

Table 15-7 Total Parenteral Nutrition Monitoring Checklist

Procedure	Time limit
Obtain portable chest x-ray.	After catheter placement
Record vital signs, being alert for elevated temperature, one of the first signs of catheter sepsis.	Every 4 hr
Observe and note physical and mental changes.	Every 4 hr
Encourage active exercise, to promote protein anabolism.	Every 4 hr
Collect double-voided urine specimen and check for glucose and acetone. If urine is 3+ or greater, obtain blood glucose through lab or glucometer. Notify physician if value is 200 mg/dl or greater.	Every 6 hr
Measure urine specific gravity and chart intake and output totals. Notify physician if urine output < 300 ml/8 hr.	Every 8 hr
Observe for dependent and generalized edema.	Every 8 hr
Provide mouth care to promote hygiene and prevent parotitis.	Every 8 hr
Record weight. Maintain weight gain at <0.5 kg (1 lb)/24 hr.	Every 24 hr and then 3 times per week
Calculate fluid and nutrient intake and output balance.	Every 24 hr
Obtain ordered daily laboratory tests (serum electrolyte levels, visceral protein measurements, and others).	Every 24 hr for first week and then biweekly or weekly
Change TPN containers.	Every 24 hr
Change TPN administration tubing.	Every 48-72 hr
Change gauze or transparent dressing.	Every 72 hr

also mandate the use of Luer-Lok or other locking connections to prevent air embolism. Table 15-7 provides a TPN monitoring checklist.

Termination of TPN should be performed gradually to prevent rebound hypoglycemia. Only when the patient is taking adequate enteral nutrition (i.e., two thirds of maintenance calories) should TPN be discontinued. The reintroduction of food into the GI tract must be slow and gradual if the patient has been without food for a prolonged period of time. Blood glucose and calorie counts should be monitored until adequate enteral intake is achieved. A patient's TPN fluids can be reduced to 85 ml/hr on the first day, 42 ml/hr on the second day, and then discontinued on the third day.

INTRAVENOUS FAT EMULSIONS

Intravenous fat emulsions are administered to provide for essential fatty acids and may also be given as a source of calories. If lipids are not given with a TPN regimen, long-chain fatty acid deficiency will appear in about 7 days with clinical findings at 4 weeks. To prevent this, 500

Skill 15-1   Changing a Central Venous Catheter Dressing, Tubing, and Injection Caps Used for TPN

TPN catheter insertion sites may be dressed with gauze covered with tape, adhesive-backed cloth (Elastoplast), occlusive foam material, or transparent occlusive dressings. One should plan to change the dressing every 72 hours or more frequently if wet, soiled, or nonocclusive. The TPN bag should be changed every 24 hours, the injection caps every 72 hours, and the TPN administration tubing every 48 to 72 hours, depending on hospital policy. The following procedure will describe a dressing change with a transparent dressing and will coincide with a new tubing, caps, and TPN solution change.

EQUIPMENT AND SUPPLIES

- Face mask, clean unsterile gloves, and sterile gloves
- Trash bag
- TPN dressing change kit; if unavailable, collect the following supplies:
    6 alcohol-acetone or alcohol or hydrogen peroxide swab sticks
    6 povidone-iodine swab sticks
    Povidone-iodine ointment
    Tincture of benzoin and cotton swab sticks or skin preps
    Sterile 2 × 2 gauze pad and clear tape
    Transparent occlusive dressing
    New TPN infusion bag with tubing and filter extension set
    New injection caps

NURSING INTERVENTIONS

1. Assemble supplies on clean worktable at bedside. Place trash bag within reach. Prime IV tubing, apply face masks to self and patient, and wash hands.
2. Open sterile supplies and put on unsterile rubber gloves.
3. Remove outdated dressing, inspect for drainage, and place in trash bag. Check position of catheter and observe site for signs of infection, inflammation, or infiltration. If necessary, obtain culture of any discharge.
4. Put on sterile gloves and obtain acetone-alcohol, alcohol, or hydrogen peroxide swab. Acetone serves to "defat" the skin, helping to prevent bacterial growth. Do not use acetone swabs with silicone catheters. Hydrogen peroxide may be used as a substitute.
5. Use first swab stick to clean catheter. Use next two swab sticks to prep area, starting at the insertion site and working outward in a circular motion, past the hub of the catheter. Remove debris, crusting, old ointment, and dried blood.
6. Repeat cleansing with three povidone-iodine swabs. Allow alcohol to dry before applying the povidone-iodine or tincture of iodine solution may form, causing skin burning and irritation.

7. Allow povidone-iodine to air dry and do not remove it since it has a combined antifungal and bactericidal action and some time-release activity.
8. Examine catheter lumens. Ensure that TPN solution will be entering distal lumen of multilumen catheter. This will prevent infiltration if slippage of catheter occurs.
9. Place sterile gauze pad under catheter hub. Clean catheter hub connection site with povidone-iodine swab stick. Allow to dry.
10. Lower patient's head of bed to flat position. Have patient perform Valsalva maneuver to prevent air from entering central venous system. Quickly change IV tubing. Tighten connection site carefully.
11. Raise head of bed. Remove gauze pad. Gauze should not be used under transparent dressings because of trapping of moisture.
12. For a catheter that has a clamp attached, close off the clamp before the new tubing is connected. This will eliminate need for Valsalva maneuver.
13. Apply povidone-iodine ointment to insertion site.
14. Apply skin prep or tincture of benzoin for dressing edges only if necessary, such as if patient is diaphoretic.
15. Apply transparent dressing in a side-to-side fashion, pinching the transparent dressing around the hub of the catheter and onto the skin. Leave the catheter hub or triple lumens out of the dressing so that the IV tubing can be changed without disturbing the dressing.
16. Secure the tubing with tape using the chevron method.
17. If it is time to change the injection caps, clamp the lumen to prevent air from entering (unless using a Groshong CV catheter). If clamps are unavailable, patient will need to perform the Valsalva maneuver.
18. Clean the connection site with povidone-iodine swab stick. Allow to dry. Quickly disconnect the old cap and screw on the new cap.
19. For catheters with large injection caps, prefill the cap with normal saline. Position the proximal end of the catheter below heart level before removing the old cap. This prevents the catheter fluid level from dropping (the manometer effect).

---

ml of 10% fat needs to be given at least twice weekly.[7] Because it is advantageous to combine fat with glucose as a source of calories, many practitioners provide 30% to 40% of caloric intake as fat. There is evidence that providing lipids continuously throughout the 24-hour period is preferable to intermittent administration.[11] This enables continual oxidation of lipids, thus minimizing carbohydrate utilization. IV lipids protect the venous endothelium from injury resulting from hypertonic dextrose solutions.[11] The slower rate also helps to prevent liver function problems. It is not recommended to exceed 60% of the caloric intake as fat or to exceed 2.5 gm/kg/24 hr in adults and 4 gm/kg/24 hr in infants and children.

Intravenous fat should not be given to patients with disturbances in normal fat metabolism, such as pathological hyperlipemia, lipoid nephrosis, or acute pancreatitis, if accompanied by hyperlipemia. An initial baseline value of plasma triglycerides should be obtained. Patients suffering from hepatic disease should not receive intravenous lipids because the liver helps to use fatty acids. They should be administered with caution when there is a risk of fat embolism, when the patient has anemia or blood coagulation disorders, or pulmonary disease. Two types of adverse reactions may occur with lipid infusions. The first occurs during the infusion and may include chest or back pain, fever, shaking chills, dyspnea, palpitations, and cyanosis.

Skill 15-2   **Administration of Intravenous Fat Emulsions**

EQUIPMENT AND SUPPLIES

- Bottle of IV lipid
- Special fat emulsion IV administration tubing
- Heparin lock
- 20-gauge needle
- IV pole
- Volumetric infusion pump, if available
- Alcohol swab
- 5-ml syringe containing saline solution
  For 24-hour continuous infusion add the following:
    Dextrose/amino acid solution
    Tubing for primary line with filter
    IV Y-connector and extension tubing
    Additional IV pole and volumetric infusion pump
    Povidone-iodine and alcohol swabs

NURSING INTERVENTIONS

1. Examine lipid emulsion bottle carefully. If creaming (separation of the emulsion into fat globules), oiling out (separation of the emulsion into layers), or frothiness is noticed, return solution to the pharmacy for a replacement.
2. Do not inject any additives into emulsion bottle or use a filter.
3. Wash hands, attach needle to end of IV tubing, clamp tubing, remove protective top from bottle, and puncture rubber top.
4. Hang bottle upright and prime tubing very slowly to prevent easily formed air bubbles and loss of large amounts of the solution. Place on volumetric infusion pump, if available.
5. Check IV adaptor plug for patency. If patent, insert needle at end of IV lipid tubing into heparin lock and administer the solution.

6. Administer patient's first fat emulsion at ordered rate. Usually this will be 0.5 gm/kg/24 hr infused over 8 to 12 hours. If the patient has no adverse reactions, the amount infused can be increased in increments of 1.0 gm/kg/24 hr according to physician's order.
7. Do not infuse the fat emulsion at a rate $>$ 0.15 gm/kg/hr or 2.5 gm/kg/24 hr. The 10% fat emulsion contains 50 gm of fat in 500 ml of solution.
8. To prevent bacterial and fungal growth, avoid letting the fat emulsion hang for more than 24 hours.
9. With intermittent infusions, change the IV tubing with each new bottle of fat emulsion.
10. If patient is to receive continual 24-hour lipid infusion, plan to administer through Y-site with amino acid/dextrose solution or, preferably, through separate lumen of multilumen catheter.
11. Place the fat emulsion as close to the catheter insertion site as possible to prevent prolonged contact with the dextrose/amino acid solution. This aids in the preservation of the fat emulsion's stability.
12. Change lipid emulsion tubing every 24 hours, according to agency protocol.
13. Hang fat emulsion bottle higher than other solution to prevent backup into primary line. Lipid emulsions have a lower specific gravity and would otherwise back flow into the amino acid/dextrose line.
14. Place both solutions on volumetric infusion pumps.
15. Ten hours after an infusion, check patient for lipemia or elevated triglycerides to determine if the lipids should be given at a reduced rate or amount.

These symptoms will generally subside if the infusion rate is slowed. The second type of reaction occurs after prolonged administration and consists of transient enzyme elevations, leukopenia, thrombocytopenia, eosinophilia, and hepatomegaly.[20]

CENTRAL VENOUS ACCESS DEVICE
Occlusion

The occlusion of a central venous access device (VAD) is a serious situation. Once a catheter becomes occluded, the patient may be at risk for infection, occlusive vascular thrombosis, and pulmonary emboli. Unless patency can be restored, the catheter will have to be removed. Not only is the patient temporarily denied administration of vital fluids and nutrition, there is also the added risk, discomfort, and expense if the VAD has to be reinserted.[29] VADs are most often occluded by fibrin or clot formation. Two types of occlusion can occur. There may be a fibrin sheath against the catheter tip creating a one-way valve effect whereby one is able to instill fluid but unable to aspirate blood. If one is unable to instill and also unable to aspirate, there may be a frank clot in the catheter. Dislodging such a clot into the right atrium could prove to be fatal, so urokinase is used to declot the catheter. Silicone central VADs may

also be occluded by crystals that form inside the lumen resulting from the interaction of certain drugs with the silicone lining. Experience has shown that phenytoin (Dilantin) and diazepam (Valium) can cause such problems.[15] When a patient's fluids do not appear to be infusing and there is no blood return, the first procedure for the nurse to attempt is to verify catheter occlusion.

Use of Urokinase for Central Venous Access Device Obstruction

Urokinase dissolves catheter clots by triggering the body's own fibrinolytic system. An inactive enzyme precursor is converted into plasmin. Plasmin is absorbed by the clot and acts to dissolve fibrin. If the proper concentration is used for clearing catheters, there will be no ill effects on systemic clotting. Most catheters can be cleared within 20 to 30 minutes with one instillation of urokinase; although some will need a second instillation. Even though the half-life of urokinase is very short (10 to 15 minutes), local thrombolytic activity will continue 12 to 24 hours following administration, so a catheter may become patent 12 hours after administration of urokinase. Before using urokinase, a chest x-ray should be performed to determine the position of the catheter tip.[4]

Skill 15-3 Assessment of Central Venous Access Device Occlusion

EQUIPMENT AND SUPPLIES

- Nonsterile gloves
- 5 ml sterile saline
- 10 ml syringe
- Adaptor caps
- Alcohol and povidone-iodine swab stick
- 5 ml syringe containing 4 ml of 10 U/ml heparin flush
- Sterile 4 × 4 sponge

NURSING INTERVENTIONS

1. Ensure that infusion pump is plugged into power outlet and is functioning properly. Check for kinks in tubing. Wash hands and put on nonsterile gloves.
2. Place sterile 4 × 4 sponge under catheter hub to absorb fluid.
3. Clamp catheter unless pulmonary artery catheter or other rigid catheter is being used. If the catheter does not have a clamp, use a stopcock and close it.
4. Cleanse catheter hub connection site with povidone-iodine swab stick. Allow to dry.
5. Remove IV line. Cover end of IV tubing with capped needle, or, if at home, wrap with packaged alcohol swab.
6. Connect 10 ml syringe with 5 ml normal saline flush. Any syringe with a smaller diameter may cause damage to the catheter tip because of increased pressure.[38]
7. Open clamp and pull back on plunger. If clot appears, attempt to aspirate but do not inject a clot back into catheter. If no clot appears, attempt to slowly inject saline, using a slight pumping action with syringe.
8. If still unable to flush, remove dressing and observe for kink or obstruction of catheter by sutures.
9. Have patient cough, turn side to side, or raise arm over head of affected side.
10. If able to instill flush, attempt to aspirate 3 ml to check for a blood return.
11. Clamp catheter and attach 5 ml syringe with 4 ml (10 U/ml) heparin flush solution. Unclamp catheter and instill heparin.
12. Reclamp catheter, disconnect syringe, cleanse hub with alcohol or povidone-iodine wipe, and reattach IV solution. Unclamp and resume infusion.
13. If you were unable to clear catheter, inform physician and obtain order for insertion of urokinase (Skill 15-5).

THE GROSHONG CENTRAL VENOUS (CV) CATHETER

Because of its three-position valve (Fig. 15-2), the Groshong CV catheter is becoming more popular, especially for long-term use. Located adjacent to the closed distal tip of the catheter, the valve remains closed when not in use. Infusion, even of highly viscous fluids, is accomplished with slight pressure causing the valve to open outwards, releasing the infusate into the superior vena cava. Aspiration with a syringe creates a negative pressure, causing the valve to open inwards to easily achieve blood withdrawal. When the catheter is not in use, the Groshong valve normally remains closed so that retrograde blood flow, air embolism, and catheter occlusion are greatly re-

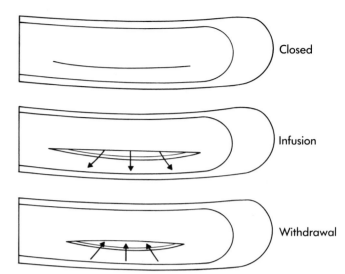

Fig. 15-2 The Groshong three-position valve is located adjacent to the closed distal tip of the catheter.

duced. When injection caps or IV tubing are changed, the catheter does not require clamping. It has to be irrigated only once per week to maintain patency when not in use.

PEDIATRIC CONSIDERATIONS
Candidates for TPN

Pediatric candidates for TPN include those with the following:

- Severe chronic diarrhea.
- GI tract anomalies, such as congenital obstruction lesions of the small intestine, omphalocele, tracheoesophageal fistulas or atresias, various short bowel syndromes, and necrotizing enterocolitis.
- Diseases, such as cancer, Crohn's disease, cystic fibrosis, acute renal failure, and congenital heart disease.
- A disorder that prevents the child from beginning enteral nutrition within a 5-day period.
- Low birth weight infants (less than 2500 gm) who are not fed enterally by the third to fifth day of life.[12]

Premature infants, especially those with respiratory distress syndrome, have extremely limited substrate reserve and a very rapid growth rate. During the last trimester of pregnancy the fetal brain grows rapidly. A neonate who is born prematurely and exposed to malnutrition will have an interruption of the brain "growth spurt" and will be at risk for permanent brain injury. Children at high nutritional risk who might require parenteral nutrition may be identified by the following criteria[14]:

- Serum albumin less than 3.0 gm/dl.
- Weight loss greater than 5% (other than weight loss caused by dehydration).
- Weight to height ratio below the fifth percentile.
- Total lymphocyte count less than 1000/mm^3 (excluding chemotherapy patients).

Skill 15-4 Administration of Urokinase for Central Venous Access Device Obstruction

EQUIPMENT AND SUPPLIES

- Urokinase 5000 U
- Heparin flush 40 U (10 U/ml)
- Alcohol and povidone-iodine swab sticks
- 1 18-gauge needle
- 1 3-ml syringe
- 2 10-ml syringes
- Luer-Lok injection cap
- Nonsterile gloves
- Sterile 4 × 4 sponge

NURSING INTERVENTIONS

1. Assemble equipment and wash hands.
2. Reconstitute urokinase according to manufacturer's directions. Avoid shaking vial to prevent precipitation. Use immediately because of short drug half-life.
3. Withdraw urokinase into 3-ml syringe. If Silastic catheter has two lumens, draw up enough urokinase to inject into both lumens, as a prophylactic measure.
4. Put on nonsterile gloves. Clamp catheter. If catheter is rigid and does not have a clamp, use a stopcock and close it.
5. Place sterile sponge under hub connection. Cleanse hub connection site with povidone-iodine swab stick. Allow to dry.
6. Remove IV line and attach syringe of urokinase to catheter hub and unclamp catheter or open stopcock.
7. Slowly inject urokinase. If urokinase is difficult to inject, use gentle, repeated push-pull action with syringe. Avoid heavy pressure that may rupture silastic catheter or cause catheter embolus.
8. Leave syringe attached to hub and allow solution to dwell for 30 minutes.
9. Aspirate urokinase and blood. If blood returns, withdraw 3 ml.
10. Clamp catheter, disconnect syringe, connect syringe containing heparin flush, and instill heparin.
11. Reclamp catheter, disconnect syringe, wipe hub with alcohol, and reattach injection cap or IV line.
12. If blood did not return in Step 9, reinstill aspirated urokinase solution. Leave syringe attached and allow solution to dwell another 90 to 120 minutes.
13. Attempt to aspirate 3 ml blood. If catheter is still occluded, repeat procedure from beginning, as ordered. Remember that once urokinase has been inserted, the local thrombolytic activity will still continue and catheter patency may be noted 12 hours later.

Skill 15-5 Irrigation of Groshong CV Catheter

The Groshong CV catheter should be irrigated as follows:
- Use 5 ml of saline every 7 days when not in use and after each use.
- Use 10 ml of saline after any blood aspiration, infusion, or transfusion or when blood is observed in the catheter.
- Use 20 ml of saline before blood sampling after infusion of TPN solutions.

EQUIPMENT AND SUPPLIES

- Injectable sodium chloride (0.9%) (normal saline)
- Alcohol or povidone-iodine wipes or swab sticks
- 19- or 20-gauge, 2.5 cm (1-inch) needle
- Appropriate syringes

NURSING INTERVENTIONS

1. For the 5 ml irrigation, swab latex top of Luer-Lok injection cap with antiseptic wipe.
2. Insert syringe needle into latex injection cap and vigorously irrigate catheter lumen with 5 ml normal saline solution.
3. Maintain positive pressure on syringe plunger as syringe is withdrawn. Do not clamp catheter following irrigation.
4. Remove syringe needle from injection cap and change injection cap if necessary. The injection cap should be replaced every 72 hours, when the cap has been removed, and as needed.
5. If it is time to replace injection cap, liberally swab around the connection site with povidone-iodine swab sticks.
6. Remove cap with a slight counterclockwise twist and pull off. Continue holding catheter with one hand and discard old cap.
7. Grasp the new injection cap by the barrel, being careful not to contaminate the latex top. Twist and insert into the connector in a clockwise direction.
8. When irrigating with as much as 10 or 20 ml normal saline, the cap will not be used. Remove the latex injection cap from connector and discard.
9. Swab connection site, making sure not to allow antiseptic solution to enter catheter connector. Maintain sterility of connector by not letting go of it.
10. Remove needle from syringe and insert the syringe barrel directly into the catheter connector. Twist slightly to ensure proper connection.
11. Vigorously irrigate lumen with the 10 or 20 ml of normal saline. Maintain positive pressure on syringe plunger as syringe is withdrawn. Do not clamp catheter following irrigation.
12. Carefully twist and remove syringe from catheter connector and then follow above procedure for applying a new injection cap.

Skill 15-6   Blood Aspiration from the Groshong CV Catheter

Blood aspiration from the Groshong CV catheter is carried out for the purpose of obtaining blood samples for laboratory specimens; thereby eliminating the need for peripheral venipunctures. This procedure should be performed only by a registered nurse or a physician. Vacutainers and other blood aspiration devices are not used with the Groshong catheter.

EQUIPMENT AND SUPPLIES

- Alcohol or povidone-iodine wipes
- 2 19- or 20-gauge, 2.5 cm (1-inch) needles
- 2 10-ml syringes
- 1 10-ml syringe with normal saline
- Appropriate blood specimen tubes

NURSING INTERVENTIONS

1. Remove and discard injection cap and swab the outside of the catheter connector with one of the antiseptic wipes. Continue holding the connector so it does not make contact with any surface. Do not clamp catheter.
2. Without a needle, insert the tip of the first 10-ml syringe directly into the connector. Twist slightly to ensure proper connection.
3. Aspirate 3 ml to 5 ml of fluid. To facilitate blood withdrawal, pull back plunger ½ ml, pausing for a 2-second count; then slowly continue aspiration.
4. Twist and remove syringe from catheter connector and set aside. Continue holding connector and do not clamp catheter.
5. Attach the second 10-ml syringe barrel directly into the catheter connector. Aspirate appropriate amount of blood.
6. Being careful not to contaminate catheter connector site, remove syringe, place needle on tip, and insert needle into blood tube. Let vacuum in tube withdraw blood from syringe.
7. Vigorously irrigate the catheter lumen with 10 ml normal saline.
8. Liberally swab around catheter connector opening and apply new injection cap.

Peripheral TPN

Peripheral delivery of TPN is always preferable to central line delivery in the neonatal intensive care unit (ICU). Because the peripheral route solutions used in infants are provided at maximal dextrose concentrations of 12.5%, the infants must be given IV lipids to provide for an adequate caloric intake.[12]

Central TPN

Candidates for central line placement include very low birth weight (VLBW) infants (less than 1500 gm) and infants with associated gastrointestinal (GI) anomalies. Generally central vein catheters are indicated when the infants:

- Have poor peripheral veins.
- Require a lengthy TPN course expected to exceed 2 weeks.
- Need increased calories, exceeding 100 kcal/kg.
- Are fluid restricted, requiring higher osmolar solutions.

Skill 15-7   Repair of Groshong CV Catheter Connector

When the catheter connector appears worn or if the connector or catheter has been damaged, the connector will need to be changed. This minimizes the potential for infection and overuse of the catheter connector.

EQUIPMENT AND SUPPLIES

- Sterile scissors
- Alcohol or povidone-iodine wipes
- Connector package with sleeve and stylet
- Sterile gloves

NURSING INTERVENTIONS

1. Open sterile packages and put on gloves.
2. Liberally swab the catheter around and well below the area that contains the old connector.
3. Cut the catheter just below the old connector. Continue to hold catheter and do not clamp. Discard old connector.
4. Remove the white connector sleeve with the French-size indicator from the body of the connector. Slide the sleeve well over the outside diameter of the catheter lumen.
5. Firmly push the catheter lumen onto the connector until it reaches the base of the connector.
6. Holding the connector firmly, slide the sleeve toward the connector, past the connector base and firmly onto the connector hub.
7. Remove the stylet from the connector and discard.
8. Apply new injection cap and irrigate catheter.

Preterm infants

Central catheters for TPN in infants and small children can be inserted by several methods. If a Broviac-type catheter with fibrous cuff is used, the catheter can be threaded into the external jugular to the right atrium and tunneled subcutaneously down the chest wall. The catheter can also be threaded into the facial vein to the right atrium and tunneled subcutaneously up behind the ear. Catheter exit sites are easier to maintain in these locations because they are away from secretions and permit the infant head and body movements without putting undue tension on the catheter. Usually a stockinette cap or a close-fitting undershirt can be used to cover the dressing and connection areas. Because Broviac catheters can cause infection and mechanical complications in neonates, tiny, noncuffed silicone catheters are also occasionally used. These catheters are limited to a flow rate of 25 ml/hr and are inserted percutaneously into the external jugular or basilica vein.

Glucose and protein

Central line TPN solutions for infants generally contain a maximum of 25% glucose. The maximum glucose level recommended by the American Academy of Pediatrics is 30 gm/kg/24 hr.[12] Nutritional solutions are gradually increased in both concentration and rate to allow the child's pancreas to adapt to the high glucose load. For neonatal use, the amino acid concentration in TPN solutions is usually 1.5% to 2.5%. Standard adult amino acid products can provide all of the essential amino acids needed for neonates except for tyrosine, cysteine, and taurine, which are not essential for adults.[25]

Vitamins and minerals

Preterm infants have different nutritional needs from term infants. Their metabolic systems are immature and their needs for protein and calories high. They require higher proportions of minerals and vitamins for their sizes than adults. The preterm infant is especially at risk for iron, zinc, and copper deficiency because of limited stores and very rapid growth. The full-term infant has accumulated stores of these trace elements during gestation.[34]

To promote bone and tissue growth, TPN solutions for infants and children contain higher concentrations of calcium, phosphorous, and magnesium than adult solutions. Infants on long-term TPN are at risk of developing metabolic bone disease, which presents as rickets, bone demineralization on x-ray, or fractures. The best treatment is to provide enteral feeding as soon as possible.

Fluids

The younger an infant is, the greater the water losses are because of the greater skin surface area. The immature infant's skin is thin and densely vascularized, enhancing heat transport and loss to the environment. Other factors that increase fluid requirements include radiant warmers, phototherapy, glycosuria, acute tubular necrosis, draining colostomies, chest tube drainage, third space losses, diarrhea, and vomiting. Small infants also run a high risk of sudden fluid overload should TPN fluids be infused too quickly. Their fluids should always be administered through a microvolumetric infusion pump.

Lipids

Infants do not have the ability to rapidly metabolize and clear lipids from their serum, so they will need to be closely observed for lipid overload. Infants especially at risk are those at less than 32 or 33 weeks gestation, small-for-gestational-age infants, and young preterm infants (those less than 1 week of age). Infants with jaundice, pulmonary hypertension, respiratory difficulties, and sepsis should receive lipids only when serum triglyceride levels can be closely monitored. Complications that could result from the use of IV lipids in LBW infants include the following:

- Danger to jaundiced infants because of the competition of resultant free fatty acids with bilirubin for albumin-binding sites.[25]
- Decreased production of complement and impaired phagocytosis of white blood cells because of their being coated by excess lipid.[34]
- Adverse effect on pulmonary diffusion capacity with impairment of oxygenation because of the deposition of lipid particles in pulmonary microcirculation.

Pediatric Assessment

Infants on TPN will need to have growth monitored. Growth in the neonate and infant will indicate the ade-

quacy of nutrition. Adequate growth is defined as that appropriate for the fetus in-utero at the same gestation. Weight acquisition in-utero is approximately 20 gm/kg/24 hr at 28 weeks gestation and 30 gm/kg/24 hr at 33 weeks gestation. Weight, recumbent length, and head circumference measurements are the most important indices of growth in this population and should be monitored as follows:

- Weight monitored daily or more frequently if infant is of LBW with marked fluid shifts.
- Length monitored weekly.
- Head circumference monitored weekly.

Sham Feedings

Developmental considerations of infants on TPN should be given careful attention. Infants who are not fed by mouth for an extended period of time should be given sham feedings. A *sham feeding* is the pretense or simulation of giving an oral feeding by holding the infant and having the baby suck on a pacifier while receiving TPN. The nurse should set aside time for regular sham feedings, for holding the baby close, and for providing eye contact and soothing vocalizations.

PSYCHOSOCIAL CONSIDERATIONS

Psychological and social problems that can be seen with long-term TPN patients include the following: delirium, drug dependency, depression, grief, and anxiety. The patient who presents with delirium should be evaluated for possible electrolyte imbalance, hypovolemia, hypervolemia, hyperosmolar states, vitamin or trace element deficiencies, sepsis, or anemia. Difficulty with drugs is most commonly seen with those patients who have had frequent hospitalizations with access to narcotics or hypnotics. Anxiety in a drug withdrawal state may be the first symptom.[13]

Most patients receiving home parenteral nutrition (HPN) have significant GI disability and over half of them have stomas. A TPN catheter and a stoma often compound a patient's perception of a mutilated body image. Single individuals, especially, have a difficult time feeling sexually attractive or desirable with a permanent catheter in place. Some HPN patients will not wear bathing suits in public; although they are allowed to swim and participate in noncontact sports. Some people also experience anxiety from their feelings of dependency on a machine.[8] The frequent presence of this infusion machine provokes a feeling of being "tied to the pump." Most HPN patients now receive cyclic TPN and are tied to an infusion pump only at night. They are bothered, though, by the problems of frequent urination disturbing their sleep and difficulty in traveling.[16]

Patients on HPN who are not allowed oral supplements are deprived of the opportunity to taste, chew, and swallow food. They feel thirst, the deprivation of taste in food, and an unsatisfied appetite for food. Some individuals express cravings for certain foods and display a preoccupation with food. For those who are still hospitalized, the loss of mealtimes has an important impact because meals break the monotony of the day. Eating is a social activity, and food has social and psychological significance for individuals. Food continues to be a source of identity, security, status, and social acceptability in society. It is in the sharing of food that one frequently experiences a sense of belonging. The centrality of the sharing of food during holidays, religious festivals, or rites of passage creates a bond among those who have eaten together. The uses of and attitudes about food are frequently bound with the religious system and social structure of culture. HPN patients who can eat orally with minimal GI discomfort are encouraged to do so if they wish so that they are not denied the religious, social, and cultural aspects of eating that have been developed over a lifetime. Many HPN individuals nibble on food and go out to dinner with family and friends. They realize, though, that if they consume food that they can expect constant diarrhea the following day.

In the case of children, it is recommended that they consume the maximum amount of food that is possible for their medical conditions. Not only does oral nutrition reduce the risk of liver dysfunction and stimulate GI villus growth and adaptation, but it allows the child to learn the social skills of eating.[31]

Studies have shown that some HPN patients feel isolated from other patients and health care providers. Because there are so few individuals on HPN, they need a means of communicating with other individuals who are also receiving HPN therapy.[19] There are newsletters available such as that published by the Oley Foundation, but these patients also need to take advantage of teleconferences, phone networks, and visits from other HPN individuals, if possible. Despite their dependency on parenteral nutrition, many patients on HPN are able to lead very productive, fulfilling lives. Some of the larger, more established HPN programs have patients who have survived over 10 years on parental nutrition therapy. Studies have shown that 50% to 60% of HPN patients are able to work part- or full-time, 15% to 20% are retired or of preschool age, and only 20% to 30% are unable to work.[18]

PATIENT AND FAMILY TEACHING

Learning to administer HPN will not be easy for the patient. It usually takes 1 to 2 weeks to train a patient to provide for HPN. Two people will need to be trained—the primary caregiver (usually the patient or parent in the case of a child) and a backup support person. The following information is needed by the patient and backup support person:

- *Nutrition concepts*—rationale for HPN.
- *Compounding of parenteral solution if not using premixed solutions*—adding medications and ordering, storing, and setting up supplies.
- *Administration of solution*—priming tubing, operating infusion pump, beginning and ending infusion, and management of cyclic schedule.

- *Catheter care*—hand washing, aseptic technique, dressing changes, and irrigation of catheter.
- *Problem solving*—troubleshooting complications, monitoring, contacting health care professionals, and agency resources.

HOME HEALTH CARE CONSIDERATIONS

Patients most commonly placed on HPN are those who are unable to sustain themselves by an oral diet.

Problems with HPN that may lead to rehospitalization include sepsis, catheter-related problems, need for change of catheter, fluid and electrolyte imbalance, organ dysfunction or failure, and metabolic bone disease. Patients often complain about bone pain after 6 months of TPN, some as early as 2 months. Spontaneous fractures of the vertebrae, ribs, and feet can occur. There are probably many factors contributing to this painful disease. In the pediatric HPN age group the most common causes of death have been sepsis and TPN-induced liver failure.[31]

Depending on the amount of lipids prescribed, the cost of HPN ranges from $100 to $300 a day, with the average cost being closer to $200 to $250 a day.[9] Most patients between the ages of 20 and 65 start this expensive therapy with private insurance. They will usually have to meet an outstanding 20% expense for TPN because insurance usually covers only 80%. Eventually private insurance will run out and the individual must then seek total disability status and accrue, after 24 months, eligibility for Medicare funding. Many HPN patients are able to work but are unemployed because they do not want to lose their Medicare funding.[18] This results in emotional, financial, and social problems.

Patients on HPN need to monitor themselves carefully. Some home monitoring parameters to follow include:

- Measuring daily weights for the first 2 weeks and then three times a week thereafter. Weight should be measured at the same time of the day wearing the same amount of clothing. A patient with excessive weight gain should be assessed for edema. A safe weight repletion regimen usually produces a weight gain of 0.5 to 1 kg (1 to 2 lbs) per week.
- Taking daily temperatures. A high temperature exceeding 38° C (100.5 ° F) may indicate catheter infection that can be confirmed by blood cultures.
- Monitoring blood glucose, especially in diabetic patients or those who have frequent episodes of hypoglycemia or hyperglycemia.
- Monitoring urine glucose to determine the body's utilization of the high glucose concentrations. Urine results of 3+ or greater for three consecutive readings should be reported so the HPN can be adjusted.
- Maintaining fluid intake and output records, including IV fluids; foods that are liquid at room temperature; and urine, ostomy, and fistula output.
- Assessing self for lethargy, mood changes, rashes, edema, sweats, and chills.

Hickman and Broviac catheter sites should always be kept covered with a sterile dressing for at least 1 week after the catheter is inserted. The external part of the catheter, exit site, and cutdown site must be cleansed and disinfected each day, using sterile technique. Once the site has healed, catheter and exit site care should be performed three times each week if using a gauze dressing and after swimming or showering. If a transparent film dressing is used instead of a conventional gauze dressing, the dressing may be changed every 5 days or if it becomes soiled or detached. The entire dressing may be removed when showering, and the exit site and catheter scrubbed with chlorhexidine or povidone-iodine scrub, followed by application of a new dressing. When swimming, the patient should cover the exit site, external catheter, and hub with a transparent film dressing. Although the use of gloves is omitted from this procedure, they should be used when a caregiver is providing catheter care to an AIDS patient.

EQUIPMENT AND SUPPLIES:

- Dressing covering: Op-Site, Tegaderm, or microfoam, micropore, or dermicel tape
- 2 alcohol swabs
- 2 povidone-iodine swabs
- 1 cotton-tipped applicator
- 1 povidone-iodine swab stick
- Hydrogen peroxide
- 1 3-ml syringe
- 2 2 × 2 split dressings
- 2 2 × 2 gauze dressings
- Povidone-iodine ointment

NURSING INTERVENTIONS

1. Wash hands thoroughly for at least 3 minutes with povidone-iodine soap.
2. Open all packages and draw up 1 ml of hydrogen peroxide into syringe.
3. Remove soiled dressing and wash hands again for 1 minute.
4. Check catheter for proper position and observe for redness, swelling, or drainage.
5. Wrap one povidone-iodine swab around the catheter at the exit site and leave it in place.
6. Holding the swab in place, take another povidone-iodine swab and wipe the remaining exposed catheter. Start at exit site and wipe to hub of catheter. Let solution dry for 2 minutes.
7. Wiping from exit site to hub, remove povidone-iodine from catheter with two alcohol swabs.
8. Remove povidone-iodine swab from exit site.
9. Place a 2 × 2 dressing under catheter exit site and squirt hydrogen peroxide onto exit site with syringe. Use the 2 × 2 dressing to remove any crusts from exit site.
10. Starting at exit site and moving outward in circular motion, use povidone-iodine swab stick to cleanse 2.5-cm (1-inch) skin area.
11. Squeeze povidone-iodine ointment onto cotton-tipped applicator and apply to exit site.
12. Cover exit site with two split dressings and 2 × 2 gauze dressing and apply occlusive tape over all of the gauze.
13. Another option is to cover exit site with a transparent film dressing without any gauze, and tape the dressing down under the catheter to close up the air pockets.
14. Tape catheter cap onto the catheter hub to prevent the cap from loosening with normal body movement.
15. Coil exposed catheter and tape to side of midchest or abdomen. A woman can coil the catheter and place it in her bra. Place piece of tape over hub of catheter to prevent catheter from catching on clothing.

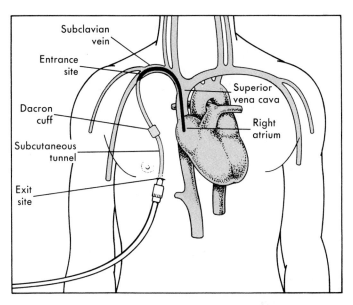

Fig. 15-3 The Hickman central venous catheter. After distal end of catheter is threaded through subclavian vein and into right atrium, proximal end is tunneled under subcutaneous tissue to increase catheter stability. A Dacron cuff on proximal portion of catheter provides a roughened surface, which encourages subcutaneous tissue to adhere to catheter and further secure it. (From Beare PG, Myers JL: *Principles and practice of adult health nursing,* St Louis, 1990, Mosby–Year Book.)

Hickman and Broviac Catheters

The Hickman (internal diameter 1.6 mm) and Broviac (internal diameter 1.0 mm) are Silastic catheters used mainly for long-term home use. The Hickman catheter is preferred if it will be necessary to infuse large quantities of fluids and to draw blood samples. The purposes of Hickman and Broviac catheters are to administer TPN, blood and blood products, chemotherapeutic agents, and antibiotic therapy and to draw blood for laboratory specimens. The tip of the catheter is placed into a large vein and advanced into the right atrium. After the catheter exits from the vein, it is tunneled under the skin so that it exits on the lower chest wall some distance from the vein insertion site (Fig. 15-3). A single Dacron cuff anchors the catheter subcutaneously and fibrous tissue forms around the cuff in 2 to 3 weeks. This tunneling and Dacron cuff help to prevent bacteria from reaching the intravascular system. Because of the cuff, sterile procedure for site care is not necessary after the site has healed, and clean technique can then be used.[9]

When solutions are not being infused through the Hickman catheter, a catheter cap or injection cap must be screwed onto the end of the hub. This prevents blood from backing into the catheter. Before opening the catheter to air, a catheter clamp must be used to occlude the catheter. Any of the long-term use catheters can be used for insertion of IV push drugs during a cardiac arrest. A 10 ml or larger syringe should be used for medications to prevent damage to the fragile catheter tip. Smaller-sized syringes

Skill 15-9   Flushing Hickman and Broviac Catheters

▼

If an infusion is not done daily, the heparin in the catheter should be changed every week. Hickman and Broviac catheters are capped with a rubber-topped plastic injection cap. This cap maintains a closed system between catheter uses. Because the cap's rubber top is punctured several times a day, it will need to be changed every 72 hours. In the home care setting, patients can save money by using alcohol sponges to keep catheter hubs and IV tubing tips sterile during procedures.[10] This is less expensive than using sterile towels, sponges, and capped needles.

EQUIPMENT AND SUPPLIES

- Bottle of isopropyl alcohol
- Bottle of povidone-iodine solution
- 4 cotton-tipped applicators
- 1 packaged alcohol swab or cotton-tipped applicator with alcohol
- Scissors
- Tape
- Tape strip (1.25 cm × 1.25 cm [½ inch × ½ inch])
- Injection cap or Luer-Lok cap
- Catheter clamp
- 3-ml syringe filled with 2½ ml heparin 100 U/ml

NURSING INTERVENTIONS

1. Assemble equipment and wash hands.
2. Cut three sides off packaged alcohol swab.
3. Open catheter cap package.
4. Remove tape from catheter and catheter cap.
5. Dip cotton-tipped applicator in povidone-iodine solution and clean the connection site at the end of the catheter hub. Let solution dry for 2 minutes.
6. Use alcohol-soaked, cotton-tipped applicators to remove the povidone-iodine.
7. Insert end of catheter into alcohol swab to keep clean.
8. Clamp catheter. Always use a catheter clamp that does not have teeth or rough edges. Rotate the clamping site every week and mark it with a piece of tape.
9. Remove needle from heparin syringe and hold upright in palm of hand, taking care not to contaminate tip.
10. Using thumb and forefinger of same hand, remove catheter cap or IV tubing from catheter hub.
11. Twist syringe tip into hub of catheter. Unclamp catheter clamp, and begin injecting 2 ml heparin into catheter.
12. Clamp catheter while still injecting heparin into catheter, leaving 0.5 ml in the syringe. This will create positive pressure in the catheter and prevent back flow.
13. Remove syringe from catheter and add several drops of heparin to catheter hub. Screw new cap onto catheter.
14. Release catheter clamp and apply tape strip around catheter cap and hub of catheter. Coil catheter on top of dressing and tape it in place.

exert too much pressure. The lines should also be flushed with saline before and after medication administration.

Implanted Venous Access Ports

The implanted venous access ports have several trade names including MediPort, Port-A-Cath, and Infuse-A-Port. They consist of a catheter connected to a chamber or port that has a self-sealing diaphragm (Fig. 15-5). The port is implanted into the subcutaneous tissue and is accessed by a specially designed Huber needle that is straight or

Skill 15-10   Temporary Repair of Broken Broviac or Hickman Catheter Hub

▼

Home care patients can obtain permanent catheter repair kits and temporary repair kits. When permanent catheter repair is needed, the patient should take the permanent repair kit to a local hospital or clinic and have a member of the health care team make the repair. The temporary repair kit contains injection caps, blunt needles, and a screw extractor (Fig. 15-4). The gauge of the blunt needle corresponds to that of the patient's catheter: 18-gauge for the Broviac, 15-gauge for the Hickman, and 22-gauge for the pediatric Broviac. The kit can be used at home to do the following:[10]

- Dislodge a broken IV tubing-tip embedded in the hub of the catheter.
- Place heparin into a catheter obstructed with an IV tubing tip or missing a catheter hub.
- Temporarily replace a catheter hub that has separated from the catheter.

EQUIPMENT AND SUPPLIES

- Blunt needle
- Injection cap
- Catheter clamp
- Alcohol swab
- Tape
- 3 ml syringe containing 2½ ml heparin 100 U/ml solution

NURSING INTERVENTIONS

1. Place catheter clamp on catheter.
2. Tear off one end of alcohol swab and insert exposed tip of catheter into swab.
3. Remove needle from heparin syringe and attach blunt needle to syringe.
4. Remove cover from blunt needle and fill needle with heparin.
5. Remove alcohol swab from catheter and insert blunt tip of needle still attached to heparin syringe into catheter lumen. With a twisting and turning motion, push needle in as far as possible.
6. Release clamp and inject 2 ml of heparin solution. Clamp catheter while still injecting heparin.
7. Remove syringe and add a few drops of heparin solution to blunt needle hub. Insert injection cap into hub of needle and tighten with a turning motion.
8. Release catheter clamp and tape junctions of blunt needle, catheter, and injection cap.
9. Contact appropriate medical personnel who will perform permanent repair.

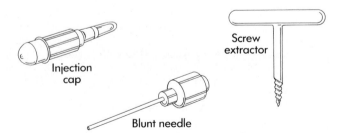

Fig. 15-4   Items in a temporary repair kit for repairing a Hickman or Broviac catheter.

Skill 15-11 Dislodgement of Broken IV Tubing Tip from Hub of Broviac or Hickman Catheter

EQUIPMENT AND SUPPLIES

- Screw extractor
- Blunt needle
- Injection cap
- Catheter clamp
- Alcohol swabs
- Tape
- 3 ml syringe filled with 2½ ml heparin 100 U/ml

NURSING INTERVENTIONS

1. Place catheter clamp on catheter and wrap alcohol swab around catheter hub.
2. Remove needle from heparin syringe and replace with blunt needle. Fill needle with heparin solution.
3. Insert blunt needle attached to heparin syringe through lodged IV tubing tip in hub of catheter. Gently rotate syringe while pushing forward on needle.
4. Release catheter clamp and inject 2 ml heparin solution. Reapply catheter clamp and remove blunt needle and syringe from catheter. Wrap catheter hub in an alcohol swab.
5. Obtain screw extractor and screw it into the IV tubing tip in a counterclockwise direction. Then pull straight out to dislodge and remove IV tubing tip.
6. Add a few drops of heparin solution to hub of catheter, place injection cap on catheter, tightening with a turning motion, and tape junctions.

Skill 15-12 Temporary Repair of Severed or Split-Hickman or Broviac Catheter

EQUIPMENT AND SUPPLIES:

- Blunt needle
- Injection cap
- Scissors
- Catheter clamp
- Alcohol swab
- Syringe with 2½ ml of heparin 100 U/ml
- Tape

NURSING INTERVENTIONS

1. Place catheter clamp on catheter between skin exit site and damaged segment.
2. Cut off damaged section of catheter and wrap newly exposed tip in an alcohol swab.
3. Remove needle from heparin syringe and attach blunt needle.
4. Remove cover from blunt needle and fill needle with heparin solution.
5. Remove alcohol swab from catheter tip and insert tip of blunt needle still attached to heparin solution syringe into catheter lumen. Push needle in as far as possible, using a twisting and turning motion.
6. Release catheter clamp and inject 2 ml heparin solution into catheter. Clamp catheter while still injecting heparin solution and then remove syringe from hub of needle.
7. Add some drops of heparin solution to hub of needle and place injection cap on hub of needle, tightening with a turning motion.
8. Release catheter clamp and tape junctions of needle, injection cap, and catheter.
9. Contact appropriate medical personnel who will perform permanent repair.

Skill 15-13 Accessing the Implanted Venous Access Port

Huber needles need to be changed every 7 days.[15] Skin preparation for insertion of these needles varies. Some procedure manuals recommend the use of sterile gloves; others have a nongloved procedure. Some procedures call for the removal of povidone-iodine solution from the skin; whereas others let the povidone-iodine remain on the skin.[24] A dressing should be applied that will support the Huber needle but will not prevent visualization of the insertion site. Otherwise, indications of a dislodged needle, such as edema, might be undetected. A T-extension tubing with a clamp may be used between the Huber needle hub and IV tubing to reduce pressure on the needle (Fig. 15-6).[30] Some companies provide a Huber needle already attached to an extension set with wings for secure taping (Fig. 15-7). More research needs to be performed to determine the proper procedures for caring for an implanted central VAD.

EQUIPMENT AND SUPPLIES

- Primed IV tubing and fluids
- 10-cm (4-inch) T-extension tubing with clamp
- Alcohol swabs
- 3 povidone-iodine swab sticks
- Huber needle with a 90 degree angle bend (20 G for drawing blood, 19 G for blood transfusion, and 22 G for IV infusion)
- 10 ml syringe containing injectable normal saline solution
- Sterile 2 × 2 gauze sponges
- 1-inch micropore tape
- Sterile gloves and sterile towel
- Clear plastic dressing

NURSING INTERVENTIONS

1. Set up equipment, wash hands, and open supplies.
2. Prepare skin over implanted device by cleansing with povidone-iodine swab in outward spiral motion, covering a 13-cm (5-inch) diameter. Repeat three times using a fresh swab each time.
3. Attach the extension tubing to the normal saline filled syringe and flush solution into the tubing, purging the air from the line. Clamp the tubing.
4. Attach Huber needle to extension tubing and flush out air in needle with the normal saline. Set aside on sterile towel.
5. Put on sterile gloves and palpate area to locate center of the septum. Stabilize it between the thumb and the index finger. (Fig. 15-7)
6. Firmly insert needle into septum through the skin until it stops at the back of the port.
7. Unclamp extension tubing and slowly inject the saline into the port. If resistance is met, do not use force. Reclamp tubing and have the patient change positions, cough, extend arms over head, and take a deep breath. If still unable to inject flush, follow procedure outlined in Skill 15-3.
8. If no resistance is met, inject 5 ml saline into the port. Aspirate the fluid back into the syringe to check for a blood return.
9. If a blood return is seen, inject the remaining saline solution into the catheter. Tape the Huber needle securely into place at a right angle, using the gauze sponges to support the needle. Apply a clear plastic dressing for visualization of the skin.
10. If no blood return is seen, follow procedure outlined in Skill 15-4.
11. If the device is patent, reclamp the extension tubing, remove the syringe, and attach the IV fluids tubing.
12. Unclamp the extension tubing and regulate the flow using an infusion pump.

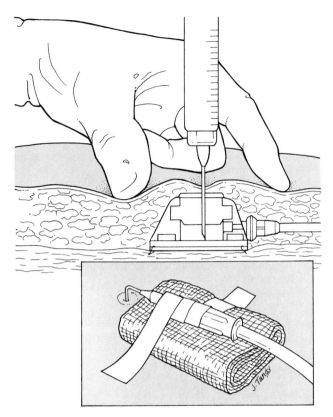

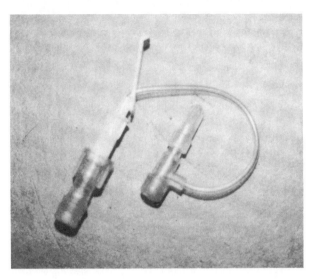

Fig. 15-6 T-extension tubing with self-clamp for use with subclavian or implanted central venous access device to reduce pressure on the Huber needle. (From Taylor JP, Taylor JE: Vascular access devices: uses and aftercare, *J Emerg Nurs* 13(3):163, 1987.

Fig. 15-5 Implanted venous access port. Stabilize between thumb and index finger when inserting needle into septum. Inset: Use a gauze sponge to support Huber needle. Secure needle using chevron taping method.

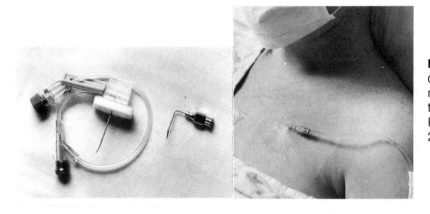

Fig. 15-7 Huber needles are noncoring and are designed for use in implantable ports. Some companies offer an infusion set with a Huber needle attached for easy access to the ports. (From Perry AG, Potter PA: *Clinical nursing skills and techniques,* ed 2, St Louis, 1990, Mosby–Year Book.)

bent at a 90 degree angle. The bevel of a Huber needle is deflected slightly to allow for slicing, not coring of the septum, which contributes to the long lifetime of the device. Needle access is generally limited to less than 2000 punctures before the device must be replaced. The implanted ports provide a venous access site for inserting highly irritating drugs, such as those used for intermittent long-term cancer chemotherapy. Other uses include TPN, chronic blood support, the need for frequent blood sampling, and use in diabetic, sickle cell anemia, and acquired immune deficiency syndrome (AIDS) patients. Double-lu-

men implantable ports are available that allow for infusion of incompatible drugs or drug infusion with parenteral nutrition. Another available device combines an implanted port with the Groshong catheter. The advantage of implanted central VADs include the following:
- Long access life with minimal required maintenance.
- Lower infection rate as compared to tunnelled right atrial catheters.
- Decrease in thrombosis as compared to tunnelled catheters.
- Improved cosmetic appearance.

- Patient can swim, shower, or bathe without wetting the device (when it is not in use).
- Dressing does not have to be worn over the site when the device is not in use.
- When not in use, the device has to be flushed only every 4 weeks.

Disadvantages of implanted central VADs include the following:

- Requires greater technical skills for nursing staff.
- Not suitable for use in cyclical TPN because daily accessing of the port may cause scar tissue build-up and discomfort for the patient.
- Not all patients are candidates because some may find accessing the device to be painful and technically difficult.
- Shifting or floating of the port may occur, or the port may be implanted too deeply, causing difficulty in palpation of the port.
- Patients will need to be careful about avoiding direct pressure over the device, such as when wearing a shoulder harness seat belt or shoulder bag.

REFERENCES

1. American Society for Parental and Enteral Nutrition: Guidelines for use of total parental nutrition in the hospitalized adult patient, *J Parenter Ent Nutr* 10(5):441, 1986.
2. Ang SD, Canham JE, Daly JM: Parenteral infusion with an admixture of amino acids, dextrose, and fat emulsion solution: compatibility and clinical safety, *J Parent Ent Nutr* 11(1):23, 1987.
3. Brendel V: Catheters utilized in delivering total parenteral nutrition, *Nat Intravenous Ther Assoc* 7:488, 1984.
4. Brown LH, Wantroba I, Simonson G: Reestablishing patency in an occluded central venous access device, *Crit Care Nurse* 9(5):114, 1989.
5. Brown R, Quercia RA, Sigman R: Total nutrient admixture: a review, *J Parenter Ent Nutr* 10(6):650, 1986.
6. Buzby KM, O'Neill L: *Parenteral nutrition solutions and additives.* In Skipper A, editor: *Dietitian's handbook of enteral and parenteral nutrition,* Rockville, Md, 1989, Aspen Publishers.
7. Cerra FB: *Metabolic support.* In Cerra FB, editor: *Manual of critical care,* St Louis, 1987, Mosby–Year Book.
8. Detsky AS et al: Quality of life of patients on long-term total parenteral nutrition at home, *J Gen Intern Med* 1:26, 1986.
9. Evans LE, DeMoss CJ: *Alterations in nutrition.* In Malloy C, Hartshorn J, editors: *Acute care nursing in the home: a holistic approach,* Philadelphia, 1989, JB Lippincott.
10. Fleming CR, Berkner S, editors: *Home parenteral nutrition: a handbook for patients,* Philadelphia, 1987, JB Lippincott.
11. Gilder H: Parenteral nourishment of patients undergoing surgical or traumatic stress, *J Parenter Ent Nutr* 10(1):88, 1986.
12. Groh-Wargo S: *Prematurity/low birth weight.* In Lang CE, editor: *Nutritional support in critical care,* Rockville, Md, 1987, Aspen Publishers.
13. Gulledge AD: Common psychiatric concerns in home parenteral nutrition, *Cleve Clin J Med* 52(3):329, 1985.
14. Haas-Beckert B: Removing the mysteries of parenteral nutrition, *Pediatr Nurs* 13(1):37, 1987.
15. Hadaway LC: Evaluation and use of advanced IV technology, part I: Central venous access devices, *J Intravenous Nurs* 12(2):73, 1989.
16. Herfindal ET et al: Survey of home nutritional support patients, *J Parenter Ent Nutr* 13(3):255, 1989.
17. Hohenbrink K: *The pediatric patient.* In Lang CE, editor: *Nutritional support in critical care,* Rockville, Md, 1987, Aspen Publishers.
18. Howard L, Heaphey LL, Timchalk M: A review of the current national status of home parenteral and enteral nutrition from the provider and consumer perspective, *J Parenter Ent Nutr* 10(4):416, 1986.
19. Ihde JK: *Metabolic response and support of the surgical patient.* In Ihde JK, Jacobsen WK, Briggs BA, editors: *Principles of critical care,* Philadelphia, 1987, WB Saunders.
20. Klein RA, Patton LR, Barbaccia DM: Peripheral intravenous nutrition: utilization of lipid as the primary caloric source, *Nutr Support Serv* 5(4):17, 1985.
21. Lang CE, Schulte CV: *The adult patient.* In Lang CE, editor: *Nutritional support in critical care,* Rockville, Md, 1987, Aspen Publishers.
22. McCrae JD: *Home parenteral nutrition.* In Skipper A, editor: *Dietitian's handbook of enteral and parenteral nutrition,* Rockville, Md, 1989, Aspen Publishers.
23. Mirtallo JM: *Parenteral therapy.* In Lang CE, editor: *Nutritional support in critical care,* Rockville, Md, 1987, Aspen Publishers.
24. Murphy LM, Lipman TO: Central venous catheter care in parenteral nutrition: a review, *J Parenter Ent Nutr* 11(2):190, 1987.
25. Pereira GR et al: Parenteral nutrition for the premature neonate—amino acid, carbohydrate, and fat sources, *Nutr Support Serv* 4(10), 1984.
26. Powell CR et al: Op-site dressing study: A prospective randomized study evaluating povidone iodine ointment and extension set changes with 7-day op-site dressings applied to total parenteral nutrition subclavian sites, *J Parenter Ent Nutr* 9(3):443, 1985.
27. Rajala M: *Formulation of parenteral solutions.* In Krey SH, Murray RL, editors: *Dynamics of nutrition support, assessment, implementation, and evaluation,* Norwalk, Conn, 1986, Appleton & Lange.
28. Sajbel TA, Dutro MP, Radway PR: Use of separate insulin infusions with total parenteral nutrition, *J Parenter Ent Nutr* 11(1):97, 1987.
29. Simonson G, Brown LH, Wantroba I: Reestablishing patency in the occluded implanted central venous access device (VAD)—part 2, *Crit Care Nurse* 9(9):13, 1989.
30. Taylor JP, Taylor JE: Vascular access devices: uses and aftercare, *J Emerg Nurs* 13(3):160, 1987.
31. Vargas JH, Ament ME, Berquist WE: Long-term home parenteral nutrition in pediatrics: ten years of experience in 102 patients, *J Pediatr Gastroenterol Nutr* 6(1):24, 1987.
32. Young CP et al: Catheter sepsis during parenteral nutrition: the safety of long-term OpSite dressings, *J Parenter Ent Nutr* 12(4):365, 1988.
33. Young LS: *Principles of parenteral nutrition: indications, administration, and monitoring.* In Krey SH, Murray RL, editors: *Dynamics of nutrition support, assessment, implementation, and evaluation,* Norwalk, Conn, 1986, Appleton & Lange.
34. Zlotkin SH, Stallings VA, Pencharz PB: Total parenteral nutrition in children, *Pediatr Clin North Am* 32(2), 1985.

CHAPTER 16

Enteral Feeding

Objectives

After completing this chapter, the reader will be able to:

- Identify the types of patients who may require enteral feeding.
- Discuss the assessment of nutritional status.
- Describe how to calculate nutritional requirements of critical care patients.
- Differentiate between the various types of enteral feeding formulas.
- Specify the various complications of enteral feeding.
- Describe the ongoing assessment of a patient receiving enteral nutrition.
- Formulate the nursing diagnoses and patient outcomes for patients receiving enteral nutrition.
- Describe the skills required to administer enteral feedings.
- Differentiate between pediatric and adult enteral nutrition patient care requirements and precautions.

Enteral feeding or *enteral nutrition* is the administration of blenderized table foods or commercially prepared liquid formulas taken by mouth or delivered into the gastrointestinal (GI) tract through orogastric, nasogastric, nasoenteric, esophagostomy, pharyngotomy, gastrostomy, or jejunostomy tubes. If the patient cannot voluntarily ingest an adequate diet, enteral feedings may be required. The use of enteral feedings has been shown to preserve gut integrity, accelerate would healing, restore cell-mediated immunity, promote positive nitrogen balance, decrease length of hospitalization, decrease mortality, and improve overall nutritional status.[10]

INDICATIONS FOR ENTERAL NUTRITION

Once food ingestion has ceased, the following can occur[10]:

- Reduction in the activity and concentration of important secretions, including the intestinal enzymes maltase, sucrase, galactokinase, Na-K-ATPase; and gastric hormones, such as secretin, gastrin, and cholecystokinin.
- Physical diminution of gut weight and protein content and impairment of absorptive capacity for nutrients.
- Structural and functional atrophy even when complete nutritional support is provided intravenously.

The provision of nutrients into the gut is the preferred method of feeding patients who have a GI tract that can be used safely and effectively and who cannot ingest adequate nutrients by mouth. Food deprivation has profound adverse effects.

The indications for enteral nutrition can be divided into four clinical situations: (1) those where enteral nutrition should be a part of routine care, (2) those where enteral nutrition would usually be helpful, and (3) those where enteral nutrition is of limited or undetermined value, and (4) those in which enteral nutrition should not be used. The following national guidelines were developed by the American Society of Parenteral and Enteral Nutrition.[2]

Clinical Situations Where Enteral Nutrition Should Be a Part of Routine Care

- Normal nutritional status with less than 50% of required nutrient intake orally for the previous 7 to 10 days.
- Protein-calorie malnutrition with inadequate oral intake of nutrients for the previous 5 days. Protein-calorie malnutrition is defined as greater than 10% loss of usual weight, or serum albumin levels less than 3.5 gm/dl.
- Major full-thickness burns.
- Severe dysphagia.
- Massive small bowel resection in combination with administration of total parenteral nutrition (TPN).
- Low output enterocutaneous fistulas (less than 500 ml/24 hr).

Clinical Situations Where Enteral Nutrition Would Usually Be Helpful

- Radiation therapy.
- Mild chemotherapy.
- Major trauma.
- Liver failure and severe renal dysfunction.

Clinical Situations Where Enteral Nutrition Is of Limited or Undetermined Value

- Intensive chemotherapy.
- Acute enteritis.
- Immediate postoperative period or poststress period.
- Less than 10% remaining small intestine.

Clinical Situations in Which Enteral Nutrition Should Not Be Used

- Severe diarrhea.
- Complete mechanical intestinal obstruction.
- Ileus or intestinal hypomotility.
- High output external fistulas (greater than 500 ml/24 hr).
- Shock. Patients in septic shock receive antibiotics that cause marked diarrhea if they are fed enterally.
- Severe acute pancreatitis.
- Prognosis not warranting aggressive nutritional support.
- Aggressive nutritional support not desired by the patient or legal guardian, and such action being in accordance with hospital policy and existing law.

DETERMINATION OF NUTRITIONAL STATUS

The determination of nutritional status is the evaluation of the adequacy of nourishment and the signs and symptoms of malnutrition. Malnutrition may be either acute or chronic and exists in the following forms (see the box on p. 368)[17]:

- Protein malnutrition (kwashiorkor).
- Protein-calorie malnutrition (marasmus).
- Stress and starvation (combined kwashiorkor and marasmus).
- Obesity (20% or more over ideal body weight).
- Vitamin deficiencies.
- Mineral deficiencies.

When losses of energy and protein exceed intake, the body draws on its own stores of fat and glycogen to meet energy needs. Somatic and visceral mass is used to supply nitrogen and essential amino acids for protein synthesis. The nutritional assessment used to measure these stores in the clinical setting are listed in the box on p. 369.

Dietary History

The dietary history should include a social and drug history pertaining to nutritional problems as follows:

- Recent oral intake.
- Previous diet prescriptions.
- Weight history.
- Mechanical feeding problems.
- Alcohol or drug addiction.
- Chronic drug use.
- Medication history.
- Food allergies.
- Food aversions.
- Who prepares meals.
- Meal setting.
- Ability for self-feeding.
- Diet supplementation.
- Previous nutritional support.
- Changes in appetite.
- Elimination pattern.
- Nausea, vomiting, or pain.
- Chronic diseases.
- Stroke or neurological diseases.
- Diseases of GI system.
- Surgery to GI system.
- Recent NPO order.
- Pregnancy or childbirth.
- Physical activity level.
- Dentures.

Medical History and Physical Assessment

During the physical assessment, each system should be examined for indicators of nutritional deficiencies or disorders (Table 15-6). The impact of the patient's disease or dysfunction on GI function, venous access, and delivery, absorption, and metabolism of nutrients should be determined.

Anthropometrics

Anthropometrics is the measurement of the body or its parts, such as height and weight. Triceps skinfolds and mid-upper arm muscle circumference may be used,[1] but rarely in the intensive care unit.

The patient's degree of malnutrition can also be assessed by determining the current weight as a percentage of ideal body weight, current weight as a percentage of usual weight, and recent weight change (see box on p. 369) The percent of recent weight change correlates best with ultimate morbidity and mortality in individual patients. Fluid shifts often mask a true change in lean body mass and fat. One liter of fluid equals approximately 1 kg (2 lbs) so a patient should be monitored for signs of overhydration, edema, and ascites. A weight gain of greater than 1/8 to 1/4 kg (1/4 to 1/2 lb)/24 hr after surgery, trauma, during nutritional support, or before dialysis may reflect changes in hydration. Frequently weight loss occurs initially in the starved patient started on nutrition therapy as serum oncotic pressure is normalized and edema is mobilized. If anabolism and weight gain are the goals, a gain of approximately 1 kg (2 lbs) a week should be achieved. In most critically ill patients, though, weight maintenance rather than weight gain should be the primary objective.

Laboratory Tests

Plasma fibronectin has been found to be very sensitive to nutritional depletion and repletion during health and critical illness. Consumed rapidly during acute illness, it peaks early during nutritional repletion but does not track positive nitrogen balance after 1 week. For the critical care patient, it has been found that the subjective global assessment (SGA) scoring system (Fig. 16-1) is easy to perform and is a predictor of nutrition-related complications.[8] The

▼ **Interpretation of the Nutrition Assessment**[17,25]

PROTEIN MALNUTRITION (KWASHIORKOR)
Dietary history
- Adequate calorie or high glucose intake.
- Inadequate protein intake or stress state with increased protein losses.

Medical history
- Frequent decubitus ulcers or wound dehiscence.
- Recent stress event (e.g., surgery, trauma, burns, infection, or sepsis).
- Chronic protein loss (resulting from burns, decubiti, fistulas, or dialysis).
- Secondary complications, including infection, sepsis, and slow wound healing.
- Elevated liver function tests, not associated with parenteral nutrition or primary liver disease.

Physical assessment
- Normal or obese appearance.
- Moist skin.
- Dull, sunken eyes.
- Edema, ascites, or CHF.

Anthropometrics and laboratory testing
- Fat stores normal or greater than normal (normal or increased weight and triceps skinfold).
- Muscle mass normal or less than normal (decreased creatinine-height index and mid-arm muscle circumference).
- Serum proteins lower than normal (greatly decreased serum albumin, transferrin, retinal-binding protein, thyroxine-binding prealbumin, fibronectin, and total lymphocyte count).
- Anergy (immunodeficient condition characterized by diminished reaction to antigens).

PROTEIN-CALORIE MALNUTRITION (MARASMUS)
Dietary history
Inadequate intake of both calories and protein because of the following:
- Inability to ingest adequate calories and protein (e.g., bowel obstruction and dysphagia).
- Chronic losses (e.g., malabsorption and dialysis).
- Unwillingness to ingest adequate calories and protein (e.g., chronic obstructive pulmonary disease, cancer cachexia, and anorexia nervosa).
- Increased needs for growth not met (e.g., pregnancy, lactation, and adolescence).
- Impaired metabolism of nutrients (e.g., cirrhosis of liver and diabetes mellitus).

Medical history
- Chronic disease (e.g., cancer, renal failure with dialysis, emphysema, cirrhosis of the liver, rheumatoid arthritis, proteinuria, Crohn's disease, and sprue).
- Disease or surgery of the GI tract.
- Chronic losses (e.g., fistulas, decubiti, and dialysis).
- Frequent tests requiring nothing by mouth (NPO) status or clear liquid diet.
- Drug-nutrient interactions (e.g., chemotherapy and corticosteroid therapy).

Physical assessment
- Thin, emaciated appearance of torso and extremities.
- Wrinkled and dry skin, appearing aged.
- Sparse, dry, easily plucked hair.
- Bright eyes.
- Delayed wound healing.

Anthropometrics and laboratory testing
- Fat stores less than normal (greatly decreased weight and triceps skinfold).
- Muscle mass less than normal (greatly decreased creatinine-height index and mid-arm muscle circumference).
- Serum proteins normal or slightly decreased (serum albumin, transferrin, thyroxine-binding prealbumin, retinol-binding protein, fibronectin, and total lymphocyte count).

STRESS AND STARVATION (COMBINED KWASHIORKOR AND MARASMUS)
Dietary history
- A stressful event with episode of starvation immediately before or following it.

Medical history
- Chronic losses caused by fistula drainage, gastrointestinal bleeding, and malabsorption.
- History of respiratory, liver, or other organ failure.

Physical assessment
- Evidence of weight loss and muscle wastage.
- Edema or ascites.
- Slow wound healing.
- Presence of infection or sepsis.

Anthropometrics and laboratory testing
- Fat stores less than normal (slightly decreased weight and triceps skinfold).
- Muscle mass less than normal (slightly decreased creatinine-height index and mid-arm muscle circumference).
- Serum proteins less than normal (greatly decreased serum albumin, transferrin, thyroxine-binding prealbumin, retinal-binding protein, fibronectin, and total lymphocyte count).

▼ **Nutrition Assessment of Protein and Fat Stores**[25]

SOMATIC PROTEIN COMPARTMENT
Physical signs and symptoms

- Muscle wastage.
- Weakness and easy fatigability.

Anthropometric assessment

- Weight loss.
- Midarm and midarm muscle circumference.
- Midarm muscle area.
- Fat-free mass derived from anthropometric estimation of body density and fat mass.

Laboratory assessment

- Creatinine-height index.
- 3-methylhistidine excretion.
- Nitrogen balance.

VISCERAL (NONSTRIATED MUSCLE AND CIRCULATORY PROTEINS) COMPARTMENT
Physical signs and symptoms

- Pallor.
- Edema and ascites.
- Infections.
- Decubitus ulcers or wound dehiscence.

Anthropometric assessment

- Radiological or computerized tomography scan evidence of atrophy of heart, kidneys, etc.

Laboratory assessment

- Nitrogen balance.
- Albumin.
- Transferrin.
- Retinol-binding protein.
- Thyroxine-binding prealbumin.
- Fibronectin.
- Total lymphocyte count.
- Cutaneous reactivity to recall antigens tests.

FAT STORES
Physical signs and symptoms

- Sunken eyes.
- Dependent skin over extremities.
- Loss of buccal fat pads, scaphoid abdomen, and fat pads in hips, thighs, and upper arms.

Anthropometric assessment

- Weight.
- Triceps, biceps, and suprailiac and subscapular skinfolds.

Laboratory assessment

- Energy expenditure measured through indirect calorimetry or estimated from Harris-Benedict equation and compared to energy intake.

▼ **Weight Formulas for Assessing a Patient's Degree of Malnutrition**

$$\% \text{ Ideal body weight} = \frac{\text{Patient's present weight}}{\text{Ideal body weight}} \times 100$$

80% to 90% = Mild caloric malnutrition
70% to 79% = Moderate malnutrition
0% to 69% = Severe malnutrition

$$\% \text{ Usual body weight} = \frac{\text{Present weight}}{\text{Usual weight}} \times 100$$

85% to 95% = Mild malnutrition
75% to 84% = Moderate malnutrition
0% to 74% = Severe malnutrition

% Recent weight change =

$$\frac{\text{Usual weight} - \text{Present weight} \% \text{ to}}{\text{Usual weight}} \times 100$$

Significant weight loss = > 1% to 2% over 1 week
> 5% over 1 month
> 7.5% over 3 months
> 10% over 6 or more months

SGA is nonsensitive, however, for following nutritional progression.

Nutritional Requirements

The goal for adequate nutrition in the critical care patient is to provide for adequate energy and nutrients to allow for the following:

- Maintenance of existing lean body mass.
- Normal needs and physiological functions.
- Usual synthesis of enzymes and hormones.
- Repair and replacement of worn-out cells.
- Extraneous losses.
- Wound healing.
- Catabolism of stress.

Anabolism, the state of rebuilding and regaining weight and lean body mass, should not be a goal during the critical phase of an illness. Attempting to have the critical care patient gain weight during stress may cause complications, such as elevation of liver enzymes, increased carbon dioxide production, and excessive glucose and fluid load.[18] All nutritional support should be supplemented with an exercise plan. Exercise promotes optimal use of nutritional intake, minimizes protein breakdown, and helps ensure that weight gain is stored as lean muscle mass rather than as adipose tissue.

Energy Requirements

The two components of the nutritional formula that need to be calculated are the total calories and the fractional percentage of those calories that are to be supplied from carbohydrates, fat, and protein. One method of estimating energy requirements in the critical care patient is shown in Table 15-1. These methods use body weight

Features of subjective global assessment (SGA)

(Select appropriate category with a checkmark, or enter numerical value were indicated by "#.")

A. History
  1. Weight change
      Overall loss in past 6 months: Amount = # _____ kg; % Loss = # _____
      Change in past 2 weeks: _____ Increase
                                _____ No change
                                _____ Decrease

  2. Dietary intake change (relative to normal)
      _____ No change
      _____ Change   _____ Duration = # _____ Weeks.
                                  _____ Type: _____ Suboptimal solid diet _____ Full liquid diet
                                                           _____ Hypocaloric liquids   _____ Starvation

  3. Gastrointestinal symptoms (that persisted for >2 weeks)
      _____ None _____ Nausea _____ Vomiting _____ Diarrhea _____ Anorexia

  4. Functional capacity
      _____ No dysfunction (e.g., full capacity)
      _____ Dysfunction _____ Duration = # _____ Weeks.
                                  _____ Type: _____ Working suboptimally
                                                           _____ Ambulatory
                                                           _____ Bedridden

  5. Disease and its relation to nutritional requirements
      Primary diagnosis (specify) _____
      Metabolic demand (stress):   _____ No stress   _____ Low stress
                                   _____ Moderate stress _____ High stress

B. Physical (for each trait specify: 0 = normal, 1 = mild, 2 = moderate, 3 = severe).
      # _____ Loss of subcutaneous fat (triceps, chest)
      # _____ Muscle wasting (quadriceps, deltoids)
      # _____ Ankle edema
      # _____ Sacral edema
      # _____ Ascites

C. SGA rating (select one)
      _____ A = Well nourished
      _____ B = Moderately (or suspected of being) malnourished
      _____ C = Severely malnourished

Fig. 16-1 Features of subjective global assessment (SGA). (From Detsky AS et al: What is subjective global assessment of nutritional status? *J Parenter Enter Nutr* 11(1):8, 1987.)

alone as the key determinant in predicting energy needs.

More precise caloric requirements, including consideration for age, sex, height, and weight can be obtained by using more complicated equations, such as the Harris-Benedict equation. This equation can be adapted for the effect of stress factors on energy requirements (Table 16-1). Caloric expenditure may be greater during the early recovery phase of critical illness, but may be less during periods of hemodynamic decompensation. During late recovery, caloric expenditure may be nearly normal. The Harris-Benedict equation for estimating caloric requirements is as follows[11]:

Male: BEE =
  $66 + (13.7 \times \text{weight}) + (5 \times \text{height}) - (6.8 \times \text{age})$
Female: BEE =
  $65 + (9.6 \times \text{weight}) + (1.8 \times \text{height}) - (4.7 \times \text{age})$

  BEE = Basal Energy Expenditure

Multiply BEE × Stress factors in Table 16-1 for critical care patient.
Weight = Present weight (dry, daily, or ideal) in kilograms.
Height = Height in centimeters.
  Age = Age in years.

Indirect calorimetry

Energy expenditure can also be calculated by measuring respiratory gas exchange. A metabolic cart can be placed at the bedside and a gas collection device adapted to the exhalation unit of the patient's ventilator. A microcomputer generates estimates of resting energy expenditure (REE), use of energy substrates, protein requirements, and the respiratory quotient (RQ). Indirect calorimetry measures oxygen consumption and carbon dioxide production. The following ratio is the respiratory quotient:

$$\frac{\dot{V}_{CO_2} \text{ (ml)}}{\dot{V}_{O_2} \text{ (ml)}}$$

Table 16-1 Stress Factors for Estimating Caloric
Requirements[31]

Condition	Stress factor
Well-nourished and unstressed	1.0
Burned (before skin grafting) Normotensive	
0%-20% Body surface area (BSA)	1.2-1.5
20%-40% BSA	1.5-2.0
>40% BSA	1.8-2.5
Burn shock period of resuscitation	.0.5
Burned (after successful grafting)	1.0-1.3
Septic (acute phase) Normotensive	1.2-1.7
Hypotensive	0.5
Septic (recovery)	1.0
Multiple trauma (acute phase) Normotensive	1.1-1.5
Hypotensive	0.8-1.0
Multiple trauma (recovery)	1.0-1.2

The RQ reflects the oxidation of a mixed fuel, fat, carbohydrate, and amino acids, and reflects whether the patient is well nourished, starved, or overfed. The following RQs would be obtained in the following situations[17]:

0.7	Starvation with ketosis; primary source of energy is fat.
0.8	Primary source of energy is protein.
0.85	Mixed carbohydrate, fat, and amino acid oxidation.
1.0	Pure glucose oxidation.
>1.0	Overfeeding, lipogenesis (conversion of glucose to fat), and increased carbon dioxide production.

Use of the pulmonary artery catheter

Many critical care patients have pulmonary artery catheters that are used to obtain a *cardiopulmonary profile.* The oxygen consumption ($\dot{V}O_2$) obtained from the profile can serve to estimate metabolic expenditure using this simple formula[29]:

$$\text{Calorie/24hr} = 7.0 \times \dot{V}O_2 \text{ (ml/min)}.$$

Protein Requirements

Protein requirements in critical illness are listed in Table 15-1. Critical care patients require a greater amount of their total calories as protein, as much as twice that required by the normal patient, because of factors such as protein depletion, old age, infection or inflammation, and

trauma (stress).[12] Head-injured[35] and burn patients especially require early nitrogen replacement because of massive nitrogen losses and increased metabolic demands. Nitrogen balance is used to determine the adequacy of protein intake and is calculated as nitrogen intake minus nitrogen excretion from all sources. Nitrogen intake is calculated from the protein intake. For standard formulas there is usually 1 gm nitrogen for each 6.25 gm protein. Total nitrogen excretion can be approximated by determining urine urea nitrogen (UUN) plus a correction factor of 20% UUN for nonurea urinary nitrogen losses (i.e., ammonia, creatinine, and uric acid) and the addition of 2 gm for small amounts lost through the skin and stool.[4]

$$\text{Nitrogen bal (NB)} = \text{Nitrogen intake} - \text{Nitrogen excretion}$$

$$NB = \frac{\text{Protein intake (gm)}}{6.25} - (UUN + 20\% \ UUN^* + 2gm\dagger)$$

The nitrogen balance is zero in healthy individuals because anabolic and catabolic rates are in equilibrium. A positive nitrogen balance of 4 to 6 gm/24 hr indicates anabolism.[33] When nutrient intake is deficient or during catabolic conditions (i.e., trauma, burns, and sepsis), the nitrogen balance will be negative. Nitrogen losses are interpreted as follows:

5 to 10 gm loss/24hr	Mildly negative nitrogen balance.
10 to 15 gm loss/24hr	Moderate loss.
>15 gm loss/24hr	Severe loss.

Fluid Requirements

Fluid requirements are calculated so that the patient receives enough water to permit excretion of the urea and electrolytes in the urine without increasing urine osmolality beyond a maximum of 600 mOsm and to provide for increased insensible losses resulting from fever or excessive sweating. The recommended intake of water is usually 1 ml of free water for each calorie provided or half of that amount in the case of a fluid-overloaded patient. To determine water supplied by a feeding formula, one should multiply the percentage of moisture content by the total volume of the feeding. The moisture content of most 1 kcal /ml formulas is 75% to 80% of the volume. A patient receiving 1000 ml of formula would have a water deficit of approximately 200 ml. If the patient is not receiving IV fluids, water requirements can be met by giving an additional amount of free water. Often this water is provided when the tube is flushed, so all extra water provided should be recorded.

When calculating a patient's fluid requirements, losses from the body, such as through drains, emesis, and loose stool, should be taken into account. The daily loss of water in a healthy person is approximately as follows:

---

*For nonurea components.

†Skin and stool.

- Urine   1400 ml (60 ml/hr but may be as high as 2 to 3 L/24hr)
- Skin   350 ml
- Sweat   100 ml
- Feces   200 ml
- Respiration   350 ml

Usual fluid requirements are 1500 ml/m^2 or as follows:

- Adults   35 ml/kg/24hr
- Adolescents   40-60 ml/kg/24hr
- Children   70-110 ml/kg/24hr
- Infants   100-150 ml/kg/24hr

Additional adult needs can be approximated as follows:

- Fever   500-1500 ml/24hr
- Moderate perspiration 500 ml/24hr
- Profuse perspiration   1000 ml/24hr
- Tracheostomy   1000 ml/24hr

Summary of Nutritional Status

Once the nutritional assessment is complete, a summary should be made of the following:

- Patient's deficiencies or excesses of nutrients.
- Risk to the patient of continuing the present nutritional condition versus the risk of instituting nutrition support.
- Patient's nutrient requirements (i.e., basal, maintenance, and repletion).

The nutrition care plan would contain the following:

- Recommended mode of nutrition therapy.
- Monitoring procedures.
- Methods of advancing and weaning patient from nutrition support.
- Suggestions for home nutrition care.

ENTERAL FEEDING FORMULAS

A wide variety of enteral formulas are available commercially. They can be classified into two main categories, modular and nutritionally complete. The *modular formulas* typically consist of one major macronutrient, either carbohydrate, protein, or fat. These enteral modules may be mixed together or added to the patient's basic formula. *Nutritionally complete formulas* contain all the necessary macronutrients, as well as vitamins, minerals, and trace elements. The nutritionally complete formulas can be further classified into either polymeric, predigested, or disease-specific formulas. *Polymeric formulas* contain protein, fat, and carbohydrate in high molecular weight form, thereby requiring complete digestive and absorptive capabilities. Within the polymeric category, there are blenderized, fiber-supplemented, milk-based, standard lactose-free, high-nitrogen, and high-calorie formulas. In the *predigested* category, one or more of the macronutrients (i.e., protein, fat, or carbohydrate) has undergone either partial digestion (hydrolysis) or has been predigested to an elemental form ready for absorption. The predigested formulas include chemically defined (monomeric) and elemental (free amino acid) formulas. The *disease-specific formulas* have been formulated to meet the needs of patients with special disease-related needs. These include re-

nal, hepatic, pulmonary, cardiac, trauma and stress, and clear liquid formulas.[5,16,32]

COMPLICATIONS OF ENTERAL FEEDING
Pulmonary Aspiration

Aspiration probably occurs routinely and may cause the lungs to become colonized with enteral organisms. Pulmonary aspiration can occur when enteral feedings are administered intragastrically to patients who have an impaired cough or gag reflex. Patients with decreased GI motility, a reduced level of consciousness, dysphagia, and an artificial airway can also aspirate feedings. This includes discontinuing gastric feedings during episodes of respiratory distress and for a few hours before and after extubation.[31] Patients with respiratory distress frequently vomit and aspirate feedings.

Gastrointestinal Complications

Impaired GI motility and diminished nutrient absorptive capacity in the intensive care unit (ICU) patient may be caused by the following factors[37]:

1. A primary GI disease, such as pancreatitis, inflammatory bowel disease, or GI fistulas.
2. Malnutrition as a complication of a disease causing the following:
   - Decreased gastric acid secretion and gastric emptying.
   - Small bowel mucosal atrophy with decreased brush border enzymes leading to malabsorption of carbohydrates and amino acids.
   - Impaired pancreatic function leading to decreased pancreatic secretion and fat malabsorption.
3. Secondary effects of surgery, drugs, and disease processes where there is a sympathetic nervous system-mediated decrease in GI blood flow. Sepsis, trauma, hypovolemic shock, respiratory insufficiency, and electrolyte disorders in the ICU patient can cause the following:
   - Paralytic ileus.
   - Stress gastritis and ulceration.
   - Gastric atony and distention.
   - Acute intestinal and colonic ischemia.
   - Pseudoobstruction of the small bowel and colon.

Diarrhea

Diarrhea is the most frequent complication of tube feedings.[10] If diarrhea continues to be a problem, the patient will lose the GI tract as the much preferred route of nutrition and drug absorption. The following are etiologies for diarrhea:

- Lactose intolerance.
- High lipid content of diet.
- Concomitant drug therapy.
- Antibiotic therapy.
- Low serum albumin.
- Too rapid administration of diet.
- High osmolar formulas.

- Contaminated feeding solutions.
- Malnutrition.
- Severe malnutrition.
- Lack of dietary fiber.

Complications Specific to the Ventilator-Dependent Patient

Malnourished ventilator patients will be difficult to wean from the ventilator because of the following effects of poor nutrition: (a) decreased respiratory muscle mass, (b) altered surfactant production, (c) pulmonary edema related to low serum albumin, (d) diminished ventilatory response to hypoxia, (e) respiratory muscle weakness caused by hypophosphatemia, and (f) increased susceptibility to infection because of impaired cell-mediated immunity.[34]

When ventilator-dependent patients are placed on enteral nutrition, precautions must be taken to avoid the following complications:

- Undernutrition caused by inaccurate estimation of caloric needs.
- Aspiration pneumonia caused by artificial airway.
- Dyspnea caused by high amino acid intake.
- Respiratory failure caused by hypophosphatemia.

ASSESSMENT

When caring for the patient receiving enteral feeding, the nurse must continually assess for the signs and symptoms of complications and for problems that might lead to complications. The following measurements should be part of the ongoing nursing assessment:

Respiratory

- Evaluate arterial blood gases (ABGs) daily, as ordered, observing for elevated $Paco_2$ levels.
- Check for tube-feeding formula in pulmonary secretions by observing for blue food coloring.
- Use glucose oxidase reagent strips to detect presence of glucose in pulmonary secretions. Secretions with greater than 130 mg/dl of glucose are significant enough to discontinue the feedings.[15] NOTE: A false positive may be obtained if blood is present in the secretions.
- Monitor for a sudden onset of respiratory distress with intense coughing, dyspnea, and wheezing. This may indicate pulmonary aspiration.
- Assess breath sounds in all lung fields every hour and observe for the following clinical signs of aspiration pneumonia with no other obvious explanation: fever, restlessness, tachycardia, tachypnea, crackles and wheezing, frothy sputum, hypoxemia, and a new infiltrate on chest x-ray.
- Assess the cuff pressures of patients with artificial airways. Ensure that the cuff is inflated to minimum occlusion volume of 20 to 25 cm H_2O or 15 to 18 mm Hg.
- Monitor RQ for excess carbon dioxide production (RQ over 0.8).

Cardiovascular, Fluids, and Electrolytes

- Monitor vital signs every 4 hours. An orthostatic drop in the blood pressure of 15 mm Hg with an increase in the pulse of 15 beats indicates a deficit of intravascular water of 15%.
- Observe for physical signs and symptoms of electrolyte, water, vitamin, and trace element imbalances (see Table 15-6).
- Evaluate total fluid intake and output, noting 24-hour trends. Determine if patient is receiving adequate free water with tube feedings.
- Monitor serum electrolytes, blood glucose, urea nitrogen, creatinine, serum magnesium, phosphorus, calcium, liver function tests, and nitrogen balance.
- Check urine specific gravity and monitor blood sugar.
- Weigh the patient at the same time each day in patient gown with as few tubes present as possible. Empty drainage bags and remove bulky dressings if able. When interpreting weight changes, be aware that 1 liter of fluid equals approximately 1 kg (2 lbs), so excess fluids can be reflected in weight changes.

Gastrointestinal

- Assess feeding tube for slippage by recording and comparing length of tubing beyond nares insertion and every 8 hours. Mark the feeding tube with permanent ink at its exit site.
- Observe the position of the patient, ensuring that the head of the bed is elevated at a 30 to 40 degree angle and patient has been placed on the right side to facilitate passage of stomach contents through the pylorus and drainage of emesis.
- Evaluate patient's tolerance to rate, osmolality, and nutrient composition of formula.
- If the patient has a large-bore nasogastric (NG) tube, monitor the degree of gastric retention by checking for gastric residuals every 4 hours or at the beginning of each intermittent feeding. Ensure that the volume of aspirate does not exceed 50% of the previous feeding for intermittent feedings or 50% of the hourly infusion rate for continuous feedings.
- With small-bore tubes, assess for gastric retention by observing for distention, palpating for tautness of abdomen, and measuring abdominal girth every 8 hours. Measure the distance from one anterior iliac crest to the other; an increase of 8 to 10 cm (3 to 4 inches) above baseline should be considered significant.
- Assess for delayed gastric emptying by observing for anorexia, nausea, and vomiting and by noting an absence of bowel sounds.
- Auscultate bowel sounds in each of the four quadrants. If the patient is complaining of abdominal pain or cramping, auscultate that area last.[6,21]
- Assess for the presence of hyperactive bowel sounds, cramping, or diarrhea, which can be defined as the passage of greater than 4 bowel movements/day or a large (> 200 gm) liquid stool.

- Record the character, consistency, and number of stools per shift.
- Review the medications that the patient is on, evaluating those that can cause diarrhea or decreased mobility, and ensuring that they are properly diluted.
- Test gastric aspirate for pH level and presence of blood. If pH < 5.0, patient will need antacids or histamine H_2 blockers in addition to the enteral feeding.

Metabolic

- Repeat nutritional assessment every 7 to 10 days or as ordered.
- Determine patient's energy expenditure by indirect calorimetry with a metabolic cart or by using an appropriate formula, as ordered.
- Check calorie and protein count for 5 days, then once weekly, ensuring that patient is receiving adequate nutrition.
- Evaluate the feeding formula to ensure that the patient is receiving proper proportions and amounts of carbohydrate, fat, and protein, based on patient's nutritional assessment.
- Evaluate serum albumin, thyroxine-binding prealbumin, transferrin, and retinol binding protein weekly (if available). Transferrin can be calculated from total iron-binding capacity (TIBC) and is less costly.

Integumentary

- Assess patient's skin around tube entry sites for irritation and excoriation.
- Assess skin for signs of edema or dehydration (see Table 15-5).

Psychosocial

- Assess patient comfort, ensuring that tube is not uncomfortable or positioned to potentially cause harm.
- Determine if patient has a need to express feelings about changes in body image or inability to eat food orally.
- Assess patient's knowledge about the tube feedings.

NURSING DIAGNOSIS

Possible nursing diagnoses for patients receiving enteral feeding include the following:

- High risk for nutritonal deficit related to loss of consciousness secondary to head injury.
- Protein nutritional deficit related to protein loss secondary to frequent decubitus ulcers.
- Protein-calorie nutritional deficit related to anorexia secondary to chronic obstructive pulmonary disease (COPD).
- Combined protein-calorie nutritional deficit related to cancer cachexia combined with sepsis.
- Nutritional alteration—less than body requirements related to hypermetabolic demands secondary to trauma.

- High risk for pulmonary aspiration related to gastric atony secondary to hypovolemic shock.
- Decreased gastric motility related to paralytic ileus secondary to massive burn wounds.
- Potential for hyperactive bowel motility related to tube feeding administration.
- Fluid volume deficit related to diarrhea secondary to tube feeding.

PATIENT OUTCOMES

Sample patient outcomes include the following:
Patient evidences:

- Normal ABG values for patient with Pao_2 > 60 mm Hg and $Paco_2$ 35 to 45 mm Hg.
- Normal respiratory rate of 12 to 20 breaths/min with normal breath sounds.
- Normal tracheal breath sounds without evidence of tracheal cuff leak.
- Normal blood pressure for patient without orthostatic changes and heart rate (HR) < 100 beats/min.
- Normal serum electrolyte, glucose, urea nitrogen, creatinine, and liver function test values.
- Weight change of < 1 kg(0.5 lb)/24 hr or no change in weight.
- Urine output greater than 30 to 50 ml/hr and urine specific gravity of 1.003 to 1.030.
- Urine glucose of 2+ or less.
- Positive nitrogen state of 4 to 6 gm/24 hr for anabolism or nitrogen balance for the critical care patient.[32]
- Adequate protein and calorie count for nutritional needs (Table 15-1).
- Four or fewer bowel movements per day with at least one soft, guaiac negative formed stool every 2 days.
- Gastric residuals < 100 ml in continuous feedings and < 150 ml in intermittent feedings.
- Gastric aspirate pH < 5.0, guaiac negative.
- Less than 8 to 10 cm (3 to 4 inches) change in abdominal girth from baseline measurement.
- Normal temperature of 36° to 38° C (97 to 100.5° F) and white blood cell (WBC) count < 11,000 μl.
- Negative stool cultures.
- Clear, dry, intact skin of normal color around tube entry sites.
- Moist mucous membranes and normal skin turgor.
- Relaxed, calm posture with restful sleep.
- Patient expresses feelings about the loss of normal oral food intake and the need for home enteral nutrition.

ADMINISTRATION OF ENTERAL NUTRITION

Tube feedings are commonly administered by the following routes: orogastric, nasogastric, nasoenteric, or transpyloric (nasoduodenal and nasojejunal), and through tube enterostomy (gastrotomy, jejunostomy, esophagostomy, and pharyngotomy) (Fig. 16-2).

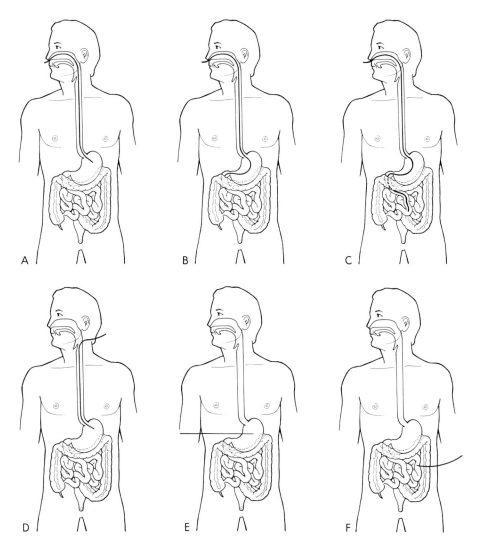

Fig. 16-2   Tube feeding routes may be surgical or nonsurgical. **A**, Nasogastric. **B**, Nasoduodenal. **C**, Nasojejunal. **D**, Esophagostomy. **E**, Gastrostomy. **F**, Jejunostomy.

The Orogastric and Nasogastric Route

Nutrients can be delivered directly into the stomach. The stomach has the advantage of reservoir capacity allowing intermittent feeding by bolus. The mixing and buffering of gastric acid by foods and the metering out of gastric contents into the small bowel minimizes GI symptoms, which sometimes occur with more distal infusion. Intragastric infusion must be undertaken with care in critically ill patients, since their stomachs may become atonic.

For patients alert enough to be fed safely by the nasogastric route, a small silicone rubber or polyurethane catheter can be passed through the nose into the stomach.

Intermittent Bolus Tube Feedings

Bolus tube feeding is the rapid delivery of formula by open syringe into a large-bore feeding tube. Generally a volume of about 350 ml of formula is given five to eight times daily, infused within a few minutes at each feeding.

Intermittent Gravity-Drip Tube Feedings

The intermittent slow gravity-drip delivery of NG tube feedings is a method by which the prescribed volume of formula (250 to 400 ml) is infused over a 20 to 30 minute period five to eight times per day.

Transpyloric (Nasoduodenal and Nasojejunal Routes)

Delivery of nutrients well down from the pylorus allows placement of three barriers between the food and the airway: the upper esophageal sphincter, the lower esophageal sphincter, and the pylorus (Fig. 16-3), thus reducing the chance of aspiration. Disadvantages of these tubes lie mainly in their small bores. Medication must be crushed or given in the liquid form. Frequent irrigation is essential to decrease the chance of occlusion. It is difficult to aspirate gastric or intestinal contents to determine accuracy of position or to measure residual feedings. Regurgitation back

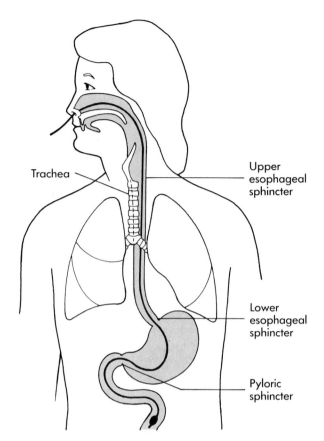

Fig. 16-3 The upper and lower esophogeal sphincters and the pyloric sphincter represent gates or barriers between the feeding site and the lungs. If these valves are competent, the feeding at the tube tip will be less likely to back up and enter the trachea.

into the stomach and into the esophagus can still occur, especially if the presence of a large-bore tube renders these sphincters incompetent. Also, critically ill patients tend to have gastric atony, which may delay or prevent passage of the tube beyond the pylorus. Nasoenteric feeding solutions are given as a continuous infusion with an infusion-control device, since the bolus administration of hyperosmolar solutions into the small intestine results in fluid and electrolyte shifts, abdominal distension, and diarrhea.

CONTINUOUS TUBE FEEDINGS BY ENTERAL FEEDING PUMP

Continuous feedings are most commonly used to deliver nutrients directly into the small intestine since it cannot tolerate bolus feedings and sudden rate changes. An advantage of continuous feeding is the decreased risk of distention and aspiration.

It is difficult to check gastric residuals, thereby making continuous feedings more dangerous in the high-risk patient who is not tolerating feedings. Continuous feedings are begun at full-strength at 25 ml/hr and gradually increased to up to 100% of the requirement. The rate of increase should be based on the residual volume or the development of diarrhea. A maximum rate of 200 ml/hr into

Skill 16-1   Administration of Intermittent Gravity-Drip Tube Feedings

EQUIPMENT AND SUPPLIES

- IV pole
- Enteral feeding container and tubing
- Feeding formula
- 50 or 60 ml syringe
- Nasogastric feeding tube or gastrostomy tube (already inserted)
- Cup of water
- Underpad
- Mild liquid soap
- Stethoscope

NURSING INTERVENTIONS

1. Wash hands. Obtain tube-feeding solution and plan to administer at either room temperature or cold (from refrigerator). If the patient has not been tolerating feedings, administer formula at room temperature.
2. Protect the gown with an underpad and position patient sitting upright or at a minimum angle of 30 degrees on the right side.[29]
3. Check for correct tube placement and amount of residual formula in stomach before each intermittent feeding.[23] Gently aspirate stomach contents with bulb or piston syringe. Withhold the feeding if the residual is greater than 50% of the previous feeding, or 150 ml, or subtract residual amount from feeding, as ordered. If patient continues to have large residuals (i.e., 50% of last feeding or 150 ml),[36] notify physician to evaluate for delayed gastric emptying.
4. Collect aspirated gastric contents in measuring container.
5. Reattach syringe barrel to NG or gastrostomy tube, and holding the tube at patient's head level, pour aspirated stomach contents into the syringe, back into stomach.
6. Prepare the feeding bag or bottle and tubing. Initiate feedings gradually, starting with 100 ml of formula for the first feeding and increasing up to 400 ml every 3 hours by the second day, or as ordered.
7. Adjust the rate of administration with the flow clamp, calculating the drip rate. Administer at rate of 5 to 10 ml/min, or as ordered.
8. Check gravity drip rate every 30 minutes.
9. Once the formula has infused, insert syringe into tip of feeding tube and pour in 30 ml water to clear the tubing.
10. Clamp the NG or gastrostomy tube by inserting cap into tip. Have patient remain in a sitting position for about 1 hour.
11. Wash feeding bag and tubing with dishwashing liquid and rinse well. Allow to dry and store in clean area until next feeding. In hospital setting, obtain new delivery system every 24 hours.

the jejunum may be achieved. The current trend in the initiation of tube feedings is to administer full-strength feedings at slower rates.[10,38] It has also been shown that mixing or diluting feedings represents an increased risk of contamination.[9,15] The intestine is sensitive to rate changes. A nurse should never speed up an enteral feeding to "catch up" after an interruption and should be cautious of letting accidental boluses of fluid enter the small intestine.

Skill 16-2   Insertion of Transpyloric Feeding Tube

EQUIPMENT AND SUPPLIES

- Small-bore nasoenteric tube
- Cup of water with straw
- 30 ml or larger piston syringe
- Tissues
- Water-soluble lubricant
- Towel or underpad
- Tape
- Emesis basin
- Stethoscope
- Gloves
- Penlight

NURSING INTERVENTIONS

1. Determine need for premedication. In those with suspected gastric atony, transpyloric passage of the tube can be facilitated by administering 20 mg of metoclopramide HCl intravenously 10 minutes before placing the tube.[22]
2. Explain procedure to patient. Ask if patient has ever broken nose or had nose surgery. Cover gown with towel or underpad and place in high Fowler's position. Do not have patient lean forward or extend the head and neck.
3. Place emesis basin and tissues in patient's lap.
4. Cut a 8-cm (3-inch) strip of 2.5-cm (1-inch)-wide tape. Split the tape lengthwise, leaving a small tab intact at one end. Stick the tape lightly on the patient's bed rail within reach.
5. Wash hands and wear gloves.
6. Examine nose for deformities or obstructions and ask if patient has a deviated septum. If so, plan to insert the tube through the other nostril.
7. Remove tube witn preinserted stylet from package, if tube has stylet (see Fig. 16-3).
8. Place the exit port of the tube at the tip of the nose. Extend the tube to the earlobe and then from the earlobe to the base of the xiphoid process. Total these measurements and mark this length around the tube with a pen (Fig. 16-4). For tubes destined for the duodenum or jejunum (transpyloric), add 23 cm (9 inches). The prestamped marks on the tube can also be used for a reference.
9. Flush tube through stylet hub (if appropriate) using 10 ml water. This will aid stylet removal after insertion is complete. During insertion, make sure stylet hub stays firmly anchored in tube connector.
10. Lubricate the first 15 cm (6 inches) of the tube with a water-soluble lubricant. If the tip is prelubricated, activate lubricant by dipping end in water.
11. Encourage the alert patient to hold the cup of water with a straw. Tell patient when to swallow the water. Advance the tube when the patient swallows the water.
12. Place nondominant hand gently on the patient's forehead to stabilize the head.
13. Using the dominant hand, insert the feeding tube into the patient's nostril, directing it posteriorly, aiming the tip parallel to the nasal septum.
14. As the tube approaches the nasopharynx, rotate it inward toward the other nostril. If patient has an ET tube, be careful not to let it guide the feeding tube into the trachea.
15. Gently insert 25 cm (10 inches) of the tube. This will bring the tip of the tube to about the level of the carina if the tube is inadvertently placed within the trachea.[23,29]
16. Listen for sounds of air exchange at the free end of the tube.
17. If no signs of respiratory air exchange are evident, insert another 30 to 40 cm (12 to 15 inches) of tube with the stylet.
18. Instruct the alert patient to move head forward so that chin touches chest, to bring the straw to the mouth, and to swallow the water. This will close the trachea and open the esophagus.
19. As the tube is advanced, continue to tell the patient to swallow. Observe for cyanosis, coughing, or gagging, indicating that the tube might be in the trachea. If the patient gags, check the back of the throat with a penlight for coiling of the tube in the throat or mouth. If the tube is coiled, withdraw it slightly until it is straight again; then continue with procedure.
20. Continue inserting tube until the premeasured mark is reached.
21. Insert piston syringe into end of tube. Place stethoscope over patient's left upper abdominal quadrant. While injecting 10 to 20 ml air into the tube, listen for air entering the stomach. This may not be a reliable assessment procedure because bubbling in the pleural space can produce a sound similar to that of the stomach.[29]
22. Attempt to aspirate gastric fluid, withdrawing plunger slowly. If you cannot aspirate gastric fluid, the tube may be in the patient's bronchus,[23] pressed against the stomach wall, curled in the stomach, not inserted far enough, or in the duodenum.
23. Test the aspirated gastric contents for pH measurement. If the pH is 3 or less, the sample is, in fact, gastric.[29]
24. Remove stylet if still in place.
25. Tape tube loosely to cheek, leaving a loop of about 10 to 15 cm (4 to 6 inches) between nose and tape on forehead. Transparent film dressing can be used instead of adhesive tape (Fig. 16-5).
26. Position patient on right side with head of bed elevated for 4 hours. This facilitates passage of tube through pylorus.
27. Confirm position of tube by portable x-ray. Be sure to indicate on x-ray slip that feeding tube has been inserted.
28. If tube has to be reinserted, remove tube, and reinsert stylet. Check stylet and do not use if it is bent. Never reinsert stylet when the feeding tube is in the patient.
29. If repeated attempts of tube insertion prove unsuccessful, the patient's anatomy may be abnormal, and the tube will need to be placed under laryngoscopic or fluoroscopic guidance.

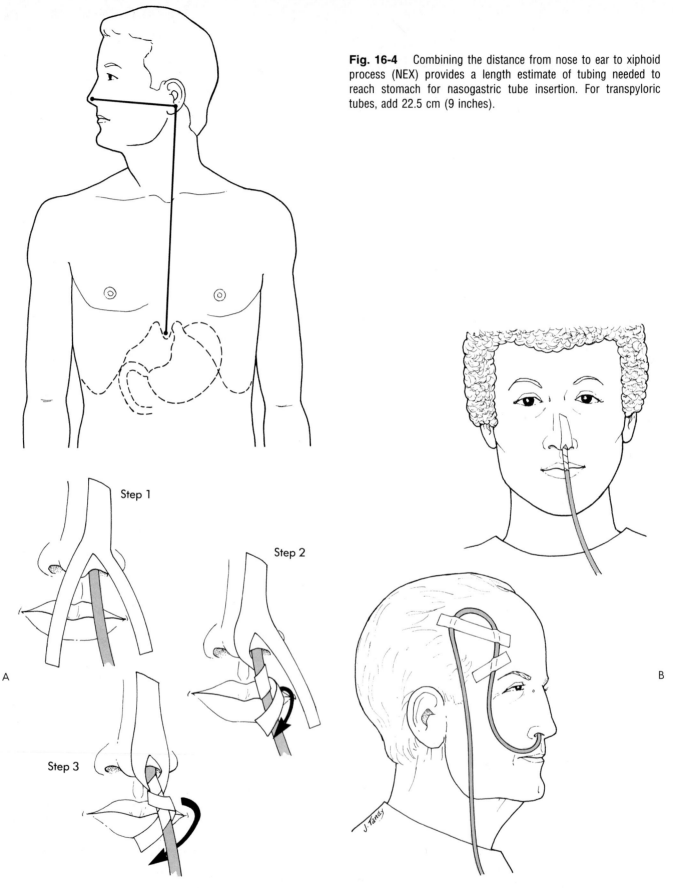

Fig. 16-4 Combining the distance from nose to ear to xiphoid process (NEX) provides a length estimate of tubing needed to reach stomach for nasogastric tube insertion. For transpyloric tubes, add 22.5 cm (9 inches).

Step 1

Step 2

Step 3

A

B

Fig. 16-5 **A,** To tape the nasogastric tube to the nose: 1) Split one half of the tape into the two tails. 2) Place the broad tab on the patient's nose and wrap one tail around the feeding tube. 3) Wrap the other tail around the tube in the opposite direction. **B,** Small bore nasogastric tubes may be taped to the forehead to allow access to the mouth and to keep the tube out of the patient's line of vision.

Skill 16-3 Administration of Continuous Tube Feedings by Enteral Feeding Pump

EQUIPMENT AND SUPPLIES

- Enteral feeding pump and pole
- Feeding formula
- Enteral nutrition infusion system (container and tubing)
- Blue food coloring according to agency policy
- 50 ml Luer-Lok syringe
- Mild liquid soap
- Small bore enteral feeding tube (in place)
- Stethoscope

NURSING INTERVENTIONS

1. If administering nasogastric feeding, place patient upright at a minimum of a 30 degree angle. For transpyloric feedings the patient may be placed in varied positions, depending on the risk of aspiration.
2. If patient has cuffed tracheostomy, deflate cuff only as much as necessary to prevent tracheal ischemia.
3. Wash hands and prepare formula aseptically in clean utility area. Currently there are prefilled, prepackaged, and ready to hang formula feedings that do not require preparation.
4. Shake the can or bottle well to mix the solution thoroughly.
5. Wipe can top and opener before opening can of ready-to-use container.
6. If not using entire amount of formula, cover can, label with patient's name and time and date opened, and place in refrigerator. The unused portion of any feeding that is in an opened can or has been made or mixed in the institution should be discarded within 24 hours.
7. Obtain new or clean feeding administration tubing and container and fill flask with enough formula to last no longer than 8 hours. If diluting formula with water, use sterile water in patients whose immune systems are compromised. These individuals may be less capable of overcoming large amounts of bacteria introduced into the GI system.[28]

8. Add 3 drops of blue food coloring into formula and shake well according to agency protocol. This helps to distinguish tube feeding lines from IV lines and helps to determine aspiration.
9. Add a time tape to the container and a label with the patient's name, name of formula, flow rate, date, and time.
10. Hang container, remove protective cap from end of tubing, squeeze drip chamber, slowly open clamp, and fill entire tubing with fluid.
11. Attach feeding line to feeding tube and connect to pump.
12. Set desired flow rate in ml/hr.
13. Open control clamp and start pump.
14. Proceed with feeding and observe for nausea, vomiting, cramping, diarrhea, and abdominal distention.
15. Check for placement and irrigate feeding tube with water or other irrigants every 4 hours to reduce accumulation of feedings within the tube. When a patient is first begun on tube feedings, check residuals frequently and hold feeding if residuals are more than twice the hourly infusion rate. Replace residual. Stop the feeding for 2 hours; recheck residual. In 2 hours, if residual is still large, notify physician. A large bore NG tube may be placed to monitor residuals. Gastric residual should be checked if the patient is distended, in pain, regurgitating, or vomiting.
16. If the feeding is temporarily discontinued, flush the tubing with 10 to 20 ml of water, using a 50 ml or larger syringe.
17. Once the feeding system is closed, it should not be reopened. New formula should never be added to formula already hanging in the system.
18. When administration of the formula is completed, carefully clean the container and tubing with liquid soap and water and rinse. Add enough formula to last for another 8 hours.
19. Within the hospital setting, hang a new enteral feeding infusion system every 24 hours.[28]
20. Provide oral and nasal hygiene every 8 hours.

IRRIGATION OF FEEDING TUBES

Occlusion of tubes results when the large proteins, sodium, calcium caseinate, or medications settle in the horizontal portions of the tube. Clogged tubes that occur during continuous feedings can be prevented by flushing with 30 to 50 ml tap water or other irrigants every 4 to 8 hours, based on fluid restrictions, whenever the feeding is interrupted and after the addition of medication. For immunosuppressed patients, such as those with AIDS, sterile water should be used in place of tap water.[28] Tubes should be irrigated before and after measuring for stomach residuals because the gastric acid brought up through the tube will cause precipitation of the formula. Current research has shown that the best substances for declogging small-bore feeding tubes are papain and distilled water.[26] Water used for flushing the tube should always be recorded on the patient's intake and output sheet, as it will need to be computed as part of the free water intake.

TUBE ENTEROSTOMIES

Tube enterostomy is the percutaneous or operative placement of a tube or catheter into any segment of the GI tract from the esophagus to the colon. Tubes specifically intended for delivery of nutrient preparations are generally placed in the stomach, jejunum, or cervical esophagus. Placement of a feeding enterostomy should be considered in the following situations:

- Patient has an inadequate oral intake and a functional GI tract.
- Enteral feeding is expected to exceed 4 weeks.
- Patient tolerance of nasoenteric tubes is poor.
- Nasal intubation of the GI tract is impossible.
- Patient experiences recurrent aspiration with nasogastric tube.

Patient conditions requiring tube enterostomy include the following: tumors of the oropharynx, esophagus, or stomach; central neurological disorders (e.g., multiple scle-

Skill 16-4   Administration of Medications by Enteral Feeding Tube

EQUIPMENT AND SUPPLIES

- 50-60 ml syringe
- 30 ml medication cup
- Cup of water
- Mortar and pestle
- Medications
- Stethoscope
- Underpad
- Extra cup

NURSING INTERVENTIONS

1. Request liquid form of medication from pharmacy. Avoid administering syrups and liquid medications with a pH value of 5.0 or less.[20] Acidic formulations cause immediate clumping of formula, including increased viscosity, particle size, and tackiness, leading to clogging of feeding tubes. Provide comparable elixirs and suspensions as viable alternatives.
2. Never add the medication to the enteral feeding, as this cannot guarantee that the patient will get the whole dose. Medications will also increase the osmolality, leading to GI irritation and diarrhea. In infants, a high osmolality could result in enterocolitis. Potassium and iron preparations are incompatible when mixed in the bag with enteral formulas and may cause feeding tube occlusion.
3. Use caution when administering antacids to patients on high-protein tube feedings, as a gelatinous mass can form.[17] Instead, ranitidine can be given as ordered to block gastric acid secretion.
4. Give medications at the proper time, based on whether or not they can be given when feeding is in the stomach. Most drugs are absorbed 1 hour before or 2 hours after a meal.
5. Flush the feeding tube and clamp it for 2 hours before and 2 hours after administering phenytoin.[30] The patient's feeding will have to be increased to take into account the loss of nutrients.
6. Check medication order and obtain medication. Wash hands and prepare the medication. Measure and pour liquid medication into 30 ml medication cup. Drugs that are hypertonic (i.e., dexamethasone) or irritating to the gastric mucosa (i.e., potassium chloride and indomethacin) should be diluted in at least 30 ml of water. Open capsules and finely crush tablets; then place them to dissolve in warm water in medication cup. Do not crush enteric-coated or sustained-release drugs.
7. Using three-way stopcock, if available, attach syringe and check placement of tube. Use 50 to 60 ml syringe.
8. Remove plunger and attach syringe to feeding tube or stopcock. A stopcock will provide for easier access to small bore tubes and decreases the risk of contamination of the system.
9. Pour or gently inject 30 ml water down tube to rinse out feeding.
10. Administer each drug separately, flushing the tube with 5 ml water between each medication. Do not mix medications together.
11. For large-bore tubes, let the medication flow by gravity drip. For small-bore tubes, apply gentle pressure with the plunger while shaking the syringe to keep particles from settling out of solution.
12. Rinse feeding tube with 30 ml water and either plug tube or reconnect to continuous feeding.
13. Record amount of free water given.

rosis and cerebral vascular accidents); and primary muscular dysfunction interfering with swallowing and preventing oral intake.

GASTROSTOMY

A *gastrostomy* is a surgical opening from the abdominal wall to the stomach. Types of gastrostomies in common use for many years are the Stamm, Witzel, and Janeway. In 1980, an alternative to operative gastrostomy was developed—percutaneous endoscopic gastrostomy (PEG) (Fig. 16-6). This procedure has greatly contributed to the advancement of enteral nutrition because it does not require general anesthesia or laparotomy.[36] Gastrostomy feedings should not

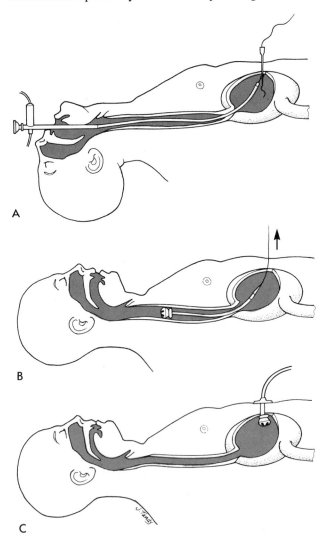

Fig. 16-6   Percutaneous gastrostomy (PEG). **A,** A catheter is insetrted through the abdominal wall into the stomach, and the stylet is removed. A silk suture is passed through the catheter into the stomach. Using the gastroscope, the suture is withdrawn through the patient's mouth. **B,** A "mushroom" catheter, which will serve as the gastrostomy tube, is pulled downward in a retrograde fashion through the esophagus and stomach and out through the abdominal wall. **C,** The gastroscope is then used to anchor the mushroom catheter and bumper firmly against the gastric wall. A second rubber bumper is positioned on the gastrostomy where it emerges from the abdominal wall.

▼

Complications Associated with Feeding Gastrostomies and Jejunostomies

GASTROSTOMY

Hemorrhage
Occlusion of tube
Displacement with gastric outlet obstruction from balloon
Migration of tube into duodenum with partial or complete obstruction
Leakage of contents intraperitoneally with peritonitis
Gastric distension
Esophageal reflux
Aspiration
Skin irritation and excoriation
Persistent fistula after tube removal
Premature or delayed closure of the stoma

JEJUNOSTOMY

Hemorrhage
Inadvertent removal or dislodgement
Intestinal obstruction from balloon with pressure necrosis of small bowel
Volvulus (twisting of bowel)
Leakage of contents into peritoneum
Occlusion of tube
Skin irritation and excoriation
Infection related to skin excoriation
Dumping syndrome
Diarrhea

be used in patients without a gag reflex, with gastric atony, gastric outlet obstruction, or gastroesophageal reflux. The feedings can be administered as bolus, continuous, or intermittent gravity drip feedings. There are many complications related to gastrostomies (see box above).

JEJUNOSTOMY

Surgeons may place feeding jejunostomy tubes following selected abdominal surgical procedures and multiple trauma.[31] These tubes enter through surgical openings from the abdominal wall into the jejunum. If feedings are to be started immediately after surgery, the jejunum is preferred. The jejunal route of access permits simultaneous gastric decompression with a nasogastric tube and intrajejunal feeding, allowing enteral nutrition in postoperative patients who would otherwise not be fed or would be receiving TPN. In as little as 8 to 24 hours after surgery, the jejunum returns to normal motility and absorptive capabilities. Jejunostomies are also performed as a primary procedure in patients who require enteral feeding for more than 6 weeks and in those for whom intragastric feeding is contraindicated. If there is symptomatic esophageal reflux, inability to protect the airway from aspiration, ulcerative or neoplastic disease of the stomach, or impaired gastric emptying, a jejunostomy is preferable to a gastrostomy. Jejunostomies have a few complications to be aware of (see the box above). Leakage of the jejunal feedings or intestinal secretions onto the skin of the abdomen is uncommon,

Skill 16-5   Gastrostomy Tube Dressing Change

▼

EQUIPMENT AND SUPPLIES

- Skin barrier: Karaya wafer, Stomahesive, or Sur-Fit wafer
- Convex insert
- Baby bottle nipple (red premature nipple for infants)
- Foley catheter (already inserted into stoma)
- Scissors
- Hemostat
- Cotton-tipped applicator
- Gloves
- Skin-prep wipe (or tincture of benzoin)
- Water-soluble lubricant
- Half-strength hydrogen peroxide
- Adhesive tape
- Paper tape

NURSING INTERVENTIONS

1. Wash hands, wear gloves, and remove old dressing.
2. Observe skin at abdominal tube exit site for redness or irritation from leaking gastric contents. Measure tube length to determine if it has gotten longer, indicating displacement out of stomach.
3. If tube slips out of the stoma, reinsert a new tube within 4 hours.
4. Cut a hole in the Stomahesive wafer ⅛ inch larger than the insertion site of the gastrostomy tube.
5. Pull the gastrostomy tube through the wafer, remove the paper backing, and apply the wafer to the skin.
6. Cut off the end of the baby bottle nipple and pull the tube through the nipple with the use of a hemostat and water-soluble lubricant.
7. Anchor the nipple to the wafer with the convex insert or adhesive tape. The nipple stabilizes the tube and eliminates irritation around the site.
8. Coat the skin bordering the wafer with a protective liquid dressing.
9. Tape wafer to skin by framing with paper tape, if desired.
10. Stabilize tube against dressing with paper tape.
11. Plan to change the wafer every week or more frequently, if necessary.
12. Every day cleanse area around the tube with ¼% to ½% hydrogen peroxide by slipping a cotton-tipped applicator down through the top of the nipple along the side of the gastrostomy tube[1] and being careful not to poke it into the tract.
13. If desired, slide nipple upward and cleanse area while viewing skin around insertion site.
14. To avoid trapping of secretions, do not use this nipple dressing if there is copious drainage around the tube. Instead, place a gauze dressing over the top of the wafer and secure with paper tape.

and if it does occur, skin excoriation is unusual. Dumping symptoms and explosive diarrhea are also rare. Jejunal intubation can be performed nonoperatively by conversion of an established gastrostomy to a feeding jejunostomy. A feeding tube is passed through the gastrostomy opening and threaded into the jejunum. The newest method of providing for jejunal intubation is through a percutaneous puncture of the stomach under endoscopic or radiographic guidance and PEG. This new procedure obviates the need for a laparotomy and general anesthesia. A jejunal catheter

Skill 16-6   Administration of Infant Gastrostomy Tube Feeding

▼

EQUIPMENT AND SUPPLIES

- 20 ml or larger catheter-tipped syringe
- Feeding formula
- Measuring cup
- Cup of water
- Tape measure
- Gauze and safety pin
- Pacifier
- Clamp
- Stethoscope

NURSING INTERVENTIONS

1. Identify the infant and communicate verbally and by touch.
2. When gastrostomy tube is first inserted, measure length of tube and repeat every 8 hours. This determines whether or not the tube has slipped into the stomach or become dislodged. Obstruction of the pylorus or duodenum may result from migration of the Foley balloon by peristalsis.
3. Measure abdominal girth at same site each shift to check for abdominal distention.
4. Change gastrostomy dressing every 3 days or more frequently as needed. Observe for skin breakdown around tube entry site. If there is an extensive amount of greenish, foul-smelling drainage, redness, swelling, or excoriation, notify physician.
5. Check for tube placement and length and amount of residual before each feeding.
6. Attach barrel of syringe to gastrostomy tube and hang it no higher than the level of the infant's head by pinning syringe to gauze strip strung over crib. If the nurse is holding infant during feeding, the syringe may be pinned to the nurse's garment. Leave gastrostomy tube open to the atmosphere to permit the escape of air, excess formula, or secretions. Change syringe every 8 hours to prevent bacterial growth.
7. In preparation for feeding, place infant on the right side, upright in an infant seat, or hold to prevent aspiration of formula.
8. Assess for residuals by observing fluid left in the suspended syringe. Never aspirate to check for residuals as suction may irritate the lining of the stomach wall. If there has been a backup of stomach contents into the syringe since the last feeding, refeed.
9. Administer formula based on amount of residual, or as ordered.
10. Administer feeding at room temperature and allow to flow in over 15 to 30 minutes, refilling syringe before it empties so as to prevent air from being forced in.
11. Provide pacifier during feeding and then provide for burping of infant to relieve distension from swallowed air.
12. If the formula is pushed back up into the syringe between feedings by the infant's crying or tensing of abdominal muscles, milk the tube to restart the flow of feeding.
13. Irrigate the tube only if it appears to be plugged, or on specific medical instructions. Use 2 to 3 ml of normal saline under low pressure.
14. Encourage parents to touch, talk to, and hold their infant.
15. Teach parents to assume more of infant's care as they become more comfortable.

is inserted through an abdominal puncture site and is guided by gastroscopy to its position within the jejunum.

At present there is available a gastrostomy-jejunal feeding tube that allows simultaneous access to the stomach and jejunum. This tube permits gastric decompression while feeding into the jejunum and also provides an easy route for administration of crushed medication through the gastric lumen. Its major advantage in patients at risk for aspiration or those who have had gastric or esophageal surgery is the ability to use the gastric port as a vent even while feeding into the small bowel.

ORAL SUPPLEMENTS

The provision of oral supplements in enteral nutrition is important in burn, trauma, and cancer critical care stepdown units. A burn or trauma patient using 5000 to 6000 kcal/24 hr will not be able to eat the amount of food needed to meet the daily caloric and protein needs. It is also important not to change patients' eating patterns, because overeating is a difficult behavior to modify once the patient has healed.

PATIENT AND FAMILY TEACHING

Before discharge, the patient or caregiver should be able to do the following:

- Discuss clean technique and bacterial contamination.
- Describe formula storage.
- Perform self-intubation of the nasogastric feeding tube, if appropriate.
- Demonstrate reinsertion of balloon-tipped Foley tube and dressing change technique, if on gastrostomy feedings.
- Check for residuals.
- Irrigate feeding tube.
- Prepare formula for administration.
- Administer formula through continuous or bolus feeding method.

Table 16-2   Daily Maintenance Fluid and Caloric Requirements for Pediatric Patients

Body weight	Fluids required per day	Baseline calories required per day
1-10 kg	100 ml/kg	100 calorie kg/24 hr
11-20	1000 ml + 50 ml/kg over 10 kg	1000 + 50 calories for each kg over 10 kg
Over 20 kg	1500 ml + 20 ml/kg over 20 kg	1500 + 20 calories for each kg over 20 kg

```
 ▼
     Pediatric Conditions in Which Enteral Tube
     Feeding May Be Indicated
```

PULMONARY

Cystic fibrosis
Bronchopulmonary
   dysplasia

NEUROLGICAL

Coma
Severe mental retardation
Dysphagia secondary to
   cranial nerve dysfunc-
   tion, muscular dystro-
   phies, or myasthenia
   gravis

GASTROINTESTINAL

Inflammatory bowel
   disease
Short-bowel syndrome
Pseudo obstruction
Glycogen storage disease
   type I
Chronic liver disease
Gastrointestinal surgery

RENAL

Chronic renal disease
Acute renal failure

CANCER AND AIDS

Terminal support care
Gastrointestinal side ef-
   fects of chemotherapy
   or radiotherapy

OTHER

Anorexia nervosa or
   bulimia
Cardiac cachexia
Multiple trauma
Burns

• Demonstrate measurement and administration of liquid medications through feeding tube.
• Demonstrate cleansing and maintenance of feeding
  equipment.
• Discuss the potential complications of tube feedings
  and actions to take.

PEDIATRIC CONSIDERATIONS
Nonnutritive Sucking and Oral Feeding

Tube fed infants often miss oral development. If the
sucking is not stimulated, it may be diminished or lost. The
normal infant learns independence when crying to signal
hunger, sucking to receive nutrition, and finishing sucking
when satisfied. A child's later learning ability comes from
having been rewarded for active, feeding-oriented behavior. Tube feedings may create passive dependence. When
infants are tube fed, they should be offered a pacifier. If
the baby is able to swallow, a piece of gauze dipped in water or milk and placed in the nipple can be used to provide
flavor and opportunity for swallowing. This nonnutritive
sucking results in stimulation of lingual and gastric lipase,
greater weight gain, and earlier nipple feedings.[7] Infants
with esophageal fistulas can be placed on "sham" oral
feedings and gastrostomy feedings simultaneously; whereby, they receive formula through a nipple and the formula
drains through the fistula.

Infants should be held in the typical eye-to-eye feeding
position and spoken to, rocked, cuddled, and burped during
tube feedings. Tube fed infants need to experience the
same types of stimulation that occur during normal feedings including the following: oral-tactile stimulation, visual
stimulation from the caregiver's face, deep tactile body
stimulation, and auditory stimulation.

There is a period in an infant's development when the
sucking reflex diminishes and oral feeding becomes a
learned rather than a reflex behavior. Infants totally deprived of oral feedings during this time may subsequently
refuse to eat and will reject food placed in the mouth. This
feeding disorder requires many months to resolve and may
be prevented by providing small oral feedings even when
the feedings are not of much nutritional significance.[24]

Children and Adolescents

Children and adolescents occasionally have to receive
enteral feeding as a result of conditions in which they will
not or cannot eat or should limit or exclude eating Nutritional support regimens must take into account not only
the child's basal and activity requirements but also requirements for growth. Children have greater caloric requirements for their weight than do adults. Normal requirements
in an adult are approximately 30 to 40 kcal/kg/24 hr, depending on activity. The healthy child has caloric requirements as listed in Table 16-2.

In a child with fever, a caloric increase of 10% is
needed for each degree Fahrenheit of temperature elevation to prevent weight loss. Children have a higher percentage of body water than do adults and so will have different fluid requirements (Table 16-2). Only 60% of
adults' body weight is water; whereas 70% to 80% of children's body weight is water. Children also have a larger
body surface area per mass than adults, resulting in a
larger insensible water loss and higher metabolic rate. Another difference is in renal function, with children less than
3 years old having a significantly lower glomerular filtration rate. The child will have more difficulty concentrating
urine than will the adult.

For the older child, the feeding time should be as normal as possible. Once the child goes home, the child
should be fed when other family members eat. Feeding
schedules should be matched to the usual times that children of a particular age group eat. Throughout a child's
hospitalization the child should be allowed to maintain activities, such as sitting, crawling, and walking while the
nurse ensures that the child's tube is not dislodged. Adolescents receiving tube feedings often have problems of alteration in body image, loss of control of normal life-style,
and fear of nonacceptance by peers. They should be encouraged to remain as active as possible and to participate
in decision making. The nurse must be nonthreatening and
nonjudgmental when caring for this age group.

Assessment

A nutritional screening form (Fig. 16-8) is useful when
assessing children at nutritional risk.

Criteria to evaluate throughout an infant's enteral feeding program, include the following:

- Growth data—serial measurements of weight, length, and head circumference. Daily weights also help to determine if the caloric and fluid intakes are excessive or insufficient.
- Intake and output records.
- Serum calcium, phosphorus, alkaline phosphatase, sodium, potassium, and blood urea nitrogen (BUN) levels.
- Vital signs—changes in pulse and respiratory rates and blood pressure might indicate dehydration, fluid overload, aspiration, or febrile episodes caused by bacterial contamination of the formula.
- Signs of feeding intolerance—spitting, vomiting, diarrhea, abdominal distension, abdominal discomfort, gastric reflux and residuals, guaiac positive stools, excess stool fat or carbohydrate, and glucosuria.

Feeding Methods

As soon as is safely possible, enteral feedings should be started. If they cannot be started by day 3 to day 5 of life,

TPN will have to be initiated. Infants receiving mechanical ventilation are not fed enterally. They are, however, fed while still on oxygen. Their first feedings are generally glucose water or sterile water. Initial formula feedings are dilute, then gradually increased, with alternating changes in volume and concentration. Close observation of pediatric patients is required because they may have difficulty adapting to minor formula changes. If the infusion is interrupted during continuous feedings, the nurse should not try to replace the lost fluid by increasing the infusion rate. The gut may respond to rate changes with profuse diarrhea and hyperglycemic episodes.

In the pediatric setting, common feeding routes and methods include giving feedings as follows:

1. On an intermittent schedule:
   - Insertion and removal after feeding of an orogastric (mouth-to-stomach) or nasogastric tube.
   - Indwelling nasogastric tube.
   - Feeding gastrostomy tube.
2. Continuous feeding using an enteral pump:

Nutritional screening

Patient's name: _____ Room: _____ Date: _____
Age: _____ Dx: _____ MD: _____
Height: _____ Percentile: _____ Weight: _____ Percentile: _____

Check conditions present in patient

Physical status
_____ Severely underweight (< 5% for wt. or > 25% difference between height & weight)
_____ Obesity (> 20% over normal weight for age/height)
_____ Recent weight loss of 10% or more of usual body weight (week to one month)
_____ Brittle hair and nails; skin changes (edema, parchment, turgor)

Low caloric/protein/nutrient intake
_____ NPO for more than 3 days (in hospital)
_____ Hypocaloric IV fluids or clear liquid diet for more than 3 days (in hospital or at home)
_____ Food rejection (for 3 days or more, in hospital or at home)

Prolonged nutrient loss
_____ Chronic emesis/diarrhea (3 days or more, in hospital or at home)
_____ Malabsorption
_____ Gastrointestinal disorder

Increased metabolic needs
_____ Persistent fever (> 100.4 PO or 101.4 R for > 3 days)
_____ Trauma (car accident, major surgery)

Drug therapy
_____ Cancer chemotherapy   _____ Steroids

Laboratory data
_____ Albumin < 3.8   _____ Total protein < 6.0
_____ Anemia, type _____
Comments: _____
_____
                    Signature _____

Dear Physician:
   Considering the patient's current medical/physical condition and its effect on his/her nutritional status, please check one of the following:
☐ A nutrition consult will not be required at this time.
☐ A nutrition consult will be needed as soon as possible.
☐ I would like the nutritional support team to follow this patient.

   Signature: _____ Date: _____

Fig. 16-8   This nutritional screening form can be used to assess children at nutritional risk. (From Bavin R, Peck M: Nutritional assessment of the hospitalized child, *Nutritional Support Services*, Nov 1985.)

- Indwelling nasogastric, nasoduodenal, or nasojejunal tube.
- Needle-catheter jejunostomy.

Once an infant who requires tube feedings develops the gag reflex, the child will tolerate nasogastric feedings better than orogastric ones. An infant's gag reflex and coordinated suck-swallow-breathe pattern appears around 32 to 34 weeks. At this age breast or nipple feedings may be started if the infant's:

- Respirations are less than 60 breaths/min.
- GI tract is intact.
- Neurological system is intact.
- Mentation is alert and vigorous.

Intragastric tube feedings

Intragastric tube feeding is the most common type of tube feeding for low birth weight (LBW) infants. The American Academy of Pediatrics recommends that intermittent intragastric feedings be used as the method of first choice in LBW infants.[37] Other indications for intragastric tube feedings include major burns, hypermetabolic states, refusal to eat, and short-term diarrhea. Gastric tubes are easier to place than transpyloric tubes and are less liable to cause perforation. Placement of formula directly into the stomach also allows for enhanced digestion of nutrients caused by the action of gastric juices, tolerance of larger osmotic loads, and lower likelihood of dumping syndrome. Infants who are extremely premature and those with delayed gastric emptying, severe gastroesophageal reflux, or severe respiratory distress may not tolerate intermittent gastric feedings well. One of the problems with intermittent gastric feeding is that vagal stimulation may occur with frequent insertion and removal of feeding tubes. This can increase the frequency of bradycardia and apnea in premature neonates. Continuous gastric feedings have a higher incidence of aspiration than intermittent feedings. They are preferred, though, for feeding neonates with short-bowel syndrome or other gastrointestinal diseases.

Transpyloric feedings

When other more traditional methods fail, transpyloric feedings are used. They are always administered as continual feedings. Smaller infants may tolerate continuous feedings better than intermittent ones. Infants experiencing continued gastric residuals, gastroesophageal reflux and aspiration, serious bradycardia and apnea with the passage of a gavage tube, persistent respiratory distress, or those on prolonged mechanical ventilation may benefit from this feeding method. Transpyloric feedings are used for infants receiving nasal continuous positive airway pressure (CPAP) where the stomach may be distended, and for those who are comatose or have a depressed gag reflex. This method is used for infants who have congenital gastrointestinal anomalies and after upper GI surgery. The advantages include the following:

- Ability to deliver a greater quantity of calories without danger of gastric distention.

- Decreased chance of aspiration.
- Increased weight gain as compared to intragastric feedings.

Disadvantages include the possibility of intestinal perforation, bypassing of the stomach's antiinfective mechanisms, bacterial overgrowth of the upper intestine, and susceptibility to dumping syndrome and diarrhea. During continuous infusions, human milk may have significant fat loss and LBW formulas have significant mineral loss. So nutrient loss is another disadvantage of this method. Jejunal tubes will require predigested formulas that have greater osmolality. Hyperosmolality can be dangerous in premature infants because it may lead to necrotizing enterocolitis.

Gastrostomy tube feedings

Gastrostomy tube feedings are reserved for infants who require extensive prolonged tube feeding for longer than 8 weeks or for those undergoing major GI surgery with the expectation of prolonged feedings. Gastrostomy is usually preferable to jejunostomy because many important phases of digestion may be bypassed when feedings are administered directly into the jejunum. Jejunostomy feedings also require a continual drip to prevent cramps and diarrhea. Gastrostomies allow for necessary nose breathing of infants, preserve the competency of the esophageal-cardiac sphincter, and are more comfortable than nasogastric tubes. Indications for gastrostomy tube feedings include the following[21]:

- Inability to suck or swallow.
- Congenital anomalies, such as esophageal atresia, tracheoesophageal fistula, and some types of cleft palate.
- Esophageal injury with obstruction or oral and esophageal burns.
- Head injury, multiple trauma, or long-term coma.
- Hypermetabolic states as in cardiac and severe respiratory disease.
- Home feeding management when parents are unable to follow nasogastric feeding regimens.

PSYCHOSOCIAL CONSIDERATIONS

Being deprived of food, liquids, and chewing, and having an unsatisfied appetite for certain foods are common distressing experiences of patients on enteral tube feeding. Also common is the experience of being deprived of socializing while eating. Whenever possible, patient preferences should be incorporated into the feeding schedule to increase the patients' feelings of control and participation in their care. Body-image disturbances can also result from the presence of a feeding tube or catheter. Many people on long-term feedings prefer enterostomy tubes that can be concealed underneath clothing. Others can be taught self-intubation for intermittent or nocturnal continuous home infusions.

Food habits are among the oldest and most entrenched aspects of many cultures. They exert deep influence on the behavior of people. A person's cultural background determines what will be eaten as well as when and how it will be eaten. Food is a symbol of sociability, warmth, friendliness, and social acceptance. Patients on tube feedings at home, tend to have fewer social relationships and activities. The inability to join with others for food at social gatherings contributes to the disengagement from social activities by the patients. Guilt feelings may be expressed by family members about eating in front of tube-fed individuals. Some home enteral nutrition (HEN) patients make their own tube feedings more of a meal than just a procedure. They blenderize food that has been prepared for the family and use that as their feeding.

HOME HEALTH CARE CONSIDERATIONS

Home health care is frequently more satisfying to the family and patient since most people would rather be at home than in the hospital setting. The most common diagnoses for HEN patients are the following: malignancy, neurological disorders of swallowing, metabolic disorders leading to nonmalignant fistulas and growth failure in inflammatory bowel disease,[13] and AIDS.

Selection of Feeding Method

The newest device for long-term gastrostomy management is the feeding gastrostomy button. This silicone device is inserted into the tract formed by the gastrostomy tube. The button is nearly flush with the skin, making it ideal for active patients. Patients may also be fed at home through a needle-catheter jejunostomy for short-term problems, or through the K-tube jejunostomy feeding tube. Another option is to daily reinsert an NG tube (e.g., 6 or 8 Fr enteric feeding tube) and administer either daytime bolus feedings or continuous nocturnal nasogastric feedings. If the patient can tolerate them, daytime bolus feedings are usually the easiest to administer. To receive continuous feedings, the patient will need an expensive enteral feeding pump with a programmable alarm system. Nocturnal feedings are often used for children who require HEN.[3] They receive feedings through a small bore nasogastric tube for 10 to 13 hours at night. The tube is then removed and they may be fed orally during the day, if possible.

Skill 16-7 Maintenance and Administration of HEN Infusion Systems

EQUIPMENT AND SUPPLIES

- IV pole or wall hook
- Enteral infusion pump for continuous feedings
- Enteral nutrition infusion system
- 60 ml Luer-Lok syringe
- Enteral feeding formula
- Measuring cup
- Cup of water
- #6 or #8 Fr enteric feeding tube with stylet
- Water-based lubricant
- Dishwashing liquid
- Micropore tape
- Stethoscope

NURSING INTERVENTIONS

1. Design a clean location for preparing enteral feedings. Wash hands with soap and scrub the area with a household cleanser before and after the formula preparation.
2. Store unopened cans or bottles of formula at room temperature and rinse top of container and can opener before opening.
3. Store opened cans or prepared formula for up to 48 hours in the refrigerator. Prepared formula bags may be stored longer in the freezer.
4. Encourage patient to get out of bed for bolus feeding meals even if only sitting in a chair by the bedside.
5. Position the patient in a Fowler's or semi-Fowler's position during and for at least 1 hour after feedings to prevent aspiration. If on a continuous drip feeding, elevate the head of the bed at all times during the feeding by placing cinder blocks under the head of the bed.
6. Place plastic or paper over the mattress and floor under the tubing to prevent soiling during the feeding.
7. Administer feeding as described in Skills 16-1 to 16-9.
8. Tape all tubing connections to prevent disconnections that may occur at night while the patient is sleeping.
9. Tape tubing to patient's forehead and ensure that tubing extends above and beyond the head so that it will not wrap around the neck when sleeping.

10. Do not allow formula poured into the administration bag to hang for longer than 12 hours. This should allow time for patients on continuous nocturnal feedings to prepare the formula and sleep through the night. The new prefilled, prepackaged, ready to hang feedings systems can hang for up to 24 hours.
11. Stop the pump every 8 hours (or slightly longer, if sleeping through the night) and irrigate the feeding tube with 30 to 60 ml water.
12. Give medications at home through the feeding tube in liquid form.
13. Flush the feeding tube with water after the administration of medication and whenever feeding is interrupted.
14. When infusion is completed, rinse enteral nutrition infusion system with at least 500 ml of tap water and drain through the tubing into the sink.
15. Wash with at least 500 ml of warm soapy tap water (use dishwashing liquid) and drain through the tubing again. Be sure to clean the threads on the container and cap thoroughly.
16. Rinse once more with tap water and drain 500 ml water through the tubing.
17. Cap tubing tip and air dry for 1 hour with the lid off.
18. Replace lid and place delivery system in a refrigerator until ready to use again later the same day.[16]
19. When administering continuous feedings for up to 12 hr per day, the enteral nutrition delivery systems may be used for up to 7 days without significant contamination.[16]
20. The feeding tube can be reused as long as it is still soft. Cost is a large consideration in HEN, so patients are taught that supplies might be utilized more economically than in the hospital setting. For example, feeding containers can be reused, and a plant hook hung over the bed or next to the dining room table may be substituted for an IV pole. After use, soak it for 1 hour in dishwashing liquid and rinse with water or dilute vinegar to dissolve crusting. Check tube for leaks by attaching the syringe to it and inserting some water.
21. Clean the exterior of the feeding pump with a cloth lightly dampened with warm, soapy water or alcohol.

Assessment

Safety factors must be stressed in home health care. The nurse should determine whether or not refrigeration is adequate so that tube feedings will not spoil and if food blenders and infusion pumps are grounded to prevent electrical shock. When a patient is first discharged home, laboratory studies should be obtained weekly for 1 month, biweekly for the next month, and then monthly. The nurse should perform the following assessments to ensure that the nutritional solutions are being administered appropriately:

- Check levels of electrolytes, BUN, creatinine, calcium, phosphate, magnesium, blood sugar, complete blood count (CBC), prothrombin time, and liver function tests, as ordered.
- Evaluate nutritional assessment measurements, such as weight and albumin and transferrin levels. Weighing the patient on a regular basis is important. If the patient does not have a scale and is unable to purchase one, the visiting nurse will supply a portable scale.
- Monitor vital signs.
- Observe for signs of aspiration and water imbalance, especially in the neurologically impaired patient.
- Have patient or caregiver keep a food diary for 3 days if the patient is able to consume food at some time, describing the food item, how it was prepared, the time and the amount consumed, and the resulting outcomes (e.g., abdominal cramping). If possible, a dietician should calculate the nutritional intake.
- Monitor any changes in feeding formulas or supplements in the event of GI distress. Suggestions can then be made to improve the nutritional intake.

REFERENCES

1. Alltop SA: Teaching for discharge: gastrostomy tubes, *RN* 5(11):42, 1988.
2. American Society for Parenteral and Enteral Nutrition: guidelines for the use of enteral nutrition in the adult patient, *J Parenteral Enteral Nutr* 11(5):435, 1987.
3. Berezin S, Medow MS, Bernarducci J et al: Home teaching of nocturnalnasogastric feeding, *J Parenteral Enteral Nutr* 12(4):392, 1988.
4. Cerra FB: *Metabolic monitoring.* In Cerra FB, editor: *Manual of critical care,* St Louis, 1987, Mosby–Year Book.
5. Cerra FB: *Metabolic support.* In Cerra FB, editor: *Pocket manual of critical care,* St Louis, 1987, Mosby–Year Book.
6. Cerrato PL: Nutritional support: your elderly patient needs attention, *RN* 53(9):77, 1990.
7. DeBear K: Sham feeding: another kind of nourishment, *Am J Nurs* 86(10):1142, 1986.
8. Detsky AS et al: What is subjective global assessment of nutritional status? *J Parenteral Enteral Nutr* 11(1):8, 1987.
9. Freedland CP et al: Microbial contamination of continuous drip feedings, *J Parenteral Enteral Nutr* 13(1):18, 1989.
10. Gottschlich MM et al: Diarrhea in tube-fed burn patients: incidence, etiology, nutritional impact, and prevention, *J Parenteral Enteral Nutr* 12(4):338, 1988.
11. Hedberg A, garcia N: *Macronutrient requirements.* In Skipper A, editor: *Dietitian's handbook of enteral and parenteral nutrition,* Rockville, Md, 1989, Aspen.
12. Heimburger DC et al: The role of protein in nutrition, with particular reference to the composition and use of enteral feeding formulas. A consensus report, *J Parenteral Enteral Nutr* 10(4):425, 1986.
13. Howard L, Heaphey LL, Timchalk M: A review of the current national status of home parenteral and enteral nutrition from the provider and consumer perspective, *J Parenteral Enteral Nutr* 10(4):416, 1986.
14. Kennedy-Caldwell C, Caldwell MD: *Pediatric enteral nutrition.* In Rombeau JL, Caldwell MD, editors: *Enteral and tube feeding,* Philadelphia, 1984, WB Saunders.
15. Kohn CL, Keithley JK: Enteral nutrition: potential complications and patient monitoring, *Nurs Clin North Am* 24(2):339, 1989.
16. Krey SH, Lockett GM: *Enteral nutrition: a comprehensive overview.* In Krey SH, Murray RL, editors: *Dynamics of nutrition support, assessment, implementation, and evaluation,* Norwalk, Conn, 1986, Appleton & Lange.
17. LaFrance RJ, Miyyagawa CI, Youngs CHF: *Pharmacotherapeutic considerations in enteral and parenteral therapy.* In Lang CE, editor: *Nutritional support in critical care,* Rockville, Md, 1987, Aspen.
18. Lang CE: *Providing nutritional support.* In Swearingen PL, Sommers MS, Miller K, editors: *Manual of critical care: Applying nursing diagnoses to adult critical illness,* St Louis, 1988 Mosby–Year Book.
19. Levenson R et al: Do weighted nasoenteric feeding tubes facilitate duodenal intubations? *J Parenteral Enteral Nutr* 12(2):135, 1988.
20. Marcuard SP, Perkins AM: Clogging of feeding tubes, *J Parenteral Enteral Nutr* 12(4):403, 1988.
21. McConnell EA: Auscultating bowel sounds, *Nursing,* 20(5):90, 1990.
22. Meer JA: Inadvertent dislodgement of nasoenteral feeding tubes: incidence and prevention, *J Parenteral Enteral Nutr* 11(2):187, 1987.
23. Merritt RJ: *Enteral feeding: who needs support?* In Balistreri WF, Farrell MK, editors: *Enteral feeding: scientific basis and clinical applications,* Columbus, Ohio, 1988, Ross Laboratories.
24. Metheny N, Dettenmeier P, Hampton K et al: Detection of inadvertent respiratory placement of small-bore feeding tubes: a report of 10 cases, *Heart Lung* 19(6):631, 1990.
25. Murray RL: *Interpreting the nutrition assessment.* In Krey SH, Murray RL, editors: *Dynamics of nutrition support: assessment, implementation, evaluation,* Norwalk, Conn, 1986, Appleton & Lange.
26. Nicholson LJ: Declogging small-bore feeding tubes, *J Parenteral Enteral Nutr* 11(6):594, 1987.
27. Pereira GR, Barbosa NM: Controversies in neonatal nutrition, *Pediatr Clin North Am* 33(1):65, 1986.
28. Perez SK, Brandt K: Enteral feeding contamination: comparison of diluents and feeding bag usage, *J Parenteral Enteral Nutr* 13(3):306, 1989.
29. Raff MH, Cho S, Dale R: A technique for positioning nasoenteral feeding tubes, *J Parenteral Enteral Nutr* 11(2):210, 1987.
30. Saklad JJ, Graves RH, Sharp WP: Interaction of oral phenytoin with enteral feedings, *J Parenteral Enteral Nutr* 10(3):322, 1986.
31. Schlichtig R, Ayres SM: *Nutritional support of the critically ill,* St Louis, 1988, Mosby–Year Book.
32. Schwartz DB: *Enteral therapy.* In Lang CE, editor: *Nutritional support in critical care,* Rockville, Md, 1987, Aspen.
33. Shronts EP, Fish JA: *Surgery, sepsis, and trauma.* In Skipper A, editor: *Dietitian's handbook of enteral and parenteral nutrition,* Rockville, Md, 1989, Aspen.
34. Spector N: Nutritional support of the ventilator-dependent patient, *Nurs Clin North Am* 24(2):407, 1989.
35. Sriram K: Home enteral hyperalimentation catheter: surgical technique and problem-solving, *Nutr Supp Serv* 6(2A):35, 1986.
36. Starkey JF, Jefferson PA, Kirby DF: Taking care of percutaneous endoscopic gastrostomy, *AJN* 88(1):42, 1988.
37. Wilson JA: gastrointestinal dysfunction in the critically ill: nutritional implications, *Nutr Comp Ther* 11(8):45, 1985.
38. Zarling EJ, Parmar JR, Mobarhan S et al: Effect of enteral formula infusion rate, osmolality, and chemical composition upon clinical tolerance and carbohydrate absorption in normal subjects, *J Parenteral Enteral Nutr* 10(6):588, 1986.

CHAPTER 17

Infection Control

Objectives

After completing this chapter, the reader will be able to:

- Apply the principles of infection control to critical care.
- Discuss the phases of septic shock.
- Explain why the critical care patient is a susceptible host.
- Assess the subjective, objective, and diagnostic findings in the patient with an infection or septic shock.
- Formulate nursing diagnoses and patient outcomes for patients with infections or in septic shock.
- Specify isolation precautions used in critical care units for patients with various types of infections.
- List the communicable diseases to which intensive care unit (ICU) nurses may become exposed within the work setting.
- Discuss the types of nosocomial infections found in ICUs.
- Explain the infection control precautions necessary for the prevention of nosocomial infections in the ICU.
- Discuss antimicrobial therapy in critical care.
- Compare and contrast pediatric and adult infection control requirements and precautions.
- Describe the potential psychosocial responses of patients to the stress of having a communicable or lethal disease.
- Discuss the infection control precautions used in home health care.

Between 5% and 10% of hospitalized patients in the United States will develop a nosocomial (hospital-associated) infection. Twenty-five percent of all nosocomial infections in hospitals occur in intensive care units (ICU).[3] According to the Centers for Disease Control (CDC), death related to nosocomial infections is among the 10 leading causes of death in the United States. If critical care nurses do not take protective measures, patients in critical care units can quickly become colonized by the hospital micro-

flora. Actual infections can then follow with the potential for lethal outbreaks of pathogens in the ICU.

Although staphyloccocal infections are no longer the epidemic threat that they were in the 1960s, they still account for 10% to 20% of nosocomial infections. In some areas a portion of these organisms are resistant to methicillin and other penicillinase-resistant antibiotics. Strains of methicillin-resistant *S. aureus* (MRSA) have become an increasing problem in hospitals.[25] Presently, about 70% of hospital-associated infections are caused by gram-negative bacteria, and the CDC has estimated that as many as 140,000 cases of gram-negative bacteremias occur annually. Approximately 50% of these progress to septic shock. There is also a current trend back to gram-positive infections, especially in cardiovascular surgery. The leading cause of death in ICU patients is now multiple organ systems failure as a result of sepsis.

PRINCIPLES OF INFECTION CONTROL

Each element in the infectious process must occur sequentially to produce an infection (Fig. 17-1):

- *Causative agents* are endogenous flora, such as microorganisms carried on the host either as transient flora or resident flora, or exogenous flora, microorganisms from a source other than the host.
- *Reservoirs* harbor the infectious agent.
- *Portals of exit* provide the pathogen with a way out of the reservoir.
- *Mode of transmission* of infection is by four primary routes: contact, airborne, vehicle, and vectorborne.
- *Portals of entry* provide a way into the new host for the infectious agent and are the same as the portals of exit.
- The presence of a *susceptible host* is the final component in the chain of infection, enabling the maturation and multiplication of the infectious agent.

The introduction of disease-producing organisms to the host can progress from simple contamination to life-threatening septic shock. *Contamination* refers to organisms that are transiently present on body surfaces (e.g., hands) or on inanimate objects (e.g., respiratory equipment). *Colonization* occurs when organisms are present in or on the host with growth and multiplication but without tissue invasion or damage. Colonization with *resident flora* (relatively

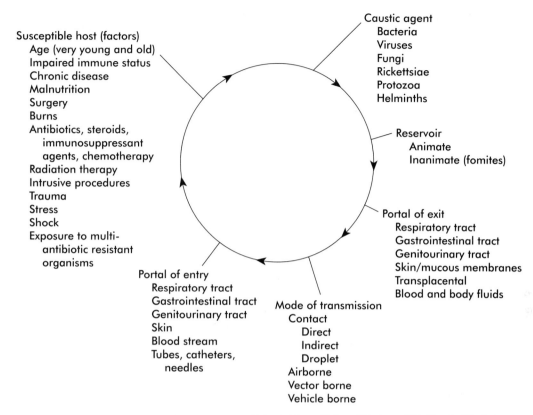

Fig. 17-1 The infectious disease process. (Adapted from Phipps WJ, Long BC, Woods NF et al: *Medical-surgical nursing: concepts and clinical practice,* ed 4, St Louis, 1991, Mosby–Year Book.)

fixed types of microorganisms also known as *normal flora*) is a nonspecific host defense. Colonization may also occur with *transient flora,* which may be present on the skin or mucous membranes, but do not establish themselves permanently on or in the host. Patients in ICUs have severe illnesses and are on antibiotics that alter the normal flora that reside in the upper airways, in the bowel, and on the skin. When these normal flora are eradicated, patients become colonized with large numbers of flora, such as *Candida, S. epidermidis,* and enterococcus. They may also be colonized with potential nosocomial pathogens, such as antibiotic-resistant *Enterobacteriaceae* and *Pseudomonas.*

Bacteremia, the presence of bacteria in the bloodstream, is detected by blood cultures. Some, but not all, bacteremic patients develop sepsis. *Septicemia* is a blood-borne infection associated with clinical signs and symptoms including fever, chills, nausea, headache, petechiae, pustules, and abscesses. The pathogens in the bloodstream have spread from an infection elsewhere in the body. *Sepsis* is an acute, systemic, inflammatory response to the invasion of microorganisms or to the toxins produced by the microorganisms. Sepsis precedes septic shock. *Septic shock* is characterized by hemodynamic instability, alterations in cellular metabolism, coagulation abnormalities, and organ failure syndromes precipitated by the interaction between the body's defense systems and bacterial toxins.

SEPTIC SHOCK

About 25% of patients who develop gram-negative bacteremia go into septic shock unless the signs and symptoms of sepsis are quickly noted and treatment is instituted. Septic shock can rapidly progress to death (often within several hours) in up to 80% of these patients. The incidence of septic shock has increased 10-fold over the last 30 years and is rapidly becoming a major problem in ICUs.[29]

Although septic shock has been associated with fungal infections, particularly in neutropenic patients, most cases are commonly caused by aerobic, gram-negative, endotoxin-producing bacilli including *Escherichia coli,* the *Klebsiella-Enterobacter-Serratia* group, *Proteus,* and *Pseudomonas aeruginosa.* Pathogens from the gram-positive bacteria include *Streptococcus pneumoniae, S. pyogenes,* and rarely, *Actinomyces.*

Phases of Septic Shock

There are two basic stages of septic shock. These stages vary in both pathophysiology and symptomatology. The first (early) stage is known as the *warm phase* (hyperdynamic). The second (late) phase is considered the *cold phase* (hypodynamic), with extreme vasoconstriction and low cardiac output (CO).

The hyperdynamic phase

The cell membranes of bacteria contain endotoxins. As bacteria are destroyed, the endotoxins are released into the blood. Endotoxins stimulate the body's immune system and activate complement, the primary chemical mediator in sepsis. During the hyperdynamic phase of septic shock the following consequences occur:

- Attraction of leukocytes to the injured area, causing further bacterial destruction and more release of endotoxin.
- Circulation of endorphins and prostaglandins, contributing to decreased systemic vascular resistance.
- Release of bradykinin, histamine, and serotinin, causing peripheral vasodilatation and increased capillary permeability.[19]
- Fluid shifts from the capillaries into the interstitial spaces with loss of circulating blood volume.
- Compensatory increase in CO and heart rate with widened pulse pressure.
- Occurrence of fever caused by release of pyrogens (e.g., prostaglandins) that affect the thermoregulatory center.

The hypodynamic phase

The cold phase indicates that many of the body systems are compromised by the chemical reactions initiated by the endotoxins. The lungs, heart, and liver are the major systems involved. The following consequences indicate that the patient has moved from warm to cold septic shock:

- Marked constrictive effects of catecholamines and of prostaglandins released from damaged tissue.
- Decreased perfusion of organs caused by hypotension and vasoconstriction.
- Widespread ischemic cellular damage.
- Disseminated intravascular coagulation (DIC), renal failure, gastrointestinal ulcers, abnormal hepatic function, and adult respiratory distress syndrome (ARDS).
- Myocardial depression with decreased CO, hypotension, and narrowed pulse pressure.

FEVER

Fever or hyperthermia implies an abnormal elevation of body temperature despite the body's attempt to lower it. Both infectious and noninfectious diseases produce fever by increasing the hypothalamic set point mediated by pyrogens and certain prostaglandins.

Critical care nurses often want to administer drugs and provide baths to reduce fever, but fever is an important host defense mechanism. Unless a patient has cardiac disease, precipitously lowering the temperature has no beneficial effects. A rapid decrease from an elevated temperature to normal range, by whatever means, regularly produces shaking chills, making the patient more uncomfortable and increasing energy expenditures. Furthermore, because chills suggest a bacteremic process, assessment of the patient's febrile response becomes difficult. An elevation in body temperature of only a few degrees results in the inhibition or death of several microorganisms. Fever also causes increased breakdown of the lysosomes in cells. This causes autodestruction of infected body cells, thereby preventing further viral replication. Another possible benefit of fever is the theorized link between fever and antibody formation.[14]

The higher thermoregulatory set point responsible for fever may allow a patient to be comfortable and unaware of a high body temperature. If the patient is complaining of febrile chills, headache, fatigue, and malaise, the nurse may want to provide an antipyretic drug. Rather than providing cool sponge baths that might induce shivering, a cooling blanket can be used to reduce fever gradually. Fever is a classic sign of infection, yet it is not always indicative of an infection. Normal temperature values do not necessarily rule out infection. The following facts may help the critical care nurse to assess fever appropriately:

- An oral temperature above 37.2° C (99° F) in a person on bedrest is a probable indication of disease. Fevers under 38.9° C (102° F) are generally the result of noninfectious disease origin. Acute infectious disease processes usually cause temperature elevations between 38.9° C (102° F) and 41.1° C (106° F).[13]
- Once the body's temperature exceeds 41° C (105.8° F), thermal injury begins. Deranged thermoregulation, convulsions, and permanent brain damage can occur.
- Rectal temperatures are normally 0.4° to 0.6° C (0.5° to 1.0° F) higher than oral or axillary temperatures. In very hot weather the body temperature may be elevated by 0.4° to 0.6° C (0.5° to 1.0° F).
- Circadian thermal rhythm varies an individual's temperature according to the time of day. Normal temperatures can reach 37.2° C (99° F) or higher between 5:00 to 7:00 PM and reach a low of 36.1° C (97° F) between 2:00 to 6:00 AM. The febrile pattern of most diseases also follows this normal diurnal pattern.
- Septic episodes frequently seen in an ICU patient usually result in intermittent fever curves or fevers that return to normal once in a 24-hour period.[13]
- Sustained or continuous fevers lasting more than 24 hours are common in scarlet fever and pneumococcal pneumonias.
- The elderly, infants, and those who are immunocompromised may not respond, even when infected, with the typical temperature patterns.
- Massive doses of steroids, such as those used in septic shock, will transiently alter the fever curve.
- Usually the pulse rate will increase 10 points for each degree of fever. For example, a patient with a temperature of 40° C (104° F) would have a pulse rate of 130 beats per minute (bpm).
- A disproportionately slow pulse is seen in certain infections, such as *Mycoplasma pneumoniae* pneumonia, blackwater fever, typhoid fever, and disseminated infection with enteric bacteria. Drug-induced fevers higher than 38.9° C (102° F) also involve a relative bradycardia.

ISOLATION PRECAUTIONS IN CRITICAL CARE

Isolation precautions for infected patients in the ICU are directed at preventing the spread of infectious diseases by the following:

- Controlling or eliminating the infectious agent.
- Controlling or eliminating the reservoir.
- Interrupting transmission.
- Protecting the largest number of susceptible persons in the ICU.

The Centers for Disease Control has developed two systems for isolation precautions: category-specific isolation precautions and disease-specific isolation precautions. *Category specific* isolation precautions group diseases and infections for which similar precautions are indicated (Table 17-1). *Disease-specific* isolation precautions consider each disease or infection individually (Table 17-2).

Table 17-1   Category Specific Isolation Precautions

Category	Example of disease or infection	Infective material	How long to apply precautions	Private room	Mask	Gown	Gloves
Strict isolation	Chickenpox, Herpes Zoster	Lesion, respiratory secretions	Until all lesions are crusted	X (Door closed)	X	X	X
Contact isolation	Acute respiratory infections in infants and young children	Respiratory secretions	Duration of illness	X	X	X*	X†
	Antibiotic-resistant bacteria, infection, or colonization	Respiratory secretions; excretions	Until off antibiotics and culture negative	X	X	X*	X†
	Major skin, wound, and burn infections	Pus	Duration of illness	X	X	X	X
	Scabies, pediculosis	Infested areas	24 hr after start of effective therapy			X†	X†
Respiratory isolation	*Haemophilus influenzae*	Respiratory secretions	24 hr after start of effective therapy	X	X (Close contact)		
	Meningococcal infections (e.g., sepsis, meningitis)			X	X (Close contact)		
Acid-fast bacillus (AFB) isolation	Pulmonary or laryngeal tuberculosis	Airborne droplet nuclei	Usually within 2-3 wk after chemotherapy begun	X (Special ventilation)	X‡		
Enteric precautions	Gastroenteritis, diarrhea	Feces	Duration of illness			X*	X†
	Viral meningitis		7 days after onset			X*	X†
	Hepatitis A	Feces	7 days after onset of jaundice			X*	X†
Drainage/secretion precautions	Minor or limited skin, wound, or burn infections (if dressing contains drainage), unless covered under another category	Drainage	Duration of illness			X*	X†
Blood/body fluid precautions	Hepatitis B	Blood and certain body fluids	Until hepatitis B surface antigen (HB$_s$Ag) negative	X*		X*	X†
	Hepatitis, non-A, non-B	Blood and certain body fluids	Duration of illness	X*		X*	X†
	HIV infections	Blood and certain body fluids	Duration of illness	X*		X*	X†
	AIDS	Blood and certain body fluids	Duration of illness	X*		X*	X†

*Recommended if splashing or soiling is likely.
†Worn when handling infective material.
‡Worn if patient is coughing and unable to cover mouth.
Adapted from Garner J, Simmons B: CDC guidelines for isolation precautions in hospitals, *Infect Control* 4:245, 1983.

Table 17-2   Sample of Disease-Specific Isolation Precautions

Example of disease or infection	Infective material	How long to apply precautions	Private room	Mask	Gown	Gloves
Acute respiratory infections in infants and young children	Respiratory secretions	Duration of illness	X	X (Close contact)	X*	X†
AIDS/HIV	Blood and certain body fluids	Duration of illness		X*	X*	X†
Antibiotic-resistant bacteria, infection, or colonization	Respiratory secretions; excretions	Until off antibiotics and culture negative	X	X (Close contact)	X*	X†
Chickenpox	Respiratory, lesion secretions	Until all lesions are crusted	X (Door closed)	X	X	X
Diarrhea	Feces	Duration of illness			X*	X†
Major skin, wound, and burn infections	Pus	Duration of illness	X		X*	X†
Meningococcal infections (e.g., sepsis, meningitis)	Respiratory secretions	24 hr after start of effective therapy	X	X (Close contact)		
Tuberculosis (pulmonary, laryngeal)	Airborne droplet nuclei	Usually within 2-3 wk after chemotherapy begun	X (Special ventilation)	X‡		

*Recommended if soiling or splashing is likely.
†Worn if patient is coughing and unable to cover mouth.
‡Worn when handling infective material.
Adapted from Garner J, Simmons B: CDC guideline for isolation precautions in hospitals, *Infect Control* 4:245, 1983.

Determining Type of Isolation Needed

- Review laboratory data, including culture reports.
- Determine if infection or colonization (e.g., multiresistant microorganisms) is present.
- Determine if isolation precautions are to be implemented.
- Consider the following factors to decide whether to isolate a patient: causative agent, reservoir of agent, portal of exit of agent from reservoir, mode of transmission of agent, portal of entry into host, and susceptibility of host.
- Choose the type of isolation precautions to implement. Is a private room necessary? Are gowns and gloves needed? Should masks be worn? Often individual nursing judgment is required.

UNIVERSAL PRECAUTIONS

Universal precautions were designed and recommended by the CDC in 1987 and were revised in 1988, based on epidemiological evidence regarding the transmission of hepatitis B virus (HBV) and human immunodeficiency virus (HIV).[4,5] Under universal precautions, blood and certain body fluids of all patients are considered potentially infectious for HIV, HBV, and other blood-borne pathogens. Physical examinations and a medical history cannot reliably identify all patients infected with HIV or other blood-borne pathogens. In the emergency care setting especially the risk of blood exposure is increased, and the infection status of the patient is usually not known. Universal precautions are intended primarily to prevent parenteral, mucous membrane, and nonintact skin exposures of health care workers to blood-borne pathogens, therefore they apply to blood and to other body fluids containing visible blood (see Guidelines box). Blood is the most important source of HIV, HBV, and other blood-borne pathogens in the occupational setting. Universal precautions also apply to the following:

- Tissues
- Semen
- Vaginal secretions
- Cerebrospinal fluid
- Pleural fluid
- Synovial fluid
- Pericardial fluid
- Peritoneal fluid
- Amniotic fluid

Universal precautions do not apply to the following list of substances unless they contain visible blood. The risk of transmission of HIV and HBV from these following fluids and materials is extremely low or nonexistent:

- Feces
- Nasal secretions
- Sputum
- Sweat
- Tears
- Urine
- Vomitus
- Human breast milk
- Saliva

Guidelines for Universal Precautions

1. Immediately and thoroughly wash hands and other skin surfaces that are contaminated with blood, body fluids containing blood, or other body fluids to which universal precautions apply. Wash hands immediately after gloves are removed.
2. Use protective barriers to prevent skin and mucous membrane exposure to blood, body fluids containing blood, and other fluids to which universal precautions apply. The type of protective barrier should be appropriate for the procedure being performed and the type of exposure anticipated.
   - Wear gloves when touching blood or body fluids, (to which universal precautions apply) mucous membranes, or nonintact skin of all patients.
   - Wear gloves when handling items or surfaces soiled with blood or body fluids (to which universal precautions apply).
   - Wear gloves when performing venipuncture and other vascular access procedures.
   - Wear gloves for performing phlebotomy if cuts, scratches, or other breaks in the skin are present.
   - Wear gloves in situations in which contamination with blood may occur, for example, when performing phlebotomy on an uncooperative patient.
   - Wear gloves for performing finger or heel sticks on infants and children.
   - Change gloves after contact with each patient.
   - Do not wash or decontaminate disposable gloves for reuse.
   - Wear masks and protective eyewear or face shields during procedures that are likely to generate splashing or droplets of blood or other body fluids (to which precautions apply) to prevent exposure of mucous membranes of the mouth, nose, and eyes.
   - Wear gowns or aprons when you anticipate splashing of blood or other body fluids to which universal precautions apply.
3. Take care to prevent injuries when using, handling, or cleaning needles, scalpels, and other sharp instruments or devices.
   - Do not recap used needles by hand.
   - Do not remove used needles from disposable syringes by hand.
   - Do not bend, break, or otherwise manipulate used needles by hand.
4. Place used disposable syringes and needles, scalpel blades, and other sharp items in puncture-resistant, leak-proof, labeled, or color-coded containers for disposal. Locate these containers close to the use area, and replace routinely.
5. To minimize exposure during emergency mouth-to-mouth resuscitation, ensure that protective mouthpieces or manual resuscitator bags are available for use in areas in which the need for resuscitation is predictable.
6. Refrain from direct patient care or handling of patient-care equipment if one has exudative lesions or weeping dermatitis.
7. For laboratory specimens, consider all blood and other body fluids from all patients to be infective. Put these specimens in a well-constructed container with a secure lid to prevent leakage during transport. Avoid contaminating the outside of the container, and place laboratory requisitions outside of the container.

Infection Control Precautions for Care of the Patient with AIDS

1. Patients with AIDS or AIDS-related complex (ARC) are at risk to acquire infection; therefore do not place them in a room with an infected patient.
2. A single room is not required unless the AIDS patient is immunocompromised, has poor hygiene, is incontinent, or has diarrhea.
3. Isolation procedures beyond universal precautions are not warranted for patients with AIDS or ARC unless they have another infection that requires isolation precautions (e.g., tuberculosis, herpes simplex, and *Cryptosporidia*).
4. Handwashing before and after patient contact and after being soiled with any body secretions or excretions is the most important means of preventing infection among patients and staff.
5. Visitors should be advised not to share razors, lip balm, cosmetics, or toothbrushes with the patient.

EXPOSURE OF ICU NURSING STAFF TO INFECTIOUS DISEASES

Nursing staff in the ICU are at some risk for iatrogenic infection. *Iatrogenic* disorders are conditions caused by medical personnel or procedures or through exposure to the environment of a health-care facility. The infections most common in ICU personnel are hepatitis B virus (HBV) and herpes simplex. The most common type of occupational injury for nurses, surpassing even sprains and strains, are injuries that occur as a result of being stuck by a needle. ICU nurses will need to be familiar with the following list of communicable diseases to which they may be exposed at work[23,31]: hepatitis B virus, hepatitis simplex virus, cytomegalovirus, chickenpox, rubella, meningitis, petussis, tuberculosis, infectious diarrhea, human immunodeficiency virus, and methicillin-resistant *S. aureus* (MRSA).

ASSESSMENT

The presence of an infection or septic shock within the human body leads to a number of specific and generalized manifestations[19,28]:

Respiratory Infection
- Assess upper respiratory tract for pain, redness, swelling, "cotton mouth", and purulent drainage.
- Assess lower respiratory tract for pain, cough, fever, chills, tachypnea, dyspnea, crackles, rhonchi, purulent sputum, infiltrates on chest x-ray, and positive culture (transtracheal or direct aspirate).

Early septic shock
- Measure respiratory rate, observing for hyperventilation. Since the body attempts to augment tissue oxygenation in impending shock the patient will usually become tachypneic (>20 breaths/min). In the nonmechanically ventilated patient, tidal volume may be as much as double to meet increased oxygen demands.

- Evaluate arterial blood gases. Initially, respiratory alkalosis (low $Paco_2$, normal bicarbonate level, and elevated pH) and hypoxemia occur.
- Auscultate lungs for crackles and/or decreased breath sounds in the bases caused by interstitial edema related to increased vascular permeability.

Late septic shock

- Evaluate peak inspiratory pressures for high values, indicating that lung compliance is decreasing, since sepsis increases the work of respiration.
- Measure pulmonary artery pressure for an increase; pulmonary hypertension occurs, since regional areas of vasoconstriction reduce the supply of oxygen in the pulmonary capillaries.
- Calculate pulmonary shunt. Pulmonary shunting occurs because of pulmonary capillary vasoconstriction.
- Observe for decreased respiratory rate (<12 breaths/min) and depth if compensatory mechanisms fail.
- Monitor for the necessity of an increased inspired oxygen (Fio_2) to maintain a normal Pao_2, indicating the development of ARDS.
- Observe for an increased $Paco_2$ (> 45 mm Hg) indicating respiratory failure.

Cardiovascular
Infection

- Compare extremities for presence of pain, warmth, swelling, or redness, indications of phlebitis.
- Observe IV sites for purulent drainage, and check for positive cultures from fluid or tissue aspirate.

Bacteremia

- Assess for presence of fever, swollen lymph nodes, chills, positive blood cultures, and positive semiquantitative culture of IV catheter, all signs of bacteremia secondary to IV devices.

Early septic shock

- Measure hemodynamic parameters, observing for high cardiac output (CO > 7 L/min and cardiac index (CI) > 4.0 L/min/m²).
- Evaluate mixed venous oxygen saturation (Svo_2) for an increase (>80%), indicating that the tissues are unable to extract oxygen as normal. During high-flow sepsis, oxygen extraction may decrease because of the high blood flow through the capillary beds.
- Palpate pulse, observing for bounding pulse with tachycardia (>100 beats/min), indicating sympathetic stimulation caused by loss of effective circulating blood volume.
- Measure blood pressure, observing for low-to-normal blood pressure with widened pulse pressure and decreasing systolic pressure (<90 mm Hg) as sepsis worsens. Low mean arterial pressure below 70 mm Hg indicates peripheral vasodilation and progressive inadequate cardiac output.
- Calculate systemic vascular resistance (SVR), noting

a decrease (<900 dynes/sec/cm⁻⁵) caused by vasodilation.

Late septic shock

- Observe for low CO (CO <4.0 L/min; CI <2.5 L/min/m²) caused by failure of compensatory mechanisms.
- Measure heart rate, and note extreme tachycardia with S_3 heart sound caused by heart's attempt to maintain CO.
- Calculate SVR, noting extreme vasoconstriction (>1200 dynes/sec/cm⁻⁵) caused by sympathetic overactivity.
- Palpate peripheral pulses, observing for weak or absent pulses caused by decreased peripheral perfusion.
- Evaluate Svo_2 for decrease (<60%) caused by decreased oxygen binding to hemoglobin secondary to acidosis, decreased CO, and decreased arterial oxygenation.

Neurological
Infection

- Evaluate for positive gram stain/culture of cerebral spinal fluid (CSF); cell count (lymphocytes) of CSF <500 mm³ indicates viral infection; >500 mm³ indicates purulent infection.
- Observe patient for alterations in mental function, disorientation, fatigue, malaise, stiff neck, headache, nausea, vomiting, delirium, drowsiness, lethargy, stupor, and coma, indicating possible neurological infection.

Early septic shock

- Assess patient for any changes in level of consciousness; as septic shock progresses, confusion will occur because of decrease in oxygen transport to the brain.

Late septic shock

- Assess patient for restlessness and anxiousness alternating with progressive lethargy; condition proceeds to lack of response to verbal stimuli and deteriorating response to painful stimuli, related to severe cerebral hypoxia.

Blood Components
Infection

- Observe platelet count for thrombocytopenia (decreased platelet count); endotoxin binds to receptors on the platelets, causing decreased thrombopoiesis.
- Evaluate white blood cell (WBC) count for leukocytosis (WBC above 10,000 mm³), which can be caused by acute infections. Stress and use of certain drugs may transiently increase the leukocyte count so that the acutely traumatized patient may have leukocytosis without infection.
- Assess for leukopenia (WBC count below 5000 mm³), which may be caused by viral infections, malaria, and overwhelming bacterial infection. WBCs are bound by endotoxins and then removed from the circulation.
- Monitor WBC differential to evaluate antibiotic ther-

apy and etiology of sepsis. Total neutrophils > 70% or > 10,000/mm^3 indicates acute inflammatory process may be occurring.

- Monitor number of immature neutrophils (called *band neutrophils* or *nonsegmented neutrophils*) released as the body attempts to fight infection; *left shift* means an increased number of immature neutrophils are in peripheral blood; > 500/mm^3 indicates infection.[30]
- Evaluate erythrocyte sedimentation rate (ESR), observing for a marked elevation that can occur in severe bacterial infections and viral pneumonia.

Early septic shock
- Observe for leukocyte count > 12,000/mm^3, an increase of 3000/mm^3 from baseline, or a shift to immature granulocyte forms.
- Evaluate for thrombocytopenia; falling platelet counts may occur before hemodynamic instability.

Late septic shock
- Monitor clotting factors. As they are consumed, fibrin degradation products and clotting times will be elevated (increased prothrombin time [PT], partial thromboplastin time [PTT], bleeding time, and fibrin split products). Fibrinogen levels will fall because of widespread clotting in capillaries.
- Observe for oozing from previous venipuncture sites caused by disseminated intravascular coagulation that eventually develops.
- Check the WBC, which may be normal or low, particularly with gram-negative sepsis.
- Assess for a complete lack of response to the standard delayed hypersensitivity skin test antigen caused by anergy.

Fluid and Electrolytes
Infection
- Check for increased serum potassium level; severe infections cause damage to a large number of body cells, resulting in release of intracellular potassium into serum.

Early septic shock
- Monitor for increased fluid requirements.
- Assess for signs of hypovolemia during high output sepsis.
- Monitor urine output for progressive tendency to oliguria caused by decreased kidney perfusion.
- Observe urine sodium for decrease, since sodium is conserved because of aldosterone and stress response.
- Measure urine specific gravity for increase; glomerular filtration rate falls in diminished perfusion.
- Check urine glucose for glycosuria caused by glucose intolerance.

Late septic shock
- Evaluate arterial blood gases. As septic shock progresses, the initial respiratory alkalosis becomes

metabolic acidosis with increased serum lactate, because cellular demands exceed oxygen supply. In the final stages of shock, there will be a combined metabolic and respiratory acidosis.
- Monitor blood urea nitrogen (BUN) and serum creatinine levels for an increase, since decreased renal perfusion and renal dysfunction develop.
- Observe for increased urinary nitrogen caused by sepsis proteolysis.

Metabolism
Infection
- Evaluate serum glucose for elevated levels caused by glucose intolerance. During infection-initiated stress, circulating adrenaline causes stimulation of gluconeogenesis and glycogenolysis, and insulin release is blocked.
- Monitor oxygen consumption for an increase caused by the hypermetabolic response. The demand may eventually exceed the supply.

Early septic shock
- Assess temperature for hyperthermia caused by release of pyrogens secondary to invading microorganisms and increased metabolic activity.
- Monitor for decreased oxygen consumption caused by blood flow through capillary beds being too rapid.

Late septic shock
- Assess body temperature for hypothermia caused by decreased metabolic activity.
- Monitor for decreased oxygen consumption, since tissues are no longer able to extract and use oxygen secondary to cellular defects.
- Check serum glucose level; hypoglycemia occurs when glucose stores become depleted.
- Monitor serum triglyceride levels for a rise caused by adipose tissue catabolism for energy production.
- Note fall in serum albumin level caused by increased gluconeogenesis, impaired hepatic function, and movement of albumin into interstitial fluid space.
- Calculate nitrogen balance, noting that even with adequate calories and protein, it tends to be negative because of tissue catabolism.
- Assess for signs of hepatic failure with rising serum glutamic-oxaloacetic transaminase (SGOT), serum glutamate pyruvate transaminase (SGPT), and lactaste dehydrogenase (LDH) levels, with eventual hyperbilirubinemia.

Gastrointestinal
Infection
- Observe for cramps, pain, distention, malaise, diarrhea, nausea, vomiting, fever, and positive culture for a known pathogen (e.g., *Salmonella, Shigella,* and *Clostridium difficile*). Obtain clostridial cytotoxin to rule out antibiotic-associated *C. difficile* colitis in patients with persistent diarrhea. In viral gastroenteritis, the main criteria will be disclosed in the history.

Septic shock

- Auscultate bowel sounds, noting absence, indicating paralytic ileus secondary to shunting of blood away from the splanchnic region and air swallowing.
- Observe abdomen, noting distention.
- Obtain gastric pH level, noting inability to control the gastric pH level, with level remaining below 3.0 despite treatment.
- Check abdominal x-ray film (flat plate) to rule out perforated viscus as the cause of the sepsis.
- Observe for signs of hepatic encephalopathy (increased serum ammonia level) causing drowsiness, muscular hypertonicity, and hyperventilation).[15]

Genitourinary
Infection

- Inspect genital area for signs of itching, inflammation, purulence, heavy discharge, and distention.
- Assess for foul odor of urine or secretions around meatus. Fever may or may not be present.
- Ask if patient has frequent and/or painful urination, back or suprapubic pain, or incontinence. Patients with indwelling urinary catheters may be asymptomatic.
- Check for positive urine culture (10^2 to 10^5 organisms/ml) or pyuria (>10 WBCs on urinalysis).
- Test for alkaline urine, caused by bacteria (such as *Proteus* and *Pseudomonas*), which cause urea-splitting.

Early septic shock

- Monitor urine output, noting less than 0.5 ml/kg/hr, which indicates decreased renal perfusion.

Late septic shock

- Monitor urine output for oliguria down to 400 ml/day or less, indicating acute renal failure caused by tubular necrosis secondary to ischemia.
- Determine fractional excretion of urine sodium, noting decrease caused by activation of the aldosterone mechanism and release of antidiuretic hormone.

Musculoskeletal
Infection

- Assess for pain, swelling, heat, inflammation, arthralgia, loss of bone continuity on radiographs, and positive cultures with aspiration of site (quantitative biopsy may be necessary for accurate culture).
- Note loss of or restricted joint movement, fever, chills, and purulent drainage.

Skin and Wounds
Infection

- Observe integument for cellulitis without pus, inflamed lumps, local pus pockets, black nails, loss of nails, dry, red skin patches, and moist, weepy skin.
- Inspect wounds for foul-smelling drainage or exudate; hemorrhagic or ecchymotic areas; ulceration into surrounding normal tissue; wound breakdown after closure; punctated ulcerated areas; and sloughing grafts.

Early septic shock

- Assess for warm, flushed skin secondary to vasodilation.

Late septic shock

- Note cold, clammy, pale skin or cyanosis caused by sustained vasoconstriction.
- Observe for interstitial edema that may develop because of capillary leakage caused by cellular disruption.

Immunosuppressed Host
Infection

- Note that pus, redness of wounds, and other signs and symptoms that require WBCs may not be present.
- Observe for change in eating habits, mental state, and disposition.
- Be alert for only 0.5° or 1.0° C (1° or 2° F) changes in temperature. Fever may be the only sign of infection.
- Observe for hyperventilation and hypotension.

NURSING DIAGNOSIS

Sample nursing diagnoses appropriate for patients with infection or septic shock include the following:

Infection

- Ventilation-perfusion imbalance related to pulmonary infection.
- Impaired coagulation related to infection.
- Disturbance in acid-base balance related to increased cellular demands secondary to infection.
- Altered patterns of urinary elimination related to urinary tract infection.
- Potential nutritional deficit related to increased cellular metabolism secondary to infection.
- Ineffective thermoregulation related to infection.

Septic Shock

- Ineffective breathing pattern: hyperventilation related to impending septic shock.
- Decrease in arterial blood pressure and widened pulse pressure related to vasodilation secondary to early septic shock.
- Elevated cardiac output related to gram-negative bacteremia.
- Decreased level of consciousness related to septic shock.
- Disruption in hematological status: thrombocytopenia and leukocytosis related to septic shock.
- Impaired glucose metabolism: hyperglycemia related to sepsis.
- Impaired skin integrity: edema related to capillary leakage secondary to sepsis.
- Oliguria secondary to septic shock.

PATIENT OUTCOMES

Possible outcomes for patients with infection include the following:

Patient Evidences:

- Respiratory rate of 12 to 20 breaths/min and minute volume of 6 to 8 L/min.
- Patent airway with normal arterial blood gases for patient: $Pao_2 > 60$ mm Hg, $Paco_2$ 35 to 45 mm Hg, pH 7.35 to 7.45, Hco_3^- 24 to 28 mEq/L, and BE +2 mEq/L).
- Adequate lung compliance: peak inspiratory pressures (PIP) of 25 to 35 mm Hg and static compliance 50 to 100 ml/cm H_2O.
- Mean pulmonary artery pressure 10 to 15 mm Hg, pulmonary vascular resistance of 150 to 250 dynes/sec/cm^{-5}, and pulmonary shunt (a/A ratio) > 0.80 to 0.85.
- Lungs clear to bases on auscultation, after pulmonary hygiene.
- Clear-to-white pulmonary secretions with negative sputum cultures and negative chest x-ray.
- Pink, slightly moist mucous membranes of the upper respiratory tract.
- Strong, steady pulse ranging from 60 to 100 beats/min.
- Mean arterial blood pressure ranging from 70 to 90 mm Hg and systemic vascular resistance of 900 to 1200 dynes/sec/cm^{-5}.
- Cardiac output of 5 to 6 L/min, cardiac index of 2.5 to 4.0 $L/min/m^2$, stroke volume 60 to 130 ml/beat.
- Negative blood and IV catheter cultures.
- WBC count of 5000 to 11,000 μl with 50% to 70% total neutrophils.
- Platelet count of 150,000 to 250,000, PT < 35 sec, fibrinogen level of 150 to 200 mg/dl, fibrin degradation products < 10.
- Erythrocyte sedimentation rate (ESR) of 0 to 15 mm/hr for men and 0 to 20 mm/hr for women.
- Adequate fluid and electrolyte levels with normal potassium levels of 3.5 to 5.0 mEq/L, central venous pressure of 0 to 6 mm Hg, and pulmonary artery wedge pressure of 6 to 15 mm Hg.
- Adequate renal function with urinary output of at least 0.5 ml/kg/min, urine specific gravity of 1.003 to 1.030, urine Na^+ level of 130 to 260 mEq/L, urinary nitrogen of < 299 mg/dl, serum BUN level of < 20 mg/dl, and serum creatinine level of < 1.5 mg/dl.
- Metabolic rate within normal limits for patient with oxygen extraction of 4 to 5 vol% and oxygen consumption of 225 to 275 ml/min.
- Temperature of 36° to 38° C (97° to 100.5° F) rectally.
- Adipose tissue metabolism within normal limits for patient with serum triglyceride levels of 35 to 200 mg/dl.
- Adequate liver functioning and glucose and cellular metabolism with total bilirubin level of 1.0 mg/100 ml, serum glucose level of 80 to 120 mg/dl, serum albumin levels of 3.5 to 5.0 g/dl, and serum lactate level of 5 to 25 mg/dl.
- Glasgow Coma score of 15 and negative gram stain/cultures of cerebral spinal fluid.
- Full range of motion of neck with normal sensation of head and neck.
- Patient voids clear straw-colored urine, negative urine cultures, urine pH of 4.5 to 8, in adequate amounts, with normal sensation, and within reasonable time periods.
- Moist, clean, and intact mucous membranes of genital areas.
- Soft, formed, brown stools with negative stool cultures.
- Normal bowel sounds and gastric pH 4.0 to 4.5.
- Size, color, temperature, range of motion, weight-bearing ability, and sensation of joints within normal limits for patient.
- Clear, intact skin of normal color, temperature, and turgor.
- Clean, moist wounds with healthy granulation tissue, beginning epithelial coverage from wound margins and negative cultures.

SURVEILLANCE OF NOSOCOMIAL INFECTIONS

Surveillance consists of continuous scrutiny of patterns and trends of infections in patients. *Incidence* defines the number of new cases of an infection (or disease) within a specified time period. *Prevalence* indicates the number of all cases of infection (or disease) in the population at a given point in time. Since 1976 the Joint Commission on the Accreditation of Health Care Organizations has required that each hospital perform infection control and surveillance (Fig 17-2).[22]

NOSOCOMIAL INFECTIONS IN THE ICU

The frequency of nosocomial infection in ICUs depends on the type of unit and patient length of stay in the unit.

Nosocomial infection rates are two to nine times higher in surgical intensive care unit (SICU) patients than in medical intensive care unit (MICU) patients. Urinary tract infections (UTIs) also occur more often in SICUs. Indwelling bladder catheters and other invasive devices are used more frequently in SICUs than in MICUs.[6]

Gram-negative organisms (e.g., *Klebsiella* and *Pseudomonas*) are more prevalent in ICUs than are gram-positive organisms (e.g., *Staphylococcus*). In addition, as the result of extensive antibiotic use, hospitals in general and ICUs in particular have become reservoirs of antibiotic-resistant bacteria. MRSA and coagulase-negative staphylococci (CN-S) have now emerged as significant nosocomial pathogens. Once MRSA is introduced into an ICU, outbreaks may occur with subsequent endemic retention of the organism, despite attempts at eradication. While CN-S are not as virulent as MRSA, they are frequently etiologic agents associated with infections involving prosthetic de-

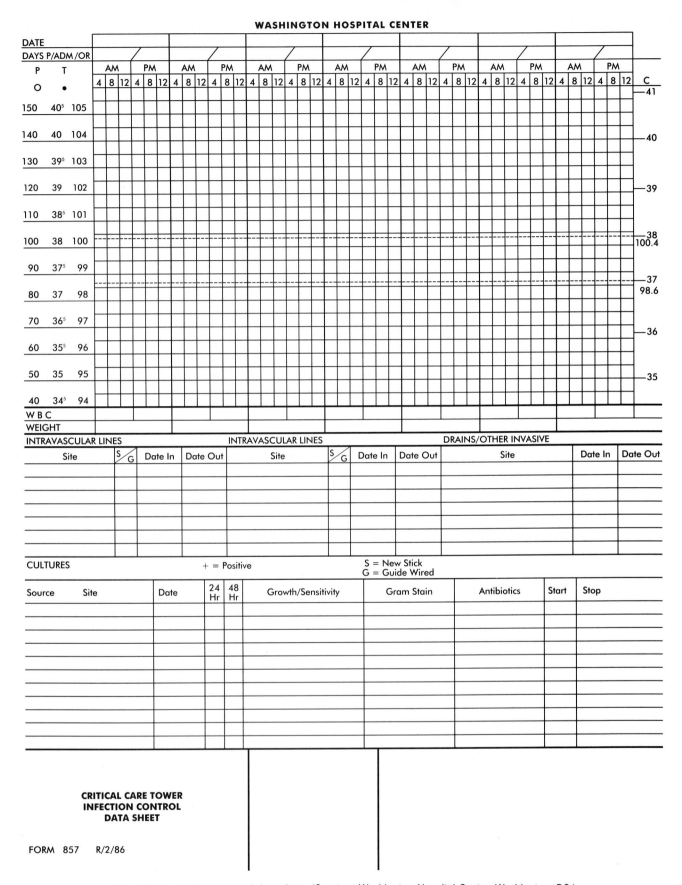

Fig. 17-2 Infection control data sheet. (Courtesy Washington Hospital Center, Washington, DC.)

vices, such as heart valves. They are also emerging as major bloodstream pathogens because of long-term use of intravascular devices.[25]

The widespread use of broad-spectrum antibiotics and indwelling vascular catheters has also dramatically increased the frequency of disseminated nosocomial opportunistic fungal infections and fungemia. Candidiasis is the cause of more case fatalities than any other systemic fungal infection. Patients at highest risk of acquiring serious life-threatening *Candida* infections include the following:

- Debilitated surgical patients who have received broad-spectrum antibiotics, prolonged total parenteral nutrition, and have undergone surgical procedures that have violated the integrity of the alimentary canal.
- Granulocytopenic patients, particularly those with hematological malignancies receiving mucosal-disrupting chemotherapy and broad-spectrum antibiotics.
- Post-transplantation patients receiving immunosuppressive drugs, primarily those with bone marrow transplants.

Handwashing is the single most important procedure for preventing nosocomial infections. The major reservoir of resistant organisms in ICUs is most commonly colonized patients. Therefore, the most significant patient-to-patient transmission, or *cross-infection,* of antibiotic-resistant microorganisms is through transient carriage on the hands of ICU personnel. Bacteria have been found on nurses' unwashed hands over 3 hours after dressing changes. Nurses may not perceive colonized patients as being at risk for transmitting infection because they are regarded as uninfected clinically. Studies have found that the major reason for infrequent handwashing among health care personnel was being too busy.

Infection rates have been significantly reduced when ICU staff use antimicrobial-containing products rather than plain soap.[9,18] These products should be used between patients in high-risk units because patients in these units are often infected or colonized with virulent or multiply-resistant microorganisms.

Nosocomial Pneumonia

It is estimated that 5 to 10 patients/1000 hospital admissions will develop pneumonia.[7] The mortality rate for nosocomial pneumonia is 20% to 50%. Most nosocomial pneumonias are caused by aerobic gram-negative bacilli (e.g., *Klebsiella pneumoniae, E. coli,* and *P. aeruginosa*).

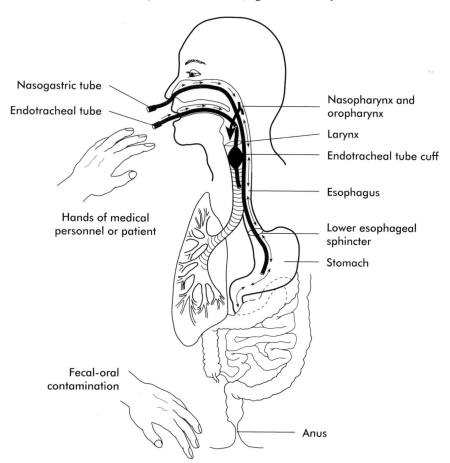

Fig. 17-3 Oropharyngeal colonization in an intubated patient with a nasogastric tube in place. Small arrows represent potential routes of oropharyngeal colonization. The large arrow depicts aspiration of oropharyngeal contents with migration of gram-negative bacilli from the stomach to the lung. (From Craven DE, Driks MR: Nosocomial pneumonia in the intubated patient, *Sem Respir Infect* 2:20-33, 1987.)

Skill 17-1   Handwashing

EQUIPMENT AND SUPPLIES

- Soap or antiseptic
- Running water
- Paper towels
- Orangewood stick or brush
- Receptacle for soiled towels

NURSING INTERVENTIONS

1. Wash hands before and after the following:
   - Patient care.
   - Taking care of susceptible patients (e.g., immunocompromised and newborns).
   - Performing invasive procedures.
   - Care of wounds (surgical, traumatic, or intravascular site).
2. Wash hands after the following:
   - Contact with mucous membranes, blood or body fluids, secretions, or excretions.
   - Taking care of an infected or colonized patient.
   - Touching inanimate sources that are likely to be contaminated (e.g., urine-measuring devices, secretion-collection apparatuses).
   - Removing gloves.
3. Remove all hand jewelry. Bacteria may become lodged under any jewelry.
4. Stand in front of sink. Keep hands and uniform away from sink.
5. Turn on water. Adjust temperature to one of comfort, and avoid splashing water.
6. Wet hands and lower arms thoroughly under running water. Keep hands lower than elbows.
7. Apply soap. If using bar soap, change bars frequently, and keep on rack to allow drainage. If using liquid soap, clean dispensers, and fill with fresh product on a regular basis.
8. Wash hands with antiseptics when providing direct care to patients who are compromised because of an invasive procedure or immune defect. Antiseptics reduce numbers of colonizing microorganisms, as well as transient flora on skin. Antiseptics have persistent antimicrobial activity.
9. Make more than one antimicrobial soap available on the unit. Different antimicrobial agents may be appropriate for various clinical situations. Also, some persons may be sensitive to certain products.
10. Wash hands vigorously using friction for at least 10 seconds.
11. Wash between fingers, palms, backs of hands, and wrists.
12. Clean under fingernails with orangewood stick or brush.
13. Rinse hands thoroughly, keeping elbows up.
14. Dry hands thoroughly with paper towel and then turn off water with paper towel.
15. Inspect hands for skin integrity. Use lotion, if needed at end of shift only.
16. Wear gloves as an adjunct to handwashing when contamination with body substances is anticipated. Change gloves between patients.
17. Use latex gloves when excessive stress to gloves is expected. Vinyl gloves have been shown to leak more frequently than latex gloves, particularly with manipulation of equipment used in ICUs.[16,17]
18. Wash hands after removing gloves. Gloves may leak or become perforated during use. Also, bacteria can multiply rapidly under gloved hands, and powder in gloves will need to be removed from hands to prevent skin irritation.

Skill 17-2   Sputum Specimen Collection by Suctioning

EQUIPMENT AND SUPPLIES

- Sterile suction kit
- Sterile normal saline solution
- Sputum trap
- Tissues

NURSING INTERVENTIONS

1. Check the suction outlet to ensure it is working and set on 120 mm Hg constant suction.
2. Wash hands, and give tissues to patient.
3. Open sterile suction kit and specimen trap, and remove lid from sterile saline.
4. Don sterile gloves, and keep dominant hand sterile.
5. Open sterile cup, and pour in saline with unsterile hand.
6. Pick up sputum trap with sterile hand, and obtain suction machine's tubing with unsterile hand, inserting the trap's rigid connector into the suction tubing.
7. Grasp the trap's latex tubing with unsterile hand; pick up the suction catheter's distal end, and insert into the trap's latex tube.
8. With sterile hand, dip end of catheter into saline to provide lubrication.
9. Insert suction catheter into airway; as patient coughs, rotate catheter and apply suction for 5 to 10 seconds, collecting 2 to 10 ml sputum; ensure that the trap is in upright position.
10. Disconnect the suction catheter and tubing; push the latex tubing over rigid connector; label specimen, and send to laboratory immediately.

Although seen less frequently than in the past, *S. aureus* may also cause nosocomial pneumonia. In about 33% of cases, anaerobic bacteria have been isolated, and *Legionella pneumophila* is common in some geographical areas.[8]

Approximately 30% to 40% of noncritically ill patients have colonization of the pharynx with gram-negative bacilli within 24 to 48 hours of hospital admission. Colonization of critically ill patients approaches 70%. Virtually 100% of patients intubated with endotracheal tubes for over 48 hours become colonized with gram-negative bacilli.[21] Patients with an endotracheal tube connected to mechanical ventilation have a 10-fold increased risk for developing pneumonia over patients without respiratory therapy devices.[7] Risk factors associated with nosocomial pneumonia are listed in the box on the right. The following are infection control precau-

---

▼ **Risk Factors Associated with Nosocomial Pneumonia**[1,8]

Nasopharyngeal colonization
Aspiration/reflux of stomach contents
Surgery (especially thoracicoabdominal, thoracic)
Severe underlying disease (e.g., cardiovascular disease, respiratory disease, malignancies, immunosuppression, neurological disorders, alcoholism, and renal failure)
Respiratory instrumentation
Prolonged broad-spectrum antimicrobial therapy
Stress ulcer prophylaxis
Prolonged hospital stay (> 40 days)
Presence of other infection

Table 17-3 Recommended Infection Control Standards for Changing Venous and Arterial Access Devices, Tubing, and Dressings[10,11,12,33]

Items to change	Frequency	Items to change	Frequency
Peripheral IV therapy		**Long-term central VAD—cont'd**	
Catheters and needles for IV fluid administration (Rotate IV site)	Every 72 hr	Central VAD gauze dressings	Every 48-72 hr
Peripheral IV fluid administration tubing	Every 72 hr	Central VAD injection caps	Every 72 hr
		Total parenteral nutrition (TPN) therapy	
Blood or blood-product administration tubing	Every 24 hr	Catheters for peripheral TPN administration	Every 24-48 hr
IV lipid emulsion tubing	Every 24 hr	Short-term central VADs used for TPN only	Every wk unless placed in operating room; then can be left in until infection supervenes
Heparin locks (Intermittent infusion devices)	Every 72 hr		
IV fluid containers that are hanging	Every 24 hr		
IV lipid emulsion containers that are hanging	Every 24 hr	TPN administration tubing	Every 48-72 hr
		TPN containers that are hanging	Every 24 hr
Peripheral IV dressing	Every 48-72 hr	Dressings over central VADs used for TPN	Every 72 hr
Central venous therapy		**Arterial pressure monitoring**	
Short-term central venous access devices (VAD)		Arterial catheter site	Every 4-5 days
Central VAD	Every wk	Arterial catheter site dressing	Every 24-48 hr
Central IV fluid administration tubing	Every 72 hr	Transducer system	Every 2-4 days
Central VAD transparent dressing	Every 5 days	Flush solution and tubing	Every 48 hr
Central VAD gauze dressings	Every 48-72 hr	**Pulmonary artery pressure monitoring**	
Central VAD injection caps	Every 72 hr	Catheter site	Every 4 days
Long-term central VAD		Transducer system	Every 2-4 days
Central VAD	Can be left in indefinitely until infection supervenes	Flush solution and tubing	Every 24-48 hr
		Central dressing site	Every 48 hr
Central VAD transparent occlusive dressings	Every 5 days		

tions for nosocomial pneumonia:

- Prevent aspiration.
- Wash hands before and after patient contact.
- Provide patients with oral hygiene.
- Check high-risk patient's immunization status.
- Isolate patients with potentially contagious diseases.
- Monitor laboratory culture reports.
- Prevent retention of secretions.
- Ensure sterility of respiratory therapy equipment.
- Avoid room air humidifiers.
- Collect sputum specimens with suction catheters and sputum traps.

Nosocomial Urinary Tract Infections

A UTI is a general term referring to any type of urinary infection (e.g., cystitis, pyelonephritis, or asymptomatic bacteriuria). One of the most important urinary tract infection control measures is to limit the use of urinary catheters to carefully selected patients, since bladder catheterization causes 66% to 86% of UTIs.[32] Fifty percent of hospitalized patients who have indwelling urinary catheters in place for more than 7 to 10 days will develop bacteriuria.[33] After 30 days, nearly all catheterized patients become infected. Some of the pathogenic organisms causing catheter-associated UTIs include: *Klebsiella, E. coli, Enterobacter, Enterococcus, Serratia, Pseudomonas,* and *Candida.* UTIs can develop into urosepsis with gram-negative septicemia, leading to septic shock and death. The urinary tract is not a frequent source of systemic sepsis in ICU patients, however, unless there is an obstruction of the renal system or a decrease in host defenses.[21,33]

Infecting microorganisms gain access to the urinary tract of the catheterized patient by the following methods:

- Loss of the urethral washing mechanisms usually provided with micturition.
- Introduction of microorganisms that inhabit the meatus or distal urethra directly into the bladder when the catheter is inserted.
- Migration of microorganisms to the bladder along the outside of the catheter. The infecting organism may be found on the patient's perineal area. They can also be transmitted from the hands of health care personnel.
- Migration of microorganisms to the bladder along the internal lumen of the catheter, if the catheter and drainage tube junction are broken. This also occurs if the collection bag has been contaminated and retrograde flow of microbes occurs.

Some of the risk factors associated with bladder catheterization include the following:

- Periurethral colonization with gram-negative rods.
- Severe underlying illness.
- Severe bladder trauma.
- Improper catheter-care techniques.
- Improper catheter insertion techniques.

Infection control precautions for catheter-associated urinary tract infections include the following:

- Insert indwelling catheters only when necessary.
- Use strict, aseptic, atraumatic insertion technique.
- Avoid meatal care with povidone-iodine solutions.
- Change catheter when obstructed or when ordered.
- Maintain a closed drainage system and unobstructed flow.
- Keep urinary drainage bag below the level of the bladder to prevent urine reflux.
- Empty urinary bag every 8 hours of more frequently if indicated.
- Do not irrigate catheter unless obstructed.
- Provide adequate fluid intake to prevent residual pooling of urine.
- Avoid using catheterization as a means of obtaining urine culture.
- If possible, separate catheterized patients from other patients to prevent cross-contamination.

Intravascular Access Infections

Intravascular systems for infusion therapy or hemodynamic monitoring are placed in over 50% of all hospitalized patients and essentially all ICU patients. Unfortunately, intravascular devices provide a potential route for microorganisms to enter the vascular system, causing bloodstream infections. Between 25% and 50% of nosocomial bacteremias occurring in ICUs originate from an intravascular device.

Microorganisms can colonize a percutaneously placed vascular catheter by several mechanisms including the following (Fig. 17-4):

- Growth of skin microorganisms along the catheter into the vein.
- Introduction of microorganisms on the catheter during venipuncture.
- Seeding of the catheter from intrinsic contamination of the infusate.
- Contamination of the catheter from a distant focus of infection in the body.

Most intravascular-related *epidemics* are caused by contamination of the infusate from a source within the hospital or manufacturing site. These infections occur much less frequently than cannula-related infections. Infections associated with contaminated solutions are almost exclusively caused by gram-negative bacilli, including *Klebsiella, Enterobacter, Serratia, Citrobacter,* and *Pseudomonas* have also been implicated in epidemics. Fungemia (fungi in the blood) has been caused by contaminated hyperalimentation fluids, particularly those containing crystalline amino acids. Sepsis unrelated to widespread outbreak is called *endemic sepsis* and originates from extrinsic (outside) contamination of the device used for intravascular fluid administration. The majority of intravascular-associated ICU infections are catheter-related.

Once a catheter site becomes contaminated, microorganisms gain access to the intravascular space by migrating along the cannula. They attach to the fibrin sheath surrounding the catheter (Fig. 17-5). *Staphylococcus epidermidis* can adhere to plastic and form biofilm, a substance

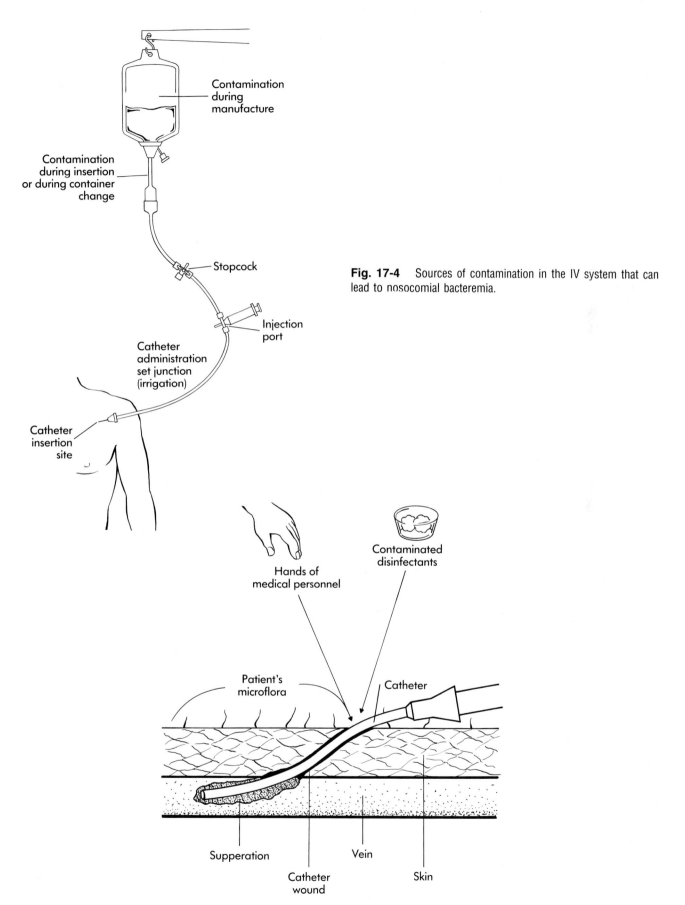

Fig. 17-4 Sources of contamination in the IV system that can lead to nosocomial bacteremia.

Fig. 17-5 Sources of contamination at the IV cannulation site. The fibrin sheath provides for bacterial multiplication and is a shield against antibiotic penetration.

that protects the organism from phagocytosis and from antibiotics. Limiting the duration peripheral venous cannulas are left in to no longer than 3 days is a critical measure for reducing infections.[11] *Staphylococcus aureus* and *Staphylococcus epidermidis* account for over 50% of all IV device-related bacteremias, followed by *Klebsiella*. In some university medical centers, however, *Candida* is now the second most common blood culture isolate. Candidemia and invasive candidiasis are most frequently seen in patients with hematological malignancies and those having organ transplantation.

Invasive pressure-monitoring systems, such as arterial lines and pulmonary artery catheters, have frequently been implicated in epidemics of septicemia. Most epidemics appear to be caused by contamination of components external to the skin, such as transducer heads or domes and stopcocks. Systems that have a reusable transducer dome are associated with a higher incidence of bacteremia. Once contaminated, these transducers act as a reservoir for microorganisms. Contaminated stopcocks have also been implicated as sources of infection.[2] Intraarterial catheters may place the patient at risk for septicemia. Several epidemics of gram-negative bacteremia have been traced to contaminated flush fluids of the intraarterial pressure monitoring systems. Half of the patients who have positive blood cultures and have been in contact with infected catheter tips have been shown to have a distant focus of infection with the same organism.

The syndrome of nonsuppurative phlebitis is another serious infection in critical care units. In nonsuppurative phlebitis the vein does not show any signs of suppuration (purulent drainage) and looks like any other phlebitic vein. It is warm, tender, and swollen and is usually the vein being used for monitoring or fluid administration. This syndrome is detected when a patient with a known bacteremia continues to be bacteremic even though the patient is receiving appropriate antibiotics. The bacteremia can be brought under control only by removing the infected vein.

Recommended infection control standards for changing intravascular access devices based on current research studies are listed in Table 17-3. Infection control precautions for intravascular access devices include the following:

- Choose upper extremity sites for IV cannulation.
- Scrub IV site with an iodophor or 70% alcohol before catheter placement, leaving on for at least 30 seconds before venipuncture.
- Insert the smallest IV cannula possible.
- Replace cannula inserted without aseptic technique during emergency situations as soon as possible.
- Use sterile guaze dressings with regular changes or transparent polyurethane dressing to cover catheter.
- Maintain a closed IV system.
- Avoid withdrawing blood specimens through peripheral IV tubing.
- Use single-dose vials for IV admixture.
- Culture the cannula (using a semiquantitative technique) for suspected IV-related infections.

- Prepare parenteral and TPN admixtures in the pharmacy in a laminar-flow hood.
- Avoid use of multilumen catheters unless patient has no other IV access sites.
- Maintain TPN administration as a closed system; in general, do not piggyback with needles into TPN lines.
- Disinfect tip of rubber diaphragm at end of Hickman-Broviac catheter with povidone-iodine or alcohol before needle puncture.
- Cleanse entry site of Hickman-Broviac catheter with hydrogen-peroxide followed by povidone-iodine or chlorhexidine gluconate; wipe antimicrobial solution off with alcohol and cover with dry dressing.
- For arterial pressure-monitoring, place catheter in the radial, not the femoral, artery.
- Do not use transparent polyurethane dressings on arterial catheter sites.
- Use heparinized or plain saline for flushing arterial catheters.
- Avoid contact between sterile and nonsterile solutions and equipment when calibrating a pressure-monitoring system.
- Use arterial pressure-monitoring systems primarily to monitor blood pressure and to obtain arterial blood gas specimens.
- Replace pressure-monitoring IV tubing and dome after use and disinfect with a high-level chemical agent, or sterilize with ethylene oxide.
- Wash hands with chlorhexidine or alcohol before central catheter insertions and cutdowns.
- To prepare skin for insertion, use povidone-iodine skin scrub and allow it to dry for at least 30 seconds; remove with 70% isopropyl alcohol, wear mask, gown, and gloves during insertion.
- Use gauze or transparent dressings over central catheter insertion sites.
- Avoid catheter changing over a guide wire.
- When thermodilution cardiac outputs are performed, use a continuous fluid system with a permanent syringe in place.
- Use an attachable sleeve device with the central catheter to reduce the rate of bacteremia.

SEMIQUANTITATIVE IV CATHETER CULTURES

Occult IV site infection does not produce inflammation or purulent drainage. However, these infections are the most common cannula-related infections and result in bacteremia more frequently than do purulent thrombophlebitis and cellulitis. Whenever a catheter site infection and/or catheter-related sepsis is suspected, the catheter should be removed and cultured. Blood cultures should also be drawn. Two techniques are used for determining if a vascular catheter is the source of the bacteria isolated from the blood. The semiquantitative method consists of rolling a catheter tip across a blood agar plate, incubating it, and reading the number of colonies that have grown at 48 hours. A total colony count of over 15, referred to as a *pos-*

itive catheter-segment culture, is significantly associated with the catheter being the source of the bacteremia. A positive culture from an external component of an IV device *(positive component culture)* may be due to contamination. The second method is to examine segments of the distal end of the IV catheter tip by light microscopy using Gram's stain.

BLOOD CULTURES

Blood cultures are performed to detect bacteremia. Gram-stain results may be obtained the same day or within 24 hours. Preliminary reports that can identify about 90% of pathogens are available in 3 days. Final reports are issued in 7 days, but cultures may be kept longer if fungi are suspected. One positive blood culture of *Staphylococcus epidermidis* among several negative cultures may be indicative of contamination from skin flora during venipuncture.

WOUND INFECTIONS

Any disruption in the skin's integrity, such as trauma, operative procedures, inadequate tissue perfusion, avascular necrosis, ischemia, hematoma, edema, or inflammation, may lead to infection.

In general a wound can be considered infected if it drains purulent material (even without confirmation by culture). Purulent material coming from a wound should be examined with a Gram's stain. One should avoid obtaining wound specimens from superficial areas, such as from decubiti and cellulitis because such sites have polymicrobial growth and are contaminated with normal skin flora. To interpret culture reports adequately, nursing staff should be aware of normal skin flora, common pathogens, and signs of wound infection. A large variety of microorganisms are part of the normal skin flora (see box). When the skin's integrity is broken, however, infections may be caused by these microorganisms.

Infection control precautions for surgical wound infections include the following:
- Observe for signs and symptoms of infection.
- For nonurgent surgical procedures in patients who are malnourished, give enternal or parenteral nutrition before the operation.
- Start parenteral anti-microbial prophylaxis shortly before the operation and discontinue promptly after the operation.

▼
Normal Skin Flora

S. epidermidis
*S. aureus**
Diptheroids
Streptococci (*viridans* group)
Enterobacter species
Other gram-negative rods*
*Candida**
Streptococcus pyrogenes (group A)*

---

*Common pathogens in surgical or traumatic wounds, lesions, deep wounds, and abscesses.

- Have patient bathe (or be bathed) with an anti-microbial soap the night before surgery. If hair removal is necessary, do it just before surgery using either clippers or a depilatory.
- Wash hands before and after caring for a surgical wound. Use only sterile gloves or instruments to handle an open or fresh wound.
- Change dressings over closed wounds if they become wet or the patient shows signs or symptoms of infection.
- Culture and Gram's stain any drainage from a wound that is suspected of being infected.
- Clean wounds of all necrotic tissue and debris through surgical or mechanical debridement with wound irrigation or wet-to-dry or wet-to-wet dressings.
- Avoid the use of povidone-iodine solution.

INFECTIONS FROM INTRAVENTRICULAR PRESSURE MONITORING

The risk of infection is related to the following:
- Insertion technique.
- Length of time the catheter remains in place.
- Capability of maintaining a closed monitoring or drainage system.
- The need to vent cerebrospinal fluid (CSF).

Infection control measures for patients with intraventricular pressure monitoring include the following:
- Use aseptic technique during insertion of monitoring equipment and during all dressing and tubing changes.
- Maintain a closed monitoring or drainage system. Assess catheter sites for signs of infection.
- Ensure that catheter is changed every 3 to 4 days or per department protocol.
- Obtain daily samples of the ventricular fluid to monitor for early signs of CNS colonization and subsequent infections.
- Use subarachnoid bolts instead of intraventricular catheters whenever possible.

GASTROINTESTINAL TRACT INFECTIONS

One of the sources of gastrointestinal (GI) tract infection in ICU patients is indwelling nasoenteric tubes and gastrostomy tubes. Bacterial contamination can be introduced via the nares, a gastrostomy tube insertion site, or the feeding solution and apparatus. Needle jejunostomy tubes can also produce localized ischemia leading to necrosis, intestinal perforation, peritonitis, and intraabdominal abscesses.

The use of antibiotics is associated with GI tract problems in ICU patients. One of these conditions, pseudomembranous colitis, can be caused by almost every antimicrobial agent and results in profuse watery diarrhea. The diarrhea occurs because of selective overgrowth of the bacterium *Clostridium difficile,* which produces a toxin that causes the lesion of pseudomembranous colitis. Antibiotic therapy can also be the cause of fungal overgrowth in the GI tract.

Skill 17-3   Collection of Wound Cultures

EQUIPMENT AND SUPPLIES

- Aerobic culture swab with culture medium (Culturette)
- Anaerobic Culturette
- Sterile package of 4 × 4 gauze
- Bottle of sterile normal saline solution
- Povidone-iodine swabs
- Sterile and clean gloves
- Dressing materials

NURSING INTERVENTIONS
Aerobic culture

1. Check physician's orders to determine if culture is to be aerobic and/or anaerobic.
2. Don clean gloves and remove all dressing materials covering site.
3. Assess wound site for swelling, erythema, purulence, odor, opening of wound edges, and presence of granulation.
4. Remove gloves, wash hands, and remove top wrapper from container of 4 × 4 gauze sponges and povidone-iodine swabs.
5. Pour saline solution into container of gauze sponges.
6. Put on sterile gloves. Obtain a gauze pad, and wring out extra moisture. Carefully wipe wound from top to bottom.
7. Observe for tenderness, and repeat this procedure until all of the gross debris has been removed.
8. Wipe wound with povidone-iodine swabs from top to bottom, dispose of gloves, and let solution dry. This removes skin flora, preventing possible contamination of specimen.

9. Remove the applicator swab from its container, position swab in the wound at the site of the most drainage, and collect drainage. Do not collect a surface specimen, which affects the accuracy of the laboratory analysis.
10. Return swab to container, crush culture-medium ampule at the base of tube, and push swab into the medium.
11. Cleanse and redress wound using sterile technique; label culture specimen, and send to laboratory. Never refrigerate specimen.

Anaerobic culture

1. After following the above steps 1 to 8, peel open the culture package.
2. Pull the culture cap (and attached swab) out of the bag.
3. Gently insert the swab into the wound, and obtain specimen.
4. Place cap back on culture tube; apply gentle fingertip pressure to the cap; push Culturette into the Bio-Bag until the top of the cap reaches the bag's line.
5. Pull the top of the Bio-Bag through the metal closure; fold the top of the bag over the metal closure at least three times; invert the Bio-Bag so that the culture cap is down.
6. With your fingers, crush the ampule closest to the swab; this will allow the medium to saturate the Culturette's pledget.
7. Invert the Bio-Bag so the culture cap is facing up; crush the bottom ampule; then hold the Bio-Bag upright until the tablet is completely dissolved. When the Bio-Bag inflates, hydrogen gas is generated. Avoid exposure to sparks or flames.
8. Label and send to laboratory immediately.

Infection control precautions for gastrointestinal infections include the following:

- Regularly assess the GI system, listening for hyperactive or absent bowel sounds, and observing for nausea, vomiting, diarrhea, cramping, and distention.
- Obtain culture and Gram's stain if patient has persistent diarrhea; obtain clostridial cytotoxin culture when indicated.
- Wash hands before handling enteral formulas and manipulating tube feeding apparatus.
- Use disposable, closed, enteral administration apparatus, and in hospital setting, hang new feeding bag and tubing every 24 hours. Do not add more feeding to enteral formulas that are already hanging. Wash formula bag and tubing, and add more formula every 8 hours in continuous enteral tube feeding.
- Discard open, refrigerated formula containers every 24 hours. Cover canned, powdered formulas tightly, and discard after 3 months.
- Switch from large-bore nasogastric feeding tube to small-bore nasoenteric feeding tube.
- Clean and moisten patient's nose, teeth, and oral cavity several times each day. Avoid inserting rectal tubes.

ANTIMICROBIAL THERAPY IN CRITICAL CARE

The widespread use of antibiotics in the ICU favors the emergence of resistant bacteria, and the hectic pace of the critical care environment enhances the opportunity for their spread. Resistance to antimicrobials occurs most commonly through the following mechanisms:

- Enzymatic inactivation of the antibiotic.
- Changes in the microorganism cell-wall permeability of cell-binding sites.
- Changes in the microorganism's metabolic pathways.
- Alterations in the microorganism's drug-receptor sites.
- Genetic resistance, occurring by spontaneous mutation and natural selection or by extrachromosomal DNA.

Multiple-resistance occurs when microorganisms become resistant to two or more unrelated antibiotics to which they are usually susceptible. Multidrug-resistant bacteria can cause potential or actual problems in the ICU (see box on Guidelines for the Prevention of the Spread of Multiple-Resistant Microorganism on p. 407).

Superinfection, secondary to antibiotic treatment, is an additional untoward effect of antibiotic therapy. A *superinfection* is a secondary infection usually caused by an opportunistic pathogen, such as when a fungal infection occurs during antibiotic treatment of another infection. In a superinfection antibiotics allow microorganisms not inhibited by them to colonize or suprainfect the patient.

Inappropriate or prolonged antimicrobial therapy with one or more antibiotics may also permit the selective emergence of more resistant pathogens. Microorganisms of particular interest are *Klebsiella,* group D streptococci (en-

terococci), *Pseudomonas aeruginosa, Bacteroides fragilis,* and *Candida albicans.* Discontinuation of all antibiotics will permit the patient's normal flora to reestablish itself and will eliminate the selective pressure on colonizing organisms. Restrictive use of antibiotics also diminishes levels of resistance and controls outbreaks of highly-resistant infections.[24]

Antibiotic Blood Serum Levels

Serum antibiotic levels are useful in adjusting doses to maximize effectiveness while minimizing toxicity. However, these levels must be interpreted in view of the patient's clinical condition.

Antibiotic serum levels can be measured at the drug's peak or trough level. The *peak* level is the highest concentration and is used when testing for toxicity. Peak levels are usually obtained about 1 to 2 hours after oral intake, about 1 hour after intramuscular (IM) administration, and about 30 minutes after IV administration. *Trough* levels are drawn at the drug's lowest concentration and are helpful

---

▼

Guidelines for the Prevention of the Spread of Multiple-Resistant Microorganisms

- Wash hands before and after patient contact.
- Wear gloves for all secretion or excretion contact.
- Separate colonized/infected patients from patients with drainage tube or urinary catheter.
- Implement isolation precautions where indicated.
- Report identified patients (colonized or infected) to hospital infection control team.

Skill 17-4   Administration of Intravenous Antibiotics
▼

Most antiinfective drugs fall into one of the following classes: sulfonamides, tetracyclines, penicillins, antifungal agents, cephalosporins, and aminoglycosides. The aminoglycosides, which include drugs such as gentamycin, neomycin, and tobramycin, can cause serious adverse reactions if given with another drug that is nephrotoxic or ototoxic. Antibiotics may be administered intravenously. Usually volume-control sets are used when the antibiotic requires a minimal amount of diluent solution and is compatible with the patient's maintenance IV solution. Most antibiotics are compatible with Ringer's lactate, dextrose, and saline solutions. Certain drugs, such as Amphotericin B and Monistat, will need to be mixed in separate IV bags and given via a piggybacked line.

EQUIPMENT AND SUPPLIES

- 12 ml syringe
- 20 g needle
- Volume-control set (Buretrol)
- IV tubing
- Bag of IV solution
- Medication vial
- Vial of sterile water
- Alcohol sponges

NURSING INTERVENTIONS

1. Check medication Kardex for time antibiotic is due. If the drug cannot be delivered on time, administer it within 30 minutes before or after it is due. This helps maintain appropriate blood levels of the antibiotic. Check all medications listed in the Kardex against the physician's orders for accuracy every 24 hours.
2. Obtain vial of medication and vial of sterile water for injection. Reconstitute drugs such as Erythromycin and Amphotericin B with sterile water without preservatives. The vial without preservatives can be used only once and then must be discarded.
3. Wipe tops of both vials with alcohol sponges. Using 12 ml syringe, withdraw approximately 10 ml sterile water. Insert water into medication vial and shake vial. Let solution dissolve totally. For Penicillin G, follow directions on vial to obtain proper concentration.
4. Withdraw correct dosage of medication from vial. If using half the dose, withdraw entire amount, measure, and cal-

culate the amount needed for half. Medication left in the vial should be labeled and can be stored for 24 hours at room temperature or placed in the refrigerator for longer storage. Check the manufacturer's recommendations.
5. Confirm the identity of patient, and assess venipuncture site for infiltration, phlebitis, or infection. When given the choice, insert toxic antibiotics through central rather than peripheral lines.
6. Fill volume-control set (Buretrol) with 20 ml solution. Wipe injection port with alcohol sponge and inject medication.
7. Open upper clamp and fill fluid chamber with the prescribed amount of solution to dilute the medication (usually 30 ml). Close clamp and gently rotate the chamber to mix the medication and solution. If cloudy precipitate appears, change entire set of IV tubing, and look up the compatibility of the drug with the IV solution.
8. Open lower clamp and adjust drip rate to deliver solution in specified time period (usually 30 minutes). Administer toxic drugs that are to be delivered over a long period of time via an infusion pump. If drugs are infused too quickly, excessively high blood levels may occur, leading to toxicity.
9. Place the name of the medication, dose, time, and date on a medication label, and attach a corner of it to the infusion set. Remove the label once the drug has infused.
10. When the infusion is completed, let 10 ml of IV solution flow into the chamber and through the tubing to flush and deliver all of the medication.
11. Assess patient for adverse effects of antibiotic therapy. Report findings and laboratory reports.

for demonstrating a satisfactory therapeutic level. They are usually obtained shortly before (30 minutes) the next scheduled dose is administered.

PEDIATRIC CONSIDERATIONS
Assessment

The following assessment guide emphasizes signs, symptoms, and laboratory data that may indicate an infection in the infant or child.

- Auscultate and observe chest for apnea, tachypnea, rapid shallow breathing, rales, rhonchi, and decreased breath sounds, indicating respiratory infection, including pleural effusion.
- Observe for productive cough and hemoptysis.
- Observe skin color for cyanosis.
- In neonate, observe for intercostal retractions, and listen for grunting.
- Measure heart rate, observing for tachycardia or bradycardia.
- Determine blood pressure, noting a decrease.
- Check laboratory reports for thrombocytopenia and abnormalities in absolute neutrophil count, absolute band count, and band/neutrophil ratio.
- Measure urine output, observing for decreased amount.
- Check laboratory reports for hypocalcemia, hypoglycemia, metabolic acidosis, and jaundice.
- Listen for shrill crying, and observe for weak sucking and unusual irritability or lethargy.
- Observe for a seizure associated with sudden increase in temperature greater than 39° C (102° F).
- In neonate, observe for seizures, hypotonia, tremors, and full fontanelle.
- Observe for anorexia, poor feeding, vomiting, or diarrhea.
- Observe for abdominal distention, guaiac- or hematest-positive stools, and increased gastric residuals, with or without bilious vomiting after feeding, all signs of necrotizing enterocolitis (NEC).
- Inspect skin for purpura, cellulitis, pustules, and abscesses.
- Measure temperature, being observant for a fever between 39.4° C (103° F) and 40.6° C (105° F) in a child 6 months to 3 years of age.
- In a premature infant and newborn note a subnormal temperature or temperature instability.

Infection control precautions for nosocomial neonatal infections include the following:

- Provide 1½ to 2 m (4 to 6 feet) distances between infants.
- Perform a 2-minute handwashing scrub before entering the unit. Wash hands for 10 to 15 seconds between infant contacts. Use an antiseptic handwashing product.
- Wear protective clothing, laundered by the hospital. Do not let personal clothing and unscrubbed skin areas touch infants. Have visitors and nonunit personnel wear cover gowns.
- Do not perform femoral blood punctures on an infant.
- Use infant formulas within 24 hours of opening and keep refrigerated. Use breast milk only for the mother's infant.

PSYCHOSOCIAL CONSIDERATIONS

Patients with infectious diseases may suffer from the fear of stigma or rejection by others.[20] Because of the stigma attached to certain infectious diseases, such as HIV, herpes, sexually transmitted diseases, hepatitis, TB, and skin lesions, patients may be shunned by family, friends, and caregivers. When staff members must wear protective garments, they tend to go into a patient's isolation room less frequently. This happens especially with HIV patients; overzealous use of isolation procedures may further isolate the patient.[26] This may lead to withdrawal and sensory deprivation when the normal sources of stimulation are removed. Nurses caring for patients on isolation must regularly assess the patient for depression and social isolation.

Individuals with HIV infection present a considerable challenge to the nurse, since they tend to have a number of psychological or internal conflicts. They have conflicts about transmission of disease, protection from infection, personal relationships, and lifestyle. These conflicts lead to anger, fear, guilt, loneliness, and feelings of abandonment. Their major psychological stress, however, is the realization that they have a lethal disease with the potential for a rapid decline to death. Although psychosocial care of the AIDS patient and family may seem overwhelming, there are many helpful resources and interventions. Many AIDS patients are enrolled in support groups and have friends or family members who will regularly visit the hospital. A variety of community referrals are available to help patients with infectious diseases to cope (see Patient and Family Teaching section).

PATIENT AND FAMILY TEACHING

Patients and families should be carefully instructed about the nature of the patient's infection and the type of isolation precautions they must take. These precautions are outlined elsewhere in the chapter. While in the ICU setting, the nurse can teach the anxious AIDS/HIV infected patient stress reduction techniques, such as relaxation or other behavioral techniques. If being sent home, the patient will need liaison with community resources. A social service referral should be made for the patient once discharge planning begins. The nurse can provide educational materials, including computer and audiovisual resources, books, directories, pamphlets, and newsletters.

HOME HEALTH CARE CONSIDERATIONS

The goals of infection control in the home setting are to reduce the following:

- Risk of transmission to the community.
- Incidence of infection.
- Cost of health care for the patient.

In home health care, it will rarely be necessary to use sterile technique, as in the hospital. Optimum clean technique is generally acceptable. The majority of household disease-producing organisms can be killed by washing equipment with household cleaning agents, such as chlorine bleach or Lysol. To prevent transmission of infective material, handwashing and the no-touch technique are the most important factors for home care of wounds, drainage secretion, and excretion control. The *no-touch technique* consists of handwashing before the dressing change and no contact with the wound or wound drainage except with sterile dressings. Gloves should be worn, if available. Handwashing involves scrubbing the hands and nails thoroughly with soap and water for at least 10 seconds.

Patients with AIDS/HIV infections will need special precautions for infection control to prevent the spread of infection to caregivers and family members. Universal precaution measures outlined earlier in the chapter can be modified for the home. However, it is important to reemphasize several of these measures, including handwashing before and after patient contact and wearing gloves when in contact with blood and body fluids. The AIDS and immunosuppressed patients will also need protection from opportunistic infections. Such protection can be provided through proper sanitation, hygiene, and nutrition.

Dressing Change Techniques

Dressing change techniques performed in the home by the nurse or other caregiver can be classified as special or standard, depending on the nature of the infected wound or lesion. Extensive wound infections that would normally require contact isolation in the hospital would receive *special dressing techniques.* Such infections include impetigo, gas gangrene, streptococcal (group A) skin infections, and staphylococcal skin wound infections.[27]

Special dressing change techniques

* Ensure that all wastebaskets have disposable plastic linings.
* Wash hands before and after patient contact.
* Wear gloves, gown, and mask during dressing changes.
* Wear gloves to remove old dressing, and then wash hands.
* Wear new pair of gloves to apply new dressing.
* Use sterile dressing change supplies.
* Use no-touch technique when handling the dressings, avoiding touching the dressing that will be applied to the wound.
* Dispose of soiled dressings and equipment in strong plastic bags.

Skill 17-5 Drawing Blood Cultures

EQUIPMENT AND SUPPLIES

* 20 g needles and 10 ml syringe for adults
* 25 g needles and 5 ml syringe for children
* Aerobic and anaerobic culture bottles with or without resin
* Antimicrobial solution soaked sponges (tincture of iodine, tincture of chlorhexidine, or povidone-iodine)
* Alcohol sponges
* Sterile gloves
* Tourniquet
* 2 x 2 gauze sponges
* Adhesive tape
* Lab slips and labels

NURSING INTERVENTIONS

1. Collect blood cultures before antibiotics are started. If patient is already receiving antibiotics, use blood culture medium with resin to provide for neutralization of antibiotic. Note on the laboratory sheet that patient is receiving antibiotics.
2. Draw at least two blood specimens from separate sites to help ensure a quality bacterial-seeded specimen; bacterial seeding occurs at different times at different sites.
3. For patients with prosthetic valve devices and/or bacterial endocarditis, draw three specimens at least 1 hour apart in a 24-hour period. For patients with intermittent bacteremias, it may be necessary to draw four to six cultures in 48 hours from different sites.
4. Do not draw blood cultures from catheters or arterial lines. Results will not be reliable because of the high rate of false-positive cultures.

5. Wash hands, and take wrappers off syringe, needles, and culture bottles. Check the instructions on the culture bottle for expiration dates and amount of blood needed. The dilution is usually 1:10 unless otherwise specified.
6. Place one set of aerobic and anaerobic blood culture bottles on table. Cleanse the tops of the culture bottles with povidone-iodine solution, and leave it on them to dry.
7. Cut strip of tape, and make adhesive bandage with 2 x 2 gauze.
8. Don gloves, choose venipuncture site, and open antiseptic sponges.
9. Cleanse skin with 2% tincture of iodine, tincture of chlorhexidine, or less desirably, povidone-iodine solution to remove transient and resident flora.
10. Use circular motion beginning at center and working outward. Wait at least 30 seconds for solution to dry and have time to disinfect area.
11. Wipe antimicrobial solution off with alcohol sponge to prevent possible irritation and allergic reaction.
12. Perform a venipuncture, and withdraw 10 ml of blood from an adult or 2 ml from a child. When withdrawing a large amount of blood, it may be easier to use a "butterfly" IV needle taped to the skin.
13. Place 2 x 2 gauze sponge with adhesive tape over site, and have patient or assistant provide pressure.
14. Replace needle on syringe with new needle, and inject 5 ml blood into each 50 ml bottle or 2 ml into a 20 ml pediatric culture bottle.
15. Label lab slip, indicating if patient is on antibiotics. Label bottles, and send to laboratory.

Standard dressing techniques

- Wash hands before and after patient contact.
- Gloves, gown, and mask are not required.
- Use sterile dressing change supplies.
- Use a plastic disposal bag over the hand like a glove to pick up soiled dressing, and then pull bag back over soiled dressing for disposal.
- Use no-touch technique when handling dressings, avoiding touching the new dressing to be applied to the wound.
- Dispose of soiled dressings and equipment using strong plastic bags.

General infection control precautions for home health care for the nurse or other caregiver include the following:

- Clean blood and contaminated body fluid spills with soap and water, then with a 1:10 solution of bleach (1 part household bleach and 9 parts water) prepared daily.
- If toys are visibly soiled with infective material, disinfect with a 1:10 bleach solution.
- Wash soiled clothing and linen with hot water, regular detergent, and 1 cup of bleach.
- Do not break, bend, or recap needles.
- Contain drainage from wounds in dressings when patient is being transported.
- Clean reusable patient-care equipment with hot, soapy water, then with a 1:10 bleach solution.
- Wash soiled surfaces with hot, soapy water. Decontaminate blood spills with a 1:10 solution of household bleach and water.
- Store thermometers in disinfection solution (70% alcohol) that completely covers the thermometer.
- Flush urine, feces, and vomitus down toilet.
- Prevent persons who are susceptible to the particular communicable disease from visiting with the patient.

REFERENCES

1. Bamberger D.: Nosocomial pneumonia. In Farber B, editor: *Infection control in intensive care*, New York, 1987, Churchill Livingstone.
2. Bronson K et al: Stopcock contamination, *Am J Nurs* 88(3):320, 1988.
3. Carpenter R: Infections and head injury: a potentially lethal combination, *Crit Care Nurs Q* 10(3):1, 1987.
4. Centers for Disease Control: Recommendations for prevention of HIV transmission in health-care settings, *Morbid Mortal Weekly Rep* 36:(Suppl 2S), 1987.
5. Centers for Disease Control: Update: universal precautions for prevention of transmission of human immunodeficiency virus, hepatitis B virus, and other bloodborne pathogens in health-care settings, *Morbid Mortal Weekly Rep* 37(24):377, 1988.
6. Craven D et al: Nosocomial infection and fatality in medical and surgical intensive care unit patients, *Arch Intern Med* 148(5):1161, 1988.
7. Craven D, Regan AM: Nosocomial pneumonia in the ICU patient, *Crit Care Nurs Q* 11(4):28, 1989.
8. Craven DE, Steger KA: Pathogenesis and prevention of nosocomial pneumonia in the mechanically ventilated patient, *Respir Care* 34(2):85, 1989.
9. Crow S: Asepsis—an indispensable part of the patient's care plan, *Crit Care Nurs Q* 11(4):11, 1989.
10. Gabriel D, Heard S: Infectious complications of indwelling arterial and venous catheters, *Curr Rev Respir Crit Care* 10(12):90, 1988.
11. Hamory BH: Nosocomial sepsis related to intravascular access, *Crit Care Nurs Q* 11(4):58, 1989.
12. Hampton AA, Sherertz RJ: Vascular-access infections in hospitalized patients, *Surg Clin North Am* 68(1):57, 1988.
13. Hart LH, Dennis SL: Two hyperthermias prevalent in the intensive care unit, *Focus Crit Care* 15(4):49, 1988.
14. Holtzclaw BJ: Temperature problems in the postoperative period, *Crit Care Nurs Clin North Am* 2(4):589, 1990.
15. Hotter AN: The pathophysiology of multi-system organ failure in the trauma patient, *AACN Clin Issues Crit Care Nurs* 1(3):465, 1990.
16. Korniewicz DM, Laughon BE, Cyr WH, et al: Leakage of virus through used vinyl and latex examination gloves, *J Clin Microbiol* 28(4):787, 1990.
17. Korniewicz DM, Laughon BE, Butz A, et al: Integrity of vinyl and latex procedure gloves, *Nurs Res* 38(3):144, 1989.
18. Larson E: Guidelines for use of topical antimicrobial agents, *Am J Infect Control* 16(6):253, 1988.
19. Littleton M: Pathophysiology and assessment of sepsis and septic shock, *Crit Care Nurs Q* 11(1):30, 1988.
20. Meisenhelder J, LaCharite C: Fear of contagion: the public response to AIDS, *Image* 21(1):7, 1989.
21. Norwood S: Diagnosing nosocomial infection in ICU patients. I. *Curr Rev Respir Crit Care* 9(9):71, 1987.
22. Rasley DA: Surveillance of nosocomial infections, *Crit Care Nurs Q* 11(4):75, 1989.
23. Rhinehart E: Employee health for critical care duty, *Crit Care Nurs Q* 11(4):66, 1989.
24. Spitzer P, Eliopoulaulos G: Antibiotic resistance in the intensive care unit and mechanisms of spread. In Farber B, editor: *Infection control in intensive care*, New York, 1987, Churchill Livingstone.
25. Stillman R et al: Emergence of coagulase negative staphylococci as major nosocomial bloodstream pathogens, *Infect Control* 8(3):108, 1987.
26. Strawn J: The psychosocial consequences of AIDS. In Durham J, Cohen F, editors: *The person with AIDS: nursing perspectives*, New York, 1987, Springer Publishing.
27. Sutton S: *Home health nursing procedures*, Baltimore, 1988, Williams & Wilkins.
28. Swearingen PL, Sommers MS, Miller K: *Manual of critical care. Applying nursing diagnoses to adult critical illness*, St Louis, 1988, Mosby–Year Book.
29. Wahl SC: Septic shock: how to detect it early, *Nurs 89* 19(1):53, 1989.
30. Wasserman, MR, Keller EL: Fever, white blood cell count, and culture and sensitivity; their value in the evaluation of the emergency patient, *Top Emerg Med* 10(4):81, 1989.
31. Williamson KM et al: Occupational health hazards for nurses: infection, *Image* 20(1):48, 1988.
32. Wong E: New aspects of urinary tract infections. In Farber B, editor: *Infection control in intensive care*, New York, 1987, Churchill Livingstone.
33. Yannelli B, Gurevich I: Infection control in critical care, *Heart Lung* 17(6):596, 1988.

CHAPTER 18

Burn Wound Therapy

Objectives

After completing this chapter, the reader will be able to:

- Discuss the types of injuries requiring burn wound therapy and the pathophysiology, wound healing process, and treatment phases of burn injury.
- Delineate the potential problems that may occur during the resuscitative and acute care phases of burn injury.
- Formulate nursing diagnoses and patient outcomes for the burn patient.
- List the nursing interventions required to provide initial prehospital and inpatient treatment to patients with acute thermal, chemical, and electrical burns.
- Specify burn unit infection control protocols and the proper method for obtaining wound cultures.
- Describe the nursing interventions required to provide hydrotherapy and wound debridement.
- Describe the technique of application of topical antimicrobial agents, using the open and occlusive wound care methods.
- Discuss the application of biological and synthetic skin dressings.
- Specify the actions required in the care of autograft skin and donor sites.
- Discuss positioning, ambulation, and range of motion exercise for burn patients.
- Discuss major complications of inadequate nutritional support of the critically burned patient.
- List essential components of an effective patient and family teaching protocol for acute burn injury.
- Describe physiological differences related to age that affect the treatment of the critically burned patient.
- Specify some of the home health skills that the patient can perform to provide less discomfort and fewer skin problems once the patient returns home.

PATHOPHYSIOLOGY OF ACUTE BURN INJURY
Loss of Normal Skin Function

The skin is the largest organ in the body and is considered vital because of its crucial functions. There are many agents that can cause burn injuries (Table 18-1).[15,18] As a result of a burn injury, skin integrity will be impaired, and the patient will have many physiological and psychological alterations. These include the following:

- Loss of body heat and temperature control.
- Destruction of sweat and sebaceous glands.
- Loss of protective covering of sensory receptors.
- Loss of protective barriers against infection.
- Decrease in number of sensory receptors.
- Loss of presentable cosmetic appearance.

BURN SEVERITY AND DEPTH OF INJURY

Burn injuries have been classified traditionally from first through third degree. Currently second and third degree burns are classified as either partial-thickness or full-thickness injuries. Partial-thickness injuries can be further categorized as superficial or deep (Table 18-2).

Three zones of thermal injury have been described. These relate tissue effects to severity of injury and ultimate viability of the injured tissue[20] (Fig. 18-1). The central area of the wound, having the greatest contact with the heat source, is characterized by coagulation necrosis of the cells and is termed the *zone of coagulation.* Peripheral to this area is the *zone of stasis* where vascular damage and potentially reversible tissue injury have occurred. Within 24 to 48 hours following injury, this area may progress to tissue death without adequate resuscitation. Lying farther peripherally is the *zone of hyperemia,* similar to a superficial partial-thickness burn in which an inflammatory response has occurred. This area has sustained minimal injury and will recover over a period of approximately 5 days. Immediately after burn injury, it may be difficult to differentiate partial-thickness from full-thickness injury particularly in children and the elderly. One goal of therapy is to prevent a zone of stasis from developing into a zone of coagulation.[20]

Table 18-1   Agents Causing Burn Injury

Agent	Characteristics
Thermal	Destruction of tissue secondary to flames, scalding liquids, or steam; systematic effects are proportional to extent of injury and depth; greatest percentage of admissions to burn units.
Chemical	Destruction of tissue secondary to coagulation or dessication of tissue protein; action continues until agent is removed; skin penetration by many chemicals leads to systemic toxicity; injury is generally deeper than it appears; small percentage of admissions to burn units.
Electrical	Destruction of tissue secondary to heat generated by electric current passing through tissues; arc burn; or thermal injury from ignition of clothing; injury is generally more extensive than it appears to be on the basis of surface injury; cardiac conduction system may be affected leading to sudden death or dysrhythmias; severe muscle contraction can produce long bone or vertebral fractures; severe msucle destruction leads to release of myoglobin that can affect kidney function.
Cold liquids/gases	Results in frostbite that is the actual freezing of tissues; freezing of tissue results in ice crystal formation that draws water out of the cells into the extracellular space. The crystals expand causing mechanical destruction of cell walls and organelles; electrolyte imbalances that result contribute to further cell destruction.
Radiation	Damage occurs primarily by gamma/x-ray particles; radiation damages the reproductive mechanisms of tissue cells leading to cellular death; wound appearance is the same as that of a thermal injury.
Toxic epidermal necrolysis syndrome (TENS)	Multiple etiologies; most common are drug reactions and staphylococcal toxin; exfoliative dermatitis occurs usually associated with mucosal involvement of conjuctiva, oronasal or anogenital areas; TENS Type I (Staphylococcal Scalded Skin syndrome) usually occurs in children; intracellular damage results in subgranular intra-epidermal cleavage plane; TENS Type II (Stevens-Johnson syndrome) usually occurs in adults; epidermal split is at the dermal/epidermal junction.

Table 18-2   Depth of Burn: Clinical Assessment

Burn	Skin area involved	Clinical picture	Healing time
First degree	Epidermal layer only.	Red, dry, painful.	Approximately 5 days.
Superficial partial-thickness	Epidermis with some dermis	Moist, pink or mottled; red, painful, blisters.	Within 21 days.
Deep partial-thickness	Destruction of epidermis with most of the dermis, epidermal cells lining hair follicles and sweat glands remain intact, may convert to full-thickness injury.	Pale, mottled, pearly white, mostly dry, often insensate, difficult to differentiate from full-thickness burn.	Heal by wound contraction and reepithelialization within 3-6 weeks; often excised and grafted to provide a better functional and cosmetic result and to decrease length of healing time.
Full-thickness	Destruction of all layers of skin down to or past the subcutaneous fat; sometimes involving fascia, muscle, and bone; the nerves are also destroyed.	Thick, dry, leathery eschar; white, cherry red or brown/black in color; insensate; blood vessels thrombosed.	Requires skin grafting.

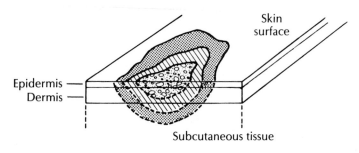

Epidermis
Dermis

Skin surface

Subcutaneous tissue

▨ Zone of hyperemia
◳ Zone of stasis
⊡ Zone of coagulation

Fig. 18-1   Zones of thermal injury. Thermal energy produces concentric zones of decreasingly severe tissue injury. In full-thickness or third-degree burns, the zone of coagulation involves the entire thickness of the dermis, but in partial-thickness, or second-degree burns (as shown here), the zone of coagulation involves only a portion of the dermis. (From Davis JH et al: *Clinical surgery,* St Louis, 1987, Mosby–Year Book.)

PHYSIOLOGICAL ALTERATIONS SECONDARY TO BURN INJURY
Local response

Cellular injury by heat results in the release of cellular enzymes and vasoactive substances, such as histamine, kinins, serotonin, prostaglandins, leukotrienes and interleukin-I. The activation of complement also occurs. As a result, vascular permeability is altered and significant hemodynamic, metabolic, and immunological effects occur locally and systemically. The magnitude of the response is proportionate to the extent of injury[17,20] (Fig. 18-2).

At the capillary level, there is a significant shift of protein molecules, fluid, and electrolytes from the intravascular space to the extravascular space. Lymph flow increases initially but subsequently decreases or ceases because of blockage of lymphatic vessels by the serum proteins leaking through the walls of the damaged capillaries. In extensive burn injury (> 25% total body surface area [TBSA]), edema forms in both burned and unburned areas because of a generalized increase in capillary permeability and hy-

poproteinemia[1] or as a result of the volume and oncotic pressure effects of the large fluid resuscitation volumes.[11] Maximum edema is seen 18 to 24 hours after burn injury.

A decrease in cell transmembrane potential also occurs in extensive burns causing a shift of extracellular sodium and water into the cell resulting in cellular swelling. It is believed this process occurs because of a decrease in adenosine triphosphatase (ATPase). With adequate resuscitation, the membrane potential is restored within 24 to 36 hours.[4]

Systemic Response

The response of all organ systems to burn injury occurs in a biphasic pattern of hypofunction followed by hyperfunction. The degree of physiological change is proportionate to the extent of burn and appears to reach a maximum response in patients with burns over 50% of the TBSA.[20] As the burn wound heals or is closed, organ function returns to normal.

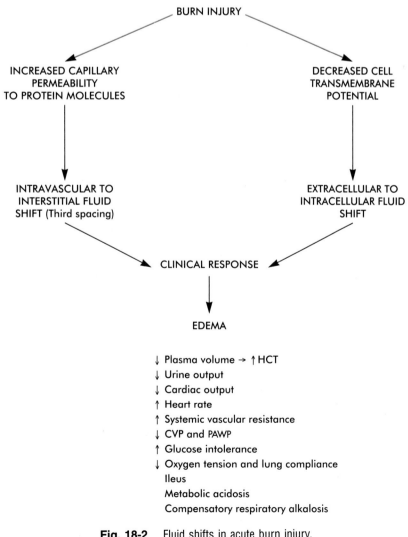

BURN INJURY

INCREASED CAPILLARY PERMEABILITY TO PROTEIN MOLECULES

DECREASED CELL TRANSMEMBRANE POTENTIAL

INTRAVASCULAR TO INTERSTITIAL FLUID SHIFT (Third spacing)

EXTRACELLULAR TO INTRACELLULAR FLUID SHIFT

CLINICAL RESPONSE

EDEMA

↓ Plasma volume → ↑ HCT
↓ Urine output
↓ Cardiac output
↑ Heart rate
↑ Systemic vascular resistance
↓ CVP and PAWP
↑ Glucose intolerance
↓ Oxygen tension and lung compliance
  Ileus
  Metabolic acidosis
  Compensatory respiratory alkalosis

Fig. 18-2 Fluid shifts in acute burn injury.

Cardiovascular Response

The cardiovascular response to burn injury is manifested by a decreased cardiac output and increased peripheral resistance. Blood flow is redistributed early in the postburn period to perfuse essential viscera rather than the peripheral areas of the body. The decreased cardiac output leads to a vasoconstrictive response, which is the body's mechanism for increasing arterial pressure and shunting blood centrally to vital organs, such as the heart and brain. With adequate fluid resuscitation, cardiac output returns to normal in the latter part of the first 24 hours postburn and becomes supranormal thereafter and remains so until the burns are closed.[20]

Host Defense Mechanisms Response

Alterations in host defense mechanisms after an extensive burn injury result from complex interactions of several factors including nutrition, hypermetabolism, and immunological alterations. With the loss of skin, the primary barrier to microorganisms is gone. There is a new portal of entry, and necrotic tissue provides an excellent medium for microbial growth.

Pulmonary Vasculature Response

Initial changes in the pulmonary vasculature as a result of the release of vasoconstriction agents after injury cause a transient pulmonary hypertension and possible decrease in oxygen tension and lung compliance.[20] Additional injury from the inhalation of smoke and products of incomplete combustion cause pulmonary changes, leading to increased mortality that varies with age and burn size.[23]

Renal Response

The renal response is also biphasic. Initially, oliguria results from a decreased plasma flow and glomerular filtration rate. When the resuscitation fluid is reabsorbed after capillary integrity is restored, the increase in cardiac output leads to increased renal blood flow and a diuresis occurs. It is a modest diuresis because of the slow mobilization of edema fluid and the excessive evaporative water loss that occurs because of the loss of skin.[20]

Gastrointestinal Response

The gastrointestinal response to severe burn injury results in the development of an ileus secondary to hypovolemia and neurological and endocrine responses to injury. A decrease in gastric mucosal blood flow may lead to mucosal erosion and eventual ulceration if not protected with antacids or H_2-histamine receptor antagonists.[20]

Metabolic Response

The metabolic response is one of the most significant alterations after burn injury. Hypermetabolism begins as resuscitation is completed and is probably mediated by the secretion of catecholamines. The extensive healing process requires a rapid metabolic rate to support tissue anabolism and reaches its peak between the sixth and tenth days after burn injury. When the wound is closed, oxygen consumption slowly returns to normal. Protein wasting and weight loss are other elements of the metabolic response. Skeletal muscle is catabolized with the rate being affected by several of the following factors: percent body surface area (BSA) burned, age, sex, preburn nutritional status, other health problems, and nutrient intake. Increases in body protein mass and weight generally do not occur until the wound is closed.[27]

WOUND HEALING

When a burn injury disrupts the integumentary system, the body automatically responds with a series of overlapping physiological changes to repair and restore epithelial continuity. Although different terms are used to describe the phases of healing, there is consensus on the actual events occurring.[3]

The *inflammatory response* begins at the moment of injury and lasts from 3 to 4 days after injury. After a brief period of vasoconstriction, increased vascular permeability ensues, and vasodilation increases blood flow to the injury site. White blood cells flood the injured area, and phagocytosis of wound debris begins. Localized edema, erythema, heat, and tenderness are characteristic signs of the inflammatory response.

During the *fibroblastic phase,* which occurs approximately 4 to 20 days after the injury, cells needed for tissue repair and reconstruction proliferate. To establish nutrition for the new tissue, the vascular endothelium proliferates and capillary budding occurs within the wound. Fibroblasts at the wound site migrate over the new capillary network, laying down a bed of granulation tissue (collagen) to fill the wound space. During *wound contraction,* which occurs as granulation tissue forms, myofibroblasts cause the wound edges to pull toward the center. The amount of contraction varies with the elasticity of the tissues and the location of the wound. Once the wound space is filled with granulation tissue, epithelial cells from the burn margins migrate across the wound and eventually reproduce to form a protective barrier between the burn wound and the external environment. This process is called *epithelialization.* Epithelial cells also migrate from the hair follicles and sweat glands present in the wound, forming small islands of cells known as epithelial buds. Newly forming epithelial cells are easily damaged by mechanical trauma and desiccation. If allowed to dry, the wound will form a neoeschar, retarding the healing process. The epithelial cells must secrete enzymes to dissolve the eschar in their path.

The *maturation phase* occurs when immature granulation tissue is highly organized and serves to restore tissue strength. This phase may begin approximately 20 days after burn injury and continues beyond 1 year. Contractures can occur if a burn wound heals with extensive scar tissue formation over a joint. A contracture is the fixation of a joint or area of skin into a flexed or fixed position caused by atrophy and shortening of muscle fibers or by scar for-

Table 18-3 Factors Affecting Wound Healing

Factor	Effect on wound healing
Moisture	Moist environment allows epithelial cells to migrate from wound edges. Dehydration delays healing.
Necrosis	Presence of necrotic tissue, such as eschar, will delay epithelialization.
Oxygen	Decreased oxygen supply to wound inhibits repair and increases potential for wound infection.
Temperature	Hypothermia decreases blood supply and available oxygen to wound and also inhibits leukocyte activity.
Wound infection	Delays healing process as bacteria compete with normal cells for limited oxygen and nutrition.
Age	As an individual ages, respiratory, immune, and cardiovascular systems are less efficient. The dermis is thinner, and its vascularity is decreased. Healing time is delayed.
Nutrition	Increased calories and protein are required for all phases of wound healing.
Health status	Problems, such as psychological stress, smoking, obesity, preexisting health problems, associated injuries, and steroid use, adversely affect wound healing.

mation and the loss of the normal elasticity of the skin.

Under optimum environmental and physiological conditions, a partial-thickness burn heals in 2 to 6 weeks. The persistence of an eschar on a full-thickness burn may delay healing and give rise to life-threatening complications. As bacteria proliferate beneath the eschar, there is a possibility of infection. Approximately 2 weeks after burn injury, the eschar begins to separate from underlying tissue as a result of microbial and leukocytic action on subeschar collagen fibers. Separation generally occurs from the wound margins inward but may occur in patches. An eschar may also be removed earlier by surgical excision. Table 18-3 describes factors that may influence the process of wound healing.

TREATMENT PHASES OF BURN INJURY

There are three phases of treatment for burn injury—resuscitative, acute, and rehabilitative.[22] In the first, or *resuscitative,* phase, the primary goal is to prevent shock secondary to changes in capillary dynamics and cardiac function and to maintain organ function. This period lasts approximately 48 hours and is the most crucial time for the burn-injured patient. Initial care must begin at the scene of injury, continue in the emergency department, and become definitive in the critical care burn unit.

The *acute phase* starts 48 hours after the burn injury when diuresis occurs and continues until the wound has been covered. This period may last weeks or even months. Burn wound care becomes the primary focus during this phase of treatment. The ultimate goal is burn wound closure, whether by spontaneous reepithelialization or by definitive autografting. Nursing care will focus not only on actions to promote wound healing but also on prevention of complications. The nurse's role is critical in the management of the patient's physiological and psychological needs during these two phases.

Restoring the patient's ability to function in society and to return patients to their family role and vocation receives primary emphasis in the third or *rehabilitative phase.* Rarely do critical care nurses participate in this final phase, but the care provided in the previous phases can determine the outcome of rehabilitation. Rehabilitation and discharge planning begin on the day of admission when the critical care nurse provides for patient teaching, emotional support, proper positioning, range of motion, early ambulation, and attentive wound care.

ASSESSMENT
Resuscitative Phase

During the initial phase of injury, the nurse should monitor the indexes of essential organ function hourly or more frequently to prevent complications and detect potential problems early.

Respiratory
- Assess lung sounds, listening for stridor or other signs of respiratory difficulty (see box below).
- Check for edema in airway or security of artificial airway and need for suctioning; airway may not have been stabilized well during transport.
- Assess adequacy of ventilation through arterial blood gas (ABG) or pulse oximeter values, since pulmonary insufficiency may occur during this phase.
- Check carboxyhemoglobin level, if indicated.
- Assist with bronchoscopic examination if there has been an inhalation injury.

▼ Clinical Findings Suggestive of Respiratory Injury

Facial burns.
Presence of soot around mouth and nose and in sputum.
Singed nasal hairs.
Signs of hypoxemia, such as tachycardia, dysrhythmias, anxiety, or lethargy.
The following are signs of respiratory difficulty:
- Increased or decreased respiratory rate.
- Increased use of accessory muscles for breathing.
- Intercostal or sternal retractions.
- Stridor.
- Hoarseness.
Abnormal breath sounds.
Abnormal ABG values.

- Assist with Xenon 133 lung scan to rule out small airways inhalation injury if there is an index of suspicion.
- Measure lung compliance, being alert for decreased compliance.
- Ensure that a daily chest x-ray is evaluated.

Cardiovascular
- Measure vital signs, to include rectal temperature. Significant alterations in vital signs are reflective of hypovolemia and the neuroendocrine response to injury common during this phase.
- Measure and record hemodynamic variables, being aware that a decreased cardiac output is common during the first 24 hours.
- Observe for a possible low central venous pressure and pulmonary artery wedge pressure.
- Palpate for peripheral pulses in extremities with circumferential burns.
- Perform serial ECG if there is a high voltage electrical injury.

Neurological
- Assess sensorium for decreased LOC, reflective of hypoxemia or hypovolemia.

Blood, fluid, and electrolytes
- Assess blood count and serum electrolyte values.

Renal
- Measure urine output, specific gravity, sugar, and acetone levels, observing for oliguria (without adequate resuscitation)—urine output is adequate at 30 to 50 ml/hr in adults and 1 ml/kg/hr in children weighing less than 30 kg (66 lbs).
- Evaluate urinalysis and urine electrolyte levels, as required.

Gastrointestinal
- Measure nasogastric (NG) tube output, pH of gastric contents, and presence of occult blood.
- Auscultate bowel sounds; absent bowel sounds may indicate an ileus.

Integumentary
- Assess level of edema in burned and nonburned tissues—maximum edema occurs between 18 to 24 hours after burn injury.

Psychosocial
- Assess comfort level—severe pain will occur in partial-thickness injury.
- Observe for anxious and combative behavior.
- Assess family for anxiety and need for repetition of information.

Acute Phase

The acute phase extends from 48 hours after burn injury until the burn wound is closed. Usually serum electrolytes, complete blood count (CBC), blood urea nitrogen (BUN), creatinine, prothrombin time/partial thromboplastin time (PT/PTT), and urinalysis are monitored at least twice a week until most of the wounds are covered. Cultures of the wound, sputum, urine, and rectal and nasogastric contents are usually obtained three times per week. During this phase the nurse will need to assess the patient with a major burn injury for the following potential problems.

Respiratory
- Observe for tachypnea, dyspnea, and signs of possible pulmonary infection.
- Check for purulent pulmonary secretions.

Cardiovascular
- Measure cardiac outputs, noting that they will be normal or increased during this phase.
- When measuring vital signs, note that heart rate will normally be between 80 to 120 beats/min.

Neurological
- Observe for restlessness, confusion, or lethargy.

Blood, fluid, and electrolytes
- Review serum laboratory reports.

Renal
- Evaluate urine output for moderate diuresis initially, then normal urine output.
- Test glucose in urine for glycosuria—sign of early sepsis or preclinical diabetes.

Gastrointestinal
- Test NG drainage and stool for occult blood; stress ulcers can occur in this phase.
- Check gastric pH levels; the inability to control gastric pH levels is a sign of impending sepsis.

Integumentary
- Check temperature; if it is beyond the range of 36°-38° C (97° to 100.5° F), hyperthermia or hypothermia may indicate sepsis or extensive loss of heat from open wounds or those in wet dressings.
- Check wound biopsy results for microbial status of wound and invasion of microbes into viable tissue.

Psychosocial
- Observe patient for signs of manipulation, regression, and sleep deprivation.
- Assess comfort level for pain and pruritus.
- Evaluate family for signs of diminishing ability to cope and provide patient with support.

NURSING DIAGNOSIS

The following are possible nursing diagnoses for the patient who has sustained a burn injury:

Resuscitative Phase

- Ineffective airway clearance related to tracheal edema secondary to inhalation injury.
- Impaired gas exchange related to interstitial edema manifested by hypoxemia and hypercapnia.
- Fluid volume deficit secondary to fluid shifts to the interstitium and evaporative loss of fluids from the injured skin.
- High risk for infection related to loss of integument and invasive therapy.
- Potential for hypothermia related to injury of skin and external cooling.
- Disturbance in comfort: acute pain related to burn trauma.
- High risk for injury related to stress response manifested by GI hemorrhage and hyperglycemia.
- High risk for ineffective individual and family coping related to acute stress of critical injury and potential life-threatening crisis.

Acute Phase

- Alteration in fluid and electrolyte balance related to diuresis.
- Impaired skin integrity related to burn wound.
- High risk for nutritional deficit related to increased metabolic demands secondary to wound healing.
- Impaired physical mobility and self-care deficit related to therapeutic splinting or contractures.
- High risk for ineffective individual and family coping related to acute stress of critical injury and potential lifestyle changes.

Rehabilitation Phase

- High risk for noncompliance related to negative side effects of prescribed treatments.
- Disturbance in comfort: pruritus related to healing of new skin.
- Disturbance in self-concept related to functional disabilities, hypertrophic scarring, and disruption of vocational roles.

PATIENT OUTCOMES

Below are sample outcomes specifically for the patient requiring burn wound therapy. Following intervention, the patient will manifest:

- Clear breath sounds on auscultation, after pulmonary hygiene.
- Decreased shortness of breath and work of breathing with appropriate positioning.
- Appropriate weight gain in first 48 hours with diuresis occurring over next 8 to 10 days at the weight loss rate of no more than 10% of weight gain per day.
- Urine output in first 48 hours of 30 to 50 ml/hr (75 to 100 ml/hr in electric injuries).
- A pulse ranging from 80 to 120 beats/min.
- A cardiac output and pulmonary artery wedge pressure that is initially low (first 6 to 12 hours) followed by a normal-to-high output with normal wedge pressure.
- Urine specific gravity between 1.010 and 1.020. (During diuresis, the specific gravity may be less than 1.010.)
- A decrease in perceived pain level based on a subjective scale or change in physiological symptoms.
- Negative sputum, blood, and urine cultures. Absence of wound biopsy evidence of burn wound infection.
- Healthy granulation tissue with beginning epithelial coverage from the burn wound margins.
- Body temperature between 36° to 38° C (97° F to 100.5° F).
- Acceptable white blood cell and platelet counts, coagulation times, and serum glucose.
- Clean, dry IV catheter sites with normal skin color and temperature.
- Allograft or autograft skin adherence to granulation tissue.
- Normal serum glucose levels.
- Gastric pH greater than 5.
- Heme negative stools and gastric contents.
- Return of bowel sounds and soft, formed stools.

CHEMICAL BURNS

A chemical burn will continue to damage the tissue until the chemical has been completely removed or neutralized by an external agent. Neutralizing agents should not be employed because they produce heat when they interact with the chemical. Although this same effect may occur with water, for the majority of chemical injuries, irrigation with large volumes of water will remove the heat.

ELECTRICAL INJURIES

Electrical injuries are caused by contact with varied sources, such as household current, arc welders, car batteries, high-tension electrical lines, or lightning. The greatest injury rate is among children from infancy to four years old, primarily from electrical cord and electrical outlet injuries. The next age peak is among the 20 to 50 year olds, predominantly male, with the majority of injuries occurring in the industrial environment.

Body tissues and fluids will conduct electricity with the body acting as a volume conductor. Heat is produced as a function of voltage drop and current flow per unit cross-sectional area (current density).[19,20,21] Because of current density, electrical injuries of the trunk are less frequent in relation to the frequency of injury to extremities.

In high-voltage injury, charring of skin occurs at points of contact and is caused by current arcing across flexion surfaces of joints. Flame injury may also be associated with arcing or clothing ignition. Other serious complications related to electrical injury include severe musculoskeletal injury, such as long bone and skull fractures from falls and vertebral fractures from falls or tetanic contrac-

Text continued on p. 420.

Skill 18-1 Initial Inpatient Treatment of Acute Burn Injury[7,15,21]

EQUIPMENT AND SUPPLIES

- Clean gloves
- Clean sheets kept in warmer, if possible
- Overhead warmers
- 16- and 18-gauge IV catheters and tubing
- Blood and urine specimen tubes
- Lactated Ringer's solution
- Suction equipment, airways, bag-valve-mask device, and intubation tray
- Nonrebreathing and high humidity face mask and T-piece
- Mechanical ventilator on standby
- Tetanus toxoid and tetanus immune globulin
- Hard cervical collar, sandbags, tape, and backboard
- Heavy scissors and plastic bag for clothing
- Sutures and suture set
- No. 18 Fr NG tube and suction setup
- No. 16 Fr urethral catheter with insertion kit
- Burn chart and burn admission packet

NURSING INTERVENTIONS
Primary survey

1. Quickly don clean gloves.
2. Establish or reassess the patency of an established airway while maintaining the head and neck in a neutral position. Often an endotracheal (ET) tube placed at the scene is not adequately positioned.
3. If an spinal cord injury (SCI) is probable and the spinal cord has not been immobilized, apply a cervical collar, sandbags, and backboard as appropriate. Maintain immobilization devices in place until all vertebral components of the spinal column have been examined by x-ray.
4. Simultaneously, observe patient's skin color and auscultate the lungs to ensure bilateral effective ventilation. Note presence of thick circumferential eschar of the chest. A patient may require immediate escharotomy caused by chest restriction.
5. Assess for indications of severe inhalation injury while another team member draws blood for ABG determinations, which include a carboxyhemoglobin level, if indicated by history.
6. If the patient requires intubation, assist with nasotracheal intubation, the preferred route for prevention of hyperextension of the neck. Tracheostomy should be avoided if possible because of the high risk of infection. Secure the airway.
7. Administer oxygen therapy as ordered. This will be by high humidity face mask, T-piece, or mechanical ventilator. Patients suspected of having carbon monoxide poisoning will require 100% oxygen. Until the ventilator or high humidity mask is available, support patient with nonrebreathing mask at 10 L/min (80% oxygen) or bag-valvemask at 15 L/min (99% oxygen).
8. Place patient on cardiac monitor and observe for significant dysrhythmias.
9. Palpate for pulse, determining quality and rate. If no pulse, begin cardiac massage.
10. Inspect for uncontrolled external bleeding. If present, provide direct pressure to area with dry dressing.
11. If the burn wound is greater than 20%, insert at least one 16- or 18-gauge IV catheter in an upper extremity vein and infuse lactated Ringer's solution at an initial rate of 500 ml/hr. Avoid inserting catheters through or below circumferential burns.
12. Suture all IV catheters in place. No dressing is necessary.

13. Avoid if possible, emergency insertion of central catheters. Central line sites should be reserved for later use.
14. While inserting IV lines, draw serum for laboratory studies, including CBC, electrolytes, BUN, creatinine, and glucose.
15. Perform brief neurological examination, determining possible need for increased SCI protection, dextrose 50% for hypoglycemia, or Narcan for narcotic overdose.
16. To further assess circulatory status, insert no. 16 Fr indwelling urethral catheter and measure urinary output. Send urine for urinalysis.
17. Insert a no. 18 Fr NG tube and connect to intermittent or low continuous suction to prevent aspiration. A patient with extensive burn injury can be expected to develop an ileus.

Secondary survey

1. While performing the secondary survey, obtain a brief history from the emergency medical technicians, patient, and family.
2. Obtain portable spinal cord and chest x-rays and send them to be read by the radiologist.
3. Remove all clothing after spinal cord x-rays have been evaluated or cut off clothing. Ensure all jewelry is removed and secured in a safe place.
4. Cover patient with warm, clean, dry sheets and use overhead warmers if available. No other wound care is required until the patient reaches an intensive care unit (ICU) or burn unit.
5. Obtain a complete set of vital signs including rectal temperature.
6. Continually reassess the airway and breathing. Evaluate ABG results and adjust patient's oxygen delivery system, as ordered.
7. Perform head-to-toe systematic survey, splinting fractures that have not yet been treated.
8. Perform assessment using the Lund and Browder chart if available (Fig. 18-3). When the burns are scattered, a rule of thumb is that the size of the patient's palm is equal to approximately 1% TBSA.
9. Assess the depth and extent of burn injury. The extent of injury includes only partial-thickness and full-thickness injury, not first-degree injury. Use the "Rule of Nines" (Fig. 18-4) for initial rapid estimate of the percentage of BSA burned.
10. Weigh patient or obtain weight from patient or family member. Record in kilograms.
11. Calculate the volume of fluids required in the first 24 hours after burn injury and administer according to the consensus formula (see Skill 18-4).
12. Evaluate peripheral pulses every 15 minutes when patients have large areas of BSA burned. Observe for edema formation as fluids are administered. There is the potential for the pressure of the edema fluid to obliterate arterial blood flow. This is especially true in extremities with circumferential full-thickness burns.
13. Prepare for possible escharotomies that may be needed to relieve the pressure. If severe muscle damage has occurred, prepare for a fasciotomy.
14. Evaluate blood pressure measurements every 15 minutes. Blood pressure measurements are the least useful objective data obtained in this phase. Because of severe vasoconstriction, the measurements are often incorrect and not indicative of the therapeutic response. However, such determinations, if evaluated with other objective data, can provide some measure of the adequacy of hemodynamic response.

Continued.

Skill 18-1   Initial Inpatient Treatment of Acute Burn Injury[7,15,21]—cont'd

15. When measuring the blood pressure, take care not to cause further tissue damage to burned areas and always remove the cuff between measurements.
16. Obtain chest x-ray and ECG.
17. Administer pain medication by IV route only. Use a short-acting narcotic, such as morphine sulfate, if not contraindicated.
18. Assess need for tetanus immunization.
19. Throughout the entire initial management period, provide emotional support to both the patient and the family.

20. Assess the need for and assist in the coordination of the transfer to a burn center.
21. Have the patient's emergency room physician make the initial contact with the burn center physician.
22. Complete a transfer summary information sheet to ensure that all critical elements of the patient preparation and transportation arrangements are clearly communicated and implemented.

AREA	0-1 YEAR	1-4 YEARS	5-9 YEARS	10-14 YEARS	15 YEARS	ADULT	2°	3°
Head	19	17	13	11	9	7		
Neck	2	2	2	2	2	2		
Ant. Trunk	13	13	13	13	13	13		
Post. Trunk	13	13	13	13	13	13		
R. Buttock	2½	2½	2½	2½	2½	2½		
L. Buttock	2½	2½	2½	2½	2½	2½		
Genitalia	1	1	1	1	1	1		
R. U. Arm	4	4	4	4	4	4		
L. U. Arm	4	4	4	4	4	4		
R. L. Arm	3	3	3	3	3	3		
L. L. Arm	3	3	3	3	3	3		
R. Hand	2½	2½	2½	2½	2½	2½		
L. Hand	2½	2½	2½	2½	2½	2½		
R. Thigh	5½	6½	8	8½	9	9½		
L. Thigh	5½	6½	8	8½	9	9½		
R. Leg	5	5	5½	6	6½	7		
L. Leg	5	5	5½	6	6½	7		
R. Foot	3½	3½	3½	3½	3½	3½		
L. Foot	3½	3½	3½	3½	3½	3½		
TOTAL								

Fig. 18-3   Estimation of extent of burn by percentage of body surface: Lund and Browder chart. (From Johanson BC, Wells SJ, Hoffmeister D et al: *Standards for critical care,* ed 3, St Louis, 1988, Mosby–Year Book.)

tions; deep tissue necrosis that may require amputation of extremities; neurological deficits caused by destruction of nerves; cataracts; and cardiac dysrhythmias. Lightning injuries frequently result in cardiopulmonary arrest and transient but severe central nervous system deficits. Cutaneous injury is usually superficial.[17,19,20]

INTRAVENOUS FLUIDS

Although there are a number of burn formulas, most burn centers administer only crystalloid fluids in the first 24 hours. It is believed that colloid-containing products are unnecessary within the first 24 hours, since the protein molecules "leak" across the capillary membranes, causing more tissue edema. The resuscitation fluid most commonly used is lactated Ringer's solution unless there are associated conditions requiring blood therapy. The formula discussed in Skill 18-4 is the consensus burn fluid administration formula taught in the Advanced Burn Life Support (ABLS) course.[15]

ESCHAROTOMY/FASCIOTOMY

An *escharotomy* is an incision through circumferential eschar of a burned extremity, or trunk, down to viable subcutaneous tissue. It allows the eschar to separate, releasing constriction on arteries or the chest. If subfascial injury has occurred, a *fasciotomy* may be performed. Fasciotomies

Skill 18-2   Initial Prehospital and Emergency Department Treatment of Chemical Burns

EQUIPMENT AND SUPPLIES

- Clean, thick rubber gloves
- Protective clothing per protocol
- Access to a shower or Hubbard tank

NURSING INTERVENTIONS

1. Wear protective clothing according to policy.
2. Rapidly remove garments that are saturated with the chemical while rushing patient to irrigation area. All other garments, such as shoes, socks, and gloves, should be removed from patient before irrigation is complete.
3. If agent is a powderlike material, such as lime, brush off as much as possible before irrigating. Check the hair, under the nails, and between the toes for collections of the chemical.
4. Continue to remove clothing while irrigating a chemical burn in the shower area.
5. To provide for comfort, seat the patient on a chair in a running shower. If unstable, the patient should be horizontal during irrigation.
6. Irrigate with water for no less than 30 minutes and preferably for 60 minutes.[21] This decreases the concentration of the chemical agent and physically removes it from the wound, thus decreasing the rate and amount of the reaction between the chemical and the tissue.
7. Following irrigation on the scene and during transportation to the hospital, place the chemically burned patient under wet towels. This helps to relieve pain and continues to dilute the chemical. Caution is needed to prevent hypothermia if the burn is extensive.
8. If possible, take samples of the chemical agent with a product label to the emergency department.

Emergency department treatment

1. If hydrofluoric acid (used in glass etching) or oxalic acid are the causative agents, irrigate with water and then neutralize the area with subcutaneous injections of 10% calcium gluconate, as ordered. This should be done only after consultation with physicians at a burn center.[15]
2. If phenol (an acidic alcohol in sanitizers and disinfectants) is the causative agent, irrigate with water only if a high density shower is available. Phenol is more soluble in polyethylene glycol, therefore a 50% solution of this agent should be used for irrigation as soon as possible. It is important to remove all of the polyethylene glycol from the skin since it may cause systemic toxicity.[13]
3. Irrigate white phosphorus burns (which may be caused by certain fertilizers or fireworks) with water and then debride the remaining phosphorus particles. The particles should be kept under water. Cover the burn wound with moist dressings to occlude air. A 1% copper sulfate solution or a Wood's lamp may be used to facilitate the identification of the phosphorus particles. If the copper sulfate solution is used, it must be thoroughly rinsed from the skin to prevent systemic effects.[13,15]
4. With moderate to large tar or asphalt burns, cool area first with large volumes of water. Use petrolatum-based products to remove the tar. Dress with petrolatum-based dressing, such as Xeroform gauze. Change dressings and wash with water every 6 to 8 hours until tar dissolves.[15]
5. For a patient whose fingers are adhered together with a fast-setting epoxy glue, remove glue with acetone. If the glue is on mucous membranes or in the eyes, swab area with vegetable oil until the glue is removed.
6. All chemical injuries should be treated based on advice from physicians at a burn center.

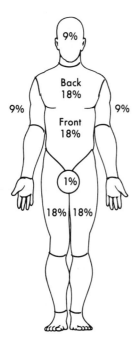

Fig. 18-4   Estimation of extent of burn (percentage of body surface involved) by Rule of Nines. (From Beare PG, Myers JL: *Principles and practice of adult health nursing,* St Louis, 1990, Mosby Year-Book.)

▼ Burn Wound Assessment Documentation Terms

Eschar - Adherent, separating, cheesy yellow, pearly white, black, presence of greenish, brown, or black spots

Granulation tissue - Beefy red, clean and pink, free bleeding, capillary budding evident, granulating well, wound contracting

Special anatomical areas - Clean and dry, purulent drainage, erythematous, edematous

Meshed grafts - Dressings damp, adherent, interstices filling in, ___% graft take, staples present, staples removed, skin intact, dry and scaly, blisters, open areas

Sheet grafts - Serosanguineous, sanguinous, or purulent drainage; intact and adherent; vesicles present; vesicles absent

Donor sites - Moist, drying, soupy, brown, red, whitish, healed, dry

Scar tissue - Red, enlarged, hypertrophic, firm, pink, hyperemic

Skill 18-3 Initial Prehospital Treatment of Electric Injuries

EQUIPMENT AND SUPPLIES

- Oxygen tank, flow meter, and face mask
- Airways, suction equipment, bag-valve-mask, or pocket mask
- Lactated Ringer's solution and IV equipment
- Spinal board, hard cervical collar, sand bags, and tape
- Musculoskeletal splints
- Gauze dressings
- Clean gloves
- Same equipment as in Skill 18-1

NURSING INTERVENTIONS
Prehospital phase

1. Remove all "live" electrical sources from the accident scene by tripping off fuses and switches controlling the source or cutting energized cables with insulated cutters. Contact the power company if necessary. "Live" wires can also be removed with a nonconductant object, such as a wooden pole.
2. Establish a patent airway with cervical-spine control.
3. Assess for adequate breathing. Apply face mask at 5 to 8 L/min if patient has normal respirations. If patient is apneic or has shallow or labored respirations, apply bag-valve-mask or pocket mask and begin ventilatory support. If necessary, intubate according to protocol.
4. Assess for pulse and adequate circulation. Provide cardiopulmonary resuscitation (CPR) if indicated.
5. Inspect for external bleeding and apply direct pressure to site with dry gauze dressing.
6. Perform rapid neurological assessment. Place patient on backboard with hard cervical collar to protect against possible SCI. Cervical spine injury, as a result of a fall, may be seen in association with electrical injury.
7. Evaluate for and stabilize any other fractures. Musculoskeletal injuries are commonly found in electrically injured patients caused by muscle tetany, falls, joint dislocations, and tendon ruptures.[19,20]
8. Connect patient to cardiac monitor.
9. Insert 16- or 18-gauge IV catheter in a peripheral vein and infuse lactated Ringer's solution at a rate of 500 ml/hr in an adult.
10. Establish radio contact with physician and monitor cardiac rhythm carefully. Respiratory arrest and ventricular fibrillation or asystole are frequent occurrences in patients with electrical injury.
11. If possible, obtain a brief history of the accident, including voltage, type of current, location of contact, and duration of contact. Transport as quickly as possible to nearest appropriate facility.

INPATIENT TREATMENT
Primary survey

1. Assess the patient's airway, breathing, and circulation on arrival at receiving facility. Keep oxygen mask on.
2. Continue to monitor cardiac rhythm. Dysrhythmias and ST segment changes are commonly found in patients with electrical injuries.
3. If the patient requires CPR, continue aggressive resuscitation in spite of dilated fixed pupils and absent vital signs. Studies have shown that patients with electrical injuries have had successful neurological recovery even after prolonged periods of apnea and asystole.[35]
4. Ensure that two 18-, 16-, or 14-g IV catheters have been inserted, and administer lactated Ringer's solution at a rate that will maintain the urine output at 75 to 100 ml/hr.[35] Do not rely on a burn formula for fluid resuscitation, because the deep tissue necrosis caused by electrical injury may not be apparent.
5. While inserting the IV lines, perform the following laboratory evaluations, as ordered: CBC, electrolytes, BUN and creatinine, type and crossmatching, serial myocardial enzymes, and ABG determinations.
6. Perform a rapid neurological assessment, looking for signs of SCI and altered LOC. Neurological injury is common.
7. Insert 18 Fr NG tube.
8. Insert 16 Fr or larger urethral catheter and assess for myoglobinuria or hemoglobinuria by observing for port wine or brownish-colored urine. Send a urine sample for urinalysis and urine hemochromogens. Severe muscle necrosis releases myoglobin and hemoglobin degradation products that when deposited in the renal tubules can cause renal failure.

Secondary survey

1. Concurrently, obtain brief history from emergency medical technicians.
2. Maintain patient on backboard with hard cervical collar until SCI has been ruled out.
3. Remove all of patient's clothing only after SCI has been ruled out. If necessary, cut the clothing away. Cover patient with sheets and light blanket.
4. Obtain complete vital signs, evaluate peripheral pulses, and observe for fascial compartment edema. The patient may require an escharotomy or fasciotomy.
5. Perform a head-to-toe systematic survey, examining the eyes for damage to the lens. Immediate burns to the eyes and development of cataracts occur in 1% to 9% of patients sustaining an electrical injury.[35]
6. Assess patient for associated injuries to bones, joints, and internal organs. This may involve preparing for a peritoneal lavage.
7. Assess the burn injury, carefully searching for multiple entry or exit wounds.
8. As the ABG values are reported, adjust the patient's oxygen delivery, as ordered.
9. Give sodium bicarbonate for acidosis, as ordered. The anaerobic metabolism occurring in large areas of ischemic muscle injury may result in lactic acidosis. Sodium bicarbonate alkalinization may also be used to prevent precipitation of hemochromogens in the renal tubules.
10. Obtain a baseline ECG.
11. Treat hemochromogens in the urine, as ordered.

Skill 18-4   Administration of Intravenous Fluids in the First 24 Hours Postburn

EQUIPMENT AND SUPPLIES

- 1000 ml bags lactated Ringer's solution
- Rapid rate volumetric infusion pump
- IV tubing and pump cassettes

NURSING INTERVENTIONS

1. When beginning fluid therapy, number all fluid containers sequentially as they are hung. Begin recording hourly intake and output as soon as possible.
2. For adults, administer 2 to 4 ml lactated Ringer's solution/kg body weight/% burn.
3. For children, administer 3 to 4 ml lactated Ringer's/kg body weight/% burn. In addition, the physician will calculate an added maintenance level of fluid (usually D5 ½ normal saline [NS]).
4. Administer one half of the calculated amount during the first 8 hours after burn injury—not after admission to the hospital.
5. Administer the remaining half of the fluid over the next 16 hours.
6. Titrate the fluid rate and provide more or less fluid to keep urine output at 30 to 50 ml/hr for adults and 1 ml/kg/hr for children less than 30 kg. For example:
   Adult patient weighing 70 kg with a 55% TBSA burn:
   2 to 4 ml × 70 kg × 55% = 7700 to 15,400 ml lactated Ringer's solution in first 24 hours after burn injury. Administer 3850 to 7700 ml in first 8 hours and the rest (3850 to 7700 ml) over the next 16 hours.
7. In patients with electrical injury, begin the fluid at a rate of 500 ml/hr and then adjust to maintain urinary output at 75 to 100 ml/hr[20] (see Skill 18-3).

are only required for relief of elevated compartmental pressure caused by muscle edema. The nurse should have an understanding of the physician's specific protocol and prepare equipment as required.

INFECTION CONTROL IN THE BURN UNIT

Control of infections in the burn unit is one of the most crucial objectives in burn care. Although there have been many advances in burn care, infection continues to be the leading cause of death in burn patients.

Infection Control Protocol for Open Method of Wound Care

1. Use reverse isolation techniques. The use of a private room is most effective in decreasing cross-contamination.[14]
2. Wash hands with a surgical detergent disinfectant for 10 to 15 seconds before the following:
   - Start of the shift.
   - Before and after any physical contact with a patient.
   - Before and after any physical contact with a patient's equipment or personal articles.

Skill 18-5   Obtaining Burn Wound Culture

Wound cultures are commonly obtained on admission and then two or three times weekly to monitor and document the changes in wound flora.

EQUIPMENT AND SUPPLIES

- Culture medium
- Requisition slip and label
- Antimicrobial solution
- Sterile normal saline

NURSING INTERVENTIONS

1. Place culture medium, laboratory requisition slip, and patient label at bedside. Dress for procedure according to dress code.
2. Cleanse area to be cultured with half-strength antimicrobial solution and rinse with sterile normal saline. Let wound air dry.
3. Place culture medium on dry wound surface using excess gauze strips on each side of the medium to lift medium out of container, place on wound, and place back in container.
4. Place lid on container and place patient's name label on lid.
5. Send culture to laboratory.
6. Document site and time of culture.

- Before and after each use of gloves.
- Whenever hands become dirty.
- After personal use of toilet.
- Before and after eating.
- At the end of a shift.
3. Wear scrub clothes, cover gown, plastic apron, hair cover, shoe covers, gloves, and mask, as appropriate. Use sterile gloves when performing direct wound care or invasive procedures.
4. Monitor environmental cleaning. Damp mop and dust all areas of the patient's room daily. Dispose of trash and infected waste properly. Remove food from the room or store properly in closed containers. Do not open windows or allow potted plants or flowers in the room.
5. Do not let staff with infectious bacterial, fungal, or viral diseases come in contact with patients.
6. Monitor visitors for the presence of infectious diseases. They must be instructed and monitored on the use of proper dress-code procedures. Children under the age of 16 pose a major risk of infection for burned patients. If allowed to visit, carefully screen them for potential presence of infectious diseases.

METHODS OF BURN WOUND TREATMENT

While allowing time for healing to occur, the burn wound must be debrided and protected to prevent infection and environmental hazards, such as hypothermia and desiccation. There are the following two main methods of treatment used to care for burn wounds:

1. *Open (exposure) method*—The wounds are covered

Skill 18-6   Cleansing Burn Wounds in Bed from Sterile Basins

Cleansing burn wounds from sterile basins with a patient in bed is indicated when the patient is hemodynamically too unstable to be safely transferred to a stretcher and transported to a hydrotherapy room.

EQUIPMENT AND SUPPLIES

- Two large sterile basins
- Antimicrobial solution
- Warmed sterile water or saline
- Gauze sponges
- Cotton-tipped applicators
- Sterile towels
- Sterile gloves
- Clean gloves
- Protective clothing according to unit protocol

NURSING INTERVENTIONS

1. Premedicate patient with pain medication, since this procedure is one of the most painful that the patient will experience.
2. Wear protective clothing according to unit protocol.
3. Assemble bath supplies at bedside. In one basin, dilute full-strength antimicrobial solution to quarter-strength with warmed sterile water or saline. In the second basin, use plain water or saline as rinse solution.
4. Ensure that the patient's vital signs are stable. The room temperature should be 29° C(85° F) with 60% humidity to prevent hypothermia caused by heat loss through open burn wounds and shivering.
5. Wearing clean gloves, remove splints or slings, (wash before reapplying) and gently remove and discard old dressings.
6. Inspect wounds for signs of healing, infection, need for debridement, and readiness for grafting.
7. Open sterile gauze sponge packs and don sterile gloves.
8. Starting with the face, bathe patient with gauze sponges and antimicrobial cleansing agent, applying only pressure needed to clean the burn wounds. Gently cleanse areas with obvious epithelial growth to prevent damage to the new tissue. Shave all hair from wounds and within a 2.5 cm (1-inch) area surrounding wounds.
9. Wet each sponge and use only once before discarding. This ensures that bacteria are not spread from one area to another.
10. Thoroughly rinse area with rinsing solution.
11. Protect eyes while cleaning face. Clean eyes gently with rinse water or saline only. Clean nares and external ear with cotton-tipped applicators.
12. Remove all previously applied topical agent.
13. Using forceps and scissors, debride any loose, necrotic tissue evident on wounds (Skill 18-7). Leave blisters intact or debride them based on unit policy; usually they are debrided in the burn unit.
14. After bathing, lay each extremity on a sterile towel to keep clean until topical agent or dressings are reapplied and linen is changed.

with a topical antimicrobial agent and then left open to air. The patient will require strict isolation. Some of the advantages of this method are that it permits continuous wound assessment and allows for movement of involved joints. The agents used in the open method often provide for better bacterial control and the patients have fewer febrile episodes. The open method is more cost effective in terms of sterile dressing supplies and labor costs (Fig. 18-5).

2. *Closed (occlusive) method*—The wound is covered with gauze dressings that have been saturated with a topical antimicrobial agent. Then thick, dry, sturdy dressings are applied. The dressings are covered with large sheets of stretch or net bandage and held together by safety pins or ties. The advantages of this method include less heat loss and more comfort for the patient. Faster eschar separation occurs and barrier isolation is not required. The occlusive dressings will need to be changed two to three times daily, requiring a great deal of time and labor for the nursing staff.

Hydrotherapy

Two important purposes of hydrotherapy in burn wound care are to prevent the buildup of microorganisms on the wound surface, and to loosen, cleanse, and debride dead

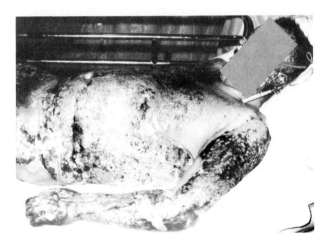

Fig. 18-5   Open or exposure method of burn wound management. A warm environment must be provided, preferably in a private room. A thin layer of topical antimicrobial agent covers the burn wounds. (From Phipps WJ, Long BC, Woods NF, and Cassmeyer VL: *Medical-surgical nursing: concepts and clinical practive,* ed 4, St Louis, 1991, Mosby–Year Book.)

tissue present on the wound. Methods for cleansing burn wounds are listed as follows:

- Bathing in bed from sterile basins.
- Having patient stand or sit in shower.
- Immersing in water in Hubbard tank (not advocated because of potential for cross-contamination).
- Spraying with water while on a plinth suspended over the Hubbard tank.
- Spraying with water while patient lies on a shower litter with a drain.

Wound Debridement

Debridement is the removal of foreign material, devitalized tissue, and cellular debris from a wound. This process is initiated in the resuscitative phase when the burn victim enters the ICU. All loose skin, including intact blisters, are removed from the wound and the area is cleansed through hydrotherapy. Later, in the acute phase, debridement becomes of primary importance to control burn wound sepsis, remove unhealthy nonviable tissue, and prepare the wound bed for coverage or grafting. If not surgically excised, all necrotic tissue should be debrided because eschar acts as a physical obstacle to epithelization and wound contraction.[16] Moist eschar is also an excellent medium for bacterial growth. Mechanical, enzymatic, and surgical debridement are three types of procedures used for burn wound management.

Mechanical debridement

Mechanical debridement should be included as part of each hydrotherapy treatment until all eschar is removed. Tissue that is loose can be gently cut away using scissors and forceps. Caution should be taken in debriding wounds of patients with low platelet counts or those on anticoagulants. If the wound requiring debridement is extensive, it may be debrided by a surgeon in the operating room.[19]

Wet-to-wet and wet-to-dry dressings

When eschar is removed, the result is a wound surface with exudate and fibrous debris. The wound must be kept clean to prevent bacterial proliferation. Debridement using wet-to-wet or wet-to-dry dressings is indicated for the removal of remnants of eschar, wound debris, adherent crusts, and exudate from the wound bed frequently in preparation for definitive skin grafting. Although wet-to-wet dressings may not accomplish as much wound debridement, they cause less damage to granulation tissue.[3]

Enzymatic debridement

Enzymatic debridement is accomplished by the use of a proteolytic substance that may shorten the time required for eschar separation from the burn wound. Applied as a topical agent, these enzymes dissolve eschar and necrotic tissue. Sutilains (Travase) is the most common enzymatic debriding agent used in burn units today.[24] Since debridement with enzymes may be incomplete, they are often used with an antimicrobial topical agent to prevent sepsis.

Skill 18-7   Mechanical Debridement with Scissors and Forceps

EQUIPMENT AND SUPPLIES

- Scissors
- Forceps
- Sterile gloves
- Coarse mesh gauze sponges
- Silver nitrate applicators (for hemostasis)
- Sutures and electrocautery unit available

NURSING INTERVENTIONS

1. Premedicate patient.
2. Assemble sterile tray at bedside.
3. Wear protective clothing according to unit protocol.
4. Clean burn wound according to hydrotherapy protocol.
5. Inspect wound for presence of loose necrotic tissue or pockets under intact eschar that might contain purulent drainage.
6. Gently lift loose eschar or tissue with forceps and cut away. Do not forcibly remove intact eschar as healthy tissue underneath may be damaged and excessive bleeding may result.
7. Assess the patient's pain tolerance throughout the procedure.
8. Control active bleeding by applying firm constant pressure with coarse mesh gauze for at least 3 minutes. If this is unsuccessful, apply silver nitrate applicator to source of bleeding and continue pressure. If bleeding continues, notify physician. Electrocautery or suturing may be indicated.
9. Once debridement is complete, clean and rinse wound and reapply antimicrobial topical agent or dressings, as indicated.
10. Document condition of wound, areas debrided, and patient's tolerance of procedure.

Advantages and Disadvantages of Biologic/Synthetic Skin Dressings

ADVANTAGES

Decrease pain.
Reduce evaporative water loss and heat loss through open burn wounds.
Allow for increased range of motion (ROM) of affected joints.
Control bacterial growth on wound surface.
Prevent further wound contamination.
Prevent damage to developing granulation tissue.
Decrease metabolic rate.

DISADVANTAGES

Expensive.
Nontransparent dressing does not permit continuous wound observation.
Inadequate supply and difficulty in collecting allograft skin.
Potential development of inflammatory reaction or submembrane infection leading to rejection of dressing and development of wound infection.

Topical Antimicrobial Agents

There are several topical antimicrobial agents that may be effective in controlling organisms in the burn wound. None of these agents will sterilize the wound. They only control the bacterial or fungal population of the wound until the body can handle the insult and until surgical management can be accomplished. The agent used will be determined by the physician based on type and depth of wound, location, laboratory and clinical assessment of the wound, and agent side effects (Table 18-4).

BIOLOGICAL AND SYNTHETIC SKIN DRESSINGS

A biological and synthetic skin dressing is human or animal tissue or synthetic material used to cover the burn wound temporarily to prevent infection or desiccation. Such dressings have assumed a greater role in burn care as more patients are undergoing early excision of eschar. Excision removes devitalized tissue before infection occurs. The wound can then be covered with autograft skin earlier so that the risk of wound infection is reduced, epithelial regeneration from surviving skin appendages is accelerated, function is restored sooner, and scar formation is lessened. Although research related to the use of cultured epithelium is promising, this wound coverage for many patients with extensive burns is not currently available. Therefore the use of biological and synthetic skin dressings is beneficial in providing wound coverage until there is sufficient autograft skin available for wound closure (see box on p. 424).[6]

Skin Grafting[20,26]

To permanently close a full-thickness or deep partial-thickness burn wound, application of autograft skin (from patient's own body) is required. In cases where extensive BSA burns limit the amount of skin that can be used as donor sites, the priority areas to be covered are the face, hands, feet, and over the joints. Any burn wound that will not heal spontaneously within 3 weeks is a candidate for grafting (Table 18-5).

Meshed autograft skin

Split-thickness meshed autograft skin is commonly used for patients with extensive burns, as the meshing allows for expansion of the graft to cover a greater area. Usually the skin grafts are only expanded 1.5 to 4 times their normal size. The skin graft is placed dermal side down on a clean wound bed and is precisely approximated at the wound margin and to adjacent skin grafts. Staples, surgical

Text continued on p. 429.

Table 18-4 Topical Antimicrobial Agents for Burn Wounds Management

Agent	Indications	Advantages	Disadvantages	Nursing Implications
Bacitracin ointment	Antimicrobial activity and lubricant for sensitive areas (i.e. lips and eyelids).	Economical; painless; easy to apply.	Limited antimicrobial activity; no penetration of eschar.	Apply to cleansed area two or three times daily.
Clotrimazole cream (Lotrimin)	Fungal colonization of wounds.	Broad antifungal spectrum of activity; ease of application; painless.	No accompanying antibacterial activity; potential skin irritation and blistering.	Apply thin coat of agent to wound and wait 20 minutes before applying any dressings ordered. Must use an antibacterial agent in addition to antifungal agent. Not for ophthalmic use.
Mafenide acetate (Sulfamylon)	Active against most gram-positive and gram-negative burn wound pathogens; drug of choice for electrical and ear burns and wounds colonized with organisms resistant to other topical agents.	Penetrates eschar better than other agents; used without dressings, thereby promoting mobility; no gram-negative resistant organisms.	Pain on application to partial-thickness burns and for 30 minutes thereafter; allergic maculopapular skin rash may occur; hyperchloremic metabolic acidosis may be produced by increased renal losses of bicarbonate and induce compensatory hyperventilation; superinfection with fungi possible; cautious use required in patients with impaired renal or pulmonary function.	Apply once or twice daily with sterile glove; do not use dressings because they reduce effectiveness of agent and may cause maceration; monitor respiratory rate closely; evaluate electrolyte values and arterial pH for acidosis; monitor intake and output; allergic skin reaction may occur.
Silver nitrate	Effective against wide spectrum of common burn wound bacterial pathogens; used in patients with sulfa allergy or epidermalogical diseases such as Toxic Epidermal Necrolysis Syndrome.	Economical; silver-resistant organisms are uncommon; painless; no sensitivity reported.	Hypotonic solution can cause leaching of sodium, potassium and other plasma solutes; methemoglobinemia may result from absorption of nitrite; poor penetration of eschar; dressings must remain moist at all times to prevent caustic concentrations of silver nitrate; requires bulky dressings limiting mobility; stains everything (including unburned skin) black.	Apply 0.5% solution wet dressings twice or three times a day; ensure that dressings remain moist by wet downs every 2 hours. Preserve solution in a light resistant container. Protect walls, floors, etc. with plastic to prevent staining from solution spills and splashes.
Silver sulfadiazine (Silvadene)	Active against wide spectrum of microbial pathogens; most frequently used topical agent for partial- and full-thickness thermal injury.	Water soluble; easily removed; painless.	With prolonged use, organisms can become resistant; transient neutropenia may occur after 2-3 days of treatment; cutaneous sensitivity reactions occur in less thatn 5% of patients; inactivates proteolytic enzymes; only moderate penetration of eschar; bone marrow depression may occur. Use with caution in patients with impaired renal or hepatic function.	Apply once or twice a day with a sterile glove with wounds left exposed or applied to gauze dressings placed over the wounds. Do not use if cream is dark in color.

Skill 18-8 Application of Topical Antimicrobial Agents

EQUIPMENT AND SUPPLIES

- Pain medication
- Sterile towels
- Bedside table space for dressing materials on a sterile field
- Antimicrobial agent
- Protective clothing according to unit protocol
- Sterile and clean gloves
- Clean bed linen and absorbent pads
- Nonadherent absorbent burn pads
- Sterile scissors
- Tubular knit dressing or expandable netting
- Coarse mesh gauze or fine mesh gauze
- Absorbent rolled-gauze
- Sterile safety pins
- Bed cradles and heat lamps

NURSING INTERVENTIONS
Closed method

1. Wear protective clothing according to unit protocol.
2. Wash hands.
3. Open sterile towel and unfold onto bedside table top.
4. Open second sterile towel package, leaving towels in package.
5. Estimate amount of dressings and agent needed. (Check care plan and shift report.)
6. Open coarse mesh gauze and remove tops from silver sulfadiazine containers or mix solutions as required. (Remember, mafenide acetate is not used with dressings.)
7. Wear sterile gloves.
8. Cut gauze into appropriate size strips for dressings as needed. (i.e., small strips for fingers whereas leg dressings can be covered with intact gauze.)
   NOTE: Steps 9 and 10 are applicable to silver sulfadiazine dressings only. If using solutions, such as silver nitrate, mix or pour in sterile basins as required.
9. Apply agent on gauze, either fine mesh gauze or coarse mesh gauze according to unit policy.
10. Stack dressings in reverse order in which they will be used and cover with sterile towel.
11. Open absorbent rolled gauze.
12. Wear new gloves and remove old dressings from patient.
13. Cleanse and debride burn wounds as discussed through Skills 18-15 to 18-17.
14. Wear new pair of sterile gloves.
15. Place impregnated gauze on burn wounds as ordered. Wrap fingers and toes separately. Do not place silver sulfadiazine dressings over grafted sites or donor sites.
16. Wrap dressings with absorbent rolled gauze, or apply tubular knit or expandable net to secure in place. Safety pins or cloth ties may be used to secure netting or knit dressings.
17. Change bed linens, protecting sheets from drainage with absorbent burn pads, as required. Cover patient with warm cotton bath blankets to prevent hypothermia. Monitor temperature closely.
   NOTE: Silver nitrate dressings must be kept moist at all times. Silver nitrate, although a clear solution, will stain all materials black (including unburned skin) when in contact with light.

Open method

1. Premedicate patient for pain 20 minutes before procedure with IV pain medication and 30 to 60 minutes when using intramuscular (IM) or by mouth (PO) medications.
2. Wear protective clothing according to unit protocol.
3. Wear sterile gloves and cleanse burn wounds according to hydrotherapy procedure (Skill 18-6).
4. Change bed linen, placing thick, absorbent burn pads under the patient to catch liquid drainage.
5. Open container of topical agent and put on new sterile gloves.
6. Spread agent evenly over wounds using aseptic technique. Creams should not be applied so close to the eye that ocular irritation will occur. Bacitracin ointment can be applied to burned eyelids. The ears should be covered with mafenide acetate only because of the high risk of chondritis.
7. Do not touch the wound or the other hand with the hand that you are using to obtain the cream unless you will be using the entire container of cream. This prevents contamination of the medication.
8. Set up bed cradles and cover them with a top sheet. Ensure adequate warmth in the room with heat lamps if necessary.
9. When using clotrimazoile cream, it must be applied and left open to air for at least 30 minutes. Thereafter, apply antibacterial topical agent or dressing, as ordered, to provide bactericidal protection.

Table 18-5 Types of Autograft Skin

Type	Description
Split-thickness sheet skin graft	Epidermis and a variable portion of the dermis that is split at a predetermined thickness allowing for transplantation to another area of the body.
Split-thickness meshed skin graft	Split-thickness sheet graft that is placed in a mesh dermatome that expands the graft from 1:15 to 1:9 times its original size before being placed on a recipient bed of granulation tissue.
Split-thickness stamp graft	A split-thickness skin graft cut into squares or rectangles of various dimensions before being placed on a recipient bed of granulation tissue.
Full-thickness skin graft	A skin graft that contains the full-thickness of the skin down to the subcutaneous tissue.
Isograft	A skin graft transplanted from the patient's identical twin and used as a permanent wound cover.
Pedicle flap	A full-thickness skin graft that is transplanted to another area of the body while maintaining a pedicle base to the original donor site. The pedicle provides a continuous blood supply to the graft until a sufficient blood supply is established at the recipient site.
Cultured epidermal sheets	Layered sheets of human epidermal cells grown in the laboratory using tissue culture techniques to expand keratinocytes derived from a small full-thickness skin biopsy.

Skill 18-9 Burn Wound Care to Special Anatomical Areas[2,16]

FACIAL BURNS

Facial burns are considered serious injuries and usually require hospitalization at a burn center. Massive facial edema often occurs because of the rich blood supply in the face and the general looseness of the skin. Facial wounds heal well using the open method.

EQUIPMENT AND SUPPLIES

- Sterile bath tray
- Prescribed ointment or antimicrobial agent
- Razor
- Protective clothing according to unit protocol.

NURSING INTERVENTIONS

1. Closely monitor the patient's respiratory status. Often patients with facial burns have sustained inhalation injury and may be at risk for respiratory compromise as edema develops.
2. Elevate the head of the bed 30 to 40 degrees to facilitate respiratory exchange and to decrease edema.
3. Locate endotracheal (ET) and tracheostomy equipment close to the patient's room.
4. Pour sterile water or saline into a basin with surgical detergent disinfectant cleansing agent to provide a quarter-strength solution. Pour plain sterile water or saline into a separate basin for rinsing.
5. Wear gloves. Wash the unburned areas of the face first and then cleanse the burned areas. Clean facial burns gently with soft foam or gauze sponges to prevent excessive bleeding. The periorbital area should be cleansed with sterile water or saline only.
6. Examine skin for areas of pressure from nasogastric and ET tubes. Change the position of the tubes and provide padding as needed.
7. Shave all facial hair in the wound.
8. Wear sterile gloves and apply a thin layer of the prescribed medication to prevent wound desiccation and infection.
9. Apply lubricant to lips. After dressing change or meals, inspect the patient's mouth and provide good oral hygiene.

BURNS OF THE EYES

Because of rapid formation of eyelid edema, the eyes should be examined as soon as possible after injury. Contact lenses are removed if present. Suspected corneal injuries are stained with fluorescein for confirmation of diagnosis. If corneal burns are suspected, the nurse should irrigate the eyes with saline. A thorough examination by an ophthalmologist is mandatory for suspected eye injuries.

EQUIPMENT AND SUPPLIES

- Gloves
- Gauze pads
- Ophthalmic ointment

NURSING INTERVENTIONS

1. Check the eyelashes to be sure they are not turning in and scratching the corneas.
2. Monitor the eyes for exudate buildup. Wear gloves and moisten a gauze pad with water and wipe exudate away from the corners of the eyes.
3. If the eyelids do not close, apply artificial tears to prevent drying of the cornea and conjunctiva. For corneal burns, apply ophthalmic antibiotic ointment as ordered to keep eyes moist and free of infection.

BURNS OF THE EARS

The ears are extremely delicate and can suffer severe damage even from a minor burn injury. Chondritis, an inflammation of the cartilage, is a potential complication of burns to the ear but may be prevented with meticulous wound care and proper positioning.[12]

EQUIPMENT AND SUPPLIES

- Cotton-tipped applicators
- Same supplies as used in facial burns
- Foam donut for positioning

NURSING INTERVENTIONS

1. Assess ears for chondritis and complaints of pain. Inspect ear canals for abnormal discharge or debris. Children are especially subject to ear infections.
2. Perform ear care during the patient's bath while cleansing the face. Cleanse the outer area of the ear canal gently with cotton-tipped applicator. After cleansing the rest of the ear with a moist gauze pad, cover superficial burns with a bland ointment or silver sulfadiazine. Cover deeper burns with mafenide acetate and leave uncovered.
3. Never apply a dressing to a burned ear.
4. Never place a pillow under the patient's head when the patient is supine. Pressure may result behind the ear, compromising blood flow to the injury site. Keep cloth tape securing tubes to the face from exerting pressure on the top of ears.
5. Use foam donut or gellike padding to protect the ear when patients are lying on their sides or in a supine position.

BURNS OF THE GENITALIA AND PERINEUM

Patients with perineal burns often require hospitalization for 24 to 48 hours to monitor patency of the lower urinary tract and treat obstruction secondary to edema should it occur. Burns of the penis require a urethral catheter to maintain urethral patency. If circumferential penile burns are present, a dorsal escharotomy may be indicated.

EQUIPMENT AND SUPPLIES

- See equipment and supplies for facial burns.

NURSING INTERVENTIONS

1. Shave the perineum if burned.
2. Protect scrotum from pressure. Do not let skin surfaces touch.
3. Check urethral catheter insertion site for drainage or erosion and carefully monitor urinary output.
4. Wash perineum meticulously and apply antimicrobial topical agent to perineal burns as ordered. Monitor for undue burning or irritation from topical agent.
5. For a more extensive burn, if silver sulfadiazine is used and a wound dressing is ordered, a diaper can be used as the wound dressing.

EQUIPMENT AND SUPPLIES

- Sterile towels
- Basin
- Sterile saline solution
- Absorbent rolled gauze or expandable meshed dressing
- Cotton-tipped applicators
- Scissors
- Coarse mesh gauze sponges
- Fine mesh gauze
- Biological or synthetic skin dressing in rolls or sheets

NURSING INTERVENTIONS

1. If using frozen allograft or xenograft, place in basin of normal saline at room temperature for at least 30 minutes to thaw (Table 18-6).
2. Rinse all dressings with saline to dilute or remove any preservative.
3. Premedicate patient for pain.
4. Wear protective clothing according to unit protocol.
5. Clean wound according to hydrotherapy protocol. Wounds must be free of necrotic debris or antimicrobial topical agents for the dressing to adhere.
6. Drape around area to be covered with sterile towels.
7. Place wet coarse mesh gauze sponges over areas to be covered until dressing is ready. Wound must be moist for dressing to adhere.
8. Wear new sterile gloves.
9. Apply dressing to wound bed, shiny (dermal) side down. Remove net backing.
10. Trim edges of dressing so it fits wound. Do not allow overlapping onto normal skin or onto adjacent pieces of dressing.
11. Using gloved hand or cotton-tipped applicator, smooth out wrinkles or bubbles in dressing. Use staples to secure dressing if indicated.
12. Cover allograft skin dressing with fine mesh gauze and absorbent rolled-gauze dressing, if indicated. Xenograft may be immobilized with expandable mesh dressing until dry.
13. Elevate covered areas on slings to decrease pressure on dressing.
14. Monitor vital signs for 24 hours. Expect a mild temperature elevation caused by coverage of wound.
15. Inspect wound daily for fluid under dressing. Puncture dressing with small needle or scalpel to drain serous fluid to prevent dressing from separating from wound bed.
16. Change xenograft skin every 3 to 5 days to prevent incorporation of collagen into wound bed. Clean wound and immediately replace xenograft dressing.
17. Allograft skin may left in place for 4 to 7 days or even longer, according to unit policy or an individual patient's wound care needs.
18. Assess the patient with a biological or synthetic skin dressing daily for the following signs of rejection: edematous granulation tissue, foul odor and suppuration, increased temperature and pulse, irritability and anxiety, and gastrointestinal (GI) malfunction.
19. Document wound assessment.
20. Store opened skin dressing in a dated and labeled container in the skin bank refrigerator. Discard according to unit policy.

Table 18-6 Biological, Biosynthetic, and Donor Site Dressings[19,38,53]

TYPE	DESCRIPTION
BIOLOGICAL DRESSING	Human or animal species tissue used to temporarily cover a wound.
Allograft skin (Homograft skin)	A graft of skin transplanted from a human cadaver and used as a temporary wound cover.
Xenograft skin (Heterograft)	A graft of skin, usually pigskin, transplanted between animals of different species. Used as a temporary wound cover.
Amniotic membranes	The amniotic and chorionic membranes collected from human placentas and used as a temporary wound dressing.
BIOSYNTHETIC DRESSING	A wound covering composed of both biological and synthetic materials.
Biobrane	A bilaminate wound dressing composed of nylon mesh enclosed in a collagen derivative with a silicon rubber membrane; permeable to some antibiotic ointments.
Integra	A bilayer wound dressing composed of 1) a "dermal" layer made of animal collagen which interfaces with an open wound surface allowing the migration of fibroblasts and vessels into the material; and 2) an "epidermal" layer made of Silastic which controls water loss from the dermis and acts as a bacterial barrier. The dermal layer is biodegraded within several months and resorbed. The epidermal layer may be removed in two to three weeks after application and replaced with autograft skin.
DONOR SITE DRESSINGS	
Op-site	A thin elastic film that is occlusive, waterproof, and permeable to moisture, vapor, and air.
DuoDerm	A hydrocolloid dressing that interacts with moisture on skin, creating a bond that makes it adhere.
N-Terface	A translucent, nonabsorbent, and nonreactive surface material used between burn wound and outer dressing.
Vigilon	A colloidal suspension on a polyethylene mesh support which provides a moist environment and is permeable to gases and water vapor.
Fine mesh gauze impregnated with scarlet red	Fine mesh gauze impregnated with a blend of lanolin, olive oil, petrolatum, and the red dye scarlet red. Promotes epithelialization of wound. Red dye stains clothing and bed linens.
Xeroform	Fine mesh gauze containing 3% bismuth tribromophenate in a petrolatum blend. Promotes epithelialization of wound and appears to be more comfortable than scarlet red gauze.
Fine mesh gauze	Cotton gauze placed directly on a donor site in the interstices of which a crust or "scab" forms. If kept clean and dry, epithelialization of the wound proceeds beneath the dressing.

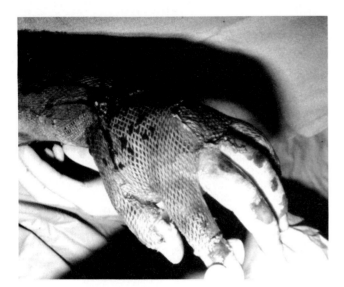

Fig. 18-6 Meshed autograft skin. (From Thelan LA, Davie JK, Urden LD: *Textbook of critical care nursing: diagnosis and management,* St Louis, 1990, Mosby–Year Book.)

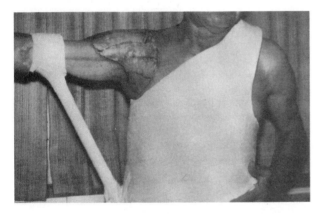

Fig. 18-7 Splint is used to prevent movement and contractures after grafting. (From Zschoche DA: *Mosby's comprehensive review of critical care,* ed 3, St Louis, 1986, Mosby–Year Book.)

tape, fibrin glue, or sutures may be used to secure the skin graft (Fig. 18-6).[8]

The graft is dressed with a layer of fine and coarse mesh gauze soaked in an antimicrobial or saline solution and wrapped in absorbent rolled gauze. Splints are applied in the operating room to prevent moving and dislodging grafted skin (Fig. 18-7). Extremities are elevated to decrease pooling of blood and pressure on grafted skin. Low air pressure or air-fluidized beds are helpful postoperatively in preventing pressure on new grafts and allowing drying of donor sites in posterior locations. They assist in preventing pressure areas from developing in unburned skin during the period of immobilization required to assure skin graft adherence.

Sheet grafts of autograft skin

Split-thickness sheet grafts of autograft skin are generally used for wounds of the face and over joints where cosmetic and functional concerns are important.

Skill 18-11 Care of Meshed Autograft Skin

EQUIPMENT AND SUPPLIES

- Basin
- Antimicrobial solution
- Fine mesh gauze
- Coarse mesh gauze sponges
- Absorbent-rolled gauze
- Expandable mesh netting
- Scissors
- Irrigation syringe
- Staple remover
- Suture removal kit
- Gloves

NURSING INTERVENTIONS

1. Educate patient and family regarding need for complete immobilization of skin grafted area. Meshed skin grafts require 3 to 5 days for epithelialization of the interstices (openings in the meshed skin) to begin. Movement during this time may cause shearing and loss of the skin graft.[10,20] Remember that during this critical time, patients may be totally dependent on the nursing staff to meet all their needs.
2. Discontinue physical therapy to skin grafted areas for 3 to 5 days. The degree of mobilization and ambulation will depend on the extent of the skin graft and its location.
3. Keep the patient comfortable and decrease anxiety to decrease movement.
4. Wear sterile gloves and protective clothing according to unit protocol.
5. Using an irrigation syringe, wet skin graft dressings with antimicrobial solution or saline every 4 to 6 hours. Dressings should be moist but not dripping. If the interstices of the new meshed skin graft become desiccated, epithelization will be delayed. If too wet, the graft may macerate.
6. The initial dressing change may occur 72 hours postoperatively and should be done by the surgeon. Assist in removing absorbent rolled-gauze and coarse mesh gauze from the skin graft and discard. The fine mesh gauze is moistened with solution and gently lifted from the skin grafts. The fine mesh gauze should not be forceably removed as skin grafts may tear.
7. Examine the skin grafts for signs of skin graft loss or infection. The skin graft should appear pink, clean, and moist; the interstices should be closing. Overlapping edges of skin grafts will appear dark brown and dry.
8. To redress the skin grafts, soak fine mesh gauze in basin containing antimicrobial solution or saline. Cut strips of fine mesh gauze and gently lay over skin grafts until completely covered.
9. Cover fine mesh gauze with coarse mesh gauze also soaked with solution and wrap with absorbent gauze and secure with expandable mesh netting. Reapply splints as required. Continue to moisten dressings as before.
10. Continue dressing changes as ordered until the interstices are completely closed. Remove staples on postoperative day 5 or when ordered. Discontinue dressings upon physician's orders.
11. Once skin grafts are healed, apply lanolin lubricant to decrease itching and cracking. The skin may feel dry because of destruction of sebaceous glands. New epidermis is fragile and must be protected from pressure and further injury.

Skill 18-12   Care of Sheet Grafts of Autograft Skin

EQUIPMENT AND SUPPLIES

- Sterile gloves and protective clothing according to unit protocol
- Cotton-tipped applicators
- Small syringe and needle or scalpel

NURSING INTERVENTIONS

1. Explain to the patient and family the need for immobilization. The patient may be fitted with a helmet device for protection of skin grafts of the face and ears. To promote adherence of sheet skin grafts applied to the anterior neck, the patient's neck should be hyperextended.
2. Assess skin graft sites for hematomas or serous blebs, which will prevent skin graft adherence. Fluid under the skin graft can be evacuated with a small syringe and needle, or a small hole may be cut near the bleb and fluid rolled to the hole with a sterile cotton-tipped applicator. Gentle rolling of the skin graft with cotton-tipped applicators to expel excess fluid through the edges of the graft or through holes should be done frequently until adherence occurs. Autograft skin that is going to adhere generally does so within 48 hours of application.
3. Sutures or staples from the skin grafts may be removed after graft adherence.
4. Document the condition of the skin graft to include type of drainage, odor, and appearance.

The Donor Site

Donor skin may be taken from almost any area of the body except the face, perineum, and palms of hands.[20] Sites may be selected for cosmetic reasons but selection may be limited by the extent of the burn. Once skin is harvested, the donor site itself becomes a superficial partial-thickness injury and must be covered with some type of dressing until healing occurs in 10 to 14 days. Various types of dressings may be used for donor sites including the following: fine mesh gauze, porcine xenograft, synthetic skin substitutes, petroleum dressings, and fine mesh gauze impregnated with scarlet red. Selection will depend on physician preference and the size and location of the donor site. Nursing care focuses on prevention of infection, prevention of tissue maceration, promotion of healing, maintenance of function, and promotion of comfort.[5]

NUTRITIONAL REQUIREMENTS OF BURN PATIENTS

An extensive burn injury causes an accelerated rate of tissue breakdown, heat production, and substrate mobilization. The degree of catabolism is dependent on the size of injury and the presence of complications, such as inhalation injury or other associated trauma. If the burn wound involves more than 30% of the TBSA, energy expenditure may be increased significantly. The larger the burn size, the greater the hypermetabolism, until a level of 60% TBSA burns is reached at which time hypermetabolism plateaus. The hypermetabolic state remains throughout the

Skill 18-13   Care of the Donor Site

EQUIPMENT AND SUPPLIES

- Heat lamp
- Scissors
- Protective clothing according to unit protocol

NURSING INTERVENTIONS

1. Remove absorbent rolled-gauze dressing from donor site when patient returns to the unit from the operating room. This dressing is used to control bleeding in the immediate postoperative period. Fine mesh gauze is placed in the operating room.
2. If bleeding continues, notify the physician.
3. Place heat lamp approximately 1 m (36 inches) from the donor site to promote drying. Ensure that heat lamp is not too close to the patient to cause burns to adjacent skin.
4. Leave donor sites open to the air with only the fine mesh gauze in place. If donor sites are on posterior surfaces of the body and the patient is unable to lie in a prone position, consider use of the air-fluidized bed to promote drying and prevent pressure. Areas that cannot be dried with heat lamps may be dried with a hand-held hair dryer.
5. Allow donor sites to remain dry for approximately 10 to 14 days for healing to occur. Do not allow them to get wet during hydrotherapy treatments.
6. Assess donor sites daily for signs of infection, such as purulent drainage, erythema, foul odor, white "soupy" appearance under fine mesh gauze, patient complaints of persistent pain, or nonadherence of fine mesh gauze. Infection of the donor site may result in conversion of the wound to a deep partial-thickness or full-thickness wound and thus delay reharvesting of the donor site. If purulence is noted, trim that area of fine mesh gauze, clean, and apply antimicrobial topical agent according to the physician's orders.
7. As the donor site heals, the fine mesh gauze will start to separate at the edges. Trim the loose edges daily until gauze fully separates from the site.
8. Do not force fine mesh gauze from the wound, as damage may occur to healing epithelium.
9. Allow patients to ambulate after fine mesh gauze has dried on lower extremity donor sites. Legs are wrapped with elastic bandages before ambulation. This will prevent pooling of blood and resultant pressure that may cause the dressing to prematurely separate from the donor site.
10. Document condition of the donor site daily. A healed donor site should appear pink and shiny. Dry areas may be treated with a lanolin lotion.

wound healing process including the period during which subsurface remodeling and scar contraction occurs.[27]

The general nutritional requirements of patients with a major burn are summarized in Table 18-7. If appropriate nutrition is not initiated and maintained, then the patient will have serious problems, such as the following:

- Significant body weight loss (may exceed 30% of preinjury weight).
- Delayed wound healing.
- Skin graft failure.
- Impaired immunological responsiveness.
- Sepsis.
- Death.

Functional Positioning for Burn Patients

AREA

Neck

Position of comfort or deformity

Pillow under neck, neck flexion, or rotation to the burned side.

Correct position

Slight extension without lateral rotation. Use extension mattress or towels under shoulders.

Precautions

Remove all pillows unless there is a posterior burn only. Keep neck neutral if there are respiratory problems.

AREA

Knee

Position of comfort or deformity

Flexion with pillows.

Correct position

Straight extension and elevation. Ambulation and tricycle riding for children is best therapy. When sitting in a chair, elevate legs and extend knees.

Precautions

Prevent prolonged direct pressure on popliteal knees.

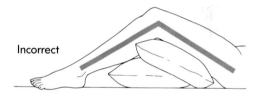

Incorrect

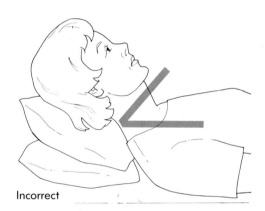

Incorrect

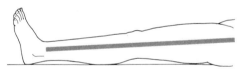

Correct

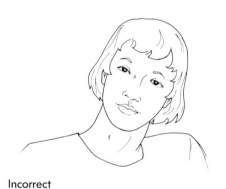

Incorrect

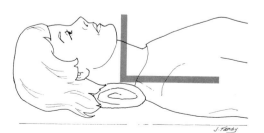

Correct

▼ Functional Positioning for Burn Patients—cont'd

AREA

Shoulder

Position of comfort or deformity

Arm positioned close to body and abduction and internal rotation.

Correct position

90-degree abduction.

Precautions

Positioning for axilla burns done early and abduction should be done with burns of chest wall even when the axilla is not involved. Must guard against brachial plexus injury from lying prone with shoulders abducted.

AREA

Elbow

Position of comfort or deformity

Arm folded across chest and flexion of elbow with pronation of forearm.

Correct position

Elevated on pillow or sling with palm up and elbow in full extension.

Precautions

Webbing of antecubital fossa often necessitates use of splints to maintain extension and avoid pressure over elbow joint to prevent ulnar nerve injury. Avoid hyperextension.

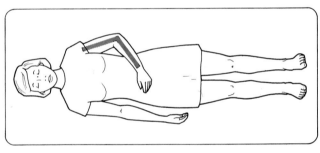

Incorrect

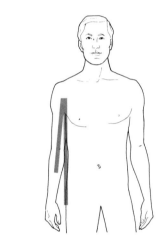

Incorrect

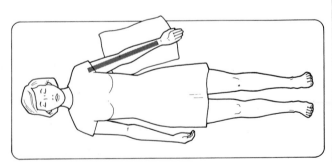

Correct

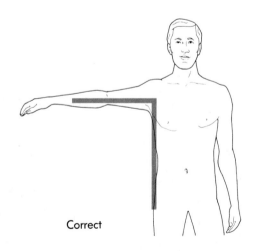

Correct

▼ Functional Positioning for Burn Patients—cont'd

AREA

Hand

Position of comfort or deformity

Claw hand position, flexion of wrist, extension of metacarpophalangeal (MCP) points, flexion of interphalangeal (IP) joints, and thumb abducted and flexed.

Correct position

Modified functional position, wrist at 25 degree extension, MCP joints flexed 50 to 70 degrees, full extension of IP joints, and thumb abducted and with slight extension.

Precautions

All flexion of IP joints is contraindicated until wound is closed. Rupture of extensor hood mechanism at the proximal interphalangeal (PIP) level can occur with flexion.

AREA

Hip

Position of comfort or deformity

"Frog legs", flexion and external rotation, and knee flexion.

Correct position

Straight body alignment and no pillows under knees. Hips and knees in full extension without internal or external rotation. Abduct 10 to 15 degrees to prevent inner thigh burn maceration.

Precautions

Without proper positioning, burns of inguinal area can result in partial subluxation.

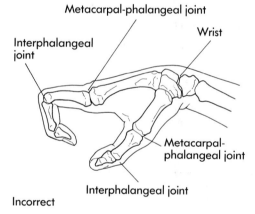

Incorrect

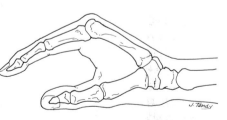

Correct

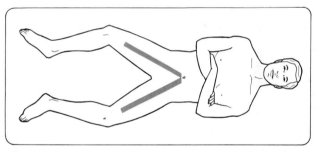

Incorrect

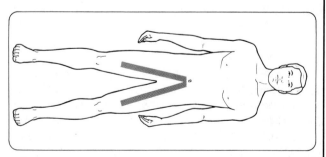

Correct

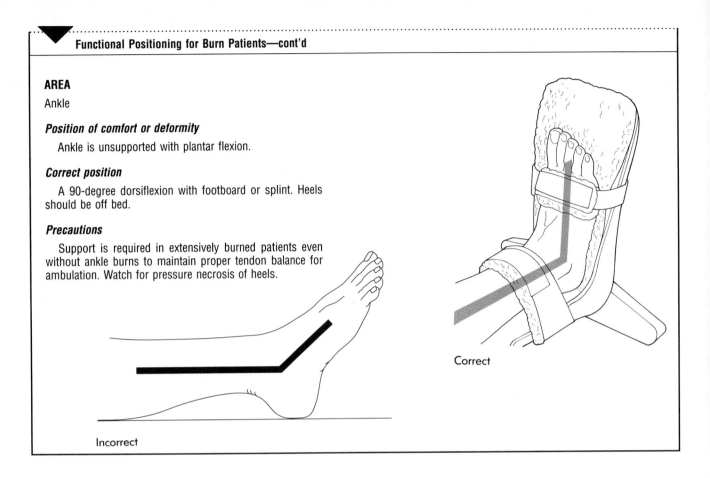

Functional Positioning for Burn Patients—cont'd

AREA

Ankle

Position of comfort or deformity

Ankle is unsupported with plantar flexion.

Correct position

A 90-degree dorsiflexion with footboard or splint. Heels should be off bed.

Precautions

Support is required in extensively burned patients even without ankle burns to maintain proper tendon balance for ambulation. Watch for pressure necrosis of heels.

Incorrect

Correct

Table 18-7 Nutritional Requirements of Patients with Major Burns

Nutrient	Suggested guideline	Monitoring parameters
Total calories	Resting energy expenditure + 25% stress factor. (Serial indirect calorimetry measures.)	Daily calorie counts, compare actual intake with goals, body weight change.
Protein	Calorie: nitrogen ratio of 100-150:1; 2-3 gm protein/kg body weight/24 hr.	Nitrogen balance, serum visceral proteins, BUN.
Carbohydrate	5 mg carbohydrate (CHO)/kg body weight/minute.	Blood sugar levels, respiratory quotient.
Fat	Provide remainder of energy requirements with fat; a combination of long chain and medium chain triglycerides. Recommend not exceeding 3 gm fat/kg body weight/24 hr.	Serum cholesterol/triglycerides, liver function tests.
Fluid and electrolytes ($K+$ and $Na+$)	Based on serum concentrations and urinary losses.	Intake and output records, serum and urinary sodium and potassium levels, weight changes for fluid balance.
Vitamins and minerals	Based on National Academy of Sciences recommended dietary allowances (RDA) with the following adjustments: • Fat soluble vitamins (A,D,E,)—RDA levels. • Water soluble vitamins (B_1, B_2, B_3, B_6, B_{12}, folate, biotin, pantothenic acid)—2 times the RDA levels. • Vitamin C—5-10 times the RDA levels. • Minerals (iron, iodine, copper, chromium, manganese)—RDA levels. • Zinc—2 times the RDA levels.	

From Carson D: *US Army Institute of Surgical Research,* Ft Sam Houston, Tx, 1989.

PEDIATRIC CONSIDERATIONS

Anatomical and physiological differences in children present challenges and concerns in the management of pediatric burn injuries.[15,20,21] Children under the age of 2 have a thinner dermis; therefore, burns that initially present as partial-thickness injury may evolve into full-thickness injury. Any burn greater than 10% BSA in a young child (< 10 years of age) should be treated in a burn center. The chest wall of a child is more pliable. Children with circumferential burns of the chest are more susceptible to restriction of the chest wall by edema. Chest wall escharotomy may be needed. Scar tissue in children does not grow like normal skin. During the rehabilitative phase, children having growth spurts may develop complications caused by having inadequate tissue.

Special consideration must be given to the airway in children because the airway diameter is narrower than an adult's and more prone to occlusion from edema. Early intubation is indicated for any child with significant respiratory distress or potential airway edema. An infant requires a different angulation of the head and neck during intubation to prevent occlusion of the airway. Cuffed ET tubes are not used on small infants. Because it is difficult to keep the uncuffed tube in place for a burned infant, a tracheostomy may be indicated for mechanical ventilation.

The Lund and Browder Chart (see Fig 18-3) or a pediatric burn chart (Fig. 18-8) must be used to calculate burn size in pediatric patients because of the differences in surface area represented by various body parts. Young children require more resuscitation fluid/kg body weight/ percent burn than adults because they have a greater ratio of BSA to mass (see Skill 18-4). Children also require more maintenance fluid than adults, particularly if they are small and have minor burns. IV fluids need to be administered through a pediatric infusion pump through a volumetric chamber to carefully control the amount of fluid being delivered. Children under the age of 2 receiving large amounts of resuscitation fluid are susceptible to the development of massive cerebral edema. The head of the bed should be elevated at all times and the rate of fluid administration closely monitored. A urine output of 30 to 50 ml/hr is an indication of adequate fluid resuscitation in children greater than 30 kg in weight. Smaller children should have an output of 1 ml/kg/hr. Glucose levels in the infant will also require closer monitoring to prevent hypoglycemia. Unlike the adult, glycogen stores in an infant's liver are limited.

Heat loss may be relatively greater in the infant than in an adult. A child's limited muscle mass produces less heat. An infant's scalp and face are proportionately larger than an adult's scalp and face, so that if that area is burned, the child may lose a significant portion of heat. Rectal temperatures must be monitored closely.

A small percentage of children experience the potentially life-threatening complication of pediatric burn hypertension. Patients with this condition develop a diastolic blood pressure greater than 20 mm Hg above their norm

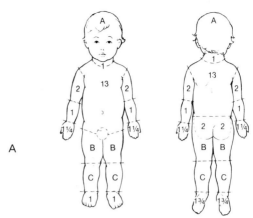

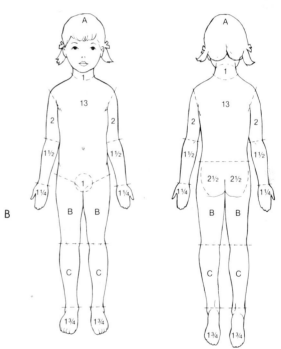

RELATIVE PERCENTAGES OF AREAS AFFECTED BY GROWTH

AREA	BIRTH	AGE 1 YR	AGE 5 YR
A = ½ of head	9½	8½	6½
B = ½ of one thigh	2¾	3¼	4
C = ½ of one leg	2½	2½	2¾

RELATIVE PERCENTAGES OF AREAS AFFECTED BY GROWTH

AREA	AGE 10 YR	AGE 15 YR	ADULT
A = ½ of head	5½	4½	3½
B = ½ of one thigh	4½	4½	4¾
C = ½ of one leg	3	3¼	3½

Fig. 18-8 Pediatric burn chart. The percent of BSA burned can be calculated from this drawing and the accompanying charts. Knowing the percent of the burn is helpful in estimating fluid requirements, nutritional requirements, and likelihood of survival. (From Whaley LP, Wong DL: *Nursing care of infants and children,* ed 4, St Louis, 1991, Mosby–Year Book.)

for a 24-hour period. There is no known cause for this and the problem may develop as early as 24 hours postburn, or as late as 2 months postburn. Once the burn wound is covered, the condition resolves.

PSYCHOSOCIAL CONSIDERATIONS

The goal in all burn therapy is to return the patient to maximum independent functioning. This goal may be complicated by psychopathology present before the burn and by the complex array of psychosocial concerns that the burn injury itself gives rise to, including fears of altered body integrity and diminished role performance. Unmet psychosocial considerations often have a detrimental effect on the patient, delaying wound closure.

There are various stages that the burn patient experiences psychologically in adapting to this devastating injury. Movement through the stages is on a continuum, although not all patients will experience every stage. The box below delineates seven adaptive stages and summarizes the behavioral manifestations that may occur, as well as interventions by staff that may facilitate the patient's resolution of each stage (also see Chapter 3).[25]

PATIENT AND FAMILY TEACHING

Rehabilitation and discharge planning begin on the day of admission and patient and family teaching is a crucial element of those processes. Burn patients often return home still requiring dressing changes, special skin care,

---

Stages of Postburn Psychological Adaptation[25]

SURVIVAL ANXIETY
Behavioral manifestations:

Tremulousness, easily startled, difficulty concentrating or following instructions, tearfulness, poor cooperation with treatment, socially withdrawn, and inappropriate behavior for hospital environment.

Interventions:

Allow verbalizations of fears, orient to prognosis, repeat instructions, and provide reality orientation.

THE PROBLEM OF PAIN
Behavioral manifestations:

Increased patient reports of pain, increased frequency of requests for analgesia, decreased cooperation with treatment because of fear of pain, and increased demanding and dependent behavior.

Interventions:

Adequately medicate patient based on an assessment, combine medication with nonpharmacological pain relief measures, and allow for adequate rest periods.

THE SEARCH FOR MEANING
Behavioral manifestations:

Detailed and repetitious recounting of events leading to injury and verbal attempts to discover a logical explanation for injury that is emotionally acceptable to the patient.

Interventions:

Avoid judging patient's reasoning or explanations of events and help the patient to validate the explanations by actively listening and participating in discussions.

INVESTMENT IN RECUPERATION
Behavioral manifestations:

Thoughts and feelings focus on a better understanding of and maximum participation in treatments, more motivated to be independent, expresses pride in small accomplishments or becomes frustrated if not satisfied with initial abilities, and if frustrated, may become depressed.

Interventions:

Educate regarding expected course of recovery, prepare the patient for physical symptoms that are likely to occur during rehabilitation, involve the patient in planning a graduated program of self-care, and praise the patient for small achievements.

ACCEPTANCE OF LOSSES
Behavioral manifestations:

Verbalizes recognition and comprehension of losses, sadness, tearfulness, decreased appetite, and sleep disturbances (depression).

Interventions:

Allow patient to verbalize losses and express emotional reactions, express that these emotions are legitimate, facilitate interactions with other patients, and facilitate interactions with family and friends.

INVESTMENT IN REHABILITATION
Behavioral manifestations:

Focuses on attaining specific personal goals related to achieving as much preburn function as possible, is more self-confident, depression may occur if new losses of function are realized, and may question professional recommendations as acceptance for responsibility increases.

Interventions:

In this stage, staff support is limited because of limited contact with the patient, praise accomplishments, continue to provide required information, and acknowledge the patient's judgment whether a preburn function that is lost is expendable or not.

REINTEGRATION OF IDENTITY
Behavioral manifestations:

Accepts losses and recognizes changes that have occurred and impact on sense of self.

Intervention:

Discontinue formal interventions with patient.

protection from environmental exposure, splints, pressure garments, exercises, and assistance in managing emotional adjustments. Providing information concerning these requirements must begin as soon as feasible in preparation for discharge.

Learning needs are determined and plans for discharge based on assessment of the patient and family in the following areas:

- *Functional disability.* Will injuries require an obvious change in lifestyle?
- *The role of the patient in the family.* Will other members have to assume responsibilities previously carried out by the patient?
- *Family support.* Does it appear that the family will be supportive? If not, who might provide support to the patient? Will the patient be able to go home or will an extended care facility be required?
- *Financial resources.* Will the patient require extensive rehabilitation? Can the patient and family adequately meet the financial demands of ongoing care?

At a minimum, satisfactorily addressing learning needs in preparation for discharge will require input from the physician, clinical nurse, occupational therapist, physical therapist, burn rehabilitation nurse, dietitian, patient, and family. Planning for discharge may also involve the social worker, chaplain, home health care nurse, financial benefits counselor, lawyer, rehabilitated burn patient, and welfare agency personnel (see box for Discharge Planning Considerations).

HOME HEALTH CARE CONSIDERATIONS

Once burn patients are discharged from the hospital, they are often started on home rehabilitation programs. The purpose of these programs is to achieve optimal physical function and a satisfactory psychological adjustment and vocational role. Rather than receive visits from a community health nurse, the patients more commonly return to an outpatient clinic and burn PT department to ensure assistance with the home program and for revision of reha-

bilitation goals. The following selected home health care procedures may be performed by the patient or family.

Skin Care for the Healed Burn

After returning home from the hospital, it is important to maintain a general cleanliness by washing hair frequently, bathing and wearing clean clothing daily, and by minimizing contact contamination until all open wounds are healed. Immediately following wound closure, the skin appears flat. Then later the skin will rise and shorten, appearing hyperemic (reddened and warm) and firm. This is when the patient must cope with skin contraction and hypertrophy. Following wound healing, it is common to experience skin dryness, itching, easy bruising and blister formation, increased sensitivity of hypertrophic skin, cold and heat hypersensitivity, and decreased sensation in grafted areas. If properly cared for, the grafted or new skin progresses to maturity in 6 to 12 months, at which time it becomes supple and the hyperemia fades.

Skill 18-14 Home Health Skin Care for the Healed Burn

EQUIPMENT AND SUPPLIES

- Hypoallergenic soap and cosmetics
- Nonperfumed lotion
- Clean washcloths
- Sterile gauze dressings
- Sterile nonadherent dressings

NURSING INTERVENTIONS

1. Wash healed skin area each day with mild soap and water. Wash gently with washcloth.
2. Rinse and dry thoroughly. Do not use deodorants or other chemicals on grafted or new skin. Use only hypoallergenic shaving cream or cosmetics.
3. Apply nonperfumed skin lubricant twice a day or more frequently if skin is dry, flaky, and itchy. If itching continues, discuss with clinical physician the need for medication to relieve the itching.
4. Do not put lotion on open wound areas.
5. If healed skin opens, cover with a sterile dressing and notify the burn clinic.
6. If blisters develop, leave them intact. If they break, allow them to dry. Apply a nonadherent dressing over these areas before reapplying a pressure garment. Blisters are a normal occurrence and heal spontaneously if kept clean.
7. Avoid even minor trauma to grafted or new skin and keep children from contact play until cleared by the physician.
8. Avoid direct sunlight to grafted or new skin.
9. Protect grafted or new skin from exposure to temperature extremes.
10. Notify the burn clinic of any signs of infection, including fever with temperature > 37.2° C (99° F), increased or foul-smelling drainage from wound, pain, swelling, redness, hardness, or warmth in or around the wound or any other part of the body.

Discharge Planning Considerations for the Burn-Injured Patient

The following factors must be considered or planned before discharge:

- Patient and family education completed.
- Follow-up appointments arranged and understood by patient and family.
- Home evaluated by family or health care worker for possible required adaptations. Arrangements made for personnel required to assist at home.
- Arrangements made with receiving facility and physician, if required.
- Vocational, physical, and emotional rehabilitation considered and arranged, if required.
- Medications and supplies prescribed and obtained.
- Financial requirements addressed.
- Transportation requirements arranged.

Skill 18-15 Care of Clothing and Pressure Garments

Pressure garments are used to improve skin appearance, improve venous return from extremities, minimize hypertrophic scarring, and protect recently healed skin (Fig. 18-9).[26] Foam padding can also be used to decrease hypertrophy of the skin within the neck contour, axillae, web spaces of fingers and toes, and the dorsum of the foot. They are used in conjunction with pressure garments.

EQUIPMENT AND SUPPLIES

- Mild laundry detergent
- Two sets of pressure garments

NURSING INTERVENTIONS

1. Launder new clothing before use by machine or hand with mild detergent.
2. Rinse clothing twice and avoid using fabric softeners and starch.
3. Wash clothing separately from those of other family members if open wounds are present.
4. If clothing dyes cause irritation, use white clothing.
5. Obtain two sets of pressure garments to provide for continuous wear and cleanliness. Pressure garments must be worn all day (except for actual bathing) until skin maturation occurs as determined by the physician.
6. Handwash pressure garments with mild detergent in cold water. Towel dry and lay flat or hang from rod, without using clothespins.
7. If the pressure garment becomes too loose, check with the burn clinic concerning the need for new garments.
8. If numbness, tingling, discomfort, and puffiness occur anywhere on the body, check with the burn clinic concerning proper garment fit.

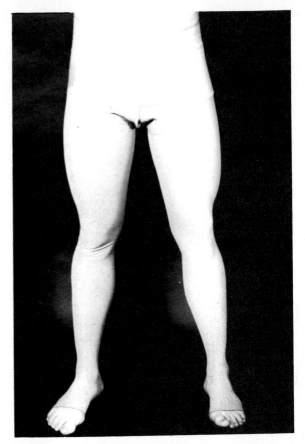

Fig. 18-9 Pressure garments are used to reduce contractures and hypertrophic scarring. (From Lewis SM, Collier IC: *Medical-surgical nursing: assessment and management of clinical problems,* ed 3, St Louis, 1992, Mosby–Year Book.)

REFERENCES

1. Arturson G: Capillary permeability in burned and nonburned areas in dogs, *Acta Chir Scand* 274:55, 1961.
2. Artz CP, Moncrief JA, Pruitt Jr BA: *Burns: a team approach,* Philadelphia, 1979, WB Saunders.
3. Cooper D: *Wound healing: a nursing responsibility.* In Kinney M et al, editors: *AACN clinical reference,* New York, 1988, McGraw-Hill.
4. Demling RH: Fluid replacement in burned patients, *Surg Clin North Am* 67(1):15, 1987.
5. Gordon MD, editor: Burn care protocols—donor site care, *J Burn Care Rehabil* 7(2):154, 1986.
6. Gordon MD, editor: Burn care protocols—synthetic and biosynthetic skin substitutes, *J Burn Care Rehabil* 9(2):209, 1986.
7. Gordon MD, editor: Burn care protocols—anchoring endotubes on patients with facial burns, *J Burn Care Rehabil* 8(3):233, 1987.
8. Gordon MD, editor: Burn care protocols—surgical fixation of skin grafts, *J Burn Care Rehabil* 9(5):516, 1988.
9. Gordon MD, editor: Burn care protocols—mechanical debridement, *J Burn Care Rehabil* 10(3):271, 1989.
10. Kravitz M: *Thermal injuries.* In Cardona VD, Hurn PD, Mason PJ et al editors: *Trauma nursing,* Philadelphia, 1988, WB Saunders.
11. Mason Jr AD: The mathematics of resuscitation, *J Trauma* 20:1015, 1980.
12. Mills II DC, Roberts LW, Mason Jr AD et al: Suppurative chondritis: its incidence, prevention, and treatment in burn patients, *Plast Reconstr Surg* 9:267, 1988.
13. Mozingo JW, Smith AA, McManus WF et al: Chemical burns, *J Trauma* 28(5):642, 1988.
14. McManus AT, McManus WF, Mason Jr AD et al: Microbial colonization in a new intensive care burn unit, *Arch Surg* 120:217, 1987.

15. Nebraska Burn Institute: *Advanced burn life support course manual,* Lincoln, Nebr, 1987, The Institute.
16. Pruitt Jr BA: The burn patient II: later care and complications of thermal injury, *Curr Probl Surg* 16(5):10, 1979.
17. Pruitt Jr BA: The universal trauma model, *Bull Amer Coll Surg* 70(10):2, 1984.
18. Pruitt Jr BA: Burn treatment for the unburned, *JAMA* 257(16):2207, 1987 (editorial).
19. Pruitt Jr BA: *Electric injury.* In Wyngaarden J, Smith L, editors: *Cecil textbook of medicine,* ed 18, Philadelphia, 1988, WB Saunders.
20. Pruitt Jr BA, Goodwin Jr CW: *Thermal injuries.* In Davis JH, Drucker WR, Foster Jr RS, editors: *Clinical surgery,* St Louis, 1987, Mosby–Year Book.
21. Pruitt Jr BA, Goodwin Jr CW: *Burn injury.* In Moore EF, editor: *Early care of the injured patient,* ed 4, St. Louis, 1990, Mosby–Year Book.
22. Robertson KE, Cross PJ, Terry JC: The crucial first days, *Am J Nurs* 1:30, 1985.
23. Shirani KZ, Pruitt Jr BA, Mason Jr AD: The influence of inhalation injury and pneumonia on burn mortality, *Ann Surg* 205(1):82, 1987.
24. Silverstein P, Maxwell P, Duckett L: *Enzymatic debridement.* In Boswick Jr JA, editor: *The art and science of burn care,* Rockville, Md, 1987, Aspen Publishers.
25. Watkins PN, Cook EL, May SR et al: Psychological stages in adaptation following burn injury: a method for facilitating psychological recovery of burn victims, *J Burn Care Rehabil* 9(4):376, 1988.
26. Waymack JP, Pruitt Jr BA: Burn wound care, *Adv Surg* 23:261, 1990.
27. Wilmore DW: *Metabolic changes after thermal injury.* In Boswick Jr JA, editor: *The art and science of burn care,* Rockville, Md, 1987, Aspen Publishers.

CHAPTER 19

Management of Radiation Exposure

Objectives

After completing this chapter, the reader will be able to:

- Describe the effect of ionizing radiation on cellular structure and function.
- Discuss methods to evaluate severity of radiation exposure.
- Describe decontamination procedures for victims of radiation accidents.
- Specify the effects of radiation on different body systems.
- Develop a plan of care for victims of acute radiation syndrome.
- Compare and contrast treatment priorities for radiation victims who have received internal versus external contamination.
- Compare and contrast nursing priorities for patients receiving sealed and unsealed internal radiation.
- Formulate a nursing care plan for patients receiving external radiation.
- Compare and contrast treatment priorities for pediatric and adult patients receiving radiation therapy.
- Formulate a plan for long-term follow-up of complications of radiation exposure.
- Evaluate nursing interventions for various radiation side effects.

Radiation exposure is often associated with anxieties and misconceptions. Nurses can allay fears and provide emotional support for patients through teaching and counseling. An understanding of the properties of various radioisotopes provides an important foundation for nursing intervention and teaching.

Radiation is the release of subatomic particles or waves of energy from atoms undergoing nuclear disintegration. Radiation can take the form of particles or fragments of disintegrating atoms (such as alpha and beta particles) or waves of energy, such as the waves of visible light, x-rays, or gamma rays. Both particulate and wave radiation are capable of penetrating and ionizing matter.[6]

Ionization is the process by which energy from a radiation source causes electrons to be dislodged from the outer shell of atoms. Freed electrons may attach themselves to other atoms. The addition of an extra electron to an atom's outer shell creates an electromagnetic negative charge. An atom that has lost an electron has a positive charge. These positively and negatively charged atoms are called *ions.*

Ionization releases energy from the atom. Energy released during this process may cause breaks in one or both strands of cellular DNA and damage to the cell membrane. The water surrounding cells may also be ionized. Ions in the water may enter cells and can cause further metabolic damage. The result is usually cellular dysfunction and death. The extent of cellular damage is dose related. Cell death may be immediate or delayed until the cell attempts to divide.[6]

Radiation affects both healthy and malignant cells in the same way, by causing breakage in one or both strands of DNA molecules inside the cells.[1] Healthy cells have a greater capability to repair the damage. Cellular repair is inhibited, however, by factors such as hypoxia, exposure to cold, and chemotherapeutic agents.[40] Radiation therapy disrupts the nuclei of the dividing cancer cells by bombarding nuclear elements with selective doses of radiation. Tissues with greater rates of cellular division are more sensitive to the effects of radiation than more slowly dividing cells. Body tissues that are highly *radiosensitive* include the lymphatic tissue, the bone marrow, epithelial tissues (such as the lining of the intestinal tract), the ovaries, and the testes. The skin, cornea, lens of the eye, esophagus, stomach, fine vasculature, growing bones, and cartilage are considered moderately radiosensitive. Slowly dividing tissues, such as muscles and nerves, are least sensitive to the effects of radiation and are relatively *radioresistant.*[2,3]

Moderate radiation exposure may result in predictable symptoms, such as nausea, vomiting, diarrhea, and anorexia. The occurrence of these symptoms following radiation exposure is sometimes termed *radiation sickness.*

Cells that escape lethal damage at the time of radiation may exhibit permanent genetic changes or mutations. Cellular mutations can result in the development of cancers that occur years later after a long latency period. Common examples are thyroid cancers and leukemias that may occur up to 30 years after exposure. Exposure of the testes or the ovaries to radiation may result in recessive genetic changes that do not manifest themselves for several generations. Whenever the gonads have been exposed to radiation it is recommended that the patient refrain from conception for at least 2 years after exposure and have genetic counseling when conception is planned.[40] Sterility, alopecia, and cataracts are additional complications of long-term exposure.

There are several types of radiation that are emitted from unstable atoms undergoing decay. Each of these has different characteristics and hazards. The most common types of radiation encountered clinically are alpha particles, beta particles, and gamma waves. Neutron particles are a fourth type of radiation with very damaging effects. Several facilities are treating patients with neutrons, although this is not common. Generally, neutrons are encountered during an industrial accident or nuclear blast.[38]

Alpha particles are slow moving, travel only short distances 5 to 7 cm (2 to 3 inches) and can be blocked by a piece of paper or the skin. Alpha particles cannot penetrate through the skin but can cause damage to surface tissues and therefore have little use in radiotherapy. Alpha particles are most damaging when a substance emitting these particles remains in direct contact with unprotected tissue for a long period of time. In this situation, the resulting radiation exposure may cause damage to tissues and potentially result in a functional disease. Alpha particles are not considered hazardous unless inhaled or ingested.

Beta particles are faster moving and more penetrating than alpha radiation. Body penetration is limited to a maximum of 8 mm (1/3 inches). Beta particles can be blocked by 2.5 cm (1 inch) of wood or a thin sheet of aluminum. They travel only a fraction of a centimeter through the body and 2 to 8 m (6.25 to 26 feet) in the air. Radioisotopes that emit beta radiation used clinically include iodine-131, gold-198, and phosphorus-32. Like alpha particles, beta particles can result in a functional disease if the patient is exposed for an extended period of time.

Gamma rays are the primary cause of acute radiation syndrome. Gamma rays are similar in nature to x-rays and can penetrate deeply into the body. Radioisotopes that emit gamma radiation are commonly used to treat many cancers.[6] These rays travel hundreds of meters in the air and can be stopped only by thick lead or concrete. Exposure to large doses of gamma rays can result in injury or destruction to body cells and tissues. Radium, cobalt-60, and cesium-137 are radioisotopes that emit gamma radiation.[6,20,37] Fig. 19-1 illustrates a comparison of the penetrating power of alpha, beta, and gamma radiation.

Neutron particles may be encountered during a radiation accident. These particles are produced by nuclear reactors used in power plants or research laboratories. Neutron radiation may also result from a nuclear blast. Neutrons are subatomic particles emitted from the nucleus of a decaying atom. When these particles come in contact with previously stable atoms they cause these atoms to become radioactive. Neutron radiation travels hundreds of meters in the air. It can be stopped by several meters of water or

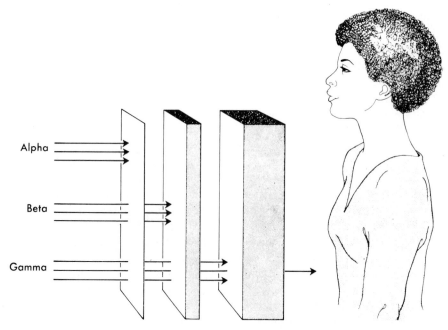

Fig. 19-1   Relative penetrating power of three types of radiation. (From Bouchard-Kurtz R, Speese-Owens N: *Nursing care of the cancer patient*, ed 4, St Louis, 1981, Mosby–Year Book.)

by special concrete. Neutron particles deeply penetrate the body tissues; exposure to neutron radiation can result in total body irradiation.[20,38]

Measurement

Radiation doses are measured in roentgens, rads, rems, and grays. The *roentgen* indicates the total amount of radiation given off in the air by a source of radiation. This measurement does not take into account the effect of radiation on the body. The amount of radiation absorbed by body tissues is measured by the *radiation absorbed dose (rad)*. The international unit, *gray (Gy)*, is commonly substituted for rad. One gray equals 100 rads. The *roentgen equivalent man (rem)* is a measurement that standardizes the effects of different types of radiation in humans. Small doses of radiation in humans are measured by the millirem. A *millirem (mrem)* is a radiation measurement that is one thousandth of a rem. For x-rays and gamma rays, 1 rem has the same biological effect as 1 rad (1 cGy). The dose of radiation received is an important determinant of illness or dysfunction. Sudden, large doses of radiation may cause more severe short-term effects on the body than smaller doses over time. However, long-term exposure to even small doses of radiation can cause certain cancers or result in illness. The symptoms of radiation exposure also vary according to whether total or partial body irradiation has occurred.[13,40]

Instruments used to measure radioactivity include film badges and survey meters.[16] *Survey meters* include the Geiger-Müller counter, ionization chambers, and dosimeters. These instruments measure radiation exposure in the air. A survey meter measures the exposure rates at any given distance from the source and should be used when exposure is a potential danger. Ring dosimeters and pen dosimeters are often used when treating a radiation accident victim. Film badges determine cumulative radiation dose. An insert within the badge is made of a thermoluminescent chip that is very sensitive to radiation. The insert is read after a specific period of time to determine cumulative dose.

Dosimetry is the measurement and calculation of radiation dosage.[6] This term is also used when dealing with therapeutic doses of radiation. *Half-life* is the length of time that it takes for a radioactive substance to decay to one half of its original activity. The active life span of radioactive substances is indicated by the half-life.

Protection of Personnel

The National Council on Radiation Protection and Measurement has established 500 mrem/yr or 125 mrem/quarter (5mGy/yr or 1.25 mGy/quarter) as the maximum exposure limit for nonoccupationally exposed workers.[5,25] Although the hospital environment contains many therapeutic and diagnostic sources of radiation, (e.g., x-rays, radioisotope studies, fluoroscopy, and cancer therapy) exposure of hospital personnel is minimal.

Excessive radiation exposure is defined as any unnecessary exposure to radiation above natural background levels.[14,15] The annual natural radiation background dose for persons living in the United States is approximately 125 mrem (1.25 mGy). Any person who may receive a dose greater than the maximum exposure limits (125 mrem/quarter) is required by law to wear a radiation film badge.[25] During an emergency, rescue personnel may receive 25 rem (25cGy) to the whole body as a one time exposure.[13] In a nonemergency situation, if exposure is expected to exceed 100 mrem (1mGy), additional staff should be substituted.[37] Studies have shown that nurses rarely receive radiation doses that approach these limits.[5,14,23] In one study of 65 critical care nurses, none received a radiation dose greater than 80 mrem (0.8 mGy) in a 36-month period.[14]

The growing fetus is very sensitive to the effects of radiation. A fetus must not receive more than 500 mrem (5 mGy) during the entire gestational period.[25] A woman who is pregnant or may be pregnant must not work with patients who are potential sources of radiation.[2,29]

Warning signs should be posted to protect personnel.[2,29] A magenta trefoil on a yellow background is the universal symbol for radiation. These signs should be placed on the patient's door, chart, and at the bedside. Any potentially contaminated area should be cordoned off. Floor markings that indicate meter distances from the patient's bed may be helpful when caring for a patient with a radioactive implant. Other protective measures will be discussed throughout this chapter.

Diagnostic Radionuclides

Occasionally, critical care nurses must accompany patients to the nuclear medicine department for diagnostic testing with radioactive isotopes. Nurses may have questions about the safety of caring for such patients. *Diagnostic radionuclides* are radioactive isotopes with short half-lives that are used medically to enhance visualization of blood circulation and body tissues. Isotopes, in small amounts, are injected intravenously, circulate in the blood stream, and may be taken up preferentially at specific body sites. A nuclear scanner is used to detect radioactivity in the blood and tissues. Common diagnostic radionuclides include technetium-99m, gallium-67, thallium-201, xenon-133, and iodine-131.[2,14]

Lung scans use radionuclides that are both inhaled and injected to study ventilation and perfusion of the lungs when a pulmonary embolus is suspected. Radionuclides are used with increasing frequency to diagnose cardiac abnormalities. Arterial blood flow, ventricular function, and cardiac wall motion may be examined with the use of radionuclides. Common cardiac studies include technetium-99m scanning, thallium-201 imaging, and the multiple-gated acquisition (MUGA) scan. The MUGA scan is a type of angiocardiography that correlates images of the motion of blood flow within the heart chambers with the ECG to evaluate cardiac function at different stages of the conduction cycle.

Radionuclides may also be used to study other body tissues, including the brain, bone, liver, and thyroid. Generally, no special precautions are necessary; however, a nurse caring for a patient who has just received a diagnostic radionuclide may want to minimize unnecessary time spent at the bedside for a few hours after injection. Since most radionuclides are excreted in the urine, the nurse should wear gloves when handling urine (and stool if gallium-67 is used) for 24 hours after injection.[14] The nuclear medicine department should be consulted regarding proper labeling of blood and urine specimens taken during the first 24 hours after injection and should be notified of any urine spills during that time period.

Classification Systems Used for Accidental Radiation Exposure

Several classification systems have been developed to assist in the diagnosis and treatment of radiation exposure. One method is to list exposure as survival probable, survival possible, and survival improbable.[20] A *survival probable* designation is assigned if exposure is 200 rads (2 Gy) or less and there are no symptoms or mild symptoms that subside in a few hours (i.e., transient nausea and vomiting). The leukocyte count remains stable. A *survival possible* designation is made if exposure has been in the range of 200 to 800 rads (2 to 8 Gy). Symptoms, such as nausea and vomiting, last only 24 to 48 hours followed by an asymptomatic period. Leukocytopenia and thrombocytopenia vary according to severity of exposure. A *survival improbable* designation is made when the radiation dose is greater than 800 rads (8 Gy). Victims experience gastrointestinal (GI) symptoms, hemorrhage, and leukocytopenia.[20]

Another classification system is based upon the relationship between symptoms and radiation dose:[37,38]

1. Doses less than 100 rads (1 Gy) generally do not cause acute symptoms.
2. Doses between 100 to 200 rads (1 to 2 Gy) may cause mild symptoms that usually subside in a few hours. Nausea and vomiting are mild. Blood counts usually do not change.
3. Doses between 200 to 400 (2 to 4 Gy) rads cause considerable GI symptomatology.
4. Doses greater than 400 rads (4 Gy) result in nausea, vomiting, cramping, and diarrhea that will begin within 2 hours. A drop in the leukocyte count will follow within 24 hours. If the dose has been greater than 450 rem (4.5 Gy), there will be a 50% mortality within 30 days often because of infection and hemorrhage secondary to bone marrow depression. Bone marrow recovery usually determines survival when the dose has been greater than 600 rem (6 Gy).
5. Doses between 600 to 1000 rem (6 to 10 Gy) result in an increased severity of GI symptoms and hemorrhage. The leukocyte count drops within 12 to 24 hours, and death usually comes within 3 weeks.
6. Doses of greater than 1000 rem (10 Gy) cause neurological symptoms, such as ataxia and confusion, to be added to the clinical picture, and death usually comes within several days. Rapid onset of confusion

Table 19-1   Classification System for Irradiated Victims[3,20,30,36]

Group	Clinical manifestations (without treatment)	Approximate exposure	Classifications	Treatment
I	Mostly asymptomatic, minimal prodromal nausea and vomiting that subsides within hours, subtle laboratory changes	150	Survival probable	Decontamination, follow-up care.
II	Mild form of acute radiation sickness, transient prodromal nausea and vomiting lasting 24-48 hours, mild hematopoietic changes including thrombocytopenia and leukopenia.	400	Survival possible, hematopoietic	Decontamination; admitted to hospital for fluid and electrolyte therapy if vomiting is severe, protective isolation, follow-up care.
III	Severe hematopoietic complications, nausea and vomiting with some evidence of gastrointestinal damage in the higher dose range.	400-600	Survival possible, hematopoietic	Decontamination, hospital admission for intense fluid and electrolyte therapy, protective isolation, transfusion of blood products as indicated, antibiotics.
IV	Accelerated form of acute radiation syndrome, fulminating nausea, vomiting, and diarrhea dominate the clinical picture, severity of the hematopoietic complications related to survival time after exposure.	600-1500	Survival improbable, gastrointestinal	Same as Group III, bone marrow transplant may be attempted, supportive care as indicated.
V	Fulminating course with marked cardiovascular or central nervous system (CNS) impairment or both, major injuries may be present.	5000+	Survival improbable, neurovascular cardiovascular cerebral	Same as Groups III and IV, radiation precautions may be necessary.

and ataxia result in a grim prognosis. The long-term effects of sudden, whole body irradiation compared to exposure to smaller doses of radiation over time are not well understood. Partial body exposure versus whole body exposure also influences the clinical picture.[38]

Radiation victims may also be grouped according to clinical manifestations and approximate dose received. This classification system delineates five groups of radiation exposure (Table 19-1).

Acute Radiation Syndrome

Acute radiation syndrome follows a sudden large dose of whole-body irradiation by neutrons, gamma rays, or a combination of both. This syndrome varies in nature and severity depending on the dose of radiation, length of exposure, pattern of distribution, and individual susceptibility. The syndrome results from exposure to intensely ionizing radiation over a short period of time and is usually associated with an industrial accident.

Acute radiation syndrome may be classified into the following four stages: prodromal, latent, manifest illness, and recovery.[37] The *prodromal* stage is characterized by the cellular release of vasoactive substances, such as histamine and bradykinin. The greater the dose, the more pronounced the clinical picture. This stage develops a few hours after exposure and lasts up to 48 hours. Presenting symptoms such as anorexia, fatigue, fever, nausea, perspiration, respiratory distress, and vomiting may be expected.

During the *latent* stage, the patient usually experiences a period of relative well-being and absence of clinical symptoms. With very high doses of radiation, the latent stage may be very short or nonexistent. With low doses of radiation, this period can last up to 2 weeks.[3]

During the *manifest illness* stage, the patient experiences a complex syndrome of symptoms that is usually dose-related. Symptoms that may present during this stage include agitation, anorexia, aspermia (nonemission of sperm), ataxia, convulsions, coma, diarrhea, disorientation, loss of body hair, erythema, fever, hemorrhage, ileus, infection, lassitude, tanning, shock, weakness, and weight loss.

The final phase, *recovery,* is determined by the dose of radiation received and the severity of the body's response. Recovery may take days, weeks, or months. There is no known treatment or medication to cure radiation syndrome. Patients who have been exposed are treated symptomatically.[20,37]

Types of Radiation Accidents

Radiation accidents may be classified in terms of exposure and contamination (Table 19-2).[3,13,20] These accident categories include the following:
- External exposure.
- External contamination.
- Internal contamination.
- Wound contamination.

Table 19-2 Types of Radiation Exposure

Type	Radioactive site	Decontamination
External exposure	None (Victim exposed but not contaminated.)	Decontamination not necessary. Assess severity of exposure. Provide treatment according to severity.
External contamination	Body surfaces and clothing	Isolation garb necessary. Monitor radiation. Remove clothing and place in leaded containers. Wash exposed body surfaces with soap and water. Collect and contain wash water. Lavage eyes, ears, and wounds with saline. Cocoon victim in sheets. Apply dosimeter to victim.
Internal contamination	Body secretions, such as emesis, urine, and feces	Isolation garb necessary. Monitor radiation. Wear gloves to handle body secretions. Place in leaded containers. Diuresis, lavage, chelating, or blocking agents may be ordered.
Wound contamination	Wound tissue	Isolation garb necessary. Monitor radiation. Lavage with saline. Debride wound as necessary. Chelating or blocking agents may be used. Collect wash solution in leaded containers.

EMERGENCY CARE OF THE VICTIM OF A RADIATION ACCIDENT

When accidental radiation exposure occurs, community emergency services and hospital-based treatments will be required. A coordinated effort involving a variety of agencies, experts, and support services is usually necessary to provide expedient care and treatment of accident victims while minimizing the radiation hazard to others.

The Prehospital Phase

The prehospital phase includes assessment and emergency care at the scene of the accident. Ambulance personnel should wear protective clothing, including gowns, rubber gloves, and shoe covers. Respirators are worn if airborne contamination is suspected. All medical response personnel should wear dosimeters and monitor the radiation levels of the site before entering. A dosimeter should be applied to the victim to monitor exposure during the decontamination.

The receiving hospital is notified that a radiation accident has occurred and preparation is begun for the victim's arrival. Notification of the hospital includes the type of injury, whether contamination is present, which radioisotopes are involved, first aid given, and decontamination measures already provided. A history is obtained as a part of the assessment of the victim at the site.

When external radiation exposure has occurred, the victim is not considered radioactive. Victims receive a potentially harmful beam of radiation that does not contaminate skin and clothing. In this situation, there is no danger to others. However, if an industrial accident is associated with an explosion or release of radioactive steam, radioactive dust or particles may cling to the clothing, hair, fingernails, and exposed skin of persons in the area. Removing the victims' clothing and washing exposed body surfaces removes many of the radioactive particles. This washing reduces further risk to both victims and rescue workers.[13,38]

Decontamination should begin at the scene of the accident if possible. All clothes should be removed and placed in labeled containers. Exposed body surfaces should be washed with soap and water. All water and waste materials should be placed in a sealed container and labeled. If necessary, eyes, ears, and wounds should be rinsed with sterile saline solution. If IV fluids must be started, the skin should be vigorously cleaned to avoid introducing radioactive particles internally. The victim should be cocooned in linen to transfer to the hospital receiving area.[22,37]

The goals of decontamination are to do the following:
1. Reduce radiation to the patient and staff by reducing surface contamination.
2. Contain and dispose of radioactive materials.
3. Monitor and document radioisotopes.

Hospital Preparation of the Radiation Emergency Area

A portion of the emergency department should be designated as a radiation treatment area. Ideally this area should be separate from the rest of the department and be accessible from outside the facility (Fig. 19-2). This area should have a closed ventilation and drainage system to prevent water and airborne radioactive contamination. If the air-conditioning is not a closed system, it should be turned off. In most hospitals closed ventilatory and drainage systems may be found in the autopsy room or the morgue, and the initial radiation decontamination may be started there.[3,13,30,36]

A radiation emergency plan should be developed and available in the emergency receiving area. This plan should include protocols for receiving the victim, handling contaminated materials, decontamination procedures, and cleanup (see the box on the right).[3,9,22]

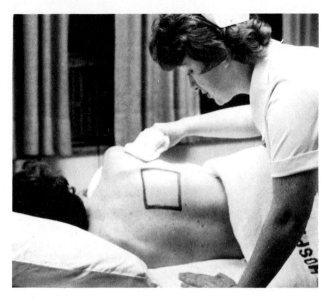

Fig. 19-2   Care must be taken not to remove skin markings used to guide radiation therapy. (From Phipps WJ, Long BC, Woods NF et al: *Medical surgical nursing,* ed 4, St Louis, 1991, Mosby–Year Book.)

▼ ....
The Radiation Emergency Plan[3,22,30]

The radiation emergency plan should include the following:
1. A list of key personnel to notify.
2. Radiation emergency supplies.
3. Protocols for the following:
   • Preparation of the area.
   • Receiving the victim.
   • Monitoring radiation levels.
   • Gowning and handling contaminated materials.
   • Decontamination of the victim.
   • Isolation and disposal of materials.
   • Cleanup.
4. Guidelines for recommended maximum radiation exposures.
5. Controlled entry into the area.
6. Care and cleanup of the ambulance or transport vehicle.

ASSESSMENT

A thorough assessment of the patient who has received excessive exposure will help determine the biological effects of radiation. The nurse should do the following:
1. Obtain the following exposure history:
   • Type of exposure.
   • Amount of radiation received.
   • Length of exposure.
   • Pattern of distribution.
   • Susceptibility of body tissue.
   • Any other injuries.
2. Assess onset, severity, duration, and character of GI symptoms, such as nausea, vomiting, and diarrhea. These symptoms can occur as early as 2 hours after exposure.

3. Monitor fluid status including decreased urine output, skin turgor, mucous membranes, weight, and intake and output.

4. Observe for the following indications of bone marrow depression: anemia, leukopenia, thrombocytopenia, infection, bleeding tendencies, fatigue, and dyspnea. Exposure to 400 or more rads (4 or more Gy) may produce signs and symptoms within 24 hours.

5. Monitor vital signs. When leukopenia exists, local evidence of infection, such as redness, swelling, heat, and pus formation, may be diminished. Fever may be the only indicator.

6. Auscultate lung fields. Inspect sputum.

7. Monitor character of urine for signs of infection.

8. Assess for signs and symptoms of bleeding; that is, bleeding from venipuncture sites, bruising, petechia, hemoptysis, hematemesis, melena, vaginal bleeding, dizziness, decreased blood pressure, increased heart rate, and changes in mental status.

9. Monitor central nervous system functioning. Alterations may indicate that high doses of radiation have been received and are a grave sign.

10. Assess for related injuries or trauma.

11. Several days after exposure, assess for bone marrow depression, skin burns, and hair loss.

NURSING DIAGNOSIS

The following are sample nursing diagnoses for patients who have experienced excessive radiation exposure:

Radiation accidents
- High risk for loss of cellular integrity related to radiation exposure.
- Impairment in nutrition related to nausea and vomiting.
- Anxiety and fear related to radiation exposure.

Bone marrow depression
- High risk for injury and infection related to bone marrow depression.
- High risk for injury and bleeding related to low platelet count.
- Decreased tissue perfusion related to low red blood count.

Radiation implants
- High risk for injury, related to implant dislodgement.
- Anxiety related to fear of radiation exposure.
- High risk for social isolation related to radiation isolation.

PATIENT OUTCOMES

Possible expected outcomes for patients receiving excessive radiation exposure include the following:

Skill 19-1 **Decontamination Following Radiation Exposure**

EQUIPMENT AND SUPPLIES[22]
- Radiation monitoring equipment, film badges, or dosimeters
- Assessment equipment (i.e., stethoscope, blood pressure cuff, etc.)
- Double sets of isolation or surgical garb, such as gowns, caps, masks, gloves, and shoe covers
- Linens (disposable, if possible)
- Plastic sheeting and bags
- Soap, shampoo, irrigating syringes, basins, and soft scrub brushes
- Containers for collection of contaminated waste
- Specimen containers
- Radiation warning signs, labels, and warning rope
- Wound dressing supplies
- Procedure and protocol manuals
- Sealing tape

NURSING INTERVENTIONS

1. Gown and glove in isolation attire and wear shoe protectors and dosimeters. Prepare the receiving area with plastic covers and cordon off the area from emergency department traffic to reduce risk to others. Collect supplies.

2. On arrival, provide life-sustaining care, as needed. Survey the victim's entire body to determine the extent of contamination.

3. Initially decontaminate the patient at the scene or in the ambulance. Remove the victim's clothing, place in leaded containers, and apply a dosimeter to the patient. Decontaminate body areas with the highest radiation levels first.

4. To decontaminate the skin, wash exposed areas with soap and water using a shower or large basin. Gently scrub body surfaces with soap or detergent. A paste of laundry detergent, cornmeal, and water can be used.[13] Take care not to cause irritation or abrasions to the skin during the scrub. Collect the wash water for analysis.

5. Irrigate the eyes, ears, and open wounds with saline solution. Debride or irrigate a contaminated wound using saline, a blocking agent, or chelating agent. An example of a blocking agent is potassium iodine, which reduces uptake of radioactive iodine by the thyroid gland.[24] Chelating agents prevent tissue uptake of radioactive substances by binding these substances into complexes that are excreted.[20] An example of a chelating agent is calcium disodium edentate.

6. To continue the decontamination process, shampoo the hair and clean and trim the fingernails. Place clipped fingernails in a container for monitoring.

7. If internal contamination is suspected, collect, contain, and monitor urine, feces, emesis, and other body fluids. Analyze nasal and oral smears and gastric washings to detect internal contamination.

8. Monitor the patient's entire body and repeat the process of decontamination as needed.

9. Cocoon the victim in hospital linen.

10. Transfer of the patient out of the emergency treatment area when surface radiation levels are close to background levels.

11. Examine all personnel for radiation levels before they leave the decontamination area. Decontaminate as necessary.

12. Dispose of equipment and supplies according to established protocols.

13. Monitor and decontaminate the entire treatment area.

Radiation accidents

Patient will evidence the following:

* Radiation levels no greater than expected background levels (approximately 0.01 to 0.1 mrad/hr) (.0001 to .001 mGy).
* Intact skin of normal color and hydration.
* Participation in own skin care.
* Minimized or controlled episodes of nausea and vomiting.
* Urine output of at least 30 ml/hr.
* A balanced fluid intake and output (less approximately 500 ml for insensible fluid loss).
* A caloric intake to meet nutritional needs.
* A stable weight as compared to baseline admission weight.

Bone marrow depression

Patient will evidence the following:

* Oral temperature between 36° to 38° C (97° to 100.5 °F).
* Pulse rate between 60 to 100 beats/min.
* Respiratory rate between 12 to 20 breaths/min.
* Clear, equal, bilateral breath sounds.
* Warm, dry, intact skin of adequate turgor and color.
* Extremities of equal size and temperature.
* Leukocyte count within 4300 to 11,000 µl.
* Hematocrit between 45% to 52% (male) and 37% to 48% (female).
* Platelet count between 200,000 to 300,000.

Radiation implants

Patient will evidence the following:

* Proper implant placement on inspection of the treatment area.
* Warm, dry, intact skin of adequate turgor and color.

RADIATION THERAPY

Radiation is used medically as a diagnostic tool and for the treatment of cancer. Clinical uses of ionizing radiation began in 1895 when Wilheim Roentgen discovered x-rays. The first cancer cure (basal cell) with the use of radiation was reported in 1899.[40,41] Early radiotherapy used single, large doses of radiation to treat superficial lesions. These doses resulted in severe side effects because the available equipment delivered virtually 100% of the dose to the skin surface. This treatment produced acceptable results for skin cancer but was poorly tolerated when deeper lesions were treated. Today, advances in medical science make it possible to treat deeper tumors while minimizing side effects. It is estimated over 50% of patients with cancer will receive radiotherapy during the course of their illnesses.[27]

Principles of Radiation Therapy

The goal of *radiotherapy* is to kill cancer cells or render them permanently unable to divide while minimizing damage to surrounding normal tissue. Ions, called *free radicals,* are produced by radiation and interact with the cell's DNA. A single or double break in the DNA chromosomes is produced and becomes lethal when the cell tries to divide.[1,2,6]

The effectiveness of radiation is determined by the age, tumor size, and radiosensitivity of tissues. A tumor is deemed radiosensitive if it is destroyed by a dose of radiation that is well-tolerated by surrounding tissues. Since radiation is most effective on cells that are dividing, a tumor that has many cells in the dividing phase is more responsive than a tumor in which a core of cells remain in the resting phase. Tumor cells usually divide at the same rate as the tissue of origin; therefore tumors that arise from tissues with rapid cell division are usually highly radiosensitive. Tumors of the bone marrow, the lymphatic tissues, epithelial cells, and the gonads are included this category. Tissues that are considered moderately high in radiosensitivity are the skin, the cornea, the lens of the eye, and the GI organs, such as the esophagus and stomach. Tissues that are affected to a moderate degree by radiation are growing cartilage, fine vasculature, and growing bones. Tumors that arise from tissues with slow generation times are relatively radioresistant. These tissues include muscles, tendons, and nerves.[1,3,6]

Dosimetry is used to calculate the radiation dose. Precise calculations are necessary to ensure an adequate radiation dose to kill the tumor and to avoid overexposure to healthy tissues.[6] Most tumors require a total of 4500 to 7500 rads (45 to 75 Gy) for treatment to be successful.[40,41] Once the total tumor lethal dose is determined, it is generally divided into smaller doses and administered in a series, a process called *fractionation.* A typical series might involve treatments on 5 days a week for a period of 2 to 8 weeks (200 rads [2 Gy]/day or 1000 rads [10 Gy]/week). A split course of therapy may also be used. This allows the patient a period of time without treatment in the middle of a series. Fractionation and split course therapy provide time for healthy cells to recover from the effects of radiation. Healthy cells have a greater capacity to recover from radiation exposure than do cancer cells. However, each type of normal tissue has a defined limit of radiation tolerance. Treatment doses above these limits will result in irreversible tissue damage.[6,41]

Radiotherapy may be external or internal. *External radiation* uses a beam of radiation to treat cancer tumors on or beneath the skin. The desired effect is to concentrate the maximum dose at the site of the tumor with minimal scatter to other areas. Radiotherapy machines in use include megavoltage machines (Cobalt-60) and supervoltage machines (linear accelerators, cyclotrons, and betatrons). These machines use gamma rays, x-rays, or electrons to irradiate the treatment field.[6,35]

Internal radiation uses radioactive materials placed within the body at the site of the tumor. In this way, radiation can be concentrated in the area of the tumor minimizing side effects to healthy tissues. Table 19-3 lists commonly used therapeutic radioisotopes. *Isotopes* are atoms of the same element that have different numbers of neutrons in their nuclei and therefore differ in atomic weight. Isotopes are frequently used in radiotherapy.

Table 19-3 Characteristics and Uses of Some Commonly Used Radioactive Agents

Radiation source	Half-life (where applicable)	Rays emitted	Appearance or form	Method of administration
X-ray	—	γ	Invisible rays	X-ray machine
Radium	1600 yr	α β	In needles, plaques, and molds	Interstitial (needles) Intracavitary (plaques and mold)
Radon	4 days	α β γ (low intensity)	In seeds and needles	Interstitial (seeds and needles)
Cesium (137-Cs)	33 yr	β γ	In needles and capsules	Interstitial (needles) Intracavitary (capsules)
Cobalt (60-Co)	5 yr	β γ	External (cobalt unit) Internal (needles, seeds, and molds)	Machine (teletherapy) Interstitial (needles and seeds)
Iodine (131-1)	8 days	β γ (low intensity)	Clear liquid	By mouth
1 Phosphorus (32-P)	14 days	β	Clear liquid	By mouth, intracavitary, and intravenous
Gold (198-Au)	3 days	β γ	Purple liquid	Intracavitary
Iridium (192-Ir)	74 days	β γ (low intensity)	In needles, wires, and seeds	Interstitial
Yttrium (90-Y)	3 days	β	Beads and needles	Interstitial

From Phipps WJ, Long BC, Woods NF et al: *Medical-surgical nursing*, ed 4, St Louis, 1991, Mosby–Year Book.

Site Specific Effects of Radiation Therapy

Radiation therapy is a local treatment, and side effects are usually limited to the treated area. General effects may be present and include fatigue and anorexia. Other adverse radiation reactions associated with radiation therapy include skin reactions, GI dysfunction, bone marrow depression, stomatitis, cystitis, and alopecia (Table 19-4). Bone marrow depression may result from radiation to bone marrow reserves, such as the sternum or iliac crest.[6,16,34,40] Site specific effects may vary depending on the dose of radiation and the area treated.

Care of the Patient Receiving External Radiation Therapy

To prepare the patient for external radiation, a procedure known as *simulation* is performed. An x-ray is taken with the patient in the treatment position to localize the area to receive radiation. This film will be used to mark the treatment field. The skin over the tumor site is marked by the physician with indelible ink. These markings are used by the radiation therapist to precisely direct the beam of radiation to the tumor site. External radiation may be directed at the tumor from several different angles. The areas through which the radiation passes are known as ports.[6] Different ports may be used on different days or during the same treatment to reduce damage to healthy tissue. The patient should be cautioned not to wash off or remove the ink markings. If the markings are inadvertently removed, the patient should inform the doctor rather than try to reconstruct them. Permanent marks or tatoos may be used to identify the borders and center of the field (Fig. 19-3). When the patient receives permanent markings, india ink and a needle are used to place a small dot along the borders of the field.[35]

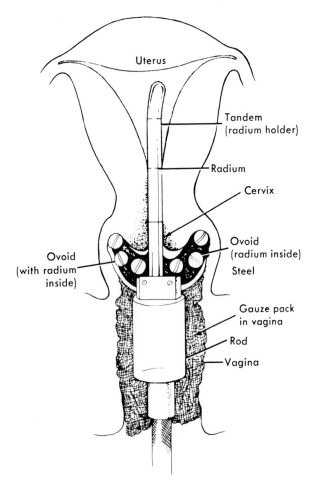

Fig. 19-3   Radiation treatment of cancer of the cervix via application with tandem and ovoids. (From Marino LB: *Cancer nursing,* St Louis, 1981, Mosby–Year Book.)

Once the treatments have begun, nothing should be used on the skin. Many soaps, lotions, and powders contain metals, such as zinc and aluminum, that can affect the radiation dose.[6] The patient should be told to avoid the use of all products on the skin unless the physician is consulted. The skin in the treatment area may undergo varying degrees of inflammation. This inflammatory response is known as *radiodermatitis.*

Skin care is of prime importance for the patient receiving external radiation therapy. Radiodermatitis reactions, which commonly occur, may range from a simple blanching or reddening of the skin to blistering and sloughing of skin tissue. Three stages of skin involvement are classified as erythema, dry desquamation with flaking, and moist desquamation with shedding.[12,16,40]

Patients who receive radiation to the skin, superficial lesions, or areas that are subjected to pressure are most likely to experience skin reactions. Treatment of relatively superficial lesions may be seen with tumors of the head, neck, and breast. Areas often subjected to pressure include the perineum, skin folds, collar area, axillae, breast, and groin. Skin reactions are characterized by itching, burning,

tingling, oozing, and sloughing of the skin. Redness may occur on or about the tenth day progressing to a dark plum color after about 3 weeks. The skin may become inelastic and peel. Skin reactions usually begin during the end of the second week of treatment. Skin care guidelines vary from institution to institution but are aimed at lubricating dry skin and minimizing trauma to irradiated skin. If moist desquamation occurs, treatment may be interrupted. When appropriately treated, healing usually begins around the fifth week of treatment and continues for approximately 4 weeks.

Care of the Patient Receiving Internal Radiation

Internal radiation involves the use of radioactive materials placed within the body to deliver radiation to the site of the tumor. Persons receiving internal radiation become a temporary source of radiation. Special precautions are needed to reduce the radiation hazard to health care personnel and visitors.

Internal radiation may be administered through sealed and unsealed methods. *Sealed sources* of radiation are radioactive substances encased in metal capsules. These radioactive substances are designed in the shape of molds, ribbons, plaques, wires, applicators, or needles. They are carefully placed within the tissue or body cavity at the site

---

Skill 19-2   Care of the Skin for Patients Experiencing Radiodermatitis

▼ ···

EQUIPMENT AND SUPPLIES

- Mild cleansing agent, such as mineral oil
- Mild skin lubricant, such as lanolin
- Sterile dressings as indicated
- Sterile saline for irrigation
- Antibiotic or steroid creams or ointments

NURSING INTERVENTIONS

1. Obtain skin care guidelines before the beginning of radiation treatments.
2. Unless contraindicated, cleanse the skin with mineral oil without removing crusts or causing irritation.
3. Apply lanolin or petroleum jelly to soothe and lubricate the skin. Other bland creams or solutions, such as A and D ointment or cod liver oil can be used as recommended.[16] Creams that contain metals, such as aluminum hydroxide, are contraindicated. Cornstarch may relieve itchiness; however, avoid use on broken skin because of increased risk of fungal growth or secondary infection.[11] All skin care products should be removed before each treatment since the patient should arrive for treatment with nothing on the skin.
4. If the skin reaction is severe, apply saline soaks, creams, or ointments as prescribed. Principles of burn therapy may be applied.[11]
5. Advise patients not to wear constricting clothing or expose themselves to friction. Launder clothing using mild, nonirritating detergent and rinse well. Avoid exposing the skin to direct sunlight and temperature extremes, such as hot and cold baths, ice packs or heating pads.[11,12]

of the tumor and left in place for a designated period of time. As with external radiation therapy, the goal of therapy is to expose the tumor to high doses of radiation while minimizing the exposure of normal body tissue. Common sources of sealed radiation include radium needles, radon seeds, gold grains, cobalt-60, cesium-137, iridium-192, radon-222, and tantalum-182.[1,6,21] Placement of sealed radiation within the body may be permanent or temporary depending upon the half-life of the isotope. Isotopes used for temporary treatment have long half-lives and are removed after the treatment period. Treatment periods usually last between 24 to 72 hours. Isotopes may be reused for multiple treatments since their radioactive effects often last for many years. A radioactive isotope with a short half-life may be used for permanent placement since the radioactivity will become clinically inert in a short period of time. Radon with a half-life of 4 days is an example of an iso-

tope that may be used for permanent internal radiation. Sealed radiation may be administered interstitially or by intracavitary placement. Interstitial placement is often used for tumors of the head and neck, tongue, breast, or muscle. Intracavity placement is used to treat cancer of the vagina, cervix, uterus, and bladder.

Unsealed sources of radiation are liquids that are administered either orally, by IV injection, or instilled into body cavities. Oral or IV isotopes are distributed throughout the body and are taken up by cancerous tissues. Intracavitary isotopes are injected into specified body cavities. They are usually color-coded to detect leakage. Unsealed radioactive isotopes have short half-lives. Their principle radioactive effects last for only a few hours or days. Oral and IV preparations are excreted from the body in body fluids. Special precautions are used when handling body fluids, such as urine, emesis, and stool. Unsealed radiation

---

Skill 19-3   Care of the Patient with an Internal Radiation Implant

▼ ....

EQUIPMENT AND SUPPLIES

- Private room
- Warning signs and labels
- Warning tape
- Dosimeters or film badges
- Protocols and calculated time limits
- Sign-in/sign out sheets
- Linen bags and trash bags
- Long-handled forceps
- Leaded containers
- Portable lead shields (optional)
- Personal supplies needed by the patient

NURSING INTERVENTIONS

1. When an implant is in place, meet patient needs as rapidly as possible. Assist patient with essential hygiene measures but do not include a complete bath.
2. Read and sign out the dosimeter. Attach the dosimeter to a belt or pocket while in the patient's room. An alternative method is to assign a film badge to each nurse who will have contact with the patient. Collect the film badges and have them read at regular intervals. Isolation attire is not necessary when a sealed radioisotope is used.
3. When possible, stand at the end of the bed opposite the implant to increase the distance from the radiation source.[12] For a cervical implant, stand at the head of the bed. For a right-sided interstitial implant of the neck, stand at the foot of the bed on the left.
4. Check the placement of the implant every 8 hours to make sure it has not become dislodged. Avoid conditions that might cause dislodgement of a sealed implant. Depending on location, the implant may be dislodged by sneezing, straining, manipulation of a Foley catheter, or undue movement.[10]

5. When ordered, change the dressings over the implant with extreme caution and check for displaced pellets. Examine all bed linen and dressings for dislodged pellets or seeds before disposal.[1,6] Never touch a dislodged pellet with bare hands and caution the patient not to handle any dislodged materials.
6. Use isolation linen bags and trash bags and store linen and trash in the patient's room until the radiation source is removed. Monitor linen and trash for radioactivity before disposal.
7. Restrict patients to bed rest with minimal head elevation to prevent dislodgement when a cervical or uterine implant is in place. Use log rolling to minimize twisting and straining. Before treatment, give enemas and insert a Foley catheter, as ordered, to reduce bladder distention. Administer a vaginal douche if ordered.
8. When a cervical or uterine implant is used, administer a bowel prep before the placement to evacuate the bowel and provide a low residue diet, as ordered, to prevent distention of the colon. An antidiarrheal medication may be prescribed to prevent defecation during the treatment period. These measures are used to minimize incidental radiation exposure to surrounding tissues.[10]
9. For patients receiving head and neck implants, provide IV fluids as needed to maintain hydration. Instruct patients regarding suctioning of the oral cavity and provide the patient with a method of communication, such as a Magic Slate. The head of the bed should be elevated 30 to 45 degrees. Report any unusual swelling or difficulty breathing to the physician immediately.
10. Return the dosimeter to its storage place outside the patient's door when leaving the room. Record the amount of radiation received during each patient contact on the sign-out sheet.
11. Following the removal of a cervical or uterine implant, remove the Foley catheter and administer a vaginal douche or enema as ordered. Dangle the patient before ambulation because prolonged bed rest may produce orthostatic hypotension.[31]

is usually administered in the nuclear medicine or radiation therapy department. Common sources used are iodine-131, phosphorus-32, and gold-198. Phosphorus-32 and gold-198 are injected into body cavities for the treatment of cancer complicated by pleural effusion or ascites. The use of these substances has decreased in recent years with the advent of chemotherapeutic agents that are as effective without the risk of radioactivity.[1,6] As with external radiation therapy, the goal of treatment is to expose the tumor to high doses of radiation while minimizing the exposure of normal tissues.

Care of the patient receiving internal sealed radiation

Common tumors treated with sealed internal radiation include cancer of the vagina, cervix, uterus, head, neck, tongue, and breast.[11,12] During treatment with sealed radiation, precautions are necessary to reduce the risk of radiation exposure to others. Sealed radiation sources are usually inserted in the operating room. Either preloading or afterloading techniques may be used to place the radioactive source. In *preloading,* the radioactive isotope is placed within an applicator that is then inserted into the tumor site. In *afterloading,* an empty applicator or capsule is placed in the patient in the operating room. This container will be used to hold the radioactive isotope during the treatments. The actual isotope is inserted, or afterloaded, later in a setting designated to minimize exposure to hospital personnel, usually the patient's room. An x-ray is performed to verify correct position of the applicator during treatment. The treatment periods usually last between 24 to 72 hours.[6,10,31]

A private room with private bath should be prepared for the patient. Radiation warning signs should be posted on the door and on the patient's chart. Radiation safety precautions or protocols should be provided by the Radiation Safety Officer and followed precisely by all caregivers.

The precautionary guidelines include specific information and instructions, as follows:

1. The type of radiation used.
2. Time of insertion.
3. Removal time.
4. Time or exposure limits for care within 1 m (3 feet) of the patient.
5. Specific precautions to be followed.
6. Phone numbers of the radiation safety personnel to be contacted if a problem arises.[1,6]

The principles of time, distance, and shielding are fundamental to the care of patients undergoing internal radiation treatments.[10,15] By reducing the time spent at the bedside, increasing the distance from the implant while in the patient's room, and using shielding, radiation exposure to nursing staff can be reduced to negligible levels. These principles are incorporated into the care and treatment guidelines for all patients with internal radiation.

Exposure rates are measured by the Radiation Safety Officer at the bedside, at various positions within the room, and at the doorway.[25] Usually a position where the exposure rate is 2.5 mrem (.025 mGy)/hr or less is located and designated by warning tape on the floor. At some institutions, the radiation dose at 1 m (3 feet) and 2 m (6 feet) is measured and indicated on the patient record. The only time a person should be within 1 m (3 feet) of the patient is when direct care is being given. At all other times, persons must remain at a distance of 2 m (6 feet) or greater from the patient, behind the warning tape or at the doorway[1,29] (Fig. 19-4).

Time spent within 1 m (3 feet) of the patient is restricted by exposure limits calculated by the Radiation Safety Officer. For example, a patient's instructions may indicate that a nurse should limit contact within 1 m (3 feet) of the patient to 10 minutes daily for a 3-day treatment period. If a patient requires more extensive care, several nurses should rotate care for the patient.

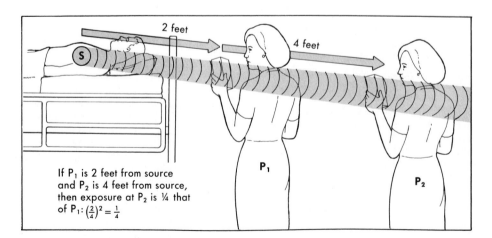

If P$_1$ is 2 feet from source and P$_2$ is 4 feet from source, then exposure at P$_2$ is ¼ that of P$_1$: $\left(\frac{2}{4}\right)^2 = \frac{1}{4}$

Fig. 19-4 Radiation levels decrease as the nurse increases her distance from the patient. (From Beare PG, Myers JL: *Principles and practice of adult health nursing,* St Louis, 1990, Mosby–Year Book.)

Table 19-4   Major Site Specific Complications of Radiation Therapy—Acute Responses[16,31-34]

Site	Response	Intervention
Skin	Erythema, radiodermatitis, dry desquamation, and moist desquamation	Avoid trauma to the site: sun burn, extremes of temperature, constricting clothing, and harsh chemicals; provide skin care as indicated.
Central nervous system	Edema, inflammation, neurological deficits, and hair loss	Monitor for neurological deficits and increased ICP; provide safety measures and physical care as necessary; administer and monitor steroid medications as indicated; cut hair short; and encourage use of wigs, hats, and scarves.
Oral cavity	Mucositis, decreased salivation, change in taste, cough, difficulty swallowing, ulceration, and dental caries	Provide oral care with a soft toothbrush or swab at least every 4 hours; encourage frequent saline washes; provide viscous xylocaine, artificial saliva, and nutritional support as necessary; encourage use of sugarless lozenges and sugarless candy to stimulate saliva; a mouthwash of one teaspoon sodium bicarbonate to one quart water or equal parts nonalcoholic containing mouthwash, peroxide and water may be used; avoid thick, dry, and difficult to chew foods; humidifiers are useful to help liquify thick secretions.
Respiratory system	Pneumonitis	Encourage coughing and deep breathing; increase fluids; prevent infections; and medicate with antibiotics as indicated.
Cardiovascular system	Myocarditis, pericarditis, and phlebitis (rare)	Provide for rest; monitor cardiovascular status and medications as necessary.
GI tract	Nausea, vomiting, ulceration, cramps, diarrhea, and anorexia	At least 30 minutes before treatment, medicate with antiemetics; avoid spicy, fatty, and fried foods; provide low residue diet and antidiarrheal medication as necessary; provide good perineal care; if nausea persists, antiemetics may be administered at regularly prescribed intervals; small, frequent, bland meals may be tolerated better than three larger meals; supplement nutrition with high caloric beverages or powders as needed; and encourage resting before and after meals.
Bladder and pelvis	Cystitis	Increase fluid intake (to 3000 ml unless contraindicated); diuretics and urinary antiseptics may be used; and avoid ingestion of coffee, tea, and alcohol since these are bladder irritants.
Bone marrow	Decreased WBCs, decreased platelets, mild anemia, shortness of breath on exertion, fatigue, bruising, and increased susceptibility to infection	Avoid exposure to pathogens; avoid raw fruits and vegetables because of their high bacterial flora; avoid trauma, prevent cuts and bruises; provide protective isolation as indicated; pace activities to cope with fatigue and dyspnea; use electric razor instead of safety razor; and monitor temperature frequently.

Visitors are usually limited to no more than 1 hour at a position where the exposure rate is equal to or less than 2.5 mrem (.025 mGy)/hr or at the doorway. Pregnant women and children should not visit the patient during the treatment period.[25]

Only essential care is given during treatment with internal radiation. Organization of care is necessary so that maximum efficiency can be achieved in the shortest periods of time. A complete bed bath is not necessary during the treatment period. The patient should be encouraged to take a complete bath before the treatment and after the source of radiation is removed. During treatment, bathing is kept to a minimum. Linen need not be changed unless it is soiled. Patients should be encouraged to collect their own urine and stool if they are ambulatory.[25,26,32]

Portable lead shields may be moved from place to place for added protection.[1,10] However, the nurse should not spend excessive time positioning shields. Emphasis should be placed upon working quickly and efficiently rather than upon the use of leaded shields and aprons that provide only partial protection.

A leaded container and long handled forceps should be kept in the room. If a pellet or radioactive seed is dislodged, it must never be picked up with bare hands or removed from the room unless placed in the leaded container. The long handled forceps must be used to place the radioactive source in the leaded container.[6,26] The Radiation Safety Officer must be notified immediately if dislodgement occurs.

The patient may exhibit symptoms related to irritation of the tissues in the treatment area. Patients frequently describe a sensation of pressure or fullness in the area of the implant. Assessment of symptoms should include the onset, severity, and duration of discomfort. Character of any drainage from the area should be noted and reported if it is excessive or unusual. Site specific assessments should be made as previously described. The patient's vital signs, intake and output, and nutritional intake should be monitored. The placement of the implant should be checked every 8 hours to make sure it has not been dislodged. The patient's psychosocial response to isolation and treatment is an important consideration. The nurse should also assess the patient's understanding of activity restrictions and ability to perform basic self-care activities.

Caring for the patient with unsealed radiation treatments

Iodine-131 is an example of an unsealed radioisotope used for cancer therapy. Iodine-131 is used to treat thyroid cancer. The patient sips liquid containing iodine-131 through a straw.[1] This form of radiation is absorbed systemically, metabolized by the body, and concentrated in the thyroid gland. As iodine-131 is metabolized, it is excreted in body fluids.

The same precautions used during the care of persons with sealed implants are followed. In addition, body fluids and excretions are considered radioactive, and special precautions are taken when handling these substances. The patient should have a private room with a private bath. A protective covering may be used in the toilet area. Urine should be stored in leaded containers and treated as radioactive waste. Occasionally, hospital protocol may allow urine to be disposed of directly into the toilet when a closed drainage system is present. In this situation, the toilet should be flushed 3 times to dilute the urine and remove residue from the toilet bowl.[1,6,41]

Vomitus may be highly radioactive, especially when vomiting occurs within the first 24 hours following administration of the isotope. If vomiting occurs, restrict the patient area and notify the Radiation Safety Officer immediately. Monitor anyone in contact with the emesis for radiation. Decontamination measures include removing contaminated clothing and cleansing of the skin. If contamination is present, linen and clothing should be stored in lead containers for 10 to 40 days, and then rechecked for radioactivity before laundering.[25,41]

Gloves are worn when handling body fluids and articles in direct contact with the patient. Hand washing is extremely important and is incorporated into the care of the patient even when gloves are used.[25] Patients are instructed to collect their urine in leaded containers, taking care that no urine is spilled. Anything contaminated with urine is washed with soap and water using friction for 5 minutes.[1]

Iodine-131 has a half life of 8 days. The time of greatest danger of radioactive contamination is in the first 1 to 4 days. Precautions are usually continued for 5 to 7 days. Iodine-131 is excreted primarily by the kidneys. Kidney function must be monitored closely. If kidney function is compromised, excretion of the isotope may take a longer period of time.[1] On discharge, the patient may be instructed to wear gloves when preparing food and to double flush the toilet. The length of time for these precautions will depend on the dose and will be calculated by the radiation physics staff.

PEDIATRIC CONSIDERATIONS

In general the younger the child, the more radiosensitive the body. Children have more body cells that are actively dividing. Bones, endocrine tissues, muscle tissue, and many body organs are increasing in size and maturing. Radiation can impair growth and development. Radiation to the growth centers of bones can retard bone growth and cause shortening of stature or uneven development. If endocrine glands are included in the radiation field, a deficiency of endocrine hormones can occur. Radiation to the gonads can result in delay of the development of secondary sex characteristics or result in sterility. Intellectual ability may be impaired if there are high doses of radiation to the head. As in adults, inflammation of body tissues may occur causing pneumonitis, pericarditis, pleurisy, and cystitis.[39] Children should be monitored closely for the development of secondary malignancies, such as leukemia and cancer of the thyroid gland. Yearly thyroid examinations following radiation exposure to the head and neck are recommended.[18]

Children who receive radiation therapy have different dose schedules than adults. The most common side effect of irradiation is malaise, which can be frustrating for an active child. Antiemetics for the treatment of nausea and vomiting should be given in oral or suppository form. Anorexia may be present. Forcing a child to eat may meet with rebellion. High calorie, nutritious foods should be encouraged while allowing the child to eat what the child wants during therapy. Later, a more balanced diet may be accepted.[39] Mucosal irritation should be soothed with saline rinses and local anesthetics, such as Chloraseptic spray. Children should be warned about the possibility of hair loss. Regrowth usually occurs within 3 to 6 months. Hair may be darker, thicker, and curlier as it grows back.[18]

Radiation exposure or therapy may be a frightening experience for a child and an emotional time for the family. A gentle, supportive approach can help establish trust and allay fears.

PSYCHOSOCIAL CONSIDERATIONS

A patient who is scheduled to receive external radiation treatments will have numerous fears and concerns regarding treatments. Nursing priorities for these patients should include providing emotional support, eliminating misconceptions, and teaching the patient to manage side effects of therapy. Some patients believe, erroneously, that they will become radioactive following treatments or that the beam of radiation will be painful. The nurse can allay these fears with simple explanations. The patient should receive information about the treatment procedures. For example, the nurse can mention that careful positioning and immobilization with sandbags or casts will be necessary to accurately direct the radiation. The teletherapy machine used may make clicking or whirling sounds; however, the beam of radiation cannot be seen or felt. Although hospital personnel must leave the room during the treatment, visual and voice contact will be maintained with the patient throughout the procedure.[6,17,35,40]

Patients may experience fatigue, depression, a sense of isolation, and altered body image during the treatment period. Patients who are already coping with a diagnosis of cancer must now deal with the isolation and side effects that are associated with radiation therapy. The nurse's concern and guidance can be a significant source of support for the patient during this difficult time.[7]

Patients receiving internal radiation are usually placed in private rooms and contact with visitors and nursing staff is limited during the treatment. These patients may experience an intense feeling of isolation and loneliness. They often have many fears and concerns about the effect and outcome of the radiation as well as the prognosis of their disease.

Nurses can help patients cope during this difficult time by allowing them to verbalize concerns, offering straight forward explanations, and providing support and comfort. Knowledge of radiation characteristics and precautions will allow the nurse to provide safe, effective, and compassionate care during the treatment period without undue risk of radiation exposure.

PATIENT AND FAMILY TEACHING

Because most persons have fears and misconceptions about radiation, the nurse should provide patients with simple explanations regarding properties of radioactive isotopes and principles of radiation therapy. To allay anxiety, it is important to provide specific information regarding the treatment sessions and the procedures that the patient will experience. Coping with the adverse effects of radiation exposure will be a major concern. Procedural details regarding therapy and the management of side effects should be included in patient teaching. Information about skin care, dietary considerations, ways to avoid infection, and how to cope with specific reactions, such as hair loss may also be included.[8]

The nurse should advise patients to avoid sunlight on irradiated skin. Irritating substances and tight clothing are contraindicated over the irradiated area. Patients cope with nausea, vomiting, and anorexia in different ways. A bland, low-residue diet with frequent small meals is usually recommended. Patients can be instructed to avoid smoking, alcohol, spices, and fatty foods. Oral ulcerations can make eating and swallowing painful. The use of viscous xylocaine as an oral analgesic is often required. One should encourage frequent mouth care and saline rinses for comfort.

During the treatment period, it is important to instruct patients to avoid persons with colds and infections, teach handwashing techniques, instruct patients to report signs and symptoms of infection, such as elevated temperature, redness, swelling, purulent drainage, and burning on urination.

Hair loss can be one of the most disturbing adverse effects of radiation therapy. Patients should be instructed to use a mild shampoo, such as baby shampoo, and to use gentle hair care. If hair loss is expected, a short haircut may minimize pulling and tangling. The use of scarves, wigs, hats, and turbans may help the patient to feel less self-conscious and develop a more positive body image. If hair returns after the treatment period it may be slightly different in texture and color. In whole brain treatment in adults with doses of 6000 rads (60 Gy), hair loss is often permanent.

The nurse should encourage patients to ask questions and express concerns during the teaching sessions. Including the family during patient teaching is important. Family members may be primary caregivers in the home setting and will have numerous concerns. Pamphlets and audiovisual aids help to explain complex ideas and allow the patient the time to go back over information at a later date. Information about community resources and support groups will be helpful when the patient begins to anticipate discharge.

One should consider learner readiness. Patients may not be able to absorb information if they are nauseated or uncomfortable. Several short sessions to present information may be more effective than providing the patient with too much information at once. This allows the patient time to mentally process the information and to formulate questions.

HOME HEALTH CARE CONSIDERATIONS

Home health care of the patient after radiation exposure should focus on assessment and treatment of the long-term effects of radiation. Most hospitals have oncology clinics that follow patient progress on an outpatient basis. Patients should be encouraged to keep clinic or doctors' office appointments to facilitate early detection of complications of radiation exposure and to monitor for possible malignancies.

Psychosocial adjustment to a diagnosis of cancer and related therapies is an important concern. There are numerous community support groups for patients who have been treated for cancer. Examples of these groups include: Reach for Recovery for breast cancer patients, the Lost Cord Group for patients who have experienced laryngectomy, and the United Ostomy Association for colostomy, ileostomy, and urostomy patients. The American Cancer Society is a good reference for the availability and location of local support groups.

Teaching patients to identify signs and symptoms of long-term complications is essential. Patients need to understand potential complications related to their type of cancer and to distinguish signs and symptoms that must be reported immediately.

Long-Term Effects of Radiation Treatments

Late effects of radiation treatment are the result of vascular damage in the treatment area and damage to tissues with slow mitotic rates, such as muscles or nerves. If a vaginal implant has been used, the patient should be instructed to inspect the nature and amount of vaginal drainage. Light spotting is normal for several weeks following the treatment. The color of vaginal drainage may change from light pink or brown to tan and then to white. Heavy bright red bleeding or a foul-smelling discharge should be reported to the physician. Good hygiene is important following treatments. Showers are recommended over tub baths. Perineal pads or sanitary napkins should be used instead of tampons. If additional cleansing is needed, a mild vinegar douche may be used unless contraindicated by the physician. One teaspoon of white vinegar is mixed with 1000 mls of water to make this solution.[11] Diarrhea or constipation may occur following treatments. However, normal bowel patterns should return within several weeks. A low-residue diet may be indicated if inflammation of the colon is present.[6,10,33]

An increase in urinary frequency may occur; however, the physician should be notified if urine becomes foul-smelling or cloudy. The patient should be instructed to drink 8 to 10 glasses of water per day.

Sexual intercourse may be resumed within 2 to 3 weeks following treatment to keep the walls of the vagina open and prevent stricture. If sexual intercourse is not possible, a dilator may be used. A water-based lubricant is recommended for added comfort and lubrication as needed by the patient.[10]

If an interstitial implant of the head or neck has been used, secretions may be thick and copious. Frequent mouth care is important. Saline rinses are preferable over commercial mouthwashes that contain alcohol and can be drying. A humidifier may be used to help liquify secretions. Portable suction may be necessary and the patient should be taught how to perform oral suctioning. Cool fluids and popsicles may be soothing. Activities should be encouraged.

REFERENCES

1. Baird SB, Donehower MG, Stalsbroten VL et al: *A cancer sourcebook for nurses,* Atlanta, 1991, American Cancer Society.
2. Beare PG, Myers JL: *Principles and practice of adult health nursing,* St Louis, 1990, Mosby–Year Book.
3. Bomberger AS: *Management of the irradiated patient.* In Garcia LM, editor: *Disaster nursing,* Rockville, Md, 1985, Aspen.
4. Deleted in proofs.
5. Burks J, Griffith P, McCormick K et al: Radiation exposure to nursing personnel from patients receiving diagnostic radionuclides, *Heart Lung* 11(3):217, 1982.
6. Burns N: *Radiotherapy, nursing and cancer,* Philadelphia, 1982, WB Saunders.
7. Dodd MJ: Efficacy of proactive information on self-care in radiation therapy patients, *Heart Lung* 16(5):538, 1987.
8. Dudjak LA: Radiation therapy nursing care record: a tool for documentation, *Oncol Nurs Forum* 15(6):763, 1988.
9. Emergency handling of radiation exposed or radioactive contaminated patients, *Emergency department policy and procedure manual,* Washington, DC, 1987, Georgetown University Medical Center.
10. Hassey K: Demystifying care of patients with radioactive implants, *Am J Nurs* 85(7):789, 1985.
11. Hassey KM, Rose CM: Altered skin integrity in patients receiving radiation therapy, *Oncol Nurs Forum* 9(4):44, 1982.
12. Haylock P: Radiation therapy, *Am J Nurs* 87(11):1441, 1987.
13. Jankowski CB: Radiation emergency, *Am J Nurs* 82(1):91, 1982.
14. Jankowski CB: Radiation exposure of nurses in a coronary care unit, *Heart Lung* 13(1):55, 1984.
15. Jankowski CB: Preventing radiation exposure in critical care, *Dimens Crit Care Nurs* 5(5):270, 1986.
16. Kelly P, Tinsley C: Planning care for the patient receiving external radiation, *Am J Nurs* 81(2):338, 1981.
17. King K, Nail L, Kreamer K et al: Patients' descriptions of the experience of receiving radiation therapy, *Oncol Nurs Forum* 12(4):55, 1985.
18. Lewis F, Levita M: Understanding radiotherapy, *Cancer Nurs* 11(3):174, 1988.
19. Deleted in proofs.
20. Markovchick VJ: *Radiation injuries.* In Rosen P, editor *Emergency medicine: concepts and clinical practice,* St Louis, 1983, Mosby–Year Book.
21. Maddock PG: Brachytherapy sources and applicators, *Semin Oncol Nurs* 3(1):15, 1987.
22. Miller KL, DeMuth WE: Handling radiation emergencies: no need to fear, *J Emerg Nurs* 9(3):141, 1983.
23. Miracle VA, Wiggenton MA: Nurses and ionizing radiation: a study of two institutions, *Crit Care Nurse* 10(5):58, 1990.
24. Murphy D: Iodide—an Rx for radiation accident, *Am J Nurs* 82(1):96, 1982.

25. National Council on Radiation Protection and Measurement, Radiation protection for medical and allied health personnel, *NCRP Report No. 48,* 1976, Bethesda, Md, NCRP Publications.

26. National Council on Radiation Protection and Measurement, Precautions in the management of patients who have received therapeutic amounts of radionuclides, *NCRP Report No. 37.* Bethesda, Md, 1978, NCRP Publications.

27. Phillips TL: *Principles of radiobiology and radiation therapy,* In Carter S, Glatstein E, Livingston R, editors: *Principles of cancer treatment,* New York, 1982, McGraw-Hill.

28. Phipps WJ, Long BC, Woods NF: *Medical-surgical nursing,* ed 4, St Louis, 1991, Mosby–Year Book.

29. Radiation safety, *Policies and procedure manual,* Washington, DC, 1982, Georgetown University Medical Center.

30. Saenger E: Radiation accidents, *Ann Emerg Med* 15(9):1061, 1986.

31. Shell JA, Carter J: The gynecological implant patient, *Semin Oncol Nurs* 3(1):54, 1987.

32. Strohl RA: Head and neck implants, *Semin Oncol Nurs* 3(1):30, 1987.

33. Strohl RA: The nursing role in radiation oncology: symptom management of acute and chronic reactions, *Oncol Nurs Forum* 15(4):429, 1988.

34. Strohl RA, Salazar OM: Management of the patient receiving hemibody irradiation, *Oncol Nurs Forum,* 9(4):44, 1982.

35. Varricchio C: The patient on radiation therapy, *Am J Nurs* 81(2):334, 1981.

36. Wagner D, editor: In the shadow of radiation, *Emerg Med* 19(2):69, 1987.

37. Weibley RE: *Understanding radiation poisoning.* In Shoemaker WC, Ayres S, Grenvok A et al, editors: *Textbook of critical care.* Philadelphia, 1989, WB Saunders.

38. Wittlake WA: *Radiation exposure.* In Burton B, Bayer M, editors: *Hazardous materials. Topics in emergency medicine* 7(1): 53, 1985.

39. Whaley L, Wong D: Nursing care of infants and children, ed 2, St Louis, 1983, Mosby–Year Book.

40. Yasko JM: Care of the patient receiving radiation therapy, *Nurs Clin North Am* 17(4):631, 1982.

41. Yasko JM: *Nursing role and management: problems with abnormal cell growth.* In Lewis S, Collier I, editors: *Medical-surgical nursing: assessment and management of clinical problems,* ed 2, New York, 1987, McGraw-Hill.

CHAPTER 20

Renal Dialysis

Objectives

After completing this chapter, the reader will be able to:

- Discuss the components of the assessment of patients requiring dialysis.
- Formulate appropriate nursing diagnoses for the patient requiring dialysis.
- List at least five patient outcomes for the patient requiring dialysis.
- Describe the administration of peritoneal dialysis and the concept of hemodialysis.
- Describe the administration of continuous arteriovenous hemofiltration and continuous arteriovenous hemodialysis.
- Discuss dialysis treatment and care of children.
- Formulate an appropriate teaching plan for the patient requiring dialysis.
- Discuss differences in home health care and hospital care for the patient requiring dialysis.

Dialysis therapy for the patient with acute renal failure (ARF) is initiated when the metabolic manifestations of the disease process affect homeostasis and more conservative treatment fails to adequately control such problems. Examples of life-threatening abnormalities include elevated serum potassium leading to cardiac rhythm disturbances, fluid volume excess leading to acute pulmonary edema and tissue hypoxia, and uncompensated metabolic acidosis. Dialysis may also be initiated to treat confusion and prevent more severe neurological manifestations that may ensue as the uremia progresses.[16]

Indications for dialysis therapy in the individual with end stage renal disease (ESRD) are not as clear. Nephrologists usually begin therapy when more conservative treatment becomes ineffective, and the symptoms of increasing uremia begin to affect the quality of the patient's life.

ASSESSMENT

A predialysis assessment is conducted before treatment to establish baseline information from which an ongoing evaluation may be made (see box on p. 457).

NURSING DIAGNOSIS

Appropriate nursing diagnoses for the patient in renal failure may be derived from the physiological effects of renal failure. Examples include the following:
- Excess potassium related to decreased renal excretion.
- Excess fluid volume related to renal failure.
- High risk for fluid volume deficit related to dialysis.
- Impaired gas exchange secondary to congestive heart failure.
- High risk for infection related to skin breakdown secondary to uremic rash.
- Dry mucous membranes related to fluid restriction secondary to ESRD.
- Sensory-perceptual alteration related to acid-base balance and uremic toxins related to ESRD.
- Impairment in skin integrity related to arteriovenous shunt.
- Confusion related to uremia.

PATIENT OUTCOMES

The following possible outcomes for the patient requiring renal dialysis are given below.

Patient evidences:
- Serum electrolytes within normal limits for patient.
- Hematocrit, hemoglobin, and coagulation studies within normal limits.
- BUN within normal limits for patient (ideally 5 to 20 mg/dl).
- Creatinine concentrations within normal limits for patient (ideally 0.5 to 1.2 mg/dl for plasma and 1 to 1.18 gm/24 hr for urine).
- Temperature between 36°-38° C (97°-100.5° F).
- Clear, clean, dry venous access site of normal temperature.

PERITONEAL DIALYSIS

Peritoneal dialysis is a method for removing fluid, electrolytes, and the toxic by-products of metabolism that accumulate in the body when the kidneys fail. This form of dialysis is especially useful when a patient can only tolerate slower rates of correction with slower removal of solutes and fluids.[18] When using this method of dialysis, dialysate solution is instilled into the peritoneal cavity

▼ **Specific Areas for Assessment of the Renal Patient**

FLUID VOLUME EXCESS

Tachycardia, S_3 (third heart sound), gallop rhythm, and pericardial friction rub
Neck vein distension and/or peripheral edema
Elevated pulmonary artery wedge pressure (PAWP) or central venous pressure (CVP)
Shortness of breath
Systolic and diastolic hypertension
Pulmonary edema
Intake in excess of output
Increase in body weight
Urine specific gravity decreased

HYPERKALEMIA

Profound muscle weakness and numbness in extremities
Apathy
ECG changes (peaked T waves, widened QRS complex, prolonged P-R interval, flattened or absent P waves, premature ventricular contractions [PVCs])
Increased serum potassium level
Complaints of intestinal colic

METABOLIC ACIDOSIS

Decrease in arterial pH
Decrease in serum bicarbonate
Drowsiness and disorientation
Seizures
Compensated acidosis
    Decreased partial pressure of carbon dioxide (P_{CO_2})
    Normal arterial pH
    Kussmaul respirations and deep sighing

UREMIA

Nausea, vomiting, diarrhea and anorexia
Muscle cramps, numbness and burning in the feet, tremors and restlessness
Asterixis, a flapping motion of the hand when it is hyperextended with the fingers extended
Pruritus
Abnormal electroencephalogram (EEG)
Fatigue, lethargy
Slurred speech
Behavior changes
Alteration in level of consciousness, confusion, seizures, coma
Altered personality, irritability
Occult blood in stool
Ecchymosis
Elevated blood urea nitrogen (BUN) and creatinine level

ANEMIA

Tachycardia, systolic murmur
High cardiac output
Dizziness and/or faintness
Weakness
Decreased hematocrit and hemoglobin level

CLOTTING ABNORMALITIES

Decreased platelet adhesion
Bruising
Pericardial, pleural or joint effusions
Subdural hematomas
Retinal hemorrhage
Epistaxis
Ecchymosis
Gastrointestinal bleeding
Bleeding at vascular access site (when shunt or fistula is in place)

COMPROMISED IMMUNE SYSTEM

Infection at access site
Pericarditis
Diverticulitis
Parotitis
Urinary tract infection
Cytomegalovirus
Non-A non-B hepatitis
Hepatitis B
Fever

MUSCULOSKELETAL ABNORMALITIES

Calcium depletion of bones
Decreased serum calcium
Elevated serum phosphate
Excess parathyroid hormone
Bone pain
Pathological fractures

NUTRITIONAL PROBLEMS

Diet restrictions (protein, potassium, sodium, calories)
Fluid restrictions
Serum albumin decreased
Supplemental feedings (enteral, nasogastric, TPN)
Loss of appetite, nausea
Weight gain
Metallic taste

<u>**Skill 20-1**</u>   **Conducting the Predialysis Assessment**

NURSING INTERVENTIONS

1. Obtain history from patient or family. Note incidences of the following:
   - Chief complaints regarding urinary disorders (output changes, urine color changes, and pain).
   - Chronic renal disease.
   - Kidney infections.
   - Ingestion of nephrotoxic substances.
   - Diabetes, collagen or vascular disease.
   - Hypertension.
   - Major blood vessel disease.
   - Lower urinary tract obstruction.
   - Wide fluctuations in urine output.
   - Hemorrhage.
   - Disseminated intravascular coagulation.
   - Cardiac disease.
   - Hepatic disease.
   - Tuberculosis.
   - Systemic lupus erythematosus.
   - Radiation therapy.
   - Nausea, vomiting, anorexia, or hiccups.
   - Shortness of breath.
   - Confusion or disorientation.
   - Visual changes.
   - Headaches.
   - Itching.
   - Lethargy or weakness.
   - Numbness or tingling.
   - Medication history (nephrotoxic drugs).
   - Nutrition history.
2. Monitor blood pressure, apical pulse, respirations, temperature, and central venous pressures. Note presence of hypertension.
3. Weigh patient. Predialysis weight is essential.
4. Assess the following:
   - General appearance including color, peripheral edema, dry skin, neck vein distention, rashes, and bruises.
   - Nails, looking for thin, brittle nails.
   - Skin and eyebrows for uremic crystals.
   - Venous access site, if in place.
   - Determine level of consciousness and mentation.
   - Note odor of breath (may smell of urine in the uremic patient, uremic fetor).
   - Note respiratory pattern (compensatory respirations, shortness of breath, or Kussmaul respirations).
   - Oral mucosa for dryness and coated tongue.
   - Retina for hypertensive changes or hemorrhage.
   - Lower abdomen for bladder distention.
   - Hyperextended hands for asterixis.
   - Extremities for tremors.

5. Palpate the following:
   - Skin temperature.
   - Extremities for edema.
   - Skin turgor.
   - Capillary refill.
   - Kidneys for size and tenderness. If pain is noted, determine characteristics. Normally, the left kidney is not palpable. Occasionally, the lower section of the right kidney is palpable. Kidneys may be palpable, however, when renal disease is present.
   - Bladder.
6. Percuss the following:
   - Heart and lungs for dullness.
   - Bladder and abdomen.
7. Auscultate the following:
   - Lungs for presence of crackles and wheezes.
   - Heart for S_3, gallop rhythm, or systolic murmur.
   - Renal artery using the bell of the stethoscope.
   - Shunt or fistula, if appropriate.
8. Monitor the following:
   - Central venous pressure (CVP) and pulmonary artery wedge pressure (PAWP) if possible
   - Urine output, noting:
     Volume.
     Color.
     Odor.
     Sediment.
     Osmolality.
     Specific gravity.
     Protein.
     Glucose.
     Hematuria.
     Pus.
     pH.
   - Review laboratory studies:
     Serum electrolytes level.
     BUN level.
     Creatinine level.
     Clotting studies.
     Complete blood count (CBC).
     Hemoglobin A (Hb A).
   - Review ECG or tracing, noting:
     Peaked T waves.
     Widened QRS complex.
     Prolonged P-R interval.
     Flattened or absent P waves.
     Premature venticular contractions (PVCs).

A   B   C

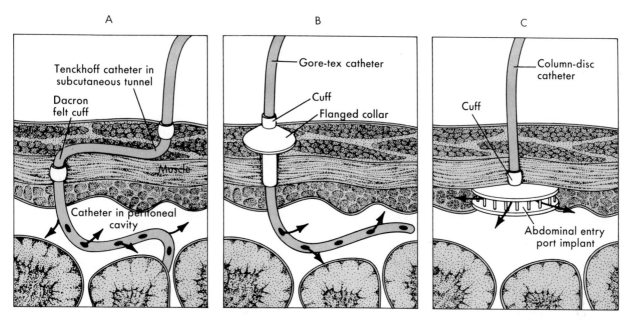

Fig. 20-1   Three types of peritoneal dialysis catheter. **A,** Tenckhoff catheter has two Dacron felt cuffs that hold the catheter in place and prevent dialysate leakage and bacterial invasion. Subcutaneous tunnel also helps prevent infection. **B,** Gore-tex catheter with Dacron cuff above a flanged collar. **C,** Column-disc catheter has cuff and large abdominal entry port implant. (From Beare PG, Myer JL: *Adult health nursing,* St Louis, 1990, Mosby–Year Book.)

through a catheter (Fig. 20-1) and the peritoneum serves as a dialyzing membrane.

This technique may be indicated in the critical care setting in several instances because it is technically easier to accomplish than hemodialysis and is more readily tolerated in unstable patients. It may be used when hemodialysis equipment and personnel are not available or when patients are healing from insertion of vascular access device. Other uses for peritoneal dialysis include the treatment of acute poisoning resulting from a dialyzable substance and as a method of elevating the temperature of hypothermia victims using warmed dialysate. Peritoneal dialysis may be contraindicated when the patient has been subjected to trauma or surgery in the abdominal area or when fibrosis or adhesions are present.

The central component of any dialysis system is a semipermeable membrane. This membrane has the ability to selectively allow the movement of smaller molecules, such as water, electrolytes, and the waste products of metabolism, to cross from one compartment to another. At the same time, it prevents the passage of larger particles, such as the formed elements of the blood and circulating plasma proteins. As blood flows by one side of the membrane, dialysate, an aqueous solution of electrolytes and glucose, is present on the other side. Small molecular weight solutes pass freely through the membrane from an area of higher concentration to an area of lower concentration. This allows the addition or removal of small molecular weight solutes to or from the serum (Fig. 20-2).

In intermittent peritoneal dialysis, the semipermeable

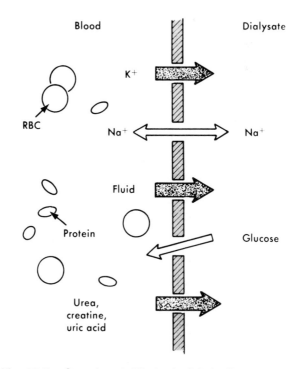

Fig. 20-2   Osmosis and diffusion in dialysis. Net movement of major particles and fluid is illustrated. (From Long BC, Phipps WJ: *Medical-surgical nursing: a nursing process approach,* ed 2, St Louis, 1989, Mosby–Year Book.)

membrane used is the peritoneal membrane. To initiate dialysis, warmed peritoneal dialysate (usually 2 L) is instilled aseptically into the peritoneal cavity through an indwelling or temporary catheter (usually over 10 minutes). During the dwell period (about 30 minutes) the exchange of electrolytes and removal of water and uremic toxins occurs. At the completion of the dwell, the dialysate fluid is allowed to drain (about 20 minutes), for a total exchange time of 1 hour. The process is repeated for the prescribed number of cycles. The composition of dialysate fluid is varied to influence the direction and rate of solute removal.

In addition, 500 to 1000 U of heparin may be added for the first 2 to 4 runs, to prevent fibrin clotting of the catheter.

Filtration, the removal of excess fluid during dialysis, is accomplished by the addition of glucose to the dialysate, making the solution hyperosmolar. A concentration of 1.5% is used to produce mild fluid removal. Filtration may be increased by using a 4.25% concentration. Because a small amount of the glucose may be absorbed, continous use of the higher percentage solution requires close monitoring of the patient.

Effective dialysis is determined by peritoneal clearance. *Peritoneal clearance* is the volume of plasma that can be completely cleared of the substance under consideration, in 1 minute of time. Urea and potassium have the highest clearance times. Clearance times for creatinine, uric acid, phosphate, and sulfate are lower. Calcium and magnesium have an even lower clearance.

The most frequent problem associated with acute peritoneal dialysis is infection or peritonitis, which tends to occur less frequently when the procedure is completed in 48 to 72 hours.[2] Meticulous care of the catheter is essential. Technical problems encountered include respiratory compromise, which occurs during the instillation and dwelling time. It can also occur if there is difficulty in draining the fluid from the patient. Some of the technical problems can be alleviated by simple maneuvers, such as repositioning the patient or slowing the infusion rate. Three classes of complications include those caused by the following:

- Mechanical problems.
- Metabolic disturbances.
- Inflammatory reactions.

HEMODIALYSIS AND HEMOFILTRATION

Hemodialysis is the most widely used form of dialysis[18] and is the treatment of choice because it is extremely efficient when compared to other methods of dialysis; the clearance of urea is nearly twice that of peritoneal dialysis. In addition, the ultrafiltration of water and correction of the electrolyte disturbances frequently encountered in ARF is more rapidly accomplished. Other uses of hemodialysis in the critical care setting include maintenance dialysis of hospitalized ESRD patients and specialized uses, such as the treatment of poisoning.

Specialized training in the operation of hemodialysis equipment is required to avoid or manage the technical problems occasionally encountered during this procedure.

For this reason, treatments are usually performed by hemodialysis nursing personnel. Critical care nurses caring for these patients must understand the principles of dialysis and hemofiltration, however, to assist the dialysis nurse in the observation and care of the intradialysis patient. The critical care nurse should be proficient in the observation and care of the hemodialysis access site.

Hemodialysis is the extracorporeal circulation of blood against dialysate separated by a semipermeable membrane. Hemodialysis functions through three principles to produce the removal of excess water, electrolytes, and nitrogenous waste products. The first principle, *diffusion,* is the movement of solutes across the semipermeable membrane from an area of higher to lower concentration, which increases as the pressure gradient between blood and dialysate increases. Diffusion results in the movement of urea, creatinine, uric acid, and potassium from the patient's blood into the dialysate solution. Protein molecules and blood cells are too large to cross the semipermeable membrane and are not diffused.

The second principle, *osmosis,* relates to the movement of fluid across a semipermeable membrane from an area of lesser concentration to one of higher concentration. Osmosis is the principle that governs the removal of fluid from the body during dialysis.

The third principle, *ultrafiltration,* is the movement of serum water and solutes across the membrane, as a result of an artificially created pressure gradient. Ultrafiltration is more efficient than osmosis for removal of fluid. The clearance of a dialyzer refers to the amount of solute removal produced, and it depends on the surface area and thickness of the membrane as well as the rate of blood flow. The ultrafiltration factor of a dialyzer refers to the rate of fluid removal produced per hour. The use of a specific dialyzer is part of the hemodialysis prescription and is based on the clearance and ultrafiltration factors described.

A typical hemodialysis system has three main components—the dialyzer, the blood path or circuit, and the dialysate path or circuit.

Blood flows from the patient's access through a compression roller blood pump, through the blood compartment of the dialyzer, and back to the patient through an air trap and air detector. A typical blood flow rate varies from 200 to 300 ml/min to ensure that waste products can be dialyzed out in the designated time. Mixed, warmed dialysate is pumped from the dialysis machine through the dialysate compartment of the dialyzer and back to the machine. Blood and dialysate flow in a countercurrent fashion, opposite to the direction in which the dialysate is being channeled, assuring that fresh dialysate and undialyzed blood are always in contact. This maximizes the efficiency of dialysis. Changes in blood flow through the dialyzer directly affect how much solute is removed.

Vascular Access Devices

A variety of vascular access devices have been developed for hemodialysis. There are two major requirements for a vascular access route—an outflow route with an ade-

The purpose of this procedure is to provide emergency access to the peritoneal cavity for the administration of peritoneal dialysis. In some institutions peritoneal dialysis solutions are available premixed, warmed, and ready for use. In other settings, the addition of potassium chloride, heparin, or antibiotics is completed by the nursing staff. Warming is also performed by nursing unit personnel.[1]

EQUIPMENT AND SUPPLIES:

- Peritoneal dialysis tray containing the following:
  Rigid peritoneal catheter
  Trocar
  Local anesthetic (Xylocaine 1%)
  Scalpel
  Syringe with needle
  Catheter connector
  Sterile cups
  Suture
- Povidone-iodine solution
- Alcohol or acetone
- Sterile gloves
- Premixed and warmed peritoneal dialysate
- Dialysate administration and drainage set
- Face masks
- Dressing materials
- Sterile drape

NURSING INTERVENTIONS

1. Check physician's order and signed consent. Follow institutional policy and procedure. Consent is necessary before treatment.
2. Monitor and record predialysis vital signs and weight. Baseline information provides a basis for on-going evaluation. Daily weights reflect fluid volume status.
3. Have patient void or empty bladder if patient is not oliguric or anuric, to prevent accidental bladder puncture.
4. Premedicate patient as ordered.
5. Put on masks (including patient).
6. Prepare tray.

7. Clean abdominal area three times with alcohol/acetone swab followed by three times with povodine-iodine swab. Use recommended preparation solution or follow institutional policy and procedure. Adequate skin preparation is essential to avoid infection.
8. Using aseptic technique, connect administration set to dialysate bag, prime tubing, and clamp.
9. Suspend dialysate on IV pole.
10. Place drainage bag below patient.
11. Close outflow clamp (Fig. 20-3).
12. Instruct patient to tighten abdominal muscles. Physician will administer local anesthetic, make small incision and insert catheter/trocar through peritoneum. After catheter placement the trocar is removed.[6]
13. Put on gloves.
14. Attach primed administration set to catheter; apply occlusive dressing material over the entry site to prevent contamination of the catheter. Betadine ointment may also be applied.
15. Infuse 1 to 2 L dialysate, as ordered.
16. Clamp tubing.
17. Physician will complete catheter placement after abdominal cavity is filled with fluid, which helps to prevent puncture of organs.
18. Drain dialysate as prescribed.
19. Record the following data:
    - Type of solution administered and any additives.
    - Patient reaction.
    - Amount and appearance of drained dialysate. (Maintain a cumulative fluid balance total.)
    - Vital signs.

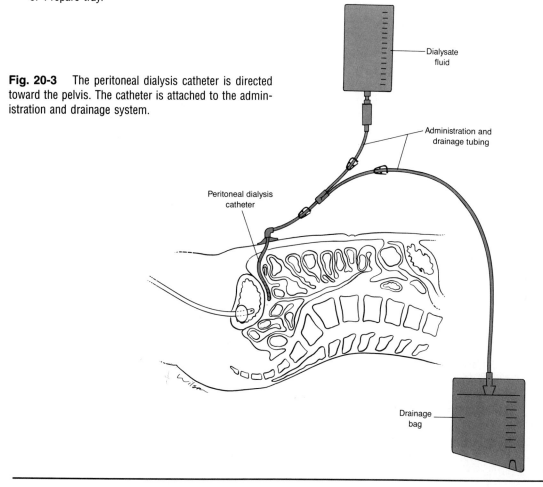

Fig. 20-3 The peritoneal dialysis catheter is directed toward the pelvis. The catheter is attached to the administration and drainage system.

Dialysate fluid

Administration and drainage tubing

Peritoneal dialysis catheter

Drainage bag

Skill 20-3   Changing a Peritoneal Catheter Dressing

The purpose of dressing changes is to prevent peritonitis by proper maintenance of the catheter and insertion site. Intact dressings should be inspected every 8 hours and changed every 48 hours; or as agency policy directs. If leakage occurs at the catheter insertion site, remove the dressing, inspect the site, and reapply a new dressing.

EQUIPMENT AND SUPPLIES

- Sterile and nonsterile gloves
- Alcohol/acetone preparations
- Povidone-iodine preparations
- Povidone-iodine ointment
- 4 × 4 fenestrated (or tracheostomy) dressing
- Cloth tape or transparent dressing material
- Face masks

NURSING INTERVENTIONS

1. Put on nonsterile gloves and masks (including patient).
2. Remove old dressing.
3. Inspect insertion site. If an exudate is present, determine if a culture should be obtained before cleansing of the site. Redness, swelling, pain, odor, warmth, or exudate may indicate infection.
4. Discard contaminated dressing materials and gloves. Wash hands.
5. Put on sterile gloves.
6. Clean catheter and insertion site area three times with alcohol/acetone preparations followed three times by povidone-iodine preparations, working from insertion site outward. Use agents listed or follow institutional policy and procedure. Adequate skin cleansing is essential to avoid peritonitis.
7. Apply sterile fenestrated dressing to provide an absorbent protective covering for insertion site (optional).
8. Secure with cloth adhesive tape or cover with transparent dressing material to provide a protective barrier to contamination.
9. Remove gloves.
10. Record any unusual findings (i.e.: redness, swelling, foul odor, pain at insertion, or exudate). Report suspected infection immediately.

Skill 20-4   Administering a Peritoneal Dialysis Exchange

Patients may experience a small amount of discomfort during infusion of the dialysate, particularly with the first few exchanges. This is related to expansion of the peritoneal cavity by dialysate and may be reduced by slowing the infusion slightly. In the case of severe discomfort, one should stop the infusion and notify the physician. Draining dialysate should appear clear and colorless or straw-colored. Pink-tinged dialysate indicates the presence of blood, and cloudy dialysate may indicate peritonitis. Thin white strands of fibrin may appear in the drainage tubing or solution. One should report continued blood in the dialysate to the physician. Routine culturing of the dialysate at regular intervals may be ordered. Specimens should be collected aseptically through the drainage sample port of the dialysate administration set.

EQUIPMENT AND SUPPLIES

- Premixed and warmed peritoneal dialysate
- Dialysate administration and drainage set
- Peritoneal dialysis flow sheet (Fig. 20-4)
- Dressing materials
- Sterile gloves
- Face masks

NURSING INTERVENTIONS

1. Check physicians order and signed consent.
2. Measure and record predialysis vital signs, monitoring pressures and weight.
3. Using aseptic technique, connect administration set to dialysate bag, prime tubing, and clamp.
4. Suspend dialysate on IV pole.
5. Remove catheter cap. Connect dialysate tubing to catheter. Repeat for drainage bag. Place drainage bag below patient.
6. Close outflow clamp. If dialysis is already in progress, the tubing will not need priming. These procedures facilitate gravity infusion and drainage.
7. Open dialysate bag clamp.
8. Infuse 1 to 2 L dialysate, as ordered (usually over 10 minutes).
9. Close clamp. See Table 20-1 for troubleshooting tips.
10. Allow solution to dwell, as ordered, (usually 20 to 30 minutes). This provides time for solutes and water to cross the semipermeable membrane.
11. Open dialysate drain clamp. Complete drainage usually takes 20 minutes. If drainage slows or stops, reposition patient forward or side to side. Repositioning patient may help to free catheter of kinks or tissue.
12. Record amount of dialysate infused, time infused and drained, and amount and type of drainage on dialysis flow sheet. Note any problems and calculate total fluid balance at the end of each exchange (Fig. 20-4).
13. Repeat steps 3 to 10 until the prescribed number of exchanges are completed.
14. At the completion of the exchanges clamp the catheter, disconnect from administration set, and cap with sterile injection cap. Cover with sterile dressing material until removed by physician.
15. Record data including vital signs, weight, amount of dialysate infused, time infused and time drained, and number of exchanges.

WASHINGTON HOSPITAL CENTER

Exchange Number	Time In	Time Out	Volume In	Volume Out	Exchange Balance	Total Balance	Solution %	MEDS/2L	Comments

Wt. Pre-dialysis_____

**PERITONEAL DIALYSIS
FLOW SHEET**

FORM 675

Fig. 20-4 Peritoneal dialysis flow sheet. (Courtesy of Washington Hospital Center, Washington, DC.)

Table 20-1   Troubleshooting Tips for Peritoneal Dialysis

Problem	Potential cause	Action
Sudden drop in blood pressure	Hypovolemia	Stop inflow and outflow; call physician; continue to monitor vital signs.
Sudden tachycardia	Hypovolemia Volume excess Electrolyte imbalance	Stop inflow and outflow; monitor apical pulse; call physician; continue to monitor vital signs; run rhythm strip.
Cardiac dysrhythmias	Electrolyte imbalance Hypotension Volume excess	Stop inflow and outflow; monitor apical pulse; call physician; continue to monitor; run rhythm strip; draw electrolytes and send to laboratory; medicate with antidysrhythmic drugs, as ordered.
Acute respiratory distress	Too much volume instilled	Stop infusion; open drainage tubing to allow free drainage; raise head of bed; call physician; provide oxygen, as needed.
Bloody drainage	Trauma (blood-tinged) Possible vessel erosion (bright blood) Overheparinization Prolonged clotting time	Observe drainage; hold heparin; call physician if it does not clear.
Sudden abdominal or back pain	Fluid too cool Too rapid filling	Check solution temperature, warm if too cool; check patency of drainage tube; slow inflow; if pain not resolved, call physician.
Sudden fever	Sepsis Bowel perforation Peritonitis	Monitor temperature; check lab cultures; draw blood and send to lab for culture; notify physician; monitor color of outflow; give antipyretic drugs as ordered; discontinue dialysis if symptoms do not subside.
Cloudy outflow	Possible infection Possible bowel perforation Possible bladder perforation	Obtain culture; continue to monitor color; call physician.
Scrotal swelling	Dislodged catheter	Notify physician.
Muscle cramps/increased weakness	Electrolyte imbalance	Draw electrolytes and send to laboratory.
Protein loss	Dialyzed out	Monitor serum protein; replace with 5% or 25% albumin, as ordered.
Leakage at exit site	Leaking around catheter Catheter may have slipped	Check drainage bag for kinks; change dressing; inspect site; monitor through next run; estimate fluid loss; notify physician.
Poor inflow	Kinked tubing Tissue in trocar	Check clamps and tubing; turn patient; raise or lower bed.
Poor outflow	Tubing over siderail Kinked tubing	Move tubing; unkink; check clamp; change bag level to increase gravity.

quate volume of blood and an inflow route of adequate diameter to accept the blood flow at a rapid rate of return. Small vessels will not be adequate because the desired rate of extracorporeal blood flow is 200 to 300 ml/min.

Initially, the selection of the type of vascular access depends on the severity of the patient's condition and the presence of a life-threatening event. When hemodialysis is anticipated, access to the patient's circulation is accomplished by the surgical creation of an arteriovenous (AV) fistula or an implanted AV graft. Both methods result in a large vessel with high blood flow that may be punctured intermittently for hemodialysis.

The *AV fistula* is an internal anastomosis of an artery to a vein (Fig. 20-5). This results in the direct flow of arterial blood into a vein. Over a period of 4 to 8 weeks the vein distends as a result of the high-pressure arterial blood flow.

The wall of the vein gradually becomes tougher and thicker. The distention, thickening, and toughening of the vein allows for the frequent puncture of the fistula for the hemodialysis procedure. Generally, two needles are used; one for outflow and one to return dialyzed blood.

AV grafts are the most frequently used access for treating chronic renal failure. The graft is a Gore-tex (or biologic material) tube, which is surgically implanted in a limb (Fig. 20-5, *B*).

An *AV shunt* is the external joining of an artery to a vein by a specially treated synthetic tubing.

AV fistulas, grafts, and shunts can collapse or clot off. To prevent damage to these access sites, blood pressure should not be taken on a limb with a fistula or shunt. A sign should be placed on the wall by the patient's bedside to alert all health care staff not to monitor blood pressure

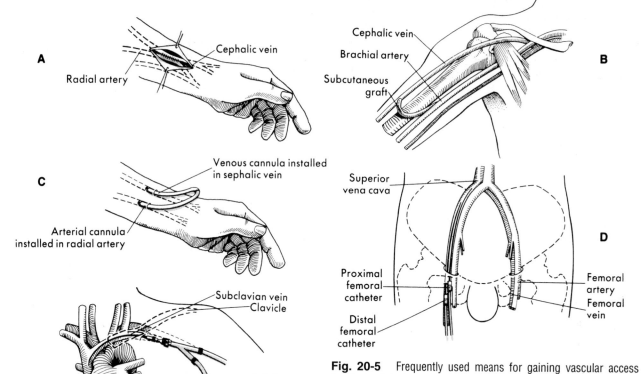

Fig. 20-5 Frequently used means for gaining vascular access for hemodialysis includes **A,** arteriovenous fistula, **B,** arteriovenous graft, **C,** external arteriovenous shunt, **D,** femoral vein catheterization, and **E,** subclavian vein catheterization. (From Long BC, Phipps WJ, Cassmeyer VL: *Medical-surgical nursing: a nursing process approach,* St Louis, 1993, Mosby–Year Book.)

Table 20-2 Advantages and Disadvantages of Venous Access Sites

Venous access route	Advantages	Disadvantages
AV fistula	Long-lasting. Minimal immobilization. No foreign material used. Safer than external shunt.	Length of time needed for fistula to mature. Can clot off. Phlebitis from puncture. Infiltration possible. May develop an aneurism. Blood pressure cannot be taken in extremity with fistula.
External shunt	Ease of placement. No puncture of the skin is necessary. Does not require time to mature. Blood samples can be obtained without venipuncture.	Can clot off. Short life span. Blood pressure cannot be taken in extremity with shunt. Infection potential. Potentially destroys blood vessel. May become dislodged. Accidental exsanguination.
AV graft	Long-lasting. Minimal immobilization. Safer than external shunt.	Requires surgical implantation. Must mature. Risk of clotting off. Risk of bleeding. False aneurysm formation. Risk of infection. Arterial or venous stenosis.
Subclavian catheter	Relatively easy to place. Dialysis may be initiated immediately.	Can clot off. Risk of infection. Some activity restrictions. Showers not permitted. X-ray needed to validate correct placement procedure to use.
Femoral catheter	Relatively easy to place. Quick insertion. Dialysis may be initiated after placement.	Immobility. Risk of infection. Risk of bleeding. Thrombophlebitis. Potential pulmonary emboli. Hematoma formation at insertion site.

or draw blood in the limb with the access. If the patient has a shunt, two bulldog clamps should be attached to the outer layer of the shunt dressing. This will enable the patient or health care provider to clamp off both sides of the shunt if it becomes dislodged and blood loss occurs.

When hemodialysis is required on an emergency basis or an existing access fails, a temporary venous access device may be inserted percutaneously into the subclavian or femoral vein[4] (See Fig. 20-5, *C* and *D*). Either the subclavian or femoral catheter can be inserted at the bedside using strict aseptic technique. After insertion, the device is heparinized until dialysis. Some devices have double lumens, allowing for the simultaneous flow of undialyzed blood into the dialyzer at the proximal lumen and the return of dialyzed blood through the distal lumen. Other devices are single lumen and therefore require a clamping device that alternately allows blood flow in and out of the circulation (Table 20-2).

Anticoagulation

Anticoagulation of the patient during hemodialysis is required to prevent clotting of the blood path and dialyzer. Systemic heparinization can be established by a single intravenous (IV) dose of heparin at the beginning of the treatment followed by an additional dose 2 hours later. More conservative heparinization is indicated when the patient is at risk for bleeding. Alternate methods include low dose heparinization, where reduced IV bolus doses are given, or heparin infusion, where a reduced amount of heparin is given continuously. Regional heparinization is a technically more difficult approach to anticoagulation. Blood entering the blood path is anticoagulated with a heparin infusion, which is subsequently reversed with a protamine infusion as it reenters the patient's circulation. The state of anticoagulation is determined quickly and inexpensively at the bedside with the use of the activated clotting time (ACT) test.

Hemofiltration

Hemofiltration is a modification of the dialysis process designed to remove serum ultrafiltrate without concurrent dialysis. Because no dialysate is used in the process, hemofiltration simply results in the removal of serum ultrafiltrate. Fluid removal in this manner is usually well-tolerated[22] and may be made more efficient by the addition of negative pressure to the dialysate compartment of the dialyzer or positive pressure to the blood compartment. Because hemofiltration is usually more easily tolerated than hemodialysis, sequential dialysis, the administration of several hours of hemofiltration followed by several hours of hemodialysis may be ordered for hemodynamically unstable patients.[22]

Complications

Complications of hemodialysis during the phase of acute illness include the following:
- Hypovolemia (from too rapid removal of fluids).
- Hypotension (related to hypovolemia), antihypertensive medications, and ultrafiltration.
- Hypertension (fluid overload).
- Infection.
- Bleeding as a result of excess anticoagulation.

CONTINUOUS ARTERIOVENOUS HEMOFILTRATION AND HEMODIALYSIS

Continuous arteriovenous hemofiltration (CAVH) is a relatively new therapy used primarily to control fluid balance but with some filtering of body wastes. *CAVH* is the continuous removal of hemofiltrate using a hemofilter system, similar to the process of hemofiltration described above. A typical CAVH system is illustrated in Fig. 20-6.

During CAVH, arterial blood flows from the patient through an arterial blood line, through the hemofilter, and back to the patient through the venous blood line. The hemofilter is a semipermeable membrane that allows for the removal of water and noncellular components of the serum while retaining the protein and cellular components in the circulation. The filtrate is collected in a drainage bag located below the filter.

There are several important differences between the hemofiltration accomplished with hemodialysis equipment and the simpler CAVH hemofilter system. In CAVH, blood flow through the hemofilter is maintained by the patient's cardiac output; no blood pump is used.[1] Because the rate of filtration depends in part on the speed of blood flow, the rate of filtration is slow and continuous. Standard hemofil-

Skill 20-5   Assessing the Patency of a Fistula or Shunt

Vascular access checks are performed to assess patency of the fistula or shunt. A suspected access failure is reported immediately. Surgically constructed fistulas are usually located on the forearm or upper arm. Surgically implanted grafts may be located on arms or legs. Report a nonfunctioning access to the nephrologist so that declotting may be attempted before the next dialysis or an alternative access may be secured. Access patency should be assessed every shift and recorded.

NURSING INTERVENTIONS

1. Locate the vascular access.
2. Examine the vessel or shunt size for bleeding, bruising, lack of pulsations, and aneurysms.
3. Palpate the access from the distal anastomosis to the proximal anastomosis. A thrill, the feeling of turbulent blood flow, should be felt along the course of the vessel. It will be stronger at the arterial end. This procedure should be conducted at least every 4 hours.
4. Auscultate the access in the same manner. A bruit, the rushing sound of turbulent blood flow, should be heard along the course of the vessel or shunt. It will be louder at the arterial end. It may be faint in shunts. Conduct this procedure every 4 hours.
5. Record the results of the examination. Report nonfunctioning accesses to the nephrologist.

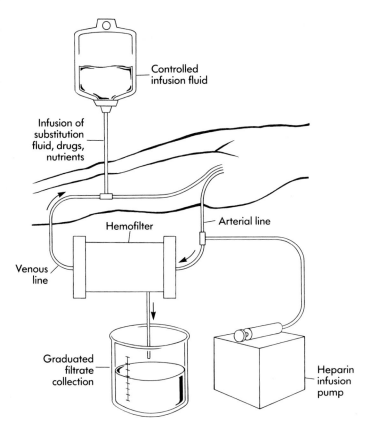

Fig. 20-6 Continuous arteriovenous hemofiltration (CAVH).

Skill 20-6 External Double Lumen Shunt Care

Strict aseptic technique is used while providing shunt care, because infection is a frequent cause of shunt failure. Dressings are usually changed every 24 hours.[10] Follow institutional policy and procedure. Should the shunt become opened or accidentally severed, clamp the arterial and venous sides immediately to stop bleeding, then reconnect them. Check for blood flow, clean and redress the site, and notify the physician.

EQUIPMENT AND SUPPLIES

- Sterile and nonsterile gloves
- Sterile sponges and tracheostomy dressing
- Povidine-iodine solution
- 3% hydrogen peroxide solution
- 2.5 to 7.5 cm (1 to 3 inches) stretch gauze
- 2 cannula clamps (Do not use hemostats on shunts.)
- Sterile towel and surgical mask

NURSING INTERVENTIONS

1. Put on surgical mask and wash hands.
2. Saturate sponges or swabsticks with povidine-iodine and saturate four sponges with hydrogen peroxide, or other solution as directed by agency policy.
3. Put on nonsterile gloves and remove old dressing.
4. Discard dressing and gloves. Avoid the use of scissors, which may cause accidental severing of the shunt.
5. Examine the insertion sites for signs of infection, such as redness, swelling, pain, warmth, or discharge.
6. Examine the shunt for patency. A thrill should be palpable and a bruit should be auscultated. Report any abnormalities to the physician. Observe the blood flow through the tubing. A layering of red cells and plasma indicates a clotted shunt.
7. Wash hands and put on sterile gloves. Place sterile towel under shunted extremity.
8. Cleanse each insertion site with hydrogen peroxide using sponges or swabsticks, beginning at the insertion site and moving outward in a circular fashion. Remove crusted exudate.
9. Clean shunt tubing with fresh sponges or swabsticks.
10. Cleanse each insertion site and shunt tubing with povidone-iodine sponges in the same manner.
11. Redress the shunt using sterile tracheostomy dressings then wrap the extremity with stretch gauze leaving the shunt exposed. Avoid wrapping too tightly; it may impede circulation in the extremity or clot the shunt.
12. Clamp two cannula clamps on the dressing.

tration is rapid but intermittent. The slower continuous hemofiltration of CAVH is usually well-tolerated in hemodynamically unstable patients.[15] Additionally, dialysate is not used in CAVH. Any metabolical wastes and electrolytes are removed by filtration alone. Because hemodialysis equipment is not required, trained hemodialysis personnel are not needed to perform the procedure.

CAVH requires a strong arterial access outflow to perfuse the hemofilter system and a venous access site to return filtered blood. Frequently, femoral arterial and venous lines are established using percutaneous large-bore catheters. Alternately, an arterial line at another access site may be used, returning blood through a separate venous site. An AV shunt may also be used for access. Blood flow must be adequate to perfuse the filter; insufficient blood flow will cause clotting and failure of the device.

The rate of filtration may range from <100 ml/hr to >1000 ml/hr depending on the rate of blood flow, the patient's mean arterial blood pressure, and the permeability of the filter.[5] Filtration may be regulated by raising or lowering the collection bag or by partially occluding the filtrate line.[12] Periodically, the system should be checked for patency using a saline bolus test. The ultrafiltration rate is guided by the patient's response, pulmonary artery pressure, central venous pressure, and changes in blood pressure.

Replacement fluids given to the patient who is being treated with CAVH are individually determined based on each patient's needs. The type and amount of replacement varies, usually depending on the amount of ultrafiltrate (see the box on p. 468 for calculation of replacement fluid).

Anticoagulation is usually accomplished with a heparin bolus before initiating therapy, followed by a heparin drip. Coagulation is usually monitored at the bedside with the ACT test.

The objective of heparinization is to keep the hemofilter free of clots. To prevent clot formation in the hemofilter, a

Skill 20-7   **Hemodialysis Venous Access Device Dressing Change**

EQUIPMENT AND SUPPLIES

- Sterile and nonsterile gloves
- Alcohol swabs or hydrogen peroxide swabs
- Povidone-iodine swabs
- Sterile sponges
- Povidone-iodine ointment
- Transparent dressing material

NURSING INTERVENTIONS

1. Wash hands; put on nonsterile gloves.
2. Remove old dressing material.
3. Discard dressing and gloves.
4. Inspect the insertion site for signs of infection, such as redness, swelling, warmth, pain, or discharge. Report any abnormal findings immediately.
5. Put on sterile gloves.
6. Cleanse area twice from the insertion site outward in a circular motion with hydrogen peroxide swabs.
7. Cleanse area in the same manner using povidone-iodine swabs.
8. Place a small amount of povidone-iodine ointment over the insertion site and cover with a sterile transparent dressing. Note the time, date, and initial on the dressing.

Calculating the Filter Replacement Fluid for Continuous Arteriovenous Hemofiltration

- Measure the ultrafiltrate (UF) produced during the previous hour.
- Measure all other types of output (O) produced during the previous hour (urine, emesis, nasogastric or chest drainage, and stool).
- Calculate the patient's IV intake during the previous hour (include all parenteral fluids, IV drips, medication, and heparin infusions).
- Add tube feedings to intake.
- Determine, from physician's order, the hourly net fluid loss (FL) desired.
- Calculate the filter replacement fluid (FRF) using the following formula:

$$(UF + O) - (IV + FL) = FRF$$

EXAMPLE:

The patient's ultrafiltrate production over the last hour was 800 ml and other outputs amounted to 45 ml. The IV intake was 120 ml. The physician wants the patient to lose 100 ml of fluid every hour. Using the above equation, $(800 + 45) - (120 + 100) = 625$ ml.

Over the next hour the patient will receive 625 ml of FRF. It is possible to receive a very low or a negative FRF if the ultrafiltrate production was very low or the IV rate was very high. In this event, the next hour FRF infusion can be held and the IV kept open at a rate of approximately 10 ml/hr.

Skill 20-8   **Flushing a Hemodialysis Access Device**

Frequent flushing of a hemodialysis access device helps to prevent clotting, a frequent cause of access failure. Individual devices require different volumes and concentrations of heparinized saline. Follow institutional policy and procedure. Avoid using a hemodialysis vascular access device for routine administration of fluid therapy and medications because this may result in difficulties with the access.

EQUIPMENT AND SUPPLIES

- Sterile saline
- Heparin solution
- 10 ml syringe with 22 g, 2.5-cm (1-inch) needle
- Alcohol wipe

NURSING INTERVENTIONS

1. Locate both ports of the access device.
2. Cleanse the injection port and insert needle, open clamp if present, and slowly inject prescribed amount of flush solution. If resistance is met, stop procedure and notify physician. Close clamp if present.
3. Repeat the procedure with the other limb of the access.
4. Record data including time, amount and concentration of flush solution, whether resistance was met, and condition of access device and surrounding tissue.

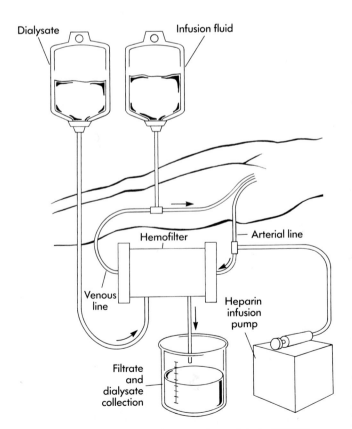

Fig. 20-7   Continuous arteriovenous hemodialysis (CAVHD).

bolus dose of 1000 to 2000 U of heparin is administered initially in the hemofilter, followed by a continuous drip administered to the arterial sleeve.[16] Because individual response to heparin is different, the rate of heparin infusion must be titrated accordingly. If clotting occurs, it can be detected quickly by frequent monitoring of the ultrafiltration rate that becomes progressively slower as clots form because clots reduce the area available for filtration in the filter. If excessive clotting occurs in the hemofilter, it should be replaced. Hemofilters have been reported to last from 12 to 144 hours.[8] If overheparinizing the patient is a potential problem, a protamine drip can be infused through the venous sleeve to reverse the effects of the heparin in the hemofilter before it reaches the patient.[11]

Continuous arteriovenous hemodialysis (CAVHD) is a process similar to CAVH, with a modification of the system to allow for the countercurrent perfusion of dialysate solution across the opposite side of the semipermeable membrane. This results in a slow exchange of electrolytes, waste products, and excess water. Because the process is slow and continuous, it is usually better tolerated in hemodynamically unstable patients[21] (Table 20-3 and Fig. 20-7).

Initiating and Monitoring CAVH

The exact procedure for set up, rinse, and priming of CAVH equipment differs slightly with the manufacturer. Refer to manufacturer's instructions before and during the set up procedure. Also, unit-based or institutional policies

---

Skill 20-9 Initiating and Monitoring Continuous Arteriovenous Hemofiltration (CAVH)

EQUIPMENT AND SUPPLIES

- Disposable CAVH system with blood tubing set
- 1000 ml NS × 2
- Solution set IV tubing
- Ultrafiltrate collection bag
- Albumin (12.5 gm)
- Heparin bolus (usually 500 U to 2000 U)
- Heparin drip with pump
- IV replacement fluid
- Sterile gloves

- Povidone-iodine swabs
- CAVH flow sheet
- Syringes (10 ml and 50 ml)
- Activated clotting time (ACT) machine and ACT tubes
- Sterile bulldog clamps
- Sterile shunt connectors
- Sterile scissors, connectors, and drapes
- Armboard

NURSING INTERVENTIONS

1. Check informed consent and physician's orders.
2. Record baseline vital signs, weight, and available hemodynamic parameters, such as mean arterial blood pressure, pulmonary artery wedge pressure, pulmonary artery diastolic pressure, and central venous pressure. This will aid in assessing fluid volume changes during the CAVH procedure. Record prefiltration lab assessments.
3. Draw up heparin and add to NS, as ordered.
4. Draw up albumin (12.5 gm) and add to first bag of NS.
5. Attach IV tubing to NS bags and prime IV line with first bag NS.[4]
6. Prepare sterile field.
7. Put on sterile gloves.
8. Assemble, inspect, rinse, and prime the system according to the manufacturer's instructions; close all clamps.
9. Attach the hemofiltrate collection bag to the hemofilter.
10. Clamp the tubing.
11. Close clamp and attach to heparin infusion line of the CAVH.
12. Determine prefiltration ACT using an ACT monitoring device. Alternately, determine the ACT manually using the procedure described in the next skill.
13. Aseptically connect the arterial and venous lines to the patient's arterial and venous accesses.
14. Open all arterial and venous blood line clamps. As arterial blood begins to enter the arterial line, administer the heparin bolus through the arterial line blood port.
15. Once blood has filled the extracorporeal circuit, measure and record vital signs, then repeat every 15 minutes for 1 hour, then every hour.
16. After 20 minutes, open the ultrafiltrate line clamp.
17. Monitor ultrafiltration rate every 30 minutes for first 2 hours, then every hour.

18. Record data on CAVH flowsheet.
19. After 30 minutes, determine the ACT.
20. Begin heparin infusion.
21. Continue to monitor the ACT every 30 minutes until stable in the desired range ordered by the physician. Notify physician for heparin infusion rate change if the ACT is out of the ordered range.
22. Keep hemofilter at heart level and drainage bag below that. Ultrafiltration may be regulated by raising and lowering the bag or by partially occluding the ultrafiltrate line with a c-clamp.
23. Replacement IV fluid may be ordered, based on the previous hourly output. Calculate the appropriate replacement rate and administer using an IV pump through the venous blood line infusion port.
24. Assess vascular access sites every 2 hours. Do not cover CAVH device with sheets or blankets.
25. If ultrafiltration rate drops suddenly, assess system patency using method described below. (Table 20-3 gives tips for troubleshooting CAVH and CAVHD.)
26. If severe hypotension develops, clamp ultrafiltrate line, leaving blood lines open. Notify physician.
27. Record the following data:
    - Vital signs.
    - Hourly intake and output.
    - Rhythm strip if irregular rhythm observed.
    - BUN, electrolytes, CBC, and clotting times.
    - Weight.
    - Site appearance.
    - Patency of hemofilter and blood lines.
    - Hematest results.
    - Amount, rate, and patency of continuous heparin infusion.

Table 20-3 Troubleshooting Tips for Continuous Arteriovenous Hemodialysis and Hemofiltration[16,21]

Problem	Potential causes	Intervention
Electrolyte imbalance	Inadequate monitoring of laboratory values Inadequate infusion of appropriate replacement therapy	Monitor serum electrolytes every 4-6 hours. Maintain careful intake and output records. Maintain prescribed infusion schedule, use infusion pump. Monitor vital signs, especially blood pressure and apical pulse at least every hour.
Dehydration or fluid overload	Inadequate infusion of replacement therapy	Maintain prescribed infusion rate. Monitor vital signs. Monitor hematocrit. Monitor skin turgor.
Exsanguination	Tubing detached from hemofilter Vascular access separation	Maintain filter in proper alignment. Secure all connections. Restrain excessive patient movement, if necessary. Avoid stress on blood lines. Call physician.
Infection/sepsis	Improper maintenance Contaminated fluid	Observe site every 4-8 hours. Monitor white blood cell (WBC) count. Monitor temperature. Use good hand washing techniques. Use sterile gloves when appropriate.
Decreased ultrafiltration rate (UFR)	Kinked tubing Hypotension Decreased cardiac output Clotting Protein coat on membrane Dehydration Placement of hemofilter above the level of the heart	Check tubing. Monitor vital signs. Monitor UFR for 1 minute every hour (normal UFR is 10-20 ml/min). Clamp arterial line and flush filter with 50 ml of heparinized saline solution (100 U/50 ml). Observe filter for clarity. Check hematocrit level every 2-4 hours. Anticipate increasing fluid replacement. Place hemofilter below level of heart.
Blood leak	Ruptured fibers	Clamp ultrafiltration line. Monitor ultrafiltrate for blood every 4 hours. Notify physician. Replace hemofilter.
Clotting of hemofilter	Obstruction Insufficient heparinization Decreased cardiac output	Monitor UFR hourly. Draw coagulation blood sample. Monitor continuous heparin infusion. Notify physician. Anticipate adjusting heparin as prescribed.

and procedures may govern the use of this device. Check with the department supervisor before beginning therapy. A physician's order stating the type of device to be used, heparinization plan, and operating parameters should be consulted before beginning.

DRUG CLEARANCE

When a patient's kidneys are not functioning properly, medication doses must be carefully monitored. The dose of medications normally excreted by the kidneys may need to be adjusted. When the patient is dialyzed, drug administration times may need to be changed to coincide with the dialysis schedule to prevent their removal. The greater the

blood's exposure to the semipermeable membrane and to fresh dialysate, the greater the amount of the drug removed. Several of the following factors determine the dialyzability of drugs:

- Surface area of the dialyzer.
- Length of each treatment.
- Blood membrane exposure.
- Thickness of the dialyzer membrane; the thinner the membrane, the faster a solute can pass through.
- Membrane pore size; the larger the pore, the more solutes that pass through.
- Rate of dialysate flow; the slower the flow, the slower the drug clearance.

Skill 20-10 Manual Determination of Activated Clotting Time (ACT)

Several automatic devices are available for determination of ACT at the bedside. If automatic equipment is not available, the test may be done manually at the bedside. The test is performed by placing a small amount of blood in a test tube containing ground diatomaceous earth. When whole blood is mixed with the particles in the tube, the clotting mechanism is activated. The tube is then agitated at regular intervals until a clot has formed, which is the activated clotting time. The normal ACT range for nonheparinized uremic patients is about 60 to 135 seconds; the usual goal of heparin therapy is to elevate the ACT to 1.5 to 2 times the baseline.[15]

EQUIPMENT AND SUPPLIES

- 3 ml syringe with needle
- Alcohol wipes
- Watch with second hand or timer
- Evacuated ACT tube

NURSING INTERVENTIONS

1. Put on gloves.
2. Draw a 2-ml specimen of whole blood from the ACT port or distal port of the venous blood line, using sterile technique.
3. Allow the specimen to flow into the ACT tube by vacuum. Note the time, then agitate the specimen by inverting it once every 10 seconds.
4. When a clot begins to form, note the number of seconds that have passed. Document the ACT on the patient's flow sheet.
5. Discard the syringe, needle, and tube in an appropriate receptical.
6. Wash hands.

Skill 20-11 Assessing the Patency of a Hemofilter

Sudden cessation of filtration may indicate that the hemofilter has clotted. To determine the condition of the hemofilter, a saline bolus test is performed.

EQUIPMENT AND SUPPLIES

- 60 ml syringe with needle
- Sterile saline for irrigation
- Alcohol wipes

NURSING INTERVENTIONS

1. Aseptically insert the needle of the filled syringe into the injection port of the arterial blood line.
2. Close the proximal arterial bloodline clamp.
3. Steadily inject the saline bolus. The fluid should pass easily through the filter; large areas of dark red discoloration in the filter or blood lines probably indicate clotting. If this is suspected, the entire system should be changed.

Skill 20-12 Discontinuing CAVH

CAVH is discontinued by clamping the arterial blood line and returning the patient's blood to the patient. Access sites must be flushed to maintain patency, discontinued, or, in the case of a shunt, reconnected.

EQUIPMENT AND SUPPLIES

- 250 ml saline for infusion
- Solution administration set
- Sterile gloves

NURSING INTERVENTIONS

1. Put on sterile gloves.
2. Prime solution administration set with saline.
3. Close clamp and connect to predilution fluid port of the arterial blood line.
4. Close arterial blood line clamp closest to the patient.
5. Open the solution administration set clamp and begin infusing saline.
6. When blood has cleared filter and venous blood line, close venous blood line clamp closest to the patient.
7. Disconnect and discard the filter system. If the patient has a shunt, reconnect it. If femoral cannulation was used, a pressure dressing is applied over the site.
8. Measure and record postfiltration vital signs, hemodynamic parameters, and weight.
9. Infuse, heparinize, discontinue, or reconnect access sites, as appropriate.
10. Assess peripheral pulses.
11. Document the following:
    - Intake and output for at least 2 hours following treatment.
    - Time of discontinuation.
    - Weight.
    - Vital signs.

Skill 20-13 Initiating and Monitoring CAVHD

EQUIPMENT AND SUPPLIES

- See equipment and supplies for Skill 20-9
- Disposable CAVHD system and tubing (Fig. 20-7)
- Dialysate solution

NURSING INTERVENTIONS

1. Follow Skill 20-9, steps 1 to 13.
2. Attach saline line to arterial end of dialyzer.
3. Connect dialysate tubing and ultrafiltrate line to appropriate parts on dialyzer.
4. Once blood flow has been established, initiate dialysate flow at the desired rate (usually 15 ml/min or 900 ml/hr).[13]
5. See Skill 20-9, steps 19 to 21.
6. Initiate fluid replacement, as ordered, (usually 5% dextrose/lactated Ringer's solution) at 50 to 100 ml/hr.
7. Measure fluid output every 30 minutes and determine replacement rate.
8. See Skill 20-9, steps 24 to 27.

- Drug bioavailability (amount of active drug absorbed into the bloodstream) is influenced by the following:

    Route of administration; IV is the most rapid, with intramuscular and oral medicine (PO) somewhat slower.

    Distribution volume; the larger the distribution area, the less the bioavailability because less remains in the bloodstream. (Fat soluble drugs are distributed through the tissues in larger volumes than water soluble drugs.)

    Distribution time; how long the drug circulates in the blood before distributed in the tissues. (Hemodialysis only filters out drugs in the blood.)

- Protein binding; drugs bound to protein cannot be significantly dialyzed out since protein molecules are too large to pass through the semipermeable membrane.

- Molecular weight; drugs with a molecular weight of less than 500 Daltons (D) usually dialyze out easily. As weight increases, dialyzability decreases. Molecules heavier than 2000 D will not be dialyzed out.

PEDIATRIC CONSIDERATIONS

The kidneys in the neonate are immature. Glomerular filtration rates (GFR) and the ability to concentrate urine, excrete acid, and reabsorb sodium, are less than in the adult. The kidneys become functionally mature when the infant is about 6 months to 1-year-old. Creatinine clearance, serum creatinine, and urinary output/kg (0.5 to 0.75 ml/kg/hr) are lower than in the adult.

Parents should provide the prenatal history and describe circumstances surrounding the labor and delivery. A growth and development history should be obtained because children with altered renal abilities often show poor growth.[7]

When examining the infant and child, the abdomen is palpated for bladder distention and kidney enlargement. The bladder in the infant can be percussed and palpated at the level of the umbilicus. The child's kidneys are generally easier to palpate than the adult's kidneys.

The physical principles for dialysis of children are the same as for adults. Dialysis is indicated for the child in ARF when other medical treatments have failed to control hypervolemia, hypertension, bleeding, acid-base balance, electrolyte imbalances, or acute poisoning.

When the decision to begin dialysis has been made, preparation of the child and parent must be prepared and informed consent must be obtained from the parents. Information is given to the child at a level the child can understand.

Peritoneal dialysis is an effective way to dialyze infants and children. This is because the relative size of the peritoneal membrane area in infants and children is two to three times larger than in adults. Peritoneal dialysis can be accomplished slowly to reduce rapid shifts in intravascular volume and electrolyte concentrations.

Procedures for catheter placement are the same as for adults. Children who are conscious may be sedated before placement. Pediatric-sized catheters should be used. These catheters have the same diameter as the adult size, but the drainage holes extend only 4.2 cm (1½ inches) from the distal end of the catheter. In the adult catheters, holes extend up to 8.4 cm (3¼ inches). Because all holes must be in the peritoneal cavity to prevent leakage, infection, and accurate inflow and outflow, it is important to use the pediatric catheters.

Initial inflow amounts should consist of 10 to 30 ml/kg of body weight of warmed 37° C (98° F) dialysate.[6] During the course of the first few runs, the dialysis fluid should be allowed to drain out within a few minutes of being introduced. This is done to check for catheter patency and bleeding. The volume is increased over subsequent runs until amounts of 25 to 100 ml/kg are reached (maximum of 2 L).

Children may experience many physical and psychological difficulties as a result of dialysis. Physical problems include decreased mobility, pain, and fatigue.[8] Psychological problems may include altered socialization, altered body image, decreased self-concept, powerlessness, helplessness, hopelessness, grief, loss, chronic sorrow, inferiority, self-rejection, and fear of technology, pain, and death.[19]

The child requiring dialysis is not the only person who experiences difficulties. The parents and other family members also experience many of the psychological problems as well as additional problems of caregiving. Many times, healthy siblings are not given as much attention and financial support because the parents are focused on the sick child.

Children and families who experience life-threatening experiences, such as renal failure, should be encouraged to discuss feelings. Teaching should be aimed at demystifying the equipment and allowing patients and families to take over a part of care.

PSYCHOSOCIAL CONSIDERATIONS

Any chronic illness or life-threatening event is stressful to both the patient and family. This is particularly true among patients who require dialysis. These patients typically experience fear of death, loss of independence, stress, anxiety, helplessness, powerlessness, anger, hostility, financial distress, altered body image, and potential change in sexual function.[19] Nurses can encourage verbalization of feelings and provide information and support for patients and their families.

PATIENT AND FAMILY TEACHING

Teaching begins with diagnosis. Basic kidney function and its role in cleaning the body of wastes needs to be stressed. Dietary restrictions of foods and fluids high in sodium, potassium, and protein require explanation, as does fluid restriction. It is also important to teach how dialysis works.

The nurse should instruct the patient and family in the

following way before and during peritoneal dialysis and hemodialysis to lessen anxiety, gain cooperation, and aid in the early detection of problems that may arise during the procedure.

- Ask patient to report feelings of nausea, cramping, weakness, diaphoresis, chest pain, shortness of breath, or pain at the access site during hemodialysis.
- After dialysis, inform patient of date and time of the next treatment.

Teaching of the patient and family is necessary for all patients receiving CAVH and CAVD. Patients and their families are most concerned about the issue of CAVH and CAVD as a life-saving device. Emotional support and encouragement will be necessary for patients and families, especially when the procedure is initiated.

HOME HEALTH CARE CONSIDERATIONS

There are three types of peritoneal dialysis for patients requiring dialysis at home. These include intermittent peritoneal dialysis (IPD), continuous ambulatory peritoneal dialysis (CAPD), and continuous cycling peritoneal dialysis (CCPD). When the patient uses IPD, approximately 40 hours a week of dialysis are required. Most patients perform this procedure at night. IPD requires an electric source for the cycler, running water, and a floor drain. The cycler has an alarm system and will alert the patient if difficulties arise. This is especially important if the patient is being dialyzed while sleeping.

With CAPD, the patient requires only dialysate and disposable tubing. The patient can be dialyzed 24 hours a day, 7 days a week. This procedure gives patients with chronic renal failure more freedom than was previously possible with the time required for hemodialysis and intermittent peritoneal dialysis.

There are several advantages of CAPD, such as the comparatively low cost when compared to that of hemodialysis; no machines, electric source, large volume of water, or floor drain are required; minimal dietary and fluid restrictions are required, and it allows better control of uremia. The main disadvantage is an increase in the potential for peritonitis.

Continuous Ambulatory Peritoneal Dialysis

Since the Food and Drug Administration approved the use of flexible plastic containers for peritoneal dialysis, CAPD has gained increasing acceptance as an alternative treatment for ESRD. CAPD consists of fewer dialysis exchanges a day with long dwell periods. Patients are taught to administer several 4- to 6-hour exchanges a day and one 8-hour exchange during sleep. To establish a permanent access, a dacron-cuffed silastic catheter is placed in the peritoneal cavity and tunneled subcutaneously to a medial-lateral exit wound. The combination of tunneling and single or double cuffs helps prevent bacterial migration along the catheter, thus decreasing the potential for peritonitis. Although the solute clearances of long dwelling exchanges are far below those obtained with more frequent ex-

changes, adequate dialysis is usually obtained because the process is continuous.

Infection is the main complication of this procedure, so patients must observe strict aseptic technique when changing bags. Manufacturers have developed several methods to prevent contamination, including antiseptic-filled connectors or ultraviolet light irradiation of the catheter junction. Other potential complications include excessive weight gain related to absorption and metabolism of dialysate glucose and chronic protein loss. Table 20-4 gives additional complications of CAPD.

CAPD is not used as a treatment for ARF because of the very low clearances of small solutes it produces. Relatively stable ESRD patients admitted to a critical care area for another reason may, however, continue to perform maintainance CAPD during their admission. Obtain a physician's order specifying the type, composition, and volume of dialysate to be used, the length of each exchange, and instructions for the type of administration system be-

Skill 20-14 Administering a CAPD Exchange
▼ ....

EQUIPMENT AND SUPPLIES

- Peritoneal dialysate, as ordered
- Povidone-iodine connection shield
- Gripper clamps
- IV pole
- Adhesive tape
- Gloves
- Disposable waterproof pad

NURSING INTERVENTIONS

1. Check physician's orders.
2. Wash hands thoroughly for 3 to 5 minutes with povidone-iodine scrub. Warm dialysate.
3. Place disposable waterproof pad on floor.
4. Place empty dialysate bag (already connected to patient) on the waterproof pad. Open tubing clamp to begin draining the exchange.
5. Check fresh dialysate bag for correct composition, clarity, leaks, and expiration date.
6. When flow into old dialysate bag stops, close tubing clamp.
7. Place both bags of dialysate on a convenient clean work area.
8. Put on gloves.
9. Place a gripper clamp on the fresh dialysate bag outlet port.
10. Remove and discard used connection shield, being careful not to touch the connection.
11. Clamp the outlet port of the old dialysate bag. Remove tubing spike from the old dialysate bag.
12. Insert tubing spike in fresh dialysate bag. Place fresh connection shield over connection. Tape connection.
13. Hang bag on pole and open clamp to infuse solution. Let dwell for prescribed time. Drain.
14. Measure outflow and inspect. If cloudy, obtain culture.
15. When dialysis procedure is complete, close clamp and roll or fold bag so that connection is protected.
16. Tape in place on patient's abdomen.

Table 20-4 Complications of CAPD

Complication	Signs and symptoms	Probable cause of complication
Peritonitis	Fever	Contamination
	Diarrhea	Break in aseptic technique
	Nausea, vomiting	Faulty equipment
	Pain	Bowel perforation
	Pus in outflow	Chemical irritation
	Blood in outflow	Exit infection
Fluid overload	Hypertension	Excessive salt/water intake
	Edema	Inadequate ultrafiltration
	Shortness of breath	Inaccurate assessment of patient's dry weight
	Increase in weight	Excessive oral intake
	Congestive heart failure	
Dehydration	Hypotension	Inadequate fluid intake
	Cramping in fingers, toes, feet	Removal of too much fluid
	Orthostatic drop in blood pressure	Inaccurate estimate of patient's dry weight
	Dizziness	Abnormal fluid intake
	Decrease in body weight	
Blood-tinged drainage	Pink fluid	Ruptured blood vessels
	Bloody fluid	Abdominal injury
		Peritonitis
Exit site inflammation	Redness	Poor skin care
	Fever	Scratching
	Purulent drainage	Irritation
	Swelling	
	Pain	
Tunnel infections	Fever	Untreated exit site infection
	Swelling	
	Discharge	
	Pain	
Protein loss	Cloudy outflow	Large amount of protein loss through the peritoneal
	Altered serum, total protein, albumin	membrane
	Weakness	
	Hypotension	
Weakness	Lethargy	Anemia
	Increased sleep	Hypotension
	Muscle weakness	Immobility
	Increased dry weight	Protein deficiency
		Fluid weight gain
Dizziness	Low blood pressure	Hypotension
	Low weight	Pulling off too much fluid
Hernia	Hernia	Increased pressure exerted by the fluid
Muscle cramps in abdomen or extremities	Cramps in hands, feet, abdomen	Improper temperature of dialysate
	Pain	Electrolyte imbalance
		Too rapid removal of fluid
		Too much fluid removal
Constipation	No bowel movement	Phosphate binders
	Poor drainage of dialysate	Intraabdominal pressure
		Immobility
		Low oral intake
Diarrhea	Hypotension	Diet
	Cramping in fingers, toes, feet	Medications
	Orthostatic drop in blood pressure	Peritonitis
	Dizziness	
	Decrease in body weight	
Nausea, vomiting	Vomiting	Inadequate dialysis
	Verbalization of feelings of nausea	Peritonitis
Lower back pain	Pain	Pressure and weight exerted by dialysate
Shoulder pain	Pain	Diaphragmatic pressure due to dialysate
		Air in peritoneal cavity
Mechanical difficulties	Pain	Kinked catheter/tubing
	Decreased outflow	Malpositioned catheter
		Fibrin clots
		Improper puncture of dialysate bag

Skill 20-15 Continuous Cycled Peritoneal Dialysis

EQUIPMENT AND SUPPLIES
- See equipment and supplies for Skill 12-14
- Cycler

NURSING INTERVENTIONS
1. Spike dialysate container with tubing.
2. Prime tubing with dialysate solution and clamp.
3. Thread tubing through cycler.
4. Connect primed tubing to peritoneal catheter using sterile technique.
5. Connect remaining tubing to weight bag near base of cycler.
6. Set time controls for infusion, dwell, and outflow.
7. Activate cycler to begin. Final infusion remains to dwell during the day.
8. Remove bag and tubing from cycler and secure to abdomen.
9. Record the following data:
   - Type and amount of dialysate infused.
   - Amount returned.
   - Vital signs.
   - Weight.

ing utilized. Patients may bring premixed solutions and equipment to the hospital with them; check with a supervisor for hospital policies and procedures related to the use of these materials.

The administration of a CAPD exchange includes the removal of dwelling peritoneal dialysate followed by the administration of fresh dialysate. Because of the risk of peritonitis, strict aseptic technique is used.

Manufacturers have developed a wide variety of peritoneal dialysis systems designed to prevent contamination during an exchange. Skill 20-14 outlines the procedure to be used with a povidone-iodine shield-type system.

CCPD combines IPD and CAPD. Solution exchanges use a cycling machine. Frequently, three exchanges are carried out during the night while the patient is sleeping, while the fourth exchange is instilled in the morning and remains in place during the day. Because this system is "opened" only twice a day, the chance of infection is reduced.

REFERENCES

1. *Amicon Diafilter-20 Hemofilter Operating Instructions,* Danvers, Mass, 1983, Amicon Corp Scientific Systems Division, Pub No 1-232.
2. Baer CL, Lancaster LE: Acute renal failure, *Crit Care Nurs Q* 14(4):1, 1992.
3. Bosworth C: SCUF/CAVH/CAVHD: Critical differences, *Crit Care Nurs Q* 14(4):45, 1992.
4. Cardonna VD, Horn PD, Mason PJB et al: *Trauma nursing,* Philadelphia, 1988, WB Saunders.
5. Dolan JT: *Critical care nursing,* Philadelphia, 1991, FA Davis.
6. Elixson, EM, Clancy GT: Neonatal peritoneal dialysis in acute renal failure, *Crit Care Nurs Q* 14(4):56, 1992.
7. Geller M: Multisystem failure in a child with HUS, *Crit Care Nurse* 10(4):56, 1990.
8. Henderson AE et al: Clinical use of the Amicon Diafilter, *Dialysis Transplant* 12(7):523, 1983.
9. Innerarity SA: Hyperkalemic emergencies, *Crit Care Nurs Q* 14(4): 32, 1992.
10. Johansen B et al: *Standards for critical care,* ed 2, St Louis, 1985, Mosby–Year Book.
11. Kaplan A, Petrillo R: Regional heparinization for continuous arteriovenous hemofiltration ASA10, *Transplant* 33:312, 1987.
12. Kiely MA: Continuous arteriovenous hemofiltration, *Crit Care Nurse* 4(4):39, 1984.
13. Lawyer LA, Velasco A: Continuous arteriovenous hemodialysis in the ICU, *Crit Care Nurse* 9(10):29, 1989.
14. Deleted in proofs.
15. Palmer L et al: Nursing management of continuous arteriovenous hemofiltration for acute renal failure, *Focus Crit Care* 13(5):32, 1988.
16. Paradiso C: Hemofiltration: an alternative to dialysis, *Heart Lung* 18(3):282, 1989.
17. Spurney RF, Fulkerson WJ, Schwab SJ: Acute renal failure in patients: prognosis for recovery of kidney function after prolonged dialysis support, *Crit Care Med* 19(1):8, 1991.
18. Stark JL: Dialysis options in the critically ill patient: hemodialysis, peritoneal dialysis, and continuous renal replacement therapy, *Crit Care Nurs Q* 14(2):40, 1992.
19. Tucker CM, Thennault SA, Ziller RC et al: Assessment of adjustment to chronic hemodialysis, *J Nephrol Nurs* 8(1):19, 1986.
20. Deleted in proofs.
21. Winkelman C: Hemofiltration: a new technique in critical care nursing, *Heart Lung* 14(3):265, 1985.
22. Wochos D: *Acute renal failure.* In Spitell J, editor: *Clinical medicine,* vol 7, Philadelphia, 1986, Harper and Row.

Organic Donation

Objectives

After completing this chapter, the reader will be able to:

- Define brain death.
- Discuss facets of brain death determination, including confirmatory studies.
- Discuss steps to obtain consent while supporting the donor family.
- Identify and discuss four areas of cerebral dysfunction that can prevent successful organ donation.
- Discuss actions and complications of aqueous Pitressin.
- List five methods of maintaining a normothermic body temperature.

Over the last 40 years the demand for organs and tissues for transplantation has increased dramatically.

Along with surgical advances, the recent development of the immunosuppressive drug cyclosporin A and better organ preservation techniques have created a growing demand for transplantable organs. In 1990 alone, 6,149 kidney, 2053 heart, 51 heart-lung blocks, 2772 liver, 946 pancreas,[19] and 35,000 corneal transplants were performed in the United States.[2]

Today almost 22,000 recipients are waiting for an organ donation to save or improve their lives.[19] Of 20,000 individuals declared brain dead each year, only 4000 become organ donors[4] largely a result of health care professionals' failure to identify potential donors. With 95% of potential organ donors dying in critical care units, the critical care nurse can play a major role in promoting organ donation. Eight out of 10 grieving families, who are asked, consent to organ or tissue donation[11]; the critical care nurse is in a position to address this issue with the family.

The enactment of required request legislation by state and federal governments directs hospitals to develop policies for informing families about the possibility of organ and tissue donation. Standardized hospital policies of routine inquiry concerning organ donation should facilitate the nurse's role in this delicate process.

The critical care nurse is the strategic link between a potential organ donor and an organ transplant recipient. Nurses in critical care units must learn the process of identifying potential donors, working with the organ procurement agency, providing support to the family, and maximizing the physiological status of the donor.

IDENTIFICATION OF POTENTIAL DONORS

Any patient who has been determined to be brain dead is a potential cadaveric organ donor. These patients may have suffered a significant neurological insult from trauma, intracranial bleeding (e.g., cerebral aneurysm), anoxia (e.g., near-drowning or overdose), or a primary brain tumor. Kidney, liver, and now lung transplants are unique because they can occur with a living related donor.

Several conditions can make a patient medically unsuitable for organ or tissue donation. Cancer, except a primary brain tumor without metastasis, rules out organ donation. Patients with any transmissible disease, such as untreated sepsis, venereal disease, hepatitis, or acquired immune deficiency syndrome (AIDS), are not suitable donors. IV drug abusers and other high-risk groups for AIDS transmission must be evaluated on a case-by-case basis. Other medical conditions, as well as age criteria for certain organs or tissues, may make a donor unsuitable, but with the present donor shortage, these criteria are changing daily. The medical team should discuss the potential donor's history with the local organ procurement agency before eliminating any patient from consideration. (Table 21-1 gives general guidelines.)

The multidisciplinary team works to the limit of its resources to save a brain-injured patient but occasionally that effort will fail. The physician must then present to the patient's family the concept of brain death and the loss of their loved one. Once a brain death evaluation has begun, the role of the critical care nurse is to contact the local organ procurement agency to involve the staff in the discussion of organ donation with the family.

Organ procurement personnel are usually responsible for obtaining consent from the next-of-kin, evaluating the donor organs for best possible use, and providing coordination of donor management and arrangements for surgical teams. Once the patient's family has consented to dona-

Table 21-1   General Criteria for Organ Donation

Organ	Contraindications	Age
General	Untreated sepsis Malignancy Communicable diseases Size	Under 70
Heart	Prior cardiac history Suboptimal function after intensive intervention	Under 70
Lungs	Positive sputum Gram stain Pulmonary edema Pulmonary contusion	Under 40
Liver	History of hepatitis B	Under 70
Pancreas	History of diabetes	Under 70
Kidneys	History of hypertension Diabetes mellitus	Under 70
Corneas	Malignancy in head and neck region	No age limit

Tissue	Untreated sepsis, human im-
	    munodeficiency virus
	    (HIV), or malignancy
	Autoimmune disease
		Under 55

tion, the organ procurement personnel are responsible for all activities involving the donor.

Throughout the process, critical care nurses remain vital members of the team, using their skills to identify potential donors and to communicate with organ procurement personnel, as well as with the families of potential donors. They must also play a key role in evaluating and managing the donor to protect the organs that will be used for transplants.

BRAIN DEATH

Medical literature has repeatedly addressed the issue of brain death because of the ethical and legal dilemmas it presents. The first hallmark statements to assist physicians in declaring a patient brain dead were the Harvard criteria published in 1968.[17] Numerous studies after the Harvard criteria have added to or amended those original judgments. The American Medical Association (AMA) and the American Bar Association jointly define *brain death* as the "irreversible cessation of all functions of the entire brain, including the brain stem." In 1981, delegates to the National Conference of Commissioners on Uniform State Laws endorsed the statement in an attempt to provide guidance to the states in developing laws that define

death.[16] The President's Commission on Ethical Problems in Medicine also published guidelines to define brain death. The key criteria were the following: (1) cerebral and brainstem functions must be absent, (2) the cause of death must be known and must exclude recovery, and (3) cessation of brain function must persist for a period of time.[18] Controversy in the medical community now focuses on the specifics of these three criteria.

In the United States, each state defines death under its own law and authorizes certain parties to determine if death has occurred, ranging from an attending physician to a specified number of neurospecialists. Each hospital can also further specify or limit the activity of its physicians. Critical care nurses must become familiar with the definition of brain death in the state in which they practice, as well as with hospital policies regarding brain death.

Determining Brain Death

The series of tests to determine brain death, usually conducted by the attending physician or neurospecialist, begins with a clinical assessment of a patient's neurological status. The physician performs two additional clinical tests—ice calorics and an apnea test. These tests evaluate lower level brain function. Hypothermia, hypoglycemia, alcohol intoxication, hypoxia, shock, drug overdose, neuromuscular blockers, central nervous system infections, and metabolic encephalopathies may suppress brain function, preventing the proper evaluation of the patient. These conditions must be assessed, treated, or eliminated before brain death can be verified.

Once the clinical examination of a patient indicates brain death, the certifying physician may request confirmatory studies. State law or hospital policy may or may not require such studies, but a physician may use them as part of personal standards of practice.

The three most common confirmatory studies are an electroencephalogram, a cerebral blood flow examination, and a cerebral angiogram. The electroencephalogram (EEG) was the initial study recommended by the Harvard criteria as helpful in confirming brain death. An isoelectric or flat EEG indicates absence of electrical activity in any of the brain cells. The appearance of false positives, however, raises questions about the accuracy of the EEG in confirming brain death.[13]

Two other studies—the cerebral angiogram and the cerebral blood flow examination—are now the preferred methods of verifying brain death. Both are used to determine if there is any perfusion of blood to the brain. When intracranial pressure (ICP) equals or surpasses mean arterial pressure (MAP), there is no perfusion of the cerebral tissue with oxygen or nutrients. Without oxygen and nutrients the brain cells die. The *cerebral blood flow examination* is a brain scan for the presence of technetium-99 that has been injected into the peripheral circulation. It is the least invasive of the two studies.

The brain may be judged functionless if nuclear imaging or cerebral angiography shows no cerebral blood flow or if the patient meets the following clinical criteria for brain death:

- Subcoma levels of narcotics, hypnotics, or alcohol.
- Definite negative history of ingestion of drugs or alcohol.
- Normothermia 35° to 38.9° C (95° to 102° F) and normotensive.
- No brainstem function as evidenced by flaccid extremities and an absence of facial grimace to pain, gag reflex, pupil reaction to light, corneal reflexes, and oculovestibular reflex.
- No evidence of motor response to deep pain in the extremities with the exception of minimal peripheral reflexes.
- Apnea in the presence of hypercarbia.

Determination of brain death for in-house and stable patients consists of two examinations based on these criteria, conducted 6 hours apart. When vital signs are rapidly deteriorating and the patient cannot be stabilized, a single determination suffices.[9]

ASSESSMENT

Nursing assessment of the potential brain-dead donor focuses first on a complete neurological assessment to evaluate brain death and then moves to those problems commonly seen in patients with fatal brain injuries (Skill 21-1).

The Oculocephalic Reflex Test (Doll's Eyes)

The oculocephalic reflex or "doll's eyes" phenomenon tests for brainstem and cranial nerve functioning. A positive or normal response indicates that the brainstem pathways are functioning and the coma is resulting from damage above the brainstem or is metabolic in nature. If the patient has a normal response, the abducens (VI), oculomotor (III), and acoustic (VIII) nerves are functioning appropriately. A negative doll's eye response or the absence of movement by both eyes, may indicate lack of brainstem functioning. This is not a definitive test, however, because a sedative drug intoxication also produces a negative doll's eyes response. Progressive loss of doll's eye response is manifested by loss of conjugate eye movement (Fig. 21-1).

The Oculovestibular Reflex (Ice Calorics)

Testing of the oculovestibular reflex determines whether the brainstem pathways to the eye muscles are intact and evaluates the integrity of the acoustic, abducens, and oculomotor nerves. The physician will check the patient's tympanic membranes before the examination, since an intact eardrum is necessary for the test (Figure 21-2).

The Apnea Test

The apnea test determines whether the patient is apneic in the presence of a high carbon dioxide blood level. In the individual with normal brainstem function, high levels of carbon dioxide induce a strong stimulus to breathe. Because inducing hypercarbia also raises ICP, this test must

be used with caution in the brain-injured patient who needs protection against herniation. It is generally used only during the brain-death evaluation. Medullary intactness can be tested by administering Atropine 1 mg IV push and observing for an increase in heart rate. Orders from a physician must be obtained for this test, and the physician will be present at the bedside.

NURSING DIAGNOSIS

The following are possible nursing diagnoses for the potential organ donor and family:

Family Diagnoses

- Compromised family coping: related to grief and loss.
- Knowledge deficit of brain death related to a lay person's medical knowledge.

Donor Diagnoses

- Decrease in cerebral tissue perfusion resulting in brain death.
- Ineffective breathing pattern related to brainstem dysfunction.
- Ventilation-perfusion imbalance related to decreased oxygen diffusion secondary to neurogenic pulmonary edema.
- Ineffective thermoregulation related to hypothalamic destruction.

PATIENT OUTCOMES

The following are sample outcomes for the potential organ donor and family:

Family Outcomes

- Family will restate the patient's condition, verbalize the word dead in referring to their loved one, and say goodbye to the patient.
- Family will articulate their decision regarding organ and tissue donation.

Donor Outcomes

- Donor will be pronounced dead based on the following:
    Local legal statutes.
    Hospital policy.
- Donor evidences the following:
    Mean BP greater than 70 mm Hg systolic.
    CVP 7 to 9 mm Hg.
    PAWP 8 to 12 mm Hg.
    Hematocrit greater than 30%.
- Donor produces the following:
    Urine output >100 ml/hr and <300 ml/hr.
    Normal serum sodium, potassium, and calcium levels.
- Donor exhibits the following:
    Pao_2 greater than 100 mm Hg.
    Clear lungs with bilateral equal breath sounds.
    Normal chest x-ray.

EQUIPMENT AND SUPPLIES

- Watch
- Stethoscope
- Sphygmomanometer
- Sterile cotton wisp
- Cotton-tipped applicator
- Flashlight or pen light
- Sterile gloves
- Scale
- Tape measure

NURSING INTERVENTIONS

1. Speak to the patient in a normal tone of voice. Explain what will be done. Use this explanation to determine if the patient will respond to voice.
2. Give simple commands, such as "Open your eyes" or "Raise your hand." If there is no response to voice, gently shake the patient to assure that the patient is not in a deep sleep or lethargic state.
3. Attempt again to determine the patient's ability to respond to commands.
4. Observe for any response, including posturing, which indicates a certain level of brain function.
5. Apply painful stimuli to determine if the patient purposely avoids that stimulus or responds in any way.
6. Observe for cough, gag, and swallow reflexes (controlled by glossopharyngeal [IX] and vagus [X] nerves), when suctioning patient.
7. Open one of patient's eyes in a darkened room, introduce a pinpoint of light, and observe pupillary response. Note pupil size, equality, reaction to light, consensual reaction, and eye movement.
8. Repeat examination on other eye.
9. Using a gloved hand, prepare a sterile, cotton-tipped applicator so that a wisp of cotton protrudes.
10. Open the patient's eyes and move the cotton-tipped applicator in a rapid, forceful stroke toward the eyes without touching them. Observe for blinking.
11. Touch the eye with the cotton-tipped applicator to determine if the patient will blink (corneal reflex controlled by the trigeminal [V] nerve).
12. Test the oculocephalic reflex or doll's eyes response. (See Skill 21-2.)
13. Test the plantar response. Using a sharp object, stroke the bottom of the foot on the lateral aspect of the sole, from the heel toward the toes, curving toward the ball of the big toe. Use as light a stimulus as possible to obtain a response.
14. Observe for dorsiflexion of the great toe with fanning of the other toes (Babinski response), indicating upper motor neuron damage.[6]
15. Weigh the donor and measure height, abdominal girth, and chest circumference.
16. Assess for hypotension resulting from the loss of vasomotor tone, diabetes insipidus, and possible posttraumatic bleeding sites.
17. Measure the heart rate, central venous pressure (CVP), blood pressure, pulmonary artery wedge pressure (PAWP), and cardiac output (CO).
18. Assess the peripheral circulation by evaluating strength of pulses, capillary refill, and skin temperature.
19. Assess all wounds for the need for pressure dressings.
20. Assess the need for increased fluid rates or inotropic drugs.
21. Monitor hemoglobin and hematocrit levels.
22. Assess the serum potassium levels repeatedly, potassium may be lost from diuresis.

23. Evaluate serum sodium and blood urea nitrogen (BUN) levels for elevation, which occur in diabetes insipidus.
24. Assess urine output for a rate less than 50 ml/hr to evaluate the need for increased fluid intake. Dehydration may have occurred from fluid restriction, osmotic diuretics, hyperglycemia, or diabetes insipidus.
25. Assess for polyuria of greater than 300 ml/hr for more than 2 hours without the prior administration of a diuretic.
26. Measure urine specific gravity. Patients with diabetes insipidus will develop a low urine specific gravity of less than 1.005.
27. Assess urine osmolarity in the polyuric patient. If urine osmolarity is less than 150 mOsm, it may be a result of diabetes insipidus. If greater than 300 mOsm, it is evidence of osmotic diuresis.
28. Monitor simultaneous urine and serum sodium levels. Decreasing urine osmolarity and sodium concentration and increasing serum osmolarity and sodium concentration indicate diabetes insipidus.
29. Calculate the osmolality of the plasma using the following formula:

$$\text{Osmolality} = 2\,\text{Na} + \frac{\text{BUN}}{2.6} + \frac{\text{Glucose}}{18}$$

Normal serum osmolality averages 290 +/− 5 mOsm/kg.[8] The above formula can predict plasma osmolality within 10 mOsm of the measured value.

30. Assess the serum osmolality of a patient who has had alcohol ingestion and mannitol administration by using the following modified formula:

$$\text{Osmolality} = 2\,\text{Na} + \frac{\text{BUN}}{2.6} + \frac{\text{Glucose}}{18} + \frac{\text{ETOH}}{4.2} + \frac{\text{Mannitol}}{18}$$

31. Auscultate breath sounds and evaluate chest x-ray for evidence of pulmonary atelectasis or infections.
32. Assess for accumulation of pulmonary secretions resulting from a loss of cough reflex, such as scattered rhonchi, wheezing, decreased or absent breath sounds in certain areas, and the sounding of the increased airway pressure alarm on the ventilator.
33. Assess for signs of neurogenic pulmonary edema evidenced by bibasilar crackles in the lungs, positive chest x-ray, PAWP greater than 25 mm Hg, poor gas exchange with a Pa_{O_2} less than 60 mm Hg, a large pulmonary shunt (Pa_{O_2}/Fi_{O_2} ratio of 200 or less), and an arterial P_{CO_2} of 45 mm Hg or greater.
34. Measure the patient's rectal temperature to ensure normothermia (between 36° to 38.6° C [97° to 101.5° F]). Hypothermia or hyperthermia may be the result of a loss of hypothalamic temperature control.
35. Assess the condition of the patient's eyes and the need for a moistening solution. Dryness may be a result of the loss of the blink reflex.
36. Check the condition of the skin and the need for cleansing or turning to prevent tissue breakdown.
37. Record data.

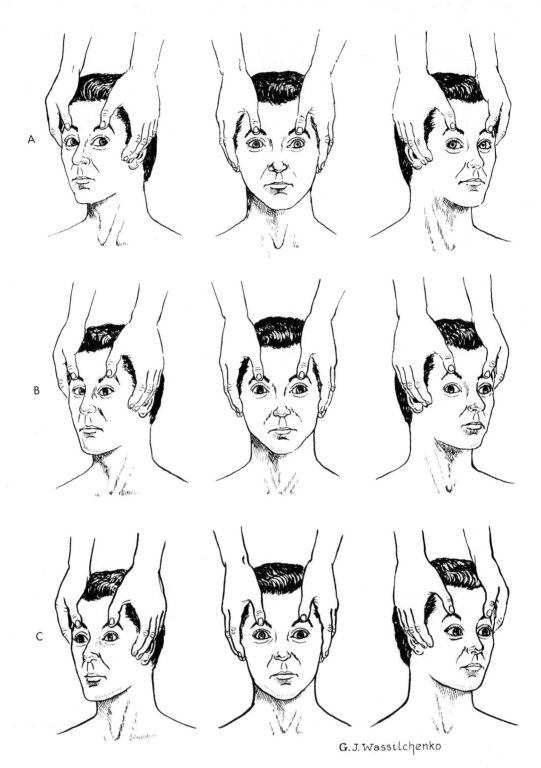

G. J. Wassilchenko

FIG. 21-1   Oculocephalic reflex (doll's eyes). **A,** Normal. **B,** Abnormal. **C,** Absent.   (From Thelan LA, Davie JK, Urden LD: *Textbook of critical care nursing: diagnosis and management,* St Louis, 1990, Mosby–Year Book.)

Skill 21-2 Oculocephalic Reflex Test[6]

NURSING INTERVENTIONS

1. Assure free movement of the head by removing any sand-bags or pillows, if the patient does not have a cervical spine injury.
2. Ensure adequate length of ventilator tubing so as not to pull or jar the endotracheal (ET) tube when the head is turned.
3. Open both eyes and hold the upper eyelids so that eye movement can be observed.
4. Turn the head briskly to one side.
5. Observe the position of the eyes. If the eyes remain fixed and move with the head, like a doll whose eyes are painted on, the nerve function is absent. If the eyes move toward a central point, like a doll whose eyes can move freely, the nerve function is present. This sideways, or parallel, movement of the eyes is called a conjugate gaze.
6. Test each side.
7. Flex the neck forward and observe.
8. Extend the head backward and observe.
9. The response should be recorded as one of the following:
   • Normal (positive) conjugate eye deviation.
   • Abnormal asymmetrical or dysconjugate eye movements.
   • Absent (negative)—no movement of either eye.

Skill 21-3 Assistance with Testing the Oculovestibular Reflex

EQUIPMENT AND SUPPLIES

• Curved basin
• Iced saline or water
• Butterfly IV catheter with needle removed
• Syringe
• Absorbent pad

NURSING INTERVENTIONS

1. Prepare patient with absorbent pad under head and shoulders.
2. Collect equipment, adding ice to saline or water only after physician arrives to ensure fluid remains cold.
3. Elevate head to 30 degrees. Attach the tubing to syringe and draw up iced saline or water.
4. Hold upper eyelids open to observe the patient's eyes.
5. Observe 3 to 5 minutes as iced fluid is injected into the ear canal. A normal response results in horizontal nystagmus (reflex sideways eye movements) with slow movement toward the irrigated ear and rapid movement away.
6. Repeat in opposite ear.
7. Allow fluid to drain from ear canal into curved basin. Remove absorbent pad and dry patient.[6]
8. Document response as follows:
   • Normal response—conjugate eye movements.
   • Abnormal response—dysconjugate or asymmetric eye movements.
   • Absent response—no eye movements.

A   B   C

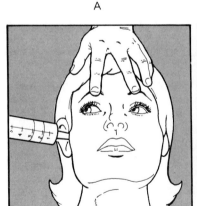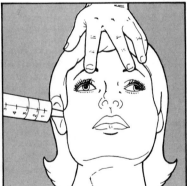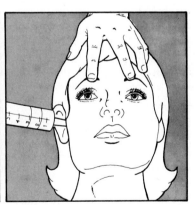

FIG. 21-2 Oculovestibular reflex (cold caloric test). **A,** Normal. **B,** Abnormal. **C,** Absent. (From Thelan LA, Davie JK, Urden LD: *Textbook of critical care nursing: diagnosis and management,* St Louis, 1990, Mosby–Year Book.)

- Donor rectal temperature remains between 36° to 38.6° C (97° and 101.5° F) rectally.
- Donor displays suitable corneal tissue for donation as assessed by eye bank technician.

FAMILY CONSENT FOR ORGAN DONATION

With the profound need for organ donors, every family of a brain dead patient should be offered the opportunity to consider donation. The Omnibus Budget Reconciliation Act of 1986 directed each hospital to develop policies to allow families this choice. This same law designated an Organ Procurement Agency (OPA) for each geographical area in the United States. It is the role of the critical care nurse to contact the staff of the local OPA as soon as evaluation of brain death begins. It is usually an OPA staff member who obtains consent for organ donation, but the critical care nurse plays an important part in the process by communicating with the OPA, sharing information about the family, and helping the OPA staff answer the family's questions. The most common concerns of families center on cost, disfigurement of the body, funeral plans, and confidentiality. Members of the family should be presented with factual information even if they cannot focus their own questions.

Consent for organ donation must be obtained from the legal next of kin. Those family members, by priority, for giving consent are spouse, adult children, parents, adult siblings, guardian, and nonrelatives providing for burial. Consent must also be accompanied by permission from the medical examiner (ME) to remove any vital organs or tissues if the patient falls into the category of an ME's case. Trauma, homicide, suicide, death before spending 24 hours in the hospital, and any unforeseen circumstances during hospitalization may require the ME's involvement. The ME needs to use accident reports or chart review to explore the circumstances of the death before allowing organ recovery surgery to alter any evidence. Once the appropriate information is collected, the donor usually is released for surgery.

The key to obtaining consent for organ donation is preparation of the family. To protect families from emotional stress, the nurse might be tempted to avoid the issue of organ donation. Personal accounts from donor families, however, indicate that it is the news of the patient's death rather than a discussion about organ donation that is stressful. When donor families were surveyed, it was found that 85% viewed organ donation as a positive aspect in their time of loss and grief.[5] They saw the benefits of donation as helping someone in need, saving a life, doing what the donor would have wanted, and knowing that their loved one lives on in another.

Nurses, who are in constant attendance of the patient, are integral in assessing the family's readiness for a conversation about organ donation. The nurse has the opportunity to discuss the following:

- The family's definition of death.
- The family's religious beliefs.
- The meaning of the illness or accident to the family.
- How the potential donor's death will affect family functioning.
- The legal next-of-kin, as well as family leaders.
- Meaningful support systems.[12]

The timing of a discussion on organ donation is critical to the family's emotional health and the success of the request. The family must first understand brain death. Any early discussion of organ donation risks alienating the family, which may feel hospital personnel are trying to "kill" their loved one for their organs. Brain death must be understood and accepted before moving on.

Nurses need to assess whether the physician's and their own message about brain death is really being heard. The nurse can do so by requesting family members to restate what was discussed and by observing for signs of acceptance. If the family is able to begin making funeral plans, say goodbye, or tell others the potential donor is dead, they are ready to discuss organ donation. Each family is unique, and a nurse needs a high level of interpersonal skills to work through this experience with them.

Donation also helps the medical personnel involved and is a benefit frequently overlooked. The nursing and physician staff who have cared for a fatally brain-injured patient experience pain and feelings of loss and failure when their efforts are unsuccessful. If their patient becomes an organ donor, they may feel their efforts were not in vain. Although they were unable to save this patient, they may assist a family to find comfort in donation and save the lives of a number of organ recipients.

The experiences of organ procurement personnel suggest the responses to organ donation will vary with cultural differences. Black and Oriental families may consent less frequently because of religious and ethnic beliefs or mistrust of the medical system. Assurances from an authoritative figure may help persuade them that donation truly benefits recipients but also that it remains their personal choice. Some Hispanic families may suspect their religious beliefs prevent donation, but in fact all of the major religions—including Jehovah's Witnesses, Islam, and Orthodox Judaism—allow organ donation.[3] Families should be encouraged to consult their religious advisers if they have questions.

EVALUATION OF DONOR

Once the next-of-kin has given legal informed consent, the nurse must turn from supporting a grieving family to preparing a cadaveric organ donor for surgery. The goal of the nurse's care is to assist the OPA staff in evaluating the organs to determine their best possible use and to manage the donor's physiological condition to promote the best organs for transplantation.

Donor evaluation requires prompt reporting of the results of a series of commonly used tests. The OPA staff depends on the critical care nurse to complete this evaluation. The information collected about the donor is communicated to the transplant surgeon for a final decision and ac-

Skill 21-4   Obtaining Legal Informed Consent

EQUIPMENT AND SUPPLIES

- Tissues
- Quiet, private conference area
- Consent forms
- Refreshments

NURSING INTERVENTIONS

1. Identify the legal next of kin for potential donor and ensure they are present to discuss organ donation and consent.
2. Provide tissues, liquid refreshments, privacy for the discussion, and other comfort and compassion measures.
3. Introduce the organ procurement staff.
4. Observe the interaction between the OPA staff and the family to act as a family advocate. Note when breaks or pauses are needed. Ask questions for the family if they cannot articulate their concerns.
5. Ensure that all organs and tissues they are willing to donate are identified on the consent form.
6. Ensure that the donation procedure is fully explained, including the need for further blood tests, obtaining tissue for human leukocyte antigen (HLA) typing, and so on.
7. Witness consent for donation.
8. Observe or witness consent for autopsy, if required by OPA.
9. Observe or witness consent for blood tests, specifically AIDS or hepatitis testing, if required by the hospital.
10. Ensure that members of the family are making their own choices or decisions and there are no significant family conflicts regarding this decision.
11. Ensure consent is obtained from the ME. (This is usually done by the OPA staff.)
12. Document the discussion.

ceptance of the organ for a specific recipient. The OPA staff uses a national computer network (United Network of Organ Sharing [UNOS]) to identify all possible recipients. To connect to the UNOS network, the OPA must know the patient's size, height, current weight, and ABO blood group. Tests for human immunodeficiency virus (HIV), hepatitis, cytomegalovirus (CMV), and syphilis, as well as blood cultures, are also common to all donors.

Other tests for the suitability for transplantation vary with each organ system. The cardiac evaluation determines if the myocardium is healthy and able to contract effectively. Blood pressure, heart rate, and the need for inotropic support can assist the transplant surgeon in assessing the heart's viability. Evaluation of the hemodynamic state determines whether inotropic support is being used to supplant fluid resuscitation in a dehydrated donor or is required to support the heart's function. The OPA staff may request placement of a pulmonary artery catheter to obtain cardiac output measurements, as well as an echocardiogram to visualize the functioning of the ventricles and rule out valvular dysfunction. An electrocardiogram (ECG), and creatine phosphokinase (CPK), creatine phosphokinase-myosin bands (CPK-MB), and lactic dehydrogenase (LDH) levels are necessary to evaluate prior cardiac dam-

age. A cardiology consult may also be a part of this evaluation process.

Pulmonary evaluation focuses on the present condition of a donor's lungs. Arterial blood gases (ABGs) are evaluated along with current pulmonary cultures. A clear chest x-ray is an absolute necessity and is also used to measure lung dimensions. Measurements from the apex to diaphragm at the midclavicular line, from the front of the spine to the sternum, a chest circumference at the axillary level, and a sternal length are also required to determine if the lungs are an appropriate size for the potential recipient. An oxygen challenge may be used to evaluate the pulmonary status. This is accomplished by placing the donor on 100% oxygen and then drawing ABGs to assess if the donor can achieve a Pao_2 of 350 mm Hg.

The hepatic evaluation consists of blood studies to determine liver function. These studies include serum glutamate oxaloacetate transaminase (AST), serum glutamate pyruvate transaminase (ALT), alkaline phosphatase, prothrombin time (PT), partial thromboplastin time (PTT), albumin, lactic dehydrogenase (LDH), and total and direct bilirubin. An abdominal circumference at the umbilicus assists in size evaluation.

The evaluation of the pancreas is based on studies of blood amylase and glucose. A careful review of bedside urine testing for glucose also assists the OPA staff and transplant surgeon in determining pancreatic function, as does information on whether the administration of insulin was required as part of the donor's treatment.[18] If the pancreas is accepted, the gut will be sterilized to allow portions of the duodenum to be removed with the pancreas.

Renal evaluation is based primarily on urinalysis, urine cultures, urine output, and blood chemistries. An appropriate fluid and electrolyte balance is required to evaluate renal function, in particular urine output. Shock states (from the cause of brain death, dehydration treatment, or herniation) can reduce renal blood flow and cause or mimic damage to the renal parenchyma. Fluid challenges, along with serial BUN and creatinine, can verify renal status.

To place the kidneys with the best possible recipient, the OPA staff must know the kidneys' full HLA type. HLA typing identifies the six major genes located on the sixth chromosome that produce antigens. These antigens identify each individual as unique. To conduct this test, a large number of white blood cells is required. They can be obtained from a blood sample, a lymph node, or separated from a portion of the spleen. The lymph node is the preferred source. The lymphocytes are mixed with an antisera and complement, incubated, and then tested with a dye to determine membrane damage. Completing HLA typing takes 6 to 8 hours and initiating this test before the nephrectomy speeds placement of the kidneys. A lymph node for tissue typing can be removed (lymphanectomy) while the donor is still in the critical care unit. Once the six antigens are identified, the OPA staff contacts UNOS either by computer or by phone to enter the antigens into the UNOS computer. Renal transplant recipients both locally and nationally are identified based on the best possible HLA match along with other medical criteria.

Donor Management Problems

The goal of donor management is to obtain the best possible physiological state in the donor before organ recovery surgery. This includes appropriate fluid and electrolyte status, adequate ABGs, a stable hemodynamic state with minimal inotropic support, and well-perfused, optimally functioning organs. Achieving that goal requires significant intervention because the brain dead donor has lost the control center for many of those functions.

The brain's control over the body ends when the brain dies and loses its protective and homeostatic mechanisms. The respiratory center, for example, no longer transmits the message to breathe. Neither lack of oxygenation nor hypercapnia create any stimulating effect. Therefore the donor must receive pulmonary support in the form of controlled ventilation to provide an oxygen supply to the viable organs. Loss of the protective cough and gag reflexes also affects the respiratory system, making it imperative that an artificial airway be maintained to ensure ventilatory support.

The brain also provides input to the body to maintain vascular tone. A brain dead donor no longer has that input, and the vascular bed tends to totally relax, causing pooling in the extremities and lungs. The result is hypotension, decreased preload, and extravasation of fluid into the airways (neurogenic pulmonary edema), which must be reversed through the use of inotropic agents. Dopamine is the agent of choice because it dilates the renal arteries at low doses. When dopamine or dobutamine are no longer effective for maintaining blood pressure, epinephrine or norepinephrine (Levophed) may be administered but such a choice requires serious consideration by the physician. Both are potent drugs with extreme vasoconstrictive effects that can damage the donor's kidneys, heart, and liver. Nonetheless, they may be necessary for short periods to vasoconstrict the blood supply to the abdominal organs and periphery and to stabilize the hemodynamic status. Conservative transplant surgeons will not accept an organ from a donor who has had epinephrine or norepinephrine drips or high doses of dopamine. More aggressive transplant surgeons will consider the organ based on its present function.

Brain death also means destruction of the hypothalamus, which has several significant effects on the donor's stability. First, body temperature may fluctuate greatly from hypothermia to hyperthermia because the hypothalamus is no longer playing its role as temperature control center of the body. To prevent damage to viable organs, normothermia must be achieved. Second, loss of the output of antidiuretic hormone (ADH) results in diabetes insipidus. Diabetes insipidus can cause an overwhelming loss of intravascular fluid through the urinary system, resulting in cardiovascular collapse if not controlled.

Diabetes insipidus follows destruction of the supraoptic nuclei of the hypothalamus or its nerve tract to the posterior pituitary. The neurons of the supraoptic nuclei are osmoreceptors that produce or withhold ADH in response to the concentration of the blood that supplies the hypothalamus. The nuclei also respond to stimuli from the atrial baroreceptors (indicating poor stretch, low preload, or hypovolemia) to cause a marked vasoconstriction of the arterioles. As a result, ADH is also known as vasopressin. ADH can also cause contraction of the smooth muscle of the intestines, bile ducts, and uterus.[14]

The major sign of diabetes insipidus is a copius amount of dilute urine, which can range from 2 to 16 L/24 hr. The lack of ADH prevents the reabsorption of free water from the renal collecting tubules. Water, low in osmolarity and sodium, is excreted in the urine. If not replaced, the loss of water decreases intravascular volume and hemoconcentration, producing significant hypernatremia. To compensate for intravascular hypovolemia, the pituitary secretes aldosterone in an effort to retain more sodium and water. This response is usually ineffective, however, and only increases hypernatremia.[14]

Compensating for the brain's lack of control clearly is a major part of donor management, but reversing the medical treatment used to preserve the brain may also be critical. The physician's attempt to save the brain may have included fluid restriction and the use of osmotic diuretics to prevent edema. Both could create relative dehydration in the donor that must be treated.

Aqueous Pitressin infusion

The treatment of diabetes insipidus consists of replacing urinary losses and supplementing ADH. ADH, also known as vasopressin or Pitressin, can be administered by intramuscular or subcutaneous injection or through an IV drip. The IV drip is the recommended procedure. Absorption occurs more quickly than with intramuscular and subcutaneous injection and negative effects can be more easily controlled because the whole dose is not given at once. Pitressin can produce anuria or significant hypertension. Should either occur, the drip can be titrated to a lower dose or discontinued. If anuria or hypertension are not reversed by discontinuing the Pitressin, treatment with diuretics or vasodilators may be necessary. Liver transplant surgeons prefer that vasopressin not be used, if it can be avoided, because it constricts the bile ducts.

Maintenance of normothermia with a hyperthermia/hypothermia blanket

The loss of body temperature control that accompanies damage to the hypothalamus can produce hyperthermia or hypothermia at extreme ranges. For example, the temperature can fluctuate up to 41.6° C (107° F) or down to 33.8° C (93° F). Both may occur, but hypothermia is more common. The greatest danger of hypothermia is decreased cardiac function, which may eventually result in fibrillation and loss of the donor.

Numerous nursing interventions can help maintain normothermia. Use of a hyperthermia/hypothermia blanket is

Skill 21-5 Maintenance of the Organ Donor

EQUIPMENT AND SUPPLIES

- Lactated Ringer's solution
- D_5 ½ NS solution
- Colloid volume expanders
- IV pressure bag
- ICU equipment

NURSING INTERVENTIONS

Cardiovascular support

1. Control bleeding sources.
2. Evaluate ability of present peripheral and central line to carry several liters of fluid simultaneously.
3. Add IV lines, if needed.
4. Assist in placement of central venous line or pulmonary artery catheter if required, especially in heart or lung donor.
5. Obtain 5 to 10 bags of lactated Ringer's solution, D_5 ½ NS, and colloid volume expanders.
6. Prepare to hang fluids and run at rapid infusion rates (i.e., 1000 to 2000 ml in an hour); regulate as ordered.
7. Add IV pressure bag, if needed, to ensure infusion.
8. Monitor hemodynamic status—heart rate, blood pressure, CVP, and PAWP every 15 minutes.
9. Maintain adequate hemodynamic status of heart rate between 60 to 100/min, CVP 10 to 12 cm H_2O, PAWP 7 to 9 mm Hg, and cardiac output 4 to 8 L/min.
10. Administer volume therapy to keep CVP greater than 10 cm H_2O.
11. Administer inotropic agents as ordered, such as dopamine and dobutamine, for hypotension uncontrolled by fluid resuscitation.
12. Maintain inotropic support, as ordered, to keep mean blood pressure >70 mm Hg.
13. Wean within parameters as fluid resuscitation continues.
14. Attempt to wean vasoconstricting agents (epinephrine and norepinephrine) first to improve perfusion to all organs. Maintain dopamine as last agent to be removed.
15. Type and crossmatch for 6 units of packed red blood cells to be available for surgery.
16. Give 2 units packed red blood cells for hematocrit less than 30%.

Fluid and electrolyte support

1. Keep accurate intake and output and report to OPA staff every half hour.
2. Obtain blood chemistries as ordered.
3. Regulate fluid intake to maintain urinary output within 100 to 300 ml/hr range. Discuss all changes with OPA staff.
4. Replace urine output ml for ml with D_5 ½ NS with potassium.
5. Start Pitressin drip if urine output is greater than 300 ml/hr (see Skill 21-6).
6. Give diuretics, as ordered, if unable to maintain adequate urinary output.
7. Be prepared to change fluid types, as ordered, based on blood chemistries.
8. Give 10 mEq KCL in 50 ml D_5W over 1 hour for serum potassium less than 3.8 mEq/L.

Respiratory support

1. Adjust ventilator settings to maintain Pao_2 of greater than 100 mm Hg and pH within normal limits (7.35 to 7.45).
2. Place patient on 5 cm PEEP to improve level of oxygenation.
3. Obtain ABGs every 4 hours and after each ventilator change.
4. Ausculate breath sounds bilaterally at least every 4 hours.
5. Suction every 2 hours and as needed to maintain a clear airway.
6. Provide chest physiotherapy to maintain normal, clear breath sounds.
7. Assess chest wall excursion at least every 8 hours.
8. Obtain a current chest x-ray (within 4 hours of brain death declaration).

General support

1. Give antibiotics, such as cephazolin sodium (Ancef) 1 gm every 8 hours IV and chloramphenicol (Chloromycetin) 1 gm every 8 hours IV, as ordered to prevent sepsis.
2. Use strict sterile technique for all procedures.
3. Measure temperature every hour.
4. Give Tylenol suppository 650 mg every 2 hours, as needed, for rectal temperature greater than 38.3° C (101° F).
5. Use warming blankets to maintain rectal temperature greater than 36° C (97° F). (see Skill 21-7).
6. Keep nasogastric (NG) tube to low suction. Irrigate to keep patent.
7. Provide eye care (see Skill 21-8).

Skill 21-6   Administration of Aqueous Pitressin Infusion

EQUIPMENT AND SUPPLIES

- Aqueous Pitressin
- Normal saline IV fluid
- Nitroprusside sodium (Nipride)
- D_5W IV fluid
- IV tubing
- IV infusion devices

NURSING INTERVENTIONS

1. Mix drip of 25 units of Pitressin in 250 ml of normal saline or as specifically ordered by the physician in charge of the case.
2. Start drip of 0.15 to 0.30 units per hour (15 to 30 ml/hr) and adjust to produce a urinary output of 100 to 300 ml/hr.
3. Observe for response by measuring the urine output every 30 min.
4. Increase dose by doubling until the desired result is achieved—urine output greater than 100 ml/hr and less than 300 ml/hr.
5. Monitor blood pressure and observe for hypertension.
6. Be prepared to wean off inotropic agents as Pitressin takes effect.
7. Mix nitroprusside drip per unit protocol or 50 mg in 250 ml D_5W to have available if extreme hypertension occurs.
8. Infuse nitroprusside to maintain blood pressure less than 170 systolic, if necessary.
9. Continue to replace urinary losses.

one. Others include providing a heavier blanket, warming linens and blankets in blanket warmer; warming fluids in fluid/blood warmer before infusing; using heat lamps or warming lights; using an overbed warmer; applying hot water bottles to the groin, axilla, trunk and extremities; and increasing the temperature on the ventilator humidifier.

Eye care

The corneas are the most commonly donated tissue. To assure quality tissue for transplantation the corneas need to receive specific care to preserve their viability. Corneas must be procured within 6 to 12 hours from the cessation of cardiac function. Eye care should be provided before death and at the time of postmortem care.

Preparation of the Donor for Organ Recovery Surgery

Transporting a critically ill donor to the surgical suite is a challenge of organization and preparation. The travel time between the critical care unit and the surgical suite are vital for maintaining the donor in a stable cardiovascular and respiratory condition. Problems during transport can lead to cardiopulmonary failure and loss of perfused organs to potential recipients. Because of the timing of organ recovery surgery, the recipient may already be in another surgical suite under anesthesia; therefore loss of the donor at this point would also risk the life of the recipient.

Skill 21-7   Maintaining Normothermia with a Hyperthermia/hypothermia Blanket

EQUIPMENT AND SUPPLIES

- Hyperthermia/hypothermia blanket control unit
- Disposable hyperthermia/hypothermia blanket
- Connecting hose
- Sheet
- Temperature probe
- Distilled water

NURSING INTERVENTIONS

1. Check the level of distilled water in the reservoir by lifting the cover off the water fill opening. The water should be touching the strainer and be visible. Add distilled water if necessary.
2. Place the hyperthermia/hypothermia blanket covered by a single sheet under the patient with the hose routed toward the control unit.
3. Connect the blanket to the control unit where the male/female couplings protrude.
4. Make certain that the blanket is flat and the hose is not twisted or kinked.
5. Place the temperature probe by either inserting into the rectum, taping to the chest (skin probe), or inserting into the esophagus (esophageal probe).
6. Allow probe to equilibrate to patient's temperature for 1 minute.
7. Insert probe into probe jack on the right side of the unit.
8. Determine if automatic or manual control is desired. Automatic control adjusts the blanket temperature to patient's temperature and is the safer method. Manual control heats or cools to a preset temperature, despite how it

affects the patient, and is best used to preheat or cool before placing the blanket under the patient.
9. Push the power on switch.
10. In automatic mode, press the red temperature set switch, then press the up or down arrows to change the setpoint display to the desired patient temperature. Next press the autocontrol switch.
11. Check the water flow indicator to confirm water is circulating and touch the blanket to confirm it is heating or cooling.
12. In manual mode, press the red temperature set switch, then press the up or down arrow to change the setpoint display to the desired temperature. Next press the manual control switch.
13. Repeat step 11.
14. Continue to monitor the patient's temperature. Monitor every 15 minutes until desired temperature is achieved. If in manual mode, continue to monitor every 30 minutes; if in automatic mode, continue to monitor every hour.
15. Periodically check the placement of the temperature probe.
16. Check skin areas frequently for signs of excessive heat.
17. To discontinue use of the blanket do the following:[9]
    - Turn the power off.
    - Allow the blanket and hose to drain water for about 10 minutes.
    - Remove probe.
    - Unplug.
    - Disconnect the hose from the unit.
    - Clean according to hospital protocol.

Skill 21-8   Providing Eye Care

EQUIPMENT AND SUPPLIES

- Tearisol
- Normal saline eye drops
- Eye pads
- Normal saline pour bottle

NURSING INTERVENTIONS

1. Elevate the head of the bed 30 degrees to prevent dependent edema of eye tissues.
2. Apply wetting agent, such as Tearisol, to eyes every hour or as needed to prevent drying.
3. Wet eye pads with normal saline and place gently on eyelids to maintain moisture and close lid.
4. Avoid greasy eye care agents, such as Lacrilube, as they make the cornea difficult to handle by the eye bank technician.

Skill 21-9   Preparation of Donor for Transport to Surgical Suite

EQUIPMENT AND SUPPLIES

- Oxygen tank
- Bag-valve-mask device
- Portable IV poles
- Portable monitor
- Methylprednisolone (Solu-Medrol)

NURSING INTERVENTIONS

1. Ensure that blood for a type and crossmatch has been drawn and that 6 units of packed red blood cells are available for surgery.
2. Obtain final set of blood chemistries and hemoglobin and hematocrit at a time when results will be available before leaving for surgery.
3. Start methylprednisolone (Solu-Medrol) 1 to 2 gm IV, at surgery. Medical studies suggest steroids stabilize cell walls and prevent any damage that may occur during the operative phase.[15]
4. Provide portable monitor and convert donor to this system.
5. Add IV poles to bed or organize portable poles at head and foot to allow ease of movement without strain on any IV lines.
6. Secure urinary drainage bag so it will not be pulled.
7. Place oxygen tank on bed, assuring a secure location.
8. Attach bag-valve-mask device and tubing to tank. Be sure to add PEEP valve to the bag, if the patient is ventilated with PEEP. Turn on oxygen when removing patient from the ventilator.
9. Give report to anesthesia personnel and surgical nurse. Include average vital signs, current chemistries, site and rate and concentration of inotropic drugs or Pitressin.

Organ and tissue recovery surgery

Most critical care nurses and donor families are unaware of the surgical procedures the donor will undergo while in surgery. This knowledge is important to nurses, not only because it helps them answer the family's questions, but more importantly because it shows them the extent of the gifts a brain-dead patient can give through donation of organs and tissues.

The organ procurement staff plays a key role in assuring that the necessary personnel are prepared and available for the surgical procedure. They arrange for the transplant teams to arrive at a designated surgery time and act as host to out-of-town surgical teams. During the organ recovery surgery, they work with the circulating nurse and anesthesiologist to ensure that all activities in surgery occur in a smooth, well-timed manner. The OPA staff will hang the cold preservation fluids, as well as provide a record of the care of the donor in surgery for each transplanting team.

With a multiorgan donor, the surgical suite needs to accommodate three to four teams: the heart, the lung, the liver and pancreas, and kidney teams. The teams may include local and out-of-town surgeons, although the kidney team is usually from the host hospital or a nearby transplant center.

After the surgery is complete, the organ procurement staff will place the kidneys and pancreas, based on local guidelines. The OPA staff are also responsible for assuring the smooth procurement of tissues by tissue bank personnel. This includes notifying the procurement personnel and arranging surgical time.

PEDIATRIC CONSIDERATIONS

The most important difference between the pediatric and adult donor populations is the more conservative approach to brain death determination in children. Physicians exercise particular caution when making the diagnosis of brain death in a child younger than 5 years old. Because young children have a great ability to recover from serious brain insults, physicians use more confirmatory tests and wait longer periods of time to allow for recovery. How much the child varies from an adult in this area is still a subject of controversy in medical literature.

The Children's Hospital of Boston's Ad Hoc Committee on Brain Death has published recommendations that brain death must include absent cerebral function based on clinical examination, as well as irreversibility. Determination of irreversibility requires identifying the cause of coma, ruling out reasons that mimic irreversible ones, and observing the patient for a period that may vary from 6 to 24 hours, depending on the cause of coma.[1]

Pediatric donor management also requires special considerations, particularly a recognition of the physiological differences between a child and an adult. The most obvious differences lie in hemodynamic normals and treatment of hypovolemia. The IV solution of choice, D_5 ¼ NS with potassium, should be used in place of lactated Ringer's solution at a rate that is consistent with the donor's size. Using the formula of 10 ml/kg to bolus the donor for fluid losses and blood replacement with packed cells prevents unnecessary fluid overload. Drug dosages must be altered for patient size as well. Appropriate urine output for a child should be based on 1 ml/kg/hr with treatment focused on appropriate output.

A child's age and size affect decisions about which tissues are appropriate for donation. Corneal or eye donation may occur at any age, but skin donation is only possible for a child weighing more than 45 kg (100 lbs). The need for fully calcified bone means that bone donation is possible only with donors over 16 years old (for women) or 21 years old (for men).

PATIENT AND FAMILY TEACHING

A key role of the critical care nurse in promoting organ donation is teaching the family of the brain-injured patient about brain death. This occurs while the patient remains in the critical care unit and becomes more focused as the medical team begins the series of tests required to declare brain death. Reinforcing explanations, the physician has already provided is the most effective approach for the nurse. Using the same words and phrases helps prevent the family from being confused by different definitions. The nurse should provide more details and be prepared to answer questions about irreversibility, the role of the ventilator, and the family's future choices. The nurse should emphasize the difference between deep coma and death and explain that the ventilator can provide oxygen but cannot keep the patient "alive." Frequent use of the phrase "legally dead" or the word "dead" instead of "brain dead" or "clinically dead" may be helpful. Discussion of death often produces a crisis response and requires repetition of the information about brain death as often as the family needs it.

After the family members understand brain death, they will need a thorough explanation of organ donation to make an informed decision about this option. Families commonly have concerns about cost, disfigurement of the body, funeral plans, and confidentiality. Teaching about organ and tissue donation should include the point that there is no cost to the donor family. The family will also need a general description of the surgical procedures involved in organ donation. The nurse should avoid using terms that connote damage to the donor's body, such as disfiguring or mutilating. Instead, provide the facts in a neutral manner, using phrases like "a central incision is made and closed again in the surgical suite as a surgical procedure." The nurse should stress that there is no pain as the patient can no longer feel pain.

Specifics in several other areas can also help to give the family an accurate picture of tissue donation. The nurse should explain that in the case of skin donation the skin is removed from the back, buttocks, and the back of the thighs at a thickness equivalent only to the skin lost from a sunburn. For bone donation, the bone is removed through surgical incisions, and prosthetics maintain the normal shape of the body. All of the incisions are covered by clothing, which is particularly important to a family that plans an open-casket viewing. Donation usually occurs between 12 and 24 hours from the time of consent and should not affect funeral plans. Donation is anonymous and confidential. There is no contact between the donor and recipient families, although the OPA provides general information in a letter of appreciation.

ETHICAL AND PSYCHOSOCIAL CONSIDERATIONS

The ethical issues surrounding organ donation are numerous and complex, raising many questions. The first and most difficult focuses on the question of life itself. What is life? What is death? In the past, lay persons equated breathing and a beating heart with life. Medical advances now allow both to continue artificially. Philosophers, in an attempt to find a better definition, focused on what makes us uniquely human. Many would say it is our ability to interact and communicate with each other. Because these are functions of the mind or brain, brain death has also been defined in terms of the total loss of function of the brain. This definition of brain death has been accepted in the medical community and allows medical teams to conduct organ recovery surgery because the surgeon is not hurting a living patient. Although these initial arguments have been resolved in the medical community, the question of the definition of life arises in each of us as we struggle with how we personally define life.

Particularly complex is the dilemma faced by parents of the infant who is born without a cerebrum (anencephalic). These infants may breathe for a while but do not live more than a few days. Clearly the tests and criteria for arriving at a determination of brain death cannot be met in this instance. Allowed to follow its natural course, anencephaly will result in the loss of potential donor organs. If taken early, the organs will save the life of another child. But is the inability to think and communicate really synonymous with death? Is the knowledge that the infant will die sufficient basis for a judgment about organ donation? Finally, is it of value to offer meaning to the life and death of one child by saving the life of another? These questions confront the family who must form a decision about organ donation, as well as the nursing staff that assists them.[10]

Nurses must also address the emotional well-being of the family. Many feel that to tell a family a loved one is brain dead and then to ask about organ donation is cruel and callous, but the record shows numerous accounts by family members who wish they had donated but were not asked. If the option of organ donation is not raised, how can the family make an informed decision? By not asking, the medical community is making this decision for them. Current legislation that requires that a family be asked about organ donation resolves part of this problem but still leaves the medical team with the questions of method, timing, and sensitivity to the family's emotional state.

It also leaves unanswered an even deeper question related to dying with respect and dignity. Is organ transplantation appropriate under any circumstances? Is it right to use a dead person's body as the "junk yard" to obtain "spare parts" for another? Or is an organ donated for transplant in fact a gift of life rather than a spare part?

Even if we accept organ donation, questions about how the system operates remain. Should a recipient be allowed to receive more than one organ transplant while others may die waiting? Many surgeons accept a less than optimal organ as a bridge to wait for a better functioning organ in the future. Should organs from high-risk patients be used as that bridge to save another's life? Should the recipient be told about the associated risk? Should those who have had a bridging transplant be precluded from a second transplant when that original organ fails? Should recipients be excluded based on prior alcohol or substance abuse? Concern has been expressed that this is partially a moral judgment about who deserves to live, not about who will achieve the best transplant outcome.

Finally, should we be expending our national medical resources on organ transplantation? Would the money be better spent on maternal child health care needs? Those who support transplantation point out that new areas of medical technology improve with experience and that with improvement the cost declines.

Clearly, there are no easy answers, but one of the greatest benefits of organ donation and transplantation may be the pressure created to explore these questions and to examine our beliefs and values.

REFERENCES

1. Ad Hoc Committee on Brain Death, Children's Hospital Boston: Determination of brain death, *J Pediatr,* 110(1):15, 1987.
2. American Council on Transplantation: *U.S. transplant stat sheet,* 1990, The Council.
3. American Council on Transplantation: *Religious views on organ donation and transplantation,* 1988, The Council.
4. Bart KJ et al: Increasing the supply of cadaveric kidneys for transplantation, *Transplantation,* 31:383, 1981.
5. Bartucci MR: Organ donation: a study of the donor family perspective, *J Neurosci Nurs* 19(12):305, 1987.
6. Bates B: *A guide to physical examination and history taking,* Philadelphia, 1987, JB Lippincott.
7. Burrell LO, Burrell ZL: *Critical care,* St Louis, 1982, Mosby–Year Book.
8. Cincinnati Sub-Zero Products: *Blanketrol II hyper-hypothermia operation and technical manual,* 1982.
9. Dunham CM, Cowley RA: *Shock trauma/critical care handbook,* Rockville, Md, 1986, Aspen.
10. Erlen JA, Holzman IR: Anencephalic infants: should they be organ donors? *Pediatr Nurs* 14(1):60, 1988.
11. Gallup Poll: *U.S. attitudes towards organ transplantation/organ donation,* 1985.
12. Gideon MD, Taylor PB: Kidney donation: care of the cadaver donor's family, *J Neurosurg Nurs* 13:248, 1981.
13. Grigg MM et al: Electroencephalographic activity after brain death, *Arch Neurol* 44(9):948, 1987.
14. Guyton AC: *Textbook of medical physiology,* Philadelphia, 1990, WB Saunders.
15. Hamilton HK, editor: *Nursing 1988 drug handbook,* Springhouse, Pa, 1988, Springhouse.
16. President's Commission for the Study of Ethical Problems in Medicine and Biomedical Research: *Defining death: medical, legal, and ethical issues in the determination of death,* Washington, DC, 1983, US Government Printing Office.
17. Report of the Ad Hoc Committee of the Harvard Medical School: A definition of irreversible coma, *JAMA* 205:337, 1968.
18. Shoemaker WC et al: *Textbook of critical care,* Philadelphia, 1989, WB Saunders.
19. United Network of Organ Sharing: Annual report of the US scientific registry for organ transplantation and organ procurement network, *US Department of Organ Transplantation* ES16, 1990.

Ventricular Fibrillation and Pulseless Ventricular Tachycardia

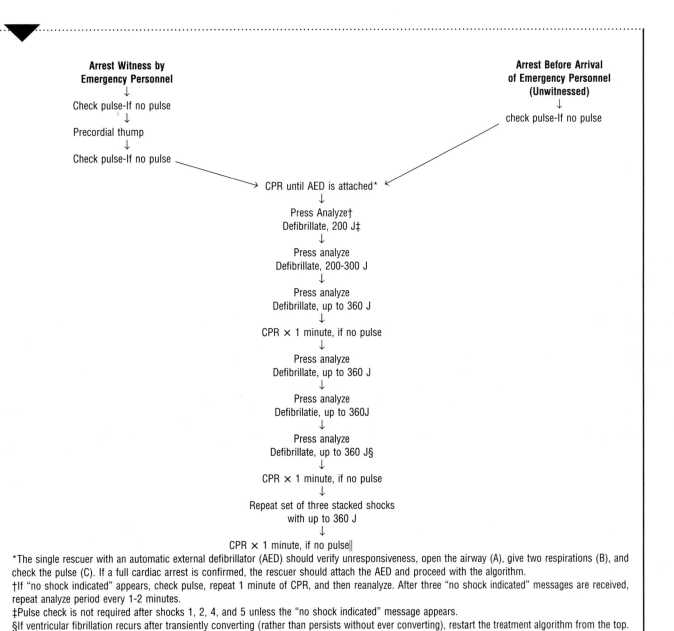

Arrest Witness by Emergency Personnel
↓
Check pulse-If no pulse
↓
Precordial thump
↓
Check pulse-If no pulse

Arrest Before Arrival of Emergency Personnel (Unwitnessed)
↓
check pulse-If no pulse

CPR until AED is attached*
↓
Press Analyze†
Defibrillate, 200 J‡
↓
Press analyze
Defibrillate, 200-300 J
↓
Press analyze
Defibrillate, up to 360 J
↓
CPR × 1 minute, if no pulse
↓
Press analyze
Defibrillate, up to 360 J
↓
Press analyze
Defibrilatie, up to 360J
↓
Press analyze
Defibrillate, up to 360 J§
↓
CPR × 1 minute, if no pulse
↓
Repeat set of three stacked shocks
with up to 360 J
↓
CPR × 1 minute, if no pulse‖

*The single rescuer with an automatic external defibrillator (AED) should verify unresponsiveness, open the airway (A), give two respirations (B), and check the pulse (C). If a full cardiac arrest is confirmed, the rescuer should attach the AED and proceed with the algorithm.

†If "no shock indicated" appears, check pulse, repeat 1 minute of CPR, and then reanalyze. After three "no shock indicated" messages are received, repeat analyze period every 1-2 minutes.

‡Pulse check is not required after shocks 1, 2, 4, and 5 unless the "no shock indicated" message appears.

§If ventricular fibrillation recurs after transiently converting (rather than persists without ever converting), restart the treatment algorithm from the top.

‖In the unlikely event that ventricular fibrillation persists after nine shocks, then repeat sets of three stacked shocks, with 1 minute of CPR between each set.

From *Textbook of Advanced Cardiac Life Support,* 1987, 1990. Copyright American Heart Association; published in Cʀɪᴛɪᴄᴀʟ Cᴀʀᴇ Nᴜʀsᴇ/June 1992

Cardiovascular Effects of Adrenergic and Dopaminergic Receptor Activation

Receptor	Location	Heart	Systemic arteries	Pulmonary arteries	Veins
Alpha	Blood vessels of skin, mucosa, skeletal muscle, and mesenteric and splanchnic beds	0	Constriction +++	Constriction +	Constriction +++
Beta 1	Sinoatrial and atrioventricular nodes	Rate ++ Automaticity +++	0	Constriction	0
	Ventricular muscle	Contractility +++			
Beta 2	Bronchial smooth muscle, blood vessels of skeletal muscle, and uterus	0	Dilation ++	Dilation +	Dilation ++
Dopaminergic	Renal, mesenteric, and splanchnic arteriolar beds	0	Dilation	0	0

0, no effect; +, increase.

Drugs Commonly Administered by Continuous IV Infusion in the ICU

Drug	Dilution (final concentration)	Indications	Actions
Aminocaproic acid (Amicar)	Initial infusion: 4-5 gm/250 ml D$_5$W over first hr Maintenance infusion: 15 gm/250 ml D$_5$W (60 mg/ml)	Hemorrhage from overactivity of the fibrinolytic system; urinary fibrinolysis resulting from trauma, shock, and surgery or cancer of genitourinary system; systemic hyperfibrinolysis from heart surgery, abruptio placentae, hepatic cirrhosis, and cancer.	Inhibits plasminogen activator substances; inhibits plasmin activity; increases fibrinogen activity in clot formation by inhibiting the enzyme required for destruction of formed fibrin.
Amrinone lactate (Inocor)	500 mg/100 ml 0.9% NaCl (2.5 mg/ml)	Short-term management of congestive heart failure in patients who have not satisfactorily responded to diuretics, digitalis, or vasodilators.	Direct relaxant effect on vascular smooth muscle causing decreased preload (venous capacitance) and afterload (arteriolar resistance); cardiac inotropic agent that increases cardiac output.
Bretylium tosylate (Bretylol)	1 gm/250 ml D$_5$W (4 mg/ml)	Treatment and prophylaxis of ventricular tachycardia and ventricular fibrillation unresponsive to lidocaine or class IA drugs.	Causes initial release of norepinephrine, followed by impaired release of norepinephrine, thereby decreasing excitability; raises ventricular fibrillation threshold by increasing action potential duration and effective refractory period; and increases cardiac contractility and occasionally heart rate.
Dobutamine hydrochloride (Dobutrex)	500 mg/250 ml D$_5$W (2000 μg/ml)	Short-term inotropic management of heart failure resulting from depressed contractility from organic heart disease or cardiac surgical procedures.	Stimulates beta 1 receptors of the heart, with inotropic effect and relatively minor effect on heart rate; minimal vasoconstrictor (alpha 1) and vasodilator (beta 2) effects; causes increased cardiac output without significant increase in heart rate.
Dopamine hydrochloride (Intropin)	800 mg/500 ml D$_5$W (1600 μg/ml)	Used to increase blood pressure, cardiac output, renal blood flow, and urine output when treating shock caused by acute myocardial infarction, trauma, septicemia, renal failure, open heart surgery, and chronic cardiac decompensation.	At small doses of 0.5-2 μg/kg/min stimulates dopaminergic receptors, producing renal vasodilation; at larger doses of 2-10 μg/kg/min stimulates dopaminergic and beta 1 adrenergic receptors, producing cardiac stimulation and renal vasodilation; at large doses greater than 10 μg/kg/min stimulates alpha-adrenergic receptors and may cause renal vasoconstriction.
Epinephrine hydrochloride 1:1000 (Adrenalin Chloride)	1 mg/250 ml D$_5$W (4 μg/ml), or 8 mg/250 ml D$_5$W (32 μg/ml)	Cardiac resuscitation, complete heart block, Stokes-Adams syndrome, carotid sinus hypersensitivity, anaphylactic shock, and refractory asthma attacks; used to increase blood pressure (mainly systolic), heart rate, cardiac contractility, and coronary blood flow.	Potent sympathomimetic; acts directly on alpha receptors causing vasoconstriction and on beta 1 receptors causing inotropic/chrontropic effects; acts on beta 2 receptors causing relaxation of bronchial smooth muscle; constricts bronchial arterioles and

Continued.

Drug	Dilution (final concentration)	Indications	Actions
Epinephrine hydrochloride 1:1000 (Adrenalin Chloride)—cont'd			inhibits histamine release, thus reducing congestion and edema; increases blood sugar and free fatty acids.
Esmolol hydrochloride (Brevibloc)	5 gm/500 ml D$_5$W (10 mg/ml)	Control of rapid ventricular response in atrial fibrillation and flutter; used for clinically important non-compensatory sinus tachycardia.	Cardioselective (beta 1) adrenergic blocker with antidysrhythmic effects; results in decreased heart rate, contractility, blood pressure, and atrioventricular conduction; causes slowing of the ventricular response in supraventricular tachydysrhythmias.
Heparin sodium	20,000 units/500 ml D$_5$W (40 units/ml)	Anticoagulant therapy for treatment and prophylaxis of thromboembolic disorders including venous thrombosis, peripheral arterial emboli, pulmonary emboli, atrial fibrillation with embolization, stroke-in-evolution, acute coronary thrombosis, unstable angina, prophylaxis during vascular and cardiac procedures, and disseminated intravascular coagulation.	Anticoagulant that inhibits the conversion of prothrombin to thrombin and fibrinogen to fibrin; reduces adhesiveness of platelets; does not dissolve well-established clots but prevents thrombus formation and extension of existing thrombi.
Isoproterenol hydrochloride (Isuprel)	1 mg/250 ml D$_5$W (4 μg/ml)	Treatment of bronchospasm, atrioventricular heart block, cardiac standstill, carotid sinus hypersensitivity, bradydysrhythmias, and shock associated with decreased cardiac output.	Sympathomimetic agent that stimulates both beta 1 receptors (myocardial) and beta 2 receptors (pulmonary); causes increased cardiac output, heart rate, systolic blood pressure, and myocardial oxygen requirements; shortens AV conduction time and refractory period in AV block; smooth muscle and peripheral vasodilator with predominant effects on GI tract, bronchial tree, and uterus.
Lidocaine hydrochloride (Xylocaine)	1 gm/250 ml D$_5$W (4 mg/ml)	Treatment and prophylaxis of ventricular dysrhythmias such as premature ventricular contractions or ventricular tachycardia.	Slows the entry of sodium through the fast channels, decreases excitability, and lengthens the effective refractory period; by slowing the rate of depolarization, it decreases excessive automaticity of ectopic pacemakers.
Magnesium sulfate	4 gm/250 ml D$_5$W (16 mg/ml)	As an anticonvulsant in convulsive states caused by severe eclampsia, pre-eclampsia, glomerulonephritis, and hypoparathyroidism; also used for severe hypomagnesemia, cerebral edema, alcohol withdrawal, and uterine tetany.	A central nervous system depressant and a depressant of smooth, skeletal, and cardiac muscle; has a mild diuretic and vasodilating effect.
Morphine sulfate	100 mg/200 ml D$_5$W (0.5 mg/ml)	Relief of severe pain such as due to cancer, myocardial infarction, renal or biliary colic, and traumatic injury; used to relieve dyspnea of pulmonary edema.	Opium-derivative narcotic analgesic that induces sleep and inhibits perception of pain by binding to opiate receptors in the central nervous system, decreasing sodium permeability, and inhibiting transmission of pain impulses; depresses respiratory center and cough reflex.
Nitroglycerine (Nitrostat)	50 mg/500 ml D$_5$W (100 μg/ml) or 100 mg/500 ml D$_5$W (200 μg/ml) or 200 mg/500 ml D$_5$W (400 μg/ml)	Treatment of acute congestive heart failure (CHF); used to control ischemic pain, limit infarct size, and treat CHF in presence of acute myocardial infarction; pro-	Vascular smooth muscle relaxant and vasodilator primarily on venous vessels with some reduction in arteriolar resistance; reduces preload and afterload, thereby

Drug	Dilution (final concentration)	Indications	Actions
Nitroglycerine (Nitrostat) —cont'd		phylaxis and management of vasospastic angina pectoris; controlled reduction of blood pressure during and after cardiovascular surgery.	improving cardiac output; dilates coronary arteries, with increase in coronary blood flow and improvement of collateral flow to ischemic regions; relieves and can prevent anginal attacks; reduces pulmonary resistance and systemic pressure while preserving coronary perfusion pressure.
Norepinephrine Bitartrate (Levophed)	8 mg/500 D_5W (16 μg/ml)	Short-term management of hypotensive states occuring during situations that include hemorrhage, trauma, surgery, septicemia, drug reactions, and blood reactions.	Potent sympathomimetic drug that stimulates alpha adrenergic receptors to produce venous and arterial vasoconstriction; provides positive beta 1 receptor (inotrophic/chronotropic) stimulation of the heart but has fewer beta effects than epinephrine and isoproterenol; increases blood pressure, pulmonary artery pressure, coronary blood flow, and cardiac output; may reduce skeletal muscle, skin, renal, and splanchnic blood flow; inhibits insulin release and enhances glycogenolysis.
Oxytocin (Pitocin, Syntocinon)	10 units/1000 ml solution (10 milliunits/ml)	Used to induce or stimulate labor, control postpartum bleeding, and treat incomplete or inevitable abortion.	Synthetic posterior pituitary derivative that stimulates uterine and mammary gland smooth muscle, producing rhythmic contractions of uterus; has weak antidiuretic and vasopressor effects.
Pentobarbital sodium (Nembutal Sodium)	2 gm/500 ml 0.9% NaCl (4 mg/ml)	In critical care units, used for induction of coma in selected patients who have cerebral ischemia and increased intracranial pressure.	Sedative, hypnotic barbiturate of short duration with anticonvulsant effects; CNS depressant; depresses motor and sensory cortex and alters cerebellar function; may decrease cerebral blood flow, intracranial pressure, and cerebral edema.
Phenylephrine hydrochloride (Neo-Synephrine)	30 mg/500 ml D_5W (60 μg/ml)	Used to increase blood pressure in the treatment of shock or drug-induced hypotension; used to control paroxysmal atrial tachycardia.	Potent alpha adrenergic agonist that produces predominantly arterial and only slight venous vasoconstriction; increases systemic and pulmonary artery pressure and coronary blood flow.
Potassium chloride	To prevent irritation to veins: 40 mEq or less/1000 ml solution For severe potassium depletion: Up to 80 mEq/1000 ml solution	Prevention or treatment of potassium depletion; treatment of some dysrhythmias due to cardiac glycoside toxicity.	Maintains isotonicity, acid-base balance, and electrophysiological characteristics of the cell; activator in many enzymatic reactions and essential to many processes.
Procainamide hydrochloride (Pronestyl)	1 gm/250 ml D_5W (4 mg/ml)	Treatment and prophylaxis of ventricular and atrial dysrhythmias, including premature ventricular contractions, ventricular tachycardia, premature atrial contractions, and paroxysmal atrial tachycardia; used to maintain normal sinus rhythm after conversion from atrial fibrillation or flutter.	Antidysrythmic that depresses myocardial excitability and slows electrical conduction in atrium, His-Purkinje system, and ventricles.
Sodium nitroprusside (Nipride)	100 mg/250 ml D_5W (400 μg/ml)	Management of hypertensive crises; treatment of cardiogenic shock or cardiac pump failure through reduction of preload and afterload.	Potent, rapid-acting antihypertensive agent producing peripheral vasodilation of both venous (capitance) and arterial (resistance) vessels; reduces preload and afterload.

Continued.

Drug	Dilution (final concentration)	Indications	Actions
Streptokinase (Streptase)	750,000 IU/250 ml D₅W (3,000 IU/ml)	Coronary thrombosis associated with acute transmural myocardial infarction; recent acute massive pulmonary emboli; recent severe or massive deep vein thrombosis; acute arterial thrombi and emboli not originating from a left heart focus; clearance of occluded arteriovenous cannulae when obstructed by clotted blood or fibrin.	Thrombolytic agent that combines with plasminogen and converts it to plasmin, which degrades fibrin clots, fibrinogen, and other plasma proteins; causes lysis of thrombi or emboli; may alter platelet function, decrease blood viscosity, and improve collateral blood flow.
Theophylline ethylenediamine (Aminophylline)	500 mg/500 ml D₅W (1 mg/ml)	Bronchodilator in reversible bronchospasm of bronchial asthma, bronchitis, or emphysema.	Inhibits phosphodiesterase, which increases cyclic AMP and fosters release of endogenous epinephrine; relaxes smooth muscle and bronchial tubes, affecting pulmonary and peripheral vasculature; cardiac output, urinary output, and sodium excretion are increased; produces CNS/respiratory stimulation; impedes uterine contractions; induces gastric acid secretion; may inhibit histamine.
Tissue plasminogen activator, TPA (alteplase [Activase])	20 mg/20 ml sterile water for injection without preservatives, or 50 mg/50 ml sterile water for injection without preservatives. Can be further diluted with equal amounts of 0.9% NaCl or D₅W to concentration of 0.5 mg/ml	Management of acute myocardial infarction (within 4-6 hours from onset of chest pain) for the lysis of thrombi obstructing coronary arteries; management of acute massive pulmonary embolism for the lysis of acute pulmonary emboli.	Produces clot lysis by binding to fibrin in a thrombus and converts plasminogen to plasmin; result is local fibrinolysis with limited systemic proteolysis.
Trimethaphan camsylate (Arfonad)	1500 mg/500 ml D₅W (3 mg/ml)	Short-term lowering of blood pressure during hypertensive crises, surgery, pulmonary edema secondary to hypertension, cardiogenic shock, and dissecting aortic aneurysm.	Ganglionic blocking agent and potent vasodilator that blocks transmission at sympathetic and parasympathetic ganglia by cholinergic receptor competition; decreases blood pressure.
Urokinase (Abbokinase)	500,000 units/125 ml 0.9% NaCl (4000 units/ml)	Lysis of acute, massive pulmonary emboli if two or more lobar arteries are involved or if hemodynamics are unstable; lysis of coronary artery thrombi; lysis of obstructed IV catheters occluded only by clotted blood or fibrin.	Enzyme that converts plasminogen to plasmin, which degrades fibrin clots, fibrinogen, and other plasma proteins; acts both within and upon the surface of thrombi and emboli; produces anticoagulant effect.
Vasopressin (Pitressin)	200 units/250 ml D₅W (0.8 units/ml)	Treatment of neurogenic diabetes insipidus due to deficient antidiuretic hormone; management of abdominal distention; management of upper GI variceal bleeding.	Synthetic vasopressin from the posterior pituitary that possesses antidiuretic action by altering the permeability of the renal collecting ducts, allowing reabsorption of water; increases GI peristalsis; vasoconstrictor, especially upon GI tract and peripheral venous and arterial vessels; reduces portal venous pressure and may reduce coronary blood flow.

Calculation of Intravenous Infusion Rates

Example:

Mr. Hart weighs 100 kg (220 lbs). He is presently in septic shock and you have started a dopamine drip to maintain his blood pressure. The pharmacy sent you an IV bag containing dopamine 400 mg/500 ml D$_5$W. You are using an intravenous infusion pump to administer the medication and have found that you can maintain his pressure if he receives 30 ml/hour. What is your reply when the physician asks you how many μg/kg/min the patient is receiving?

Hint: 1 mg = 1000 μg

Answer:

Draw a grid, as shown, and record the given values. Since the answer is expressed in μg/min, you would want to ensure that microgram values are on top of the equation, and minutes are on the bottom. In order to convert the milligrams to micrograms and hour to minutes, you will also have to insert these equivalencies into your equation.

$$\frac{400 \text{ mg}}{500 \text{ ml}} \quad \frac{30 \text{ ml}}{1 \text{ hr}} \quad \frac{1000 \,\mu\text{g}}{1 \text{ mg}} \quad \frac{1 \text{ hr}}{60 \text{ min}} = \frac{? \,\mu\text{g}}{\text{min}}$$

After setting up the equation, go through and cancel units that are the same and divide the smaller numerical values into the larger ones until you have an answer that can be expressed in micrograms per minute.

$$\frac{400 \text{ m\hspace{-0.6em}/\hspace{0.2em}g}}{500 \text{ m\hspace{-0.6em}/\hspace{0.2em}l}} \quad \frac{30 \text{ m\hspace{-0.6em}/\hspace{0.2em}l}}{1 \text{ h\hspace{-0.6em}/\hspace{0.2em}r}} \quad \frac{\overset{2}{1000} \,\mu\text{g}}{1 \text{ m\hspace{-0.6em}/\hspace{0.2em}g}} \quad \frac{1 \text{ h\hspace{-0.6em}/\hspace{0.2em}r}}{\underset{2}{60} \text{ min}} = \frac{400 \,\mu\text{g}}{1 \text{ min}}$$

Mr. Hart is receiving 400 μg of dopamine per minute, but this answer is more informative if you know the patient's weight. Therefore, you would standardize the dosage to find out how much dopamine he is receiving per each kilogram of body weight. You divide by 100 kg and get 4 μg/kg/min. This is abbreviated in the patient's chart by stating that the patient is on a 4 μg/min dopamine infusion.

Critical Care Drug Drip Charts

Amrinone Lactate (Inocor)

500 mg (100 ml) / 100 ml N/S = Total 200 ml
Concentration: 2.5 mg/ml

Patient's Weight	lbs / kg	88 / 40	99 / 45	110 / 50	121 / 55	132 / 60	143 / 65	154 / 70	165 / 75	176 / 80	187 / 85	198 / 90	209 / 95	220 / 100
Drug dose in μg/kg/min														
Infusion rate in ml/hr	5	5.2	4.6	4.2	3.8	3.5	3.2	3.0	2.8	2.6	2.4	2.3	2.2	2.1
	6	6.2	5.6	5.0	4.5	4.2	3.8	3.6	3.3	3.1	2.9	2.8	2.6	2.5
	7	7.3	6.5	5.8	5.3	4.9	4.5	4.2	3.9	3.6	3.4	3.2	3.1	2.9
	8	8.3	7.4	6.7	6.1	5.6	5.1	4.8	4.4	4.2	3.9	3.7	3.5	3.3
	9	9.4	8.3	7.5	6.8	6.2	5.8	5.4	5.0	4.7	4.4	4.2	3.9	3.8
	10	10.4	9.3	8.3	7.6	6.9	6.4	6.0	5.6	5.2	4.9	4.6	4.4	4.2
	15	15.6	13.9	12.5	11.4	10.4	9.6	8.9	8.3	7.8	7.4	6.9	6.6	6.2
	20	20.8	18.5	16.7	15.2	13.9	12.8	11.9	11.1	10.4	9.8	9.3	8.8	8.3
	25	26.0	23.1	20.8	18.9	17.4	16.0	14.9	13.9	13.0	12.2	11.6	11.0	10.4
	30	31.2	27.8	25.0	22.7	20.8	19.2	17.9	16.7	15.6	14.7	13.9	13.2	12.5

Dobutamine Hydrochloride (Dobutrex)

500 mg in 250 ml D_5W = 2000 μg/ml

Patient's weight	lbs / kg	77 / 35	88 / 40	99 / 45	110 / 50	121 / 55	132 / 60	143 / 65	154 / 70	165 / 75	176 / 80	187 / 85	198 / 90	209 / 95	220 / 100
Drug dose in μg/kg/min															
Infusion rate in ml/hr	5	4.8	4.2	3.7	3.3	3.0	2.8	2.6	2.4	2.2	2.1	2.0	1.9	1.8	1.7
	10	9.5	8.3	7.4	6.7	6.1	5.6	5.1	4.8	4.4	4.2	3.9	3.7	3.5	3.3
	15	14.3	12.5	11.1	10.0	9.1	8.3	7.7	7.1	6.7	6.3	5.9	5.6	5.3	5.0
	20	19.0	16.7	14.8	13.3	12.1	11.1	10.3	9.5	8.9	8.3	7.8	7.4	7.0	6.7
	25	23.8	20.8	18.5	16.7	15.2	13.9	12.8	11.9	11.1	10.4	9.8	9.3	8.8	8.3
	30	28.6	25.0	22.2	20.0	18.2	16.7	15.4	14.3	13.3	12.5	11.8	11.1	10.5	10.0
	35	33.3	29.2	25.9	23.3	21.2	19.4	17.9	16.7	15.6	14.6	13.7	13.0	12.3	11.7
	40	38.1	33.3	29.6	26.7	24.2	22.2	20.5	19.0	17.8	16.7	15.7	14.8	14.0	13.3
	45	42.9	37.5	33.3	30.0	27.3	25.0	23.1	21.4	20.0	18.8	17.6	16.7	15.8	15.0
	50	47.6	41.7	37.0	33.3	30.3	27.8	25.6	23.8	22.2	20.8	19.6	18.5	17.5	16.7
	55	52.4	45.8	40.7	36.7	33.3	30.6	28.2	26.2	24.4	22.9	21.6	20.4	19.3	18.3
	60	57.1	50.0	44.4	40.0	36.4	33.3	30.8	28.6	26.7	25.0	23.5	22.2	21.1	20.0
	65	61.9	54.2	48.1	43.3	39.4	36.1	33.3	31.0	28.9	27.1	25.5	24.1	22.8	21.7
	70	66.7	58.3	51.9	46.7	42.4	38.9	35.9	33.3	31.1	29.2	27.5	25.9	24.6	23.3
	75	71.4	62.5	55.6	50.0	45.5	41.7	38.5	35.7	33.3	31.3	29.4	27.8	26.3	25.0
	80	76.2	66.7	59.3	53.3	48.5	44.4	41.0	38.1	35.6	33.3	31.4	29.6	28.1	26.7
	85	81.0	70.8	63.0	56.7	51.5	47.2	43.6	40.5	37.8	35.4	33.3	31.5	29.8	28.3
	90	85.7	75.0	66.7	60.0	54.5	50.0	46.2	42.9	40.0	37.5	35.3	33.3	31.6	30.0
	95	90.0	79.2	70.4	63.3	57.6	52.8	48.7	45.2	42.2	39.6	37.3	35.2	33.3	31.7
	100	95.2	83.3	74.1	66.7	60.6	55.6	51.3	47.6	44.4	41.7	39.2	37.0	35.1	33.3

Dopamine Hydrochloride (Intropin)

800 mg in 500 ml D$_5$W = 1600 µg/ml

Patient's weight	lbs	77	88	99	110	121	132	143	154	165	176	187	198	209	220	231	242
	kg	35	40	45	50	55	60	65	70	75	80	85	90	95	100	105	110

Drug Dose in µg/kg/min

Infusion rate in ml/hr																	
5	3.8	3.4	2.9	2.6	2.4	2.2	2.0	1.9	1.8	1.6	1.55	1.5	1.4	1.3	1.25	1.2
10	7.6	6.7	5.9	5.3	4.9	4.5	4.1	3.8	3.6	3.3	3.1	3.0	2.8	2.7	2.5	2.4
15	11	10	8.9	8.0	7.3	6.6	6.1	5.7	5.3	5.0	4.7	4.4	4.2	4.0	3.8	3.6
20	15	13	12	11	9.7	8.9	8.2	7.6	7.1	6.7	6.3	5.9	5.6	5.3	5.1	4.9
25	19	17	15	13	12	11	10	9.5	8.9	8.4	7.8	7.4	7.0	6.6	6.3	6
30	23	20	18	16	15	13	12	11	11	10	9.4	8.9	8.4	8.0	7.6	7.3
35	27	23	21	19	17	16	14	13	12	12	11	10	9.8	9.3	8.9	8.5
40	31	27	24	21	19	18	16	15	14	13	13	12	11	11	10.2	9.7
45	34	30	27	24	22	20	18	17	16	15	14	13	13	12	11	11
50	38	33	30	27	24	22	21	19	18	17	16	15	14	13	13	12
55	42	37	33	29	27	24	23	21	20	18	17	16	15	15	14	13
60	46	40	36	32	29	27	25	23	21	20	19	18	17	16	15	15
70	53	47	42	37	34	31	29	27	25	23	22	21	20	19	18	17
80	61	53	47	43	39	36	33	31	28	27	25	24	23	21	20	19
90	69	60	53	48	44	40	37	34	32	30	28	27	25	24	23	22
100	76	67	59	53	49	45	41	38	36	33	31	30	28	27	25	24

Epinepherine Hydrochloride 1:1000 (Adrenalin Chloride)
Isoproterenol Hydrochloride (Isuprel)

1 mg in 250 ml D$_5$W = 4 µg/ml

X = infusion rate in drops/min or ml/hr (pump setting); O = dose in micrograms (µg)/min

1 mg in 250 ml D$_5$W = 4 µg/ml

X	O	X	O	X	O	X	O	X	O	X	O	X	O
1	0.066	21	1.4	41	2.73	61	4.06	81	5.4	101	6.73		
2	0.133	22	1.46	42	2.8	62	4.13	82	5.46	102	6.8		
3	0.2	23	1.53	43	2.86	63	4.2	83	5.53	103	6.86		
4	0.26	24	1.6	44	2.93	64	4.26	84	5.6	104	6.93		
5	0.33	25	1.66	45	3.0	65	4.33	85	5.66	105	7.0		
6	0.4	26	1.73	46	3.06	66	4.4	86	5.73	106	7.06		
7	0.466	27	1.8	47	3.13	67	4.46	87	5.8	107	7.13		
8	0.533	28	1.86	48	3.2	68	4.53	88	5.86	108	7.2		
9	0.60	29	1.93	49	3.26	69	4.6	89	5.93	109	7.26		
10	0.666	30	2.0	50	3.33	70	4.66	90	6.0	110	7.33		
11	0.733	31	2.06	51	3.4	71	4.73	91	6.06	111	7.4		
12	0.8	32	2.13	52	3.46	72	4.8	92	6.13	112	7.46		
13	0.866	33	2.2	53	3.53	73	4.86	93	6.2	113	7.53		
14	0.933	34	2.26	54	3.6	74	4.93	94	6.26	114	7.6		
15	1.0	35	2.33	55	3.66	75	5.0	95	6.33	115	7.66		
16	1.066	36	2.4	56	3.73	76	5.06	96	6.4	116	7.73		
17	1.13	37	2.46	57	3.8	77	5.13	97	6.46	117	7.8		
18	1.20	38	2.53	58	3.86	78	5.2	98	6.53	118	7.86		
19	1.26	39	2.6	59	3.93	79	5.26	99	6.6	119	7.93		
20	1.33	40	2.66	60	4.0	80	5.33	100	6.66	120	8.0		

Esmolol Hydrochloride (Brevibloc)

5 grams in 500 ml = 10 mg/ml

Patient's Weight lbs	88	99	110	121	132	143	154	165	176	187	198	209	220	231	242
kg	40	45	50	55	60	65	70	75	80	85	90	95	100	105	110

Drug Dose in μg/kg/min

Infusion rate in mL/hr:

	88/40	99/45	110/50	121/55	132/60	143/65	154/70	165/75	176/80	187/85	198/90	209/95	220/100	231/105	242/110
5	20.8	18.5	16.7	15.2	13.9	12.8	11.9	11.1	10.4	9.8	9.3	8.8	8.3	7.9	7.6
10	41.7	37.0	33.3	30.3	27.8	25.6	23.8	22.2	20.8	19.6	18.5	17.5	16.7	15.9	15.2
15	62.5	55.6	50.0	45.5	41.7	38.5	35.7	33.3	31.3	29.4	27.8	26.3	25.0	23.8	22.7
20	83.3	74.1	66.7	60.6	55.6	51.3	47.6	44.4	41.7	39.2	37.0	35.1	33.3	31.7	30.3
25	104.2	92.6	83.3	75.8	69.4	64.1	59.5	55.6	52.1	49.0	48.3	43.9	41.7	39.7	37.9
30	125.0	111.1	100.0	90.9	83.3	76.9	71.4	66.7	62.5	58.8	55.6	52.6	50.0	47.6	45.5
35	145.8	129.6	116.7	106.1	97.2	89.7	83.3	77.8	72.9	68.6	64.8	61.4	58.3	55.6	53.0
40	166.7	148.1	133.3	121.2	111.1	102.6	95.2	88.9	83.3	78.4	74.1	70.2	66.7	63.5	60.6
45	187.5	166.7	150.0	136.4	125.0	115.4	107.1	100.0	93.8	88.2	83.3	78.9	75.0	71.4	68.2
50	208.3	185.2	166.7	151.5	138.9	128.2	119.0	111.1	104.2	98.0	92.6	87.7	83.3	79.4	75.8
55	229.2	203.7	183.3	168.7	152.8	141.0	131.0	122.2	114.6	107.8	101.9	96.5	91.7	87.3	83.3
60	250.0	222.2	200.0	181.8	166.7	153.8	142.9	133.3	125.0	117.6	111.1	105.3	100.0	95.2	90.9
65	270.8	240.7	216.7	197.0	180.6	166.7	154.8	144.4	135.4	127.5	120.4	114.0	108.3	103.2	98.5
70	281.7	259.3	233.3	212.1	194.4	179.5	166.7	155.6	145.8	137.3	129.6	122.8	116.7	111.1	106.1
75	312.5	277.8	250.0	227.3	208.3	192.3	178.6	166.7	158.3	147.1	138.9	131.6	125.0	119.0	113.6
80	333.3	296.3	266.7	242.4	222.2	205.1	190.5	177.8	166.7	156.9	148.1	140.4	133.3	127.0	121.2
85	354.2	314.8	283.3	257.6	236.1	217.9	202.4	188.9	177.1	166.7	157.4	149.1	141.7	134.9	128.8
90	375.0	333.3	300.0	272.7	250.0	230.8	214.3	200.0	187.5	176.5	166.7	157.9	150.0	142.9	136.4
95	395.8	351.9	316.7	287.9	263.9	243.6	226.2	211.1	197.9	186.3	175.9	166.7	158.3	150.8	143.9
100	416.7	370.4	333.3	303.0	277.8	256.4	238.1	222.2	208.3	196.1	185.2	175.4	166.7	158.7	151.5
105	437.5	388.9	350.0	318.2	291.7	269.2	250.0	233.3	218.8	205.9	194.4	184.2	175.0	166.7	159.1
110	458.3	407.4	366.7	333.3	305.6	282.1	261.9	244.4	229.2	215.7	203.7	193.0	183.3	174.6	166.7
115	479.2	425.9	383.3	348.5	319.4	294.9	273.8	255.8	239.8	225.5	213.0	201.8	191.7	182.5	174.2
120	500.0	444.4	400.0	363.6	333.3	307.7	285.7	266.7	250.0	235.3	222.2	210.5	200.0	190.5	181.8

Heparin Sodium

20,000 units in 500 ml D$_5$W = 40 units/ml
X = infusion rate in drops/min or ml/hr (pump setting); O = dose in units/hr

X	O	X	O	X	O	X	O	X	O	X	O
1	40	21	840	41	1640	61	2440	81	3240	101	4040
2	80	22	880	42	1680	62	2480	82	3280	102	4080
3	120	23	920	43	1720	63	2520	83	3320	103	4120
4	160	24	960	44	1760	64	2560	84	3360	104	4160
5	200	25	1000	45	1800	65	2600	85	3400	105	4200
6	240	26	1040	46	1840	66	2640	86	3440	106	4240
7	280	27	1080	47	1880	67	2680	87	3480	107	4280
8	320	28	1120	48	1920	68	2720	88	3520	108	4320
9	360	29	1160	49	1960	69	2760	89	3560	109	4360
10	400	30	1200	50	2000	70	2800	90	3600	110	4400
11	440	31	1240	51	2040	71	2840	91	3640	111	4440
12	480	32	1280	52	2080	72	2880	92	3680	112	4480
13	520	33	1320	53	2120	73	2920	93	3720	113	4520
14	560	34	1360	54	2160	74	2960	94	3760	114	4560
15	600	35	1400	55	2200	75	3000	95	3800	115	4600
16	640	36	1440	56	2240	76	3040	96	3840	116	4640
17	680	37	1480	57	2280	77	3080	97	3880	117	4680
18	720	38	1520	58	2320	78	3120	98	3920	118	4720
19	760	39	1560	59	2360	79	3160	99	3860	119	4760
20	800	40	1600	60	2400	80	3200	100	4000	120	4800

Lidocaine Hydrochloride (Xylocaine)
Procainamide Hydrochloride (Pronestyl)
Bretylium Tosylate (Bretylol)

1 gm in 250 ml D_5W = 4 mg/ml
X = infusion rate in drops/min or ml/hr (pump setting); O = dose in mg/min

X	O	X	O	X	O	X	O	X	O	X	O
1	0.07	21	1.40	41	2.73	61	4.07	81	5.40	101	6.73
2	0.13	22	1.47	42	2.80	62	4.13	82	5.47	102	6.80
3	0.20	23	1.53	43	2.87	63	4.20	83	5.53	103	6.87
4	0.27	24	1.60	44	2.93	64	4.27	84	5.60	104	6.93
5	0.33	25	1.67	45	3.00	65	4.33	85	5.67	105	7.00
6	0.40	26	1.73	46	3.07	66	4.40	86	5.73	106	7.07
7	0.47	27	1.80	47	3.13	67	4.47	87	5.80	107	7.13
8	0.53	28	1.87	48	3.20	68	4.53	88	5.87	108	7.20
9	0.60	29	1.93	49	3.27	69	4.60	89	5.93	109	7.27
10	0.67	30	2.00	50	3.33	70	4.67	90	6.00	110	7.33
11	0.73	31	2.07	51	3.40	71	4.73	91	6.07	111	7.40
12	0.80	32	2.13	52	3.47	72	4.80	92	6.13	112	7.47
13	0.87	33	2.20	53	3.53	73	4.87	93	6.20	113	7.53
14	0.93	34	2.27	54	3.60	74	4.93	94	6.27	114	7.60
15	1.00	35	2.33	55	3.67	75	5.00	95	6.33	115	7.67
16	1.07	36	2.40	56	3.73	76	5.07	96	6.40	116	7.73
17	1.13	37	2.47	57	3.80	77	5.13	97	6.47	117	7.80
18	1.20	38	2.53	58	3.87	78	5.20	98	6.53	118	7.87
19	1.27	39	2.60	59	3.93	79	5.27	99	6.60	119	7.93
20	1.33	40	2.67	60	4.00	80	5.33	100	6.67	120	8.00

Nitroglycerine (Nitrostat)

| | Concentration | | | |
| | μg/ml in 500 ml D_5W | | | |
Dosage	100 μg/ml (50 mg)	200 μg/ml (100 mg)	300 μg/ml (150 mg)	400 μg/ml (200 mg)
μg/min	ml/hr	ml/hr	ml/hr	ml/hr
5	3	2	1	—
10	6	3	2	2
15	9	5	3	2
20	12	6	4	3
25	15	8	5	4
30	18	9	6	5
35	21	11	7	5
40	24	12	8	6
45	27	14	9	7
50	30	15	10	8
55	33	17	11	8
60	36	18	12	9
65	39	20	13	10
70	42	21	14	11
75	45	23	15	11
80	48	24	16	12
85	51	26	17	13
90	54	27	18	14
95	57	29	19	14
100	60	30	20	15
105	63	32	21	16
110	66	33	22	17
115	69	35	23	17
120	72	36	24	18

Norepinephrine Bitartrate (Levophed)

8 mg in 500 ml = 16 μg/ml
X = infusion rate in drops/min or ml/hr (pump setting); O = dose in μg/min

X	O	X	O	X	O	X	O	X	O	X	O	X	O
1	0.3	21	5.6	41	10.9	61	16.3	81	21.6	101	26.9		
2	0.5	22	5.9	42	11.2	62	16.5	82	21.9	102	27.2		
3	0.8	23	6.1	43	11.5	63	16.8	83	22.1	103	27.5		
4	1.1	24	6.4	44	11.7	64	17.1	84	22.4	104	27.4		
5	1.3	25	6.7	45	12.0	65	17.3	85	22.7	105	28.0		
6	1.6	26	6.9	46	12.3	66	17.6	86	22.9	106	28.3		
7	1.9	27	7.2	47	12.5	67	17.9	87	23.2	107	28.5		
8	2.1	28	7.5	48	12.8	68	18.1	88	23.5	108	28.8		
9	2.4	29	7.7	49	13.1	69	18.4	89	23.7	109	29.1		
10	2.7	30	8.0	50	13.3	70	18.7	90	24.0	110	29.3		
11	2.9	31	8.3	51	13.6	71	18.9	91	24.3	111	29.6		
12	3.2	32	8.5	52	13.9	72	19.2	92	24.5	112	29.9		
13	3.5	33	8.8	53	14.1	73	19.5	93	24.8	113	30.1		
14	3.7	34	9.1	54	14.4	74	19.7	94	25.1	114	30.4		
15	4.0	35	9.3	55	14.7	75	20.0	95	25.3	115	30.7		
16	4.3	36	9.6	56	14.9	76	20.3	96	25.6	116	30.9		
17	4.5	37	9.9	57	15.2	77	20.5	97	25.9	117	31.2		
18	4.8	38	10.1	58	15.5	78	20.8	98	26.1	118	31.5		
19	5.1	39	10.4	59	15.7	79	21.1	99	26.4	119	31.7		
20	5.3	40	10.7	60	16.0	80	21.3	100	26.7	120	32.0		

Phenylephrine Hydrochloride (Neo-Synephrine)

30 mg in 500 ml = 60 μg/ml
X = infusion rate in drops/min or ml/hr (pump setting); O = dose in μg/min

X	O	X	O	X	O	X	O	X	O	X	O	X	O
1	1.0	21	21.0	41	41.0	61	61.0	81	81.0	101	101.0		
2	2.0	22	22.0	42	42.0	62	62.0	82	82.0	102	102.0		
3	3.0	23	23.0	43	43.0	63	63.0	83	83.0	103	103.0		
4	4.0	24	24.0	44	44.0	64	64.0	84	84.0	104	104.0		
5	5.0	25	25.0	45	45.0	65	65.0	85	85.0	105	105.0		
6	6.0	26	26.0	46	46.0	66	66.0	86	86.0	106	106.0		
7	7.0	27	27.0	47	47.0	67	67.0	87	87.0	107	107.0		
8	8.0	28	28.0	48	48.0	68	68.0	88	88.0	108	108.0		
9	9.0	29	29.0	49	49.0	69	69.0	89	89.0	109	109.0		
10	10.0	30	30.0	50	50.0	70	70.0	90	90.0	110	110.0		
11	11.0	31	31.0	51	51.0	71	71.0	91	91.0	111	111.0		
12	12.0	32	32.0	52	52.0	72	72.0	92	92.0	112	112.0		
13	13.0	33	33.0	53	53.0	73	73.0	93	93.0	113	113.0		
14	14.0	34	34.0	54	54.0	74	74.0	94	94.0	114	114.0		
15	15.0	35	35.0	55	55.0	75	75.0	95	95.0	115	115.0		
16	16.0	36	36.0	56	56.0	76	76.0	96	96.0	116	116.0		
17	17.0	37	37.0	57	57.0	77	77.0	97	97.0	117	117.0		
18	18.0	38	38.0	58	58.0	78	78.0	98	98.0	118	118.0		
19	19.0	39	39.0	59	59.0	79	79.0	99	99.0	119	119.0		
20	20.0	40	40.0	60	60.0	80	80.0	100	100.0	120	120.0		

Sodium Nitroprusside (Nipride)*

100 mg in 250 ml D$_5$W = 400 µg/ml

Patient's Weight lbs	88	99	110	121	132	143	154	165	176	187	198	209	220
kg	40	45	50	55	60	65	70	75	80	85	90	95	100

Infusion rate ml/hr

Drug Dose in µg/kg/min													
0.5	3	4	4	4	5	5	6	6	6	6	7	7	8
1.0	6	7	8	9	9	10	11	12	12	13	14	15	15
1.5	9	11	11	13	14	15	16	17	18	19	21	22	23
2.0	12	14	15	17	18	20	21	23	24	26	28	29	30
2.5	15	17	19	21	23	25	27	28	30	32	34	36	38
3.0	18	20	23	25	27	30	32	34	36	38	41	43	45
3.5	21	24	27	29	32	34	37	40	42	45	48	50	53
4.0	24	27	30	33	36	39	42	45	48	51	54	57	60
4.5	27	32	34	37	41	44	48	52	54	58	61	65	68
5.0	30	34	38	41	45	49	53	56	60	64	68	72	75

*Note format change from other drip charts.

Theophylline Ethylenediamine (Aminophylline)

500 mg in 500 ml D$_5$W = 1 mg/ml

Patient's weight lbs	88	99	110	121	132	143	154	165	176	187	198	209	220	231	242
kg	40	45	50	55	60	65	70	75	80	85	90	95	100	105	110

Drug dose in mg/kg/hr

Infusion rate in mL/hr															
5	0.12	0.11	0.10	0.09	0.08	0.08	0.07	0.07	0.06	0.06	0.06	0.05	0.05	0.05	0.05
10	0.25	0.22	0.20	0.18	0.17	0.15	0.14	0.13	0.12	0.12	0.11	0.11	0.10	0.10	0.09
15	0.37	0.33	0.30	0.27	0.25	0.23	0.21	0.20	0.19	0.18	0.17	0.16	0.15	0.14	0.14
20	0.50	0.44	0.40	0.36	0.33	0.31	0.29	0.27	0.25	0.24	0.22	0.21	0.20	0.19	0.18
25	0.62	0.56	0.50	0.45	0.42	0.38	0.36	0.33	0.31	0.29	0.28	0.26	0.25	1.24	0.23
30	0.75	0.67	0.60	0.55	0.50	0.46	0.43	0.40	0.37	0.35	0.33	0.32	0.30	0.29	0.27
35	0.87	0.78	0.70	0.64	0.58	0.54	0.50	0.47	0.44	0.41	0.39	0.37	0.35	0.33	0.32
40	1.00	0.89	0.80	0.73	0.67	0.62	0.57	0.53	0.50	0.47	0.44	0.42	0.40	0.38	0.36
45	1.13	1.00	0.90	0.82	0.75	0.69	0.64	0.60	0.56	0.53	0.50	0.47	0.45	0.43	0.41
50	1.25	1.11	1.00	0.91	0.83	0.77	0.71	0.67	0.62	0.59	0.56	0.53	0.50	0.48	0.45
55	1.38	1.22	1.10	1.00	0.92	0.85	0.79	0.73	0.69	0.65	0.61	0.58	0.55	0.52	0.50
60	1.50	1.33	1.20	1.09	1.00	0.92	0.86	0.80	0.75	0.71	0.67	0.63	0.60	0.57	0.55
65	1.63	1.44	1.30	1.18	1.08	1.00	0.93	0.87	0.81	0.76	0.72	0.68	0.65	0.62	0.59
70	1.75	1.56	1.40	1.27	1.17	1.08	1.00	0.93	0.87	0.82	0.78	0.74	0.70	0.67	0.64
75	1.87	1.67	1.50	1.36	1.25	1.15	1.07	1.00	0.94	0.88	0.83	0.79	0.75	0.71	0.68
80	2.00	1.78	1.60	1.45	1.33	1.23	1.14	1.07	1.00	0.94	0.89	0.84	0.80	0.76	0.73
85	2.13	1.89	1.70	1.55	1.42	1.31	1.21	1.13	1.06	1.00	0.94	0.89	0.85	0.81	0.77
90	2.25	2.00	1.80	1.64	1.50	1.38	1.29	1.20	1.13	1.06	1.00	0.95	0.90	0.86	0.82
95	2.38	2.11	1.90	1.73	1.58	1.46	1.36	1.27	1.19	1.12	1.06	1.00	0.95	0.90	0.86
100	2.50	2.22	2.00	1.82	1.67	1.54	1.43	1.33	1.25	1.18	1.11	1.05	1.00	0.95	0.91
105	2.63	2.33	2.10	1.91	1.75	1.62	1.50	1.40	1.31	1.24	1.17	1.11	1.05	1.00	0.95
110	2.75	2.44	2.20	2.00	1.83	1.69	1.57	1.47	1.38	1.29	1.22	1.16	1.10	1.05	1.00
115	2.88	2.56	2.30	2.09	1.92	1.77	1.64	1.53	1.44	1.35	1.28	1.21	1.15	1.10	1.05
120	3.00	2.67	2.40	2.18	2.00	1.85	1.71	1.60	1.50	1.41	1.33	1.26	1.20	1.14	1.09

Classification of Antidysrhythmic Drugs

Class	Drugs	Effects on the Action Potential of Cardiac Muscle
Class I	Moricizine hydrochloride (Ethmozine)	Local anesthetic agents that depress the rate of inward flow of sodium through fast channels during the rapid depolarization phase (Phase 0) of the action potential curve. This decreases excessive automaticity of ectopic pacemakers. Most class I drugs can be further subclassified according to the intensity of their slowing effect on conduction and their effect on repolarization whereby they depress potassium flow.
Class IA	Quinidine sulfate (Quinidex) Procainamide (Pronestyl) Disopyramide (Norpace)	Have a moderate effect on depressing sodium flow into the cell during Phase 0; prolong action potential duration by prolonging repolarization, seen as a prolonged Q-T interval.
Class IB	Lidocaine (Xylocaine) Mexiletine hydrochloride (Mexitil) Tocainide (Tonocard)	Have a minimal effect on depressing the flow of sodium in Phase 0 and they shorten the action potential duration by accelerating repolarization (shorter Q-T interval).
Class IC	Encainide hydrochloride (Enkaid) Flecainide acetate (Tambocor) Propafenone (Rythmol)	Have the maximum effect on depressing sodium flow into cell during Phase 0 and have little effect on repolarization time.
Class II	Acebutolol (Sectral) Atenolol (Tenormin) Carteolol (Cartrol) Dilevalol (Unicard) Esmolol (Brevibloc) Labetolol (Normodyne) Metoprolol (Lopressor) Nadolol (Corgard) Penbutolol (Lavatol) Pindolol (Visken) Propranolol (Inderal) Timolol (Blocardren)	Beta-adrenergic blocking agents that inhibit sympathetic activity by competing with beta-adrenergic stimulators at receptor sites; decreases length of action potential and refractory period while depressing automaticity and excitability of cardiac tissues.
Class III	Amiodarone (Cordarone) Bretylium tosylate (Bretylol)	Prolong repolarization, thus decreasing the potential for premature impulse formation.
Class II & III	Sotalol	
Class IV	Verapamil (Isoptin, Calan) Nifedipine (Procardia) Isradipine (DynaCorc) Nicardipine (Cardene) Kiltiazem (Cardizem)	Calcium channel blockers-block the influx of calcium through the slow channels during Phases 1 and 2, prolonging refractory period; inhibit calcium ions in both cardiac and vascular smooth muscle, resulting in vasodilation and decreased force of cardiac contraction.
Unclassified	Adenosine triphosphate (Adenocard)	

Index

---

t indicates table; an italicized page number
indicates a figure.